Alternative Medicine: Expanding Medical Horizons

For sale by the U.S. Government Printing Office
Superintendent of Documents, Mail Stop: SSOP, Washington, DC 20402-9328
ISBN 0-16-045479-4

Alternative Medicine: Expanding Medical Horizons

A Report to the National Institutes of Health on Alternative Medical Systems and Practices in the United States

Prepared under the auspices of the
Workshop on Alternative Medicine, Chantilly, Virginia
September 14–16, 1992

To order additional copies of *Alternative Medicine: Expanding Medical Horizons*, please use the order form printed in the back of the book.

Table of Contents

Foreword

The Office of Alternative Medicine (OAM) was established in 1991, with the appropriation of $2 million for an office "to more adequately explore unconventional medical practices." The Senate Appropriations Committee report acknowledged that "many routine and effective medical procedures now considered commonplace were once considered unconventional and counterindicated. Cancer radiation therapy is such a procedure that is now commonplace but once was considered to be quackery."

One of the first goals of the OAM was to develop a baseline of information on the state of alternative medicine in the United States. To accomplish this, a series of workshops were held in 1992. The first, a public meeting on June 17–18 in Bethesda, Maryland, included presentations from more than 80 speakers who detailed issues and concerns of importance to the alternative medicine community. On September 14–16, a second workshop was convened in Chantilly, Virginia, with a total of more than 200 participants who discussed the state of the art of the major areas of alternative medicine and to direct attention to priority areas for potential future research activities. Cochairs of the workshop working groups organized writing teams to collect and synthesize the available research in their respective fields and to develop recommendations to the National Institutes of Health (NIH).

This document represents the report of these meetings to the NIH, and includes the input of more than 200 practitioners and researchers of alternative medicine from throughout the United States. The hard work of the speakers, panel members, authors of working papers, and editors in putting this report together is gratefully acknowledged.

As the Office of Alternative Medicine proceeds to carry out its congressional mandate, the recommendations for future research in the report will be carefully considered. However, it should be pointed out that **this document does not reflect endorsement of these therapies or recommendations for research by the NIH, the U.S. Public Health Service, or the U.S. Department of Health and Human Services.** It reports on a series of opinions expressed by nongovernment participants in the workshops described above and is published for the purpose of furthering the dialogue between the alternative-complementary medicine communities and the biomedical research establishment.

The NIH cautions readers not to seek the therapies described in this document for serious health problems without consultation with a licensed physician. The NIH further cautions that many of the therapies described have not been subjected to rigorous scientific investigation to prove safety or efficacy; and many have not been approved by the U.S. Food and Drug Administration.

Preface

Because of the increasing sophistication of the U.S. health care system, its increasing administrative costs, and the exponentially expanding degree of training and specialization required by the health care practitioners who administer it, health care costs in this country have skyrocketed in the past few decades. Indeed, in 1940, health care absorbed $4 billion, a mere 4 percent of the U.S. gross national product (GNP); by 1992, health care costs had ballooned to more than $800 billion, or almost 14 percent of GNP.[1] Experts predict these costs will exceed $1 trillion this year.

Despite these expenditures, many Americans currently have little or no access to adequate health care. In fact, 37 million Americans have no health insurance at all; another 22 million have inadequate health care coverage. To increase access to basic health care, individuals and organizations from many sectors of society are now calling for reform of the present health care system. To date, this debate has focused mainly on making the current system less expensive through capping the amount of damages that can be awarded because of medical malpractice, limiting physician and hospital fees, further regulating the pharmaceutical companies, and controlling the misuse of health insurance.

Unfortunately, this debate has failed to take into account the fact that the current health care crisis is primarily a crisis of chronic disease. Today almost 33 million Americans are functionally limited in their daily activities by chronic, debilitating conditions such as arthritis, allergies, pain, hypertension, cancer, depression, cardiovascular disease, and digestive problems. More than 9 million, or almost one-third, of these individuals have limitations so severe that they cannot work, attend school, or maintain a household. The U.S. Public Health Service (PHS) estimates that 70 percent of the current health care budget is spent on the treatment of these individuals; as the population grows older, such conditions will continue to consume an even larger proportion of national health care expenditures. Furthermore, the worldwide pandemic of acquired immunodeficiency syndrome is threatening to completely overwhelm the health care delivery systems in certain areas of the United States.

While the dominant system of health care in the United States—often called "conventional medicine," or biomedicine—is extremely effective for treating infectious diseases and traumatic injuries, it is often ill equipped to handle complex, multifaceted chronic conditions. One reason is that over the years, conventional medicine has increasingly emphasized finding a single "magic bullet" solution for each condition or disease it confronts. The reality is that many chronic conditions are not amenable to such one-dimensional solutions.

Rather, such complex conditions require equally multifaceted treatment approaches. Furthermore, it is far less expensive to prevent them from occurring in the first place than to attempt to treat the symptoms and consequences with surgery and expensive drugs, which often offer only short-term solutions. For example, coronary artery disease affects approximately 7 million Americans and causes about 1.5 million heart attacks and 500,000 deaths a year. Approximately 300,000 coronary artery bypass graft operations are performed in the United States each year at a cost of about $30,000 each, or $9 billion total. Yet coronary artery bypass surgery prevents premature death in only a few patients with the most serious main coronary or multiple-vessel heart disease. On the other hand, heart disease is almost entirely attributable to poor diet (i.e., high fat intake) and unhealthy lifestyle decisions (alcohol consumption and smoking), and thus can be avoided. For those who already have heart disease, an extremely low-fat diet combined with exercise and other therapies may actually start

---

[1]*Most of the statistics cited in this preface can be found in the publication* Healthy People 2000: National Health Promotion and Disease Prevention Objectives, *U.S. Department of Health and Human Services (DHHS Pub. No. PHS–91–50212), Washington, DC, 1990.* Healthy People 2000 *is the latest in a series of reports that have been developed by the U.S. Public Health Service since the early 1970s dealing with issues that affect the health of the Nation.*

unclogging blocked arteries and significantly extend life.

Thus, for health care reform truly to succeed at reducing costs and increasing access, disease *prevention* must be the ultimate focus of the primary health care system rather than disease *treatment*. This change in emphasis can be accomplished only by restructuring the current system so that people learn that they are far better off staying healthy than relying on high technology to rescue them from a lifetime of unhealthy living. In addition, to care adequately and cost-effectively for those who already have chronic illnesses, health care reform must incorporate multifaceted approaches to the treatment of these patients, approaches that control the symptoms while alleviating the underlying causes.

In 1990, PHS recognized the need to completely revamp the current approach to health and illness when it released a 700-page report called *Healthy People 2000*. This report enumerated the challenges and goals for improving the Nation's collective health by the year 2000 and challenged the Nation to move beyond merely saving lives. It explained that "the health of a people is measured by more than death rates. Good health comes from reducing unnecessary suffering, illness, and disability. It comes from an improved quality of life. Health is thus measured by citizens' sense of well-being. The health of a Nation is measured by the extent to which the gains are accomplished for all the people." To reach this goal, the report called for "mobilizing the considerable energies and creativity of the Nation in the interest of disease prevention and health promotion". as an economic imperative.

This report was developed in the spirit of *Healthy People 2000*. Its purpose is to investigate which "alternative" health care options might best be mobilized to help in the fight against the major diseases and conditions that are robbing so many Americans of their quality of life. The individuals who helped write it comprised members of systems of medicine and therapies that emphasize improving quality of life, disease prevention, and treatments for conditions for which conventional medicine has few, if any, answers. Therefore, the popular term *alternative* has been chosen to describe these medical systems and therapies. Another term for these systems and therapies, which is preferred in Europe, is *complementary* medicine.

This report establishes a baseline of information on alternative medicine, which may be used to direct future research and policy discussions. Specifically, this report will aid OAM in its mandate to establish an information clearinghouse on alternative medicine so that the public, policymakers, and public health experts can make informed decisions about their health care options. The goal of OAM is to speed the discovery, development, and validation of potent treatments that may be added to the complementary wheel of alternatives currently available to patients and practitioners. Ultimately, it may provide the foundation for the development of a whole new system of medicine, one that incorporates the best of conventional and alternative medicines.

Brian M. Berman, M.D.
David B. Larson, M.D., M.P.H.
Cochairs, Editorial Review Board
December, 1994

Executive Summary

Introduction

Medicine in the United States evolved from a mix of Native American, Eastern, and European botanical traditions. In the mid-1800s, the medical system called biomedicine began to dominate. Biomedicine was shaped by the observations that bacteria were responsible for producing disease and characteristic pathological damage and that antitoxins and vaccines could improve a person's ability to ward off the effects of pathogens. With this knowledge, biomedical investigators and clinicians began to conquer devastating infections and to perfect effective surgical procedures.

Thus biomedicine became the "conventional," or mainstream, health care system and began setting the standards for the diagnosis and treatment of every facet of illness. Several decades ago, however, consumer trust in conventional medicine began to falter, and many Americans sought alternative treatments outside conventional medicine. Today, alternative medicine constitutes a significant portion of Americans' health care expenditures.

A number of barriers are preventing promising alternative therapies from being investigated and developed. Structural barriers are caused by problems of classification, definition, culture, and language. Regulatory and economic barriers include legal and cost implications of complying with Federal and State regulations. Belief barriers have been caused by constraining ideologies, misconceptions, and myths.

In late 1992, Congress established the Office of Alternative Medicine (OAM) within the Office of the Director, National Institutes of Health (NIH), to facilitate the fair, scientific evaluation of alternative therapies that could improve many people's health and well-being. OAM, as a de facto intermediary between the alternative medical community and the Federal research and regulatory communities, seeks to reduce barriers that may keep promising alternative therapies from coming to light.

Part I of this report examines six fields of alternative medicine: mind-body interventions, bioelectromagnetics applications in medicine, alternative systems of medical practice, manual healing methods, pharmacological and biological treatments, herbal medicine, and diet and nutrition in the prevention and treatment of chronic disease. Part II deals with a number of cross-cutting issues germane to all six fields, including research infrastructure, research databases, research methodologies, the peer review process, and public information activities. The major recommendations from all chapters are included at the end of this executive summary.

Part I, FIELDS OF PRACTICE

Mind-Body Interventions

Most traditional medical systems make use of the interconnectedness of mind and body and the power of each to affect the other. During the past 30 years there has been a growing scientific movement to explore the mind's capacity to affect the body. The clinical aspect of this enterprise is called mind-body medicine. Mind and body are so integrally related that it makes little sense to refer to therapies as having impact just on the mind or the body.

Mind-body interventions often help patients experience and express their illness in new, clearer ways. Distinctions between curing and healing have little place in contemporary medical practice but are important to patients. Perceived meaning has direct consequences to health. The placebo response is one of the most widely known examples of mind-body interactions in contemporary, scientific medicine, yet it is also one of the most undervalued, neglected assets in medical practice. That the placebo response relies heavily on the relationship between doctor and patient says a great deal about the importance of the doctor-patient relationship and the need to provide further medical training on understanding and using this relationship. The therapeutic potential of spirituality as well as religion also has been neglected in the teaching and practice of medicine.

Interest in the mind's role in the cause and course of cancer has been substantially stimulated by the discovery of the complex interactions between the mind and the neurological and immune systems, the subject of the rapidly expanding discipline of psychoneuroimmunology. The profound differences in the psychological stances taken by people who survive cancer suggest that there is extreme variation both among cultures and within cultures.

Specific mind-body interventions include psychotherapy, support groups, meditation, imagery, hypnosis, biofeedback, yoga, dance therapy, music therapy, art therapy, and prayer and mental healing.

Psychotherapy directly addresses a person's emotional and mental health, which is, in turn, closely interwoven with his or her physical health. It encompasses a wide range of specific treatments from combining medication with discussion, to simply listening to the concerns of a patient, to using more active behavioral and emotive approaches. It also should be understood more generally as the matrix of interaction in which all the helping professions operate. Conventional psychotherapy is conducted primarily by means of psychologic methods such as suggestion, persuasion, psychoanalysis, and reeducation. It can be divided into general categories. All of the therapies can be undertaken either individually or in groups.

Research indicates that psychotherapeutic treatment can hasten a recovery from a medical crisis and is in some cases the best treatment for it. Psychotherapy also appears to be valuable in the treatment of somatic illnesses, in which physical symptoms appear to have no medical cause, are often improved markedly with psychotherapy. In addition, psychotherapy has been shown to speed patients' recovery time from illness. This, in turn, leads to smaller medical bills and fewer return visits to medical practitioners.

Support groups, as the research literature demonstrates, can have a powerful positive effect in a wide variety of physical illnesses, from heart disease to cancer, from asthma to strokes. Indeed, one study found that women with breast cancer who took part in a support group lived an average of 18 months longer (a doubling of the survival time following diagnosis) than those who did not participate. In addition, all the long-term survivors belonged to the therapy group.

Support groups have two other major benefits: (1) they help members form bonds with each other, an experience that may empower the rest of their lives; and (2) they are low cost or even "no cost" (e.g., Alcoholics Anonymous).

Meditation is a self-directed practice for relaxing the body and calming the mind. Most meditative techniques have come to the West from Eastern religious practices, particularly India, China, and Japan, but can be found in all cultures of the world. Until recently, the primary purpose of meditation has been religious, although its health benefits have long been recognized. During the past 15 years, it has been explored as a way of reducing stress on both mind and body. Cardiologists, in particular, often recommend it as a way of reducing high blood pressure.

Some studies have found that regular meditation reduces health care use; increases longevity and quality of life; reduces chronic pain; reduces anxiety; reduces high blood pressure; reduces serum cholesterol level; reduces substance abuse; increases intelligence-related measures; reduces post-traumatic stress syndrome in Vietnam veterans; reduces blood pressure; and lowers blood cortisol levels initially brought on by stress.

Imagery is both a mental process (as in imagining) and a wide variety of procedures used in therapy to encourage changes in attitudes, behavior, or physiological reactions. As a mental process, it is often defined as "any thought representing a sensory quality." It includes, as well as the visual, all the senses—aural, tactile, olfactory, proprioceptive, and kinesthetic.

Imagery has been successfully tested as a strategy for alleviating nausea and vomiting associated with chemotherapy in cancer patients, to relieve stress, and to facilitate weight gain in cancer patients. It has been successfully used and tested for pain control in a variety of settings; as adjunctive therapy for several diseases, including diabetes; and with geriatric patients to enhance immunity.

Imagery is usually combined with other behavioral approaches. It is best known in the treatment of cancer as a means to help patients mobilize their immune systems, but it also is used as part of a multidisciplinary approach to cardiac rehabilitation and in many settings that specialize in treating chronic pain.

Hypnosis and hypnotic suggestion have been a part of healing from ancient times. The induction of trance states and the use of therapeutic suggestion were a central feature of the early Greek healing temples and variations of these techniques were practiced throughout the ancient world.

Modern hypnosis began in the 18th century with Franz Anton Mesmer, who used what he called "magnetic healing" to treat a variety of psychological and psychophysiological disorders, such as hysterical blindness, paralysis, headaches, and joint pains. Since then, the fortunes of hypnosis have ebbed and flowed. Freud, at first, found it extremely effective in treating hysteria and then, troubled by the sudden emergence of powerful emotions in his patients and his own difficulty with its use, abandoned it.

In the past 50 years, however, hypnosis has experienced a resurgence, first with physicians and dentists and more recently with psychologists and other mental health professionals. Today, it is widely used for addictions, such as smoking and drug use, for pain controls, and for phobias, such as the fear of flying.

One of the most dramatic uses of hypnosis is the treatment of congenital ichthyosis (fish skin disease), a genetic skin disorder that covers the surface of the skin with grotesque hard, wart-like, layered crust. Hypnosis is, however, most frequently used in more common ailments, either independently or in concert with other treatment, including the management of pain in a variety of settings, reduction of bleeding in hemophiliacs, stabilization of blood sugar in diabetics, reduction in severity of attacks of hay fever and asthma, increased breast size, the cure of warts, the *production* of skin blisters and bruises, and control of reaction to allergies such as poison ivy and certain foods.

Biofeedback is a treatment method that uses monitoring instruments to feed back to patients physiological information of which they are normally unaware. By watching the monitoring device, patients can learn by trial and error to adjust their thinking and other mental processes in order to control bodily processes heretofore thought to be involuntary—such as blood pressure, temperature, gastrointestinal functioning, and brain wave activity.

Biofeedback can be used to treat a very wide variety of conditions and diseases, ranging from stress, alcohol and other addictions, sleep disorders, epilepsy, respiratory problems, and fecal and urinary incontinence to muscle spasms, partial paralysis, or muscle dysfunction caused by injury, migraine headaches, hypertension, and a variety of vascular disorders. More applications are being developed yearly.

Yoga is a way of life that includes ethical precepts, dietary prescriptions, and physical exercise. Its practitioners have long known that their discipline has the capacity to alter mental and bodily responses normally thought to be far beyond a person's ability to modulate them. During the past 80 years, health professionals in India and the West have begun to investigate the therapeutic potential of yoga. To date, thousands of research studies have been undertaken and have shown that with the practice of yoga a person can, indeed, learn to control such physiologic parameters as blood pressure, heart rate, respiratory function, metabolic rate, skin resistance, brain waves, body temperature, and many other bodily functions.

Regular yogic meditation also has been shown to reduce anxiety levels; cause the heart to work more efficiently and decrease respiratory rate; lower blood pressure and alter brain waves; increase communication between the right and left brain; reduce cholesterol levels (when used with diet and exercise); help people stop smoking; and successfully treat arthritis.

Dance therapy began formally in the United States in 1942, and in 1956 dance therapists from across the country founded the American Dance Therapy Association, which has now grown to over 1,100 members. It publishes a journal, the *American Journal of Dance Therapy*, fosters research, monitors standards for professional practice, and develops guidelines for graduate education.

Dance/movement therapy has been demonstrated to be clinically effective in the following: developing body image, improving self-concept and increasing self-esteem; facilitating attention; ameliorating depression, decreasing fears and anxieties, and expressing anger; decreasing isolation, increasing communication skills, and fostering solidarity; decreasing bodily tension, reducing chronic pain, and enhancing circulatory and respiratory functions; reducing suicidal ideas, increasing feelings of well-being, and promoting healing; and increasing verbalization.

Music therapy is used in psychiatric hospitals, rehabilitation facilities, general hospitals, outpatient clinics, day-care treatment centers, residences for people with developmental disabilities, community mental health centers, drug and alcohol programs, senior centers, nursing homes, hospice programs, correctional facilities, halfway houses, schools, and private practice.

Studies have found music therapy effective as an analgesic, as a relaxant and anxiety reducer for infants and children, and as an adjunctive treatment with burn patients, cancer patients, cerebral palsy patients, and stroke, brain injury, or Parkinson's disease patients.

Art therapy is a means for the patient to reconcile emotional conflicts, foster self-awareness, and express unspoken and frequently unconscious concerns about his/her disease. In addition to its use in treatment, it can be used to assess individuals, couples, families, and groups. It is particularly valuable with children who often cannot talk about their real concerns.

Research on art therapy has been conducted in clinical, educational, physiological, forensic, and sociological arenas. Studies on art therapy have been conducted in many areas including with burn recovery in adolescent and young patients, with eating disorders; with emotional impairment in young children, with reading performance, with chemical addiction, and with sexual abuse in adolescents.

Prayer and mental healing techniques fall into two main types. In Type I healing, the healer enters a prayerful, altered state of consciousness in which he views himself and the patient as a single entity. There need be no physical contact and there is no attempt to "do anything" or "give something" to the person in need, only the desire to unite and "become one" with him or her and with the Universe, God, or Cosmos. Type II healers, on the other hand, do touch the healee and describe some "flow of energy" through their hands to the patient's area of pathology. Feelings of heat are common in both healer and healee. These healing techniques are offered only as generalities. Some healers use both methodologies, even in the same healing session, and other healing methods could be described.

There exist many published reports of experiments in which persons were able to influence a variety of cellular and other biological systems through mental means. The target systems for these investigations have included bacteria, yeast, fungi, mobile algae, plants, protozoa, larvae, insects, chicks, mice, rats, gerbils, cats, and dogs, as well as cellular preparations (blood cells, neurons, cancer cells) and enzyme activities. In human "target persons," eye movements, muscular movements, electrodermal activity, plethysmographic activity, respiration, and brain rhythms have been affected through direct mental influence.

These studies in general assess the ability of humans to affect physiological functions of a variety of living systems *at a distance, including studies where the "receiver" or "target" is unaware that such an effort is being made.* The fact that these studies commonly involve nonhuman targets is important; lower organisms are presumably not subject to suggestion and placebo effects, a frequent criticism when human subjects are involved.

Many of these studies do not describe the psychological strategy of the influencer as actual "prayer," in which one directs entreaties to a Supreme Being, a Universal Power, or God. But almost all of them involve a state of prayerful*ness*—a feeling of genuine caring, compassion, love, or empathy with the target system, or a feeling that the influencer is "one" with the target.

In addition to preventing or curing illnesses, these therapies by and large provide people the chance to be involved in their own care, to make vital decisions about their own health, to be touched emotionally, and to be changed psychologically in the process. Many patients today believe their doctor or medical system is impersonal, remote, and uncaring. The mind-body approach is potentially a corrective to this tendency, a reminder of the importance of human connection that opens up the power of patients acting on their own behalf.

More work needs to be done, but there is already a growing amount of evidence that many of the mind-body therapies discussed in this report, if appropriately selected and wisely applied, can be clinically as well as economically cost-effective, that they work, and that they are safe.

Bioelectromagnetics Applications in Medicine

Bioelectromagnetics (BEM) is an emerging science that studies how living organisms interact with electromagnetic (EM) fields. Electrical phenomena are found in all living organisms, and electrical currents in the body can produce magnetic fields that extend outside the body. Those that extend outside the body can be influenced by external magnetic and EM fields. Changes in the body's natural fields may produce physical and behavioral changes.

Endogenous (internal) fields are distinguished from exogenous (external) fields. The latter can be natural, such as the earth's geomagnetic field, or artificial, such as power lines, transformers, appliances, radio transmitters, or medical devices. Oscillating nonionizing EM fields in the extremely low frequency (ELF) range can have vigorous biological effects that may be beneficial. Changes in the field configuration and exposure pattern of low-level EM fields can produce specific biological responses, and certain frequencies have specific effects on body tissues.

The mechanism by which EM fields produce biological effects is under increasing study. At the cutting edge of BEM research is the question of how endogenous EM fields change with consciousness. Nonionizing BEM medical applications are classified according to whether they are thermal or nonthermal in biological tissue. Thermal applications of nonionizing radiation include radio frequency (RF) hyperthermia, laser and RF surgery, and RF diathermy.

The most important BEM modalities in alternative medicine are nonthermal applications of nonionizing radiation. Major new applications of nonthermal, nonionizing EM fields are bone repair, nerve stimulation, wound healing, treatment of osteoarthritis, electroacupuncture, tissue regeneration, and immune system stimulation.

In the study of other alternative medical treatments, BEM offers a unified conceptual framework that may help explain how diagnostic and therapeutic techniques such as acupuncture and homeopathy may produce results that are hard to understand from a more conventional viewpoint.

Alternative Systems of Medical Practice

Worldwide, only an estimated 10 percent to 30 percent of human health care is delivered by conventional, biomedically oriented practitioners. The remaining 70 percent to 90 percent ranges from self-care according to folk principles to care given in an organized health care system based on an alternative tradition or practice.

Popular health care is the kind most people practice and receive at home, such as giving herbal tea to someone who has a cold. *Community-based* health care, which reflects the health needs, beliefs, and natural environments of those who use it, refers to the nonprofessionalized but specialized health care practices of many rural and urban people. *Professionalized* health care is more formalized; practitioners undergo more standardized training and work in established locations.

Professionalized health care systems. The professionalized health care practitioners often have conducted scientific studies about the causes of illness and explanations and results of treatment. Each of the major professionalized systems has certain characteristics: a theory of health and disease; an educational scheme to teach its concepts; a delivery system involving practitioners; a material support system to produce medicines and therapeutic devices; a legal and economic mandate to regulate its practice; cultural expectations about the medical system's role; and a means to confer professional status on approved providers. These professionalized medical systems include traditional oriental medicine, acupuncture, Ayurvedic medicine, homeopathy, anthroposophy, naturopathy, and environmental medicine.

Traditional oriental medicine is a sophisticated set of many systematic techniques and methods, including acupuncture, herbal medicine, acupressure, qigong, and oriental massage. The most striking characteristic of oriental medicine is its emphasis on diagnosing disturbances of qi, or vital energy, in health and disease. Diagnosis in oriental medicine involves the classical procedures of observation, listening, questioning, and palpation, including feeling pulse quality and sensitivity of body parts.

The professionalization of oriental medicine has taken diverse paths in both East Asia and the

United States. Currently, the model in the People's Republic of China, which was established after the 1949 revolution, involves the organized training of practitioners in schools of traditional Chinese medicine. The curriculum of these schools includes acupuncture, oriental massage, herbal medicine, and pharmacology, though the clinical style of making a diagnosis and then designing a treatment plan is the one traditionally associated with herbal medicine. The graduates of these colleges are generally certified in one of the four specialty areas at a training level roughly equivalent to that of a Western country's bachelor's degree.

In the United States, the professional practitioner base for oriental medicine is organized around acupuncture and oriental massage. There are about 6,500 acupuncturist practitioners in the United States. The American Oriental Body Work Therapy Association has approximately 1,600 members representing practitioners of tuina, shiatsu, and related techniques. Many American schools of acupuncture are evolving into "colleges of oriental medicine" by adding courses in oriental massage, herbal medicine, and dietary interventions. They also are offering diplomas, master's degrees, and doctor's degrees in oriental medicine. The legal sanctioning of oriental medical practice is most extensive in New Mexico, where the acupuncture community has established an exclusive profession of oriental medicine. Their legal scope of practice is currently similar to that of primary care M.D.s and D.O.s (doctors of osteopathy), and their State statute restricts other licensed New Mexico health professionals' ability to advertise or bill for oriental medicine or acupuncture services.

Extensive research has been done in China through the institutions of traditional Chinese medicine, but only in the past quarter century have biomedical scientists in China characterized and identified active agents in much of traditional medical formulary. The use of traditional oriental herbal medicines and formulas in China and Japan has been studied for therapeutic value in the following areas: chronic hepatitis; rheumatoid arthritis; hypertension; atopic eczema; various immunologic disorders, including acquired immunodeficiency syndrome (AIDS); and certain cancers. It would be useful to repeat these studies in the United States, assessing U.S. clinical populations according to high-quality research criteria.

Acupuncture involves stimulating specific anatomic points in the body for therapeutic purposes. Puncturing the skin with a needle is the usual method, but practitioners also use heat, pressure, friction, suction, or impulses of electromagnetic energy to stimulate the points. In the past 40 years acupuncture has become a well-known, reasonably available treatment in developed and developing countries. Acupuncture is used to regulate or correct the flow of qi to restore health.

Modern theories of acupuncture are based on laboratory research conducted in the past 40 years. Acupuncture points have certain electrical properties, and stimulating these points alters chemical neurotransmitters in the body. The physiological effects of acupuncture stimulation in experimental animals have been well documented, and in the past 20 years acupuncture has become an increasingly established health care practice. An estimated 3,000 conventionally trained U.S. physicians have taken courses to incorporate acupuncture in their medical practices.

Acupuncture is one of the most thoroughly researched and documented of the so-called alternative medical practices. A series of controlled studies has shown compelling evidence for the efficacy of acupuncture in the treatment of a variety of conditions, including osteoarthritis, chemotherapy-induced nausea, asthma, back pain, painful menstrual cycles, bladder instability, and migraine headaches. Studies on acupuncture also have shown positive results in the areas of chronic pain management and in the management of drug addiction, two areas where conventional Western medicine has had only a modicum of success.

Ayurveda is India's traditional, natural system of medicine that has been practiced for more than 5,000 years. Ayurveda provides an integrated approach to preventing and treating illness through lifestyle interventions and natural therapies. Ayurvedic theory states that all disease begins with an imbalance or stress in the individual's consciousness. Lifestyle interventions are a major Ayurvedic preventive and therapeutic approach. There are 10 Ayurveda clinics in North America, including one hospital-based clinic that has served 25,000 patients since 1985.

In India, Ayurvedic practitioners receive state-recognized, institutionalized training in parallel to their physician counterparts in India's state-supported systems for conventional Western biomedicine and homeopathic medicine. The research base is growing concerning the physiological effects of meditative techniques and yoga postures in Indian medical literature and Western psychological literature. Published studies have documented reductions in cardiovascular disease risk factors, including blood pressure, cholesterol, and reaction to stress, in individuals who practice Ayurvedic methods.

Laboratory and clinical studies on Ayurvedic herbal preparations and other therapies have shown them to have a range of potentially beneficial effects for preventing and treating certain cancers, treating infectious disease, promoting health, and treating aging. Mechanisms underlying these effects may include free-radical scavenging effects, immune system modulation, brain neurotransmitter modulation, and hormonal effects.

Homeopathic medicine is practiced worldwide, especially in Europe, Latin America, and Asia. However, even in the United States the homeopathic drug market is a multimillion-dollar industry. Homeopathic remedies, which are made from naturally occurring plant, animal, or mineral substances, are recognized and regulated by the Food and Drug Administration (FDA) and are manufactured by established pharmaceutical companies under strict guidelines. Homeopathy is used to treat acute and chronic health problems as well as for disease prevention and health promotion. Recent clinical trials suggest that homeopathic medicines have a positive effect on allergic rhinitis, fibrositis, and influenza.

Basic research in homeopathy has involved investigations into the chemical and biological activity of highly diluted substances. Some homeopathic medicines are diluted to concentrations as low as 10^{-30} to $10^{-20,000}$. This particular aspect of homeopathic theory and practice has caused many modern scientists to reject homeopathic medicine. Critics of homeopathy contend that such extreme dilutions of the medicines are beyond the point at which any active molecules of the medicine can theoretically still be found in the solution. On the other hand, scientists who accept the potential benefits of homeopathic theory suggest several theories to explain how highly diluted homeopathic medicines may act. Using recent developments in quantum physics, they have proposed that electromagnetic energy in the medicines may interact with the body on some level. Researchers in physical chemistry have proposed the "memory of water" theory, whereby the structure of the water-alcohol solution is altered by the medicine during the process of dilution and retains this structure even after none of the actual substance remains.

Anthroposophically extended medicine is an extension of Western biomedicine and also incorporates approaches and therapeutics from two alternative medicine movements: naturopathy and homeopathy. There are an estimated 30 to 100 M.D.s in the United States who practice anthroposophical medicine. Hundreds of uniquely formulated medications are used in anthroposophical practice, each seeking to match the key dynamic forces in plants, animals, and minerals with disease processes in humans to stimulate healing. Much research in anthroposophically extended medicine has been connected with attempts to understand the nature of disease, assess treatments qualitatively, and understand how the essential properties of the objects under investigation could be applied in therapy.

Naturopathic medicine, as a distinct American health care profession, is almost 100 years old. It was founded as a formal health care system at the turn of the century by medical practitioners from various natural therapeutic disciplines. By the early 1900s, more than 20 naturopathic medical schools existed, and naturopathic physicians were licensed in most States. Today there are more than 1,000 licensed naturopathic doctors in the United States.

As practiced today, naturopathic medicine integrates traditional natural therapeutics—including botanical medicine, clinical nutrition, homeopathy, acupuncture, traditional oriental medicine, hydrotherapy, and naturopathic manipulative therapy—with modern scientific medical diagnostic science and standards of care. The medical research base of naturopathic practice consists of empirical documentation of treatments using case history observations, medical records, and summaries of practitioners' clinical experiences.

At present, the two accredited naturopathic medical schools in the United States have active research departments. Naturopathic researchers have investigated the pharmacology and physiological effects of nutritional and natural therapeutic agents, and naturopathic physicians have been active in the investigation of new homeopathic remedies and in the natural treatment of women's health problems. The most recently completed naturopathic study in women's health tested the clinical and endocrine effects of a botanical formula as an alternative to estrogen replacement therapy. Results of this study showed a clinically significant benefit (measured as reduction in the total number of menopausal symptoms) among the treated women versus the placebo group.

Environmental medicine, like anthroposophically extended medicine, also can be viewed as an extension of modern biomedicine. Environmental medicine traces its roots to the practice of allergy treatment and the work of Dr. Theron Randolph in the 1940s, who identified a variety of common foods and chemicals that were able to trigger the onset of acute and chronic illness even when exposure was at relatively low levels.

Environmental medicine recognizes that illness in individuals can be caused by a broad range of incitant substances, including foods, chemicals found at home and in the workplace, and chemicals in the air, water, and food. Today there are 3,000 physicians worldwide practicing environmental medicine, and there are several environmental control units in the United States and one in Canada, where patients' sensitivities are unmasked through fasting and complete avoidance of potentially incitant chemicals.

Research in this field has been directed at clinical treatment of patients and at evaluation of the diagnostic and treatment techniques used by practitioners. Other studies have supported the use of the approaches of environmental medicine in treating arthritis, asthma, chemical sensitivity, colitis, depression, eczema, fatigue, and hyperactivity.

The belief that humans can get sick from cumulative low-level environmental exposure to certain incitants is not well accepted by the conventional medical community. However, because "sick building syndrome" and other chronic conditions that cannot be explained by other phenomena are being seen with greater frequency, environmental medicine offers a theoretical groundwork for dealing with such phenomena. Indeed, environmental medicine is in a position to be a leading force in the investigation of ways to reduce the incidence of these and other disorders.

Community-based health care practices. Community-based health care practices are varied and found throughout the United States. Like other health care specialists, community-based healers may emphasize naturalistic, personalistic, or energetic explanatory models or a combination. Traditional midwives and herbalists and nowadays, pragmatic weight loss specialists are probably the best known of community-based practitioners who follow the naturalistic model. In addition, the Native American medicine man or medicine woman is a community-based traditional healer with primarily naturalistic skills, that is, the skills of an herbalist in particular. Some medicine people are also shamans, in which case they are often distinguished as holy men and women.

In contrast to professionalized practitioners, community-based healers often do not have set locations such as offices or clinics for delivering care but do so in homes, at ceremonial sites, or even right where they stand. Community-based healing of the personalistic variety can also be "distant," that is, it does not require that practitioner and patient be in each other's presence. Prayers or shamanic journeys, for example, can be requested and "administered" at any time, and charm cures are sometimes delivered by telephone.

Meanwhile, community-based systems also thrive in urban areas. These systems include the popular weight loss programs and other 12-step programs. Often the practitioners rent office space and emphasize contact between client and practitioner, and they may charge considerable fees. Since these practitioners depend on their healing practice for their livelihood, they advertise and so may be easier to identify and contact for study purposes.

Native American Indian community-based medical systems all share the following rituals and practices: sweating and purging, usually done in a "sweat lodge"; the use of herbal remedies gathered from the surrounding environment and sometimes traded over long distances; and shamanic healing involving naturalistic or personalistic healing. Tribes such as the Lakota and Dineh (Navajo) also use practices such as the medicine wheel, sacred hoop, and the "sing," which is a healing ceremonial that lasts from 2 to 9 days and nights and is guided by a highly skilled specialist called a "singer."

Formal research into the healing ceremonies and herbal medicines conducted and used by bona fide Native American Indian healers or holy people is almost nonexistent, even though Native American Indians believe they positively cure both the mind and body. Ailments and diseases such as heart disease, diabetes, thyroid conditions, cancer, skin rashes, and asthma reportedly have been cured by Native American Indian doctors who are knowledgeable about the complex ceremonies.

Latin American community-based practices include curanderismo, which is a folk system of medicine that includes two distinct components: a humoral model for classifying activity, food, drugs, and illness; and a series of folk illnesses.

In the humoral component of curanderismo things could be classified as having qualitative (not literal) characteristics of hot or cold, dry or moist. According to this theory, good health is maintained by maintaining a balance of hot and cold. Thus, a good meal will contain both hot and cold foods, and a person with a hot disease must be given cold remedies and vice versa. Again, a person who is exposed to cold when excessively hot may "take cold" and become ill.

The second component, the folk illnesses, is actively in use in much of Mexico and among less educated Hispanic U.S. citizens. Studies have found that as many as 96 percent of Mexican-American households (more frequent in the less Americanized communities) treated members for Hispanic folk illnesses. Similarly high use patterns among Mexican migrant workers has been found in Florida and Mexico.

Although no formal effectiveness studies seem to have been done on this system, its wide popularity and the research suggesting the relevance of the folk diagnoses for biomedical practice indicate the need for further demographic and effectiveness studies.

Alcoholics Anonymous (AA) is an example of an urban community-based healing system for helping people whose lives are damaged by the consumption of alcohol to stop drinking. Founded in 1935 by Bob Smith, M.D., and Bill Wilson, two alcoholics, it is a patient-centered self-help fellowship of men and women. AA has burgeoned and today is widely considered the most successful existing method for supporting sobriety.

In contrast to most community-based systems, a very large literature exists analyzing AA. Several models attempt to explain its success. One popular psychometric model interprets AA as a "cult" and the achievement of sobriety as a "conversion experience." Another model, however, asserts that members recover by integrating their own experiences with alcohol with those of others in the group and by learning and practicing some new ways to behave. Through these new ways, AA members feel as if they are living apart from the urban materialist norm; that the cause of alcoholism is not at issue; that people should share, not compete; and that the individual need not rise above the rest (spiritual anonymity).

Studies have concluded that active AA membership allows up to 68 percent of alcoholics to drink less or not at all for up to a year, and 40 percent to 50 percent to achieve sobriety for many years. More active or dedicated members (those who attend meetings more often) remain sober longer.

Manual Healing Methods

Touch and manipulation with the hands have been in use in health and medical practice since the beginning of medical care. Physicians' hands were once their most important diagnostic and therapeutic tool. Today, however, many medical and health practitioners tend to retreat from physical contact with the patient, distanced by diagnostic equipment and legal and time constraints.

The manual healing methods are based on the understanding that dysfunction of a part of the body often affects secondarily the function of other discrete, not necessarily directly connected, body parts. Consequently, theories and processes have been developed for correcting secondary dysfunctions by manipulating soft tissues or realigning body parts. Overcoming misalignments and manipulating soft tissues bring the parts back to optimal function, and the body returns to health.

One of the earliest U.S. health care systems to use manual healing methods was *osteopathic medicine*. In 1993 more than 32,000 American-educated and -licensed D.O.s were practicing in the United States. More than 60 percent of osteopathic physicians are involved in primary care—family medicine, pediatrics, internal medicine, and obstetrics-gynecology. An extensive body of work supports the use of osteopathic techniques for musculoskeletal and nonmusculoskeletal problems. Nearly all osteopathically oriented research has been funded from the private sector.

Chiropractic science is concerned with investigating the relationship between structure (primarily of the spine) and function (primarily of the nervous system) of the human body to restore and preserve health. Chiropractic medicine applies such knowledge to diagnosing and treating structural dysfunctions that can affect the nervous system. Chiropractic physicians use manual procedures and interventions, not surgical or chemotherapeutic ones. In 1993 more than 45,000 licensed chiropractors were practicing in the United States.

Chiropractic specialty areas are extremely pertinent to other medical specialties, such as radiology, orthopedics, neurology, and sports medicine. Current chiropractic research interests include back and other pain, somatovisceral disorders, and reliability studies.

Massage therapy, one of the oldest methods in health care practice, is the scientific manipulation of the soft body tissues to return those tissues to their normal state. Massage consists of a group of manual techniques that include applying fixed or movable pressure and holding and causing the body to move. Primarily the hands are used, but sometimes forearms, elbows, and feet are used also. These techniques can affect the musculoskeletal, circulatory-lymphatic, and nervous systems. Massage therapy encompasses the concept of *vis medicatrix naturae*—helping the body heal itself—and is aimed at achieving or increasing health and well-being. Touch is the fundamental medium of massage therapy.

Massage therapists are licensed by 19 States and several localities. Most States require 500 or more hours of education from a recognized school program and a licensing examination. Massage therapy techniques include Swedish massage, deep-tissue massage, sports massage, neuromuscular massage, and manual lymph drainage. Other physical healing methods include reflexology, zone therapy, tuina, acupressure, Rolfing, Trager, Feldenkrais method, and Alexander technique.

Biofield therapeutics—laying on of hands—is also a very old form of healing. The earliest Eastern references are in the *Huang Ti Nei Ching Su Wên (The Yellow Emperor's Classic of Internal Medicine)*, dated between 2,500 and 5,000 years ago. The underlying rationales cluster around two views: first, that the healing force comes from a source other than the practitioner—God, the cosmos, or another supernatural entity—and second, that a human biofield directed, modified, or amplified in some way by the practitioner is the operative mechanism.

During biofield treatment, the practitioner places hands directly on or near the patient's body to improve general health or treat a specific dysfunction. Treatment sessions may take from 20 minutes to an hour or more; a series of sessions is often needed to treat some disorders. There is consensus among practitioners that the biofield permeates the physical body and extends outward for several inches. Extension of the external biofield depends on the person's emotional state and health. Biofield practitioners have a holistic focus. About 50,000 practitioners provide 18 million sessions annually in the United States.

At least three forms of biofield therapetutics are used in medical care inpatient and outpatient settings: healing touch, therapeutic touch, and SHEN therapy. No generally accepted theory accounts for the effect of these therapies.

Pharmacological and Biological Treatments

Pharmacological and biological treatments are an assortment of drugs and vaccines not yet accepted by mainstream medicine. A sampling of biological and pharmacological treatments currently being offered by alternative medical practitioners includes the following:

- Antineoplastons—peptide fractions originally derived from normal human blood and urine, presently being used to treat certain kinds of tumors as well as AIDS.
- Cartilage products derived from cattle, sheep, sharks, and chickens, which are being used to treat cancer and arthritis.
- Ethylene diamine tetraacetic acid (EDTA) chelation therapy, used to treat heart disease,

circulatory problems, and rheumatoid arthritis and to prevent cancer.

- Immunoaugmentive therapy, an experimental form of cancer immunotherapy consisting of daily injections of processed blood products.
- 714–X, a nitrogen-providing compound injected into the lymph system near the abdomen to treat cancer and AIDS.
- Coley's toxins, a mixture of killed cultures of bacteria from *Streptococcus pyogenes* and *Serratia marcescens*, used for treating cancer.
- MTH–68, a vaccine that uses an attenuated strain of the Newcastle disease virus of chickens (paramyxovirus), which may interfere with cancer-related viruses.
- Neural therapy, which involves injecting local anesthetics into nerve cell bodies, peripheral nerves, scars, and elsewhere to treat chronic pain.
- Apitherapy, the medicinal use of various products of the common honeybee to treat a variety of diseases: rheumatic diseases such as arthritis; neurological diseases such as multiple sclerosis, low back pain, and migraine; dermatological conditions (e.g., eczema, psoriasis, herpesvirus infections); chronic pain; and cancer.
- Iscador, a liquid extract from mistletoe plants used to treat tumors.
- Biologically guided chemotherapy.

A major impediment to full investigation of alternative pharmacological and biological treatments is the high expense of conducting the trials needed to meet FDA approval. Most alternative treatments lack sponsors and funding for clinical trials of safety and effectiveness. Many potentially useful alternative drugs or vaccines are supported by data indicating they may be useful in treating cancer, AIDS, heart disease, hepatitis, and other major health problems.

Herbal Medicine

All cultures have long folk medicine traditions that include the use of plants and plant products. Even in ancient cultures, people methodically collected information on herbs and developed well-defined herbal pharmacopoeias. Indeed, well into the 20th century much of the pharmacopoeia of scientific medicine was derived from the herbal lore of native peoples. Many drugs commonly used today are of herbal origin. Indeed, about one-quarter of the prescription drugs dispensed by community pharmacies in the United States contain at least one active ingredient derived from plant material.

The World Health Organization (WHO) estimates that 4 billion people, 80 percent of the world population, presently use herbal medicine for some aspect of primary health care. Herbal medicine is a major component in all indigenous peoples' traditional medicine and a common element in Ayurvedic, homeopathic, naturopathic, traditional oriental, and Native American Indian medicine.

Although during the centuries the discovery of useful therapeutics from plants has changed the face of medicine and the course of civilization, many people, especially some in the Federal Government, evaluate herbal remedies as though they were either worthless or dangerous. Today in the United States, herbal products can be marketed only as food supplements. An herb manufacturer or distributor can make no specific health claims without FDA approval. Despite FDA skepticism, a growing number of Americans are interested in herbal preparations.

Two features of European drug regulation make that market more hospitable to natural remedies. First, it costs less and takes less time in Europe to approve medicines as safe and effective. This is especially true of substances that have a long use history and can be approved under the "doctrine of reasonable certainty." European guidelines for the assessment of herbal remedies follow up on WHO's *Guidelines for the Assessment of Herbal Medicines*, which state that a substance's historical use is a valid way to document safety and efficacy in the absence of scientific evidence to the contrary.

France, where traditional medicines can be sold with labeling based on traditional use, requires licensing by the French Licensing Committee and approval by the French Pharmacopoeia Committee. Germany considers whole herbal products one active ingredient; this makes it simpler to define and approve the product. The German Federal Health Office regulates products such as ginkgo and milk thistle extracts so that potency and manufacturing processes are standardized. England generally follows the rule of prior use; that is, years of use with apparent positive effects and no evidence of detrimental side effects constitute enough evidence—in lieu of other scientific data—that the product is safe.

In Japan, China, and India, patent herbal remedies composed of dried and powdered whole herbs or herb extracts, often in tablet form, are the rule. Traditional herbals are the backbone of China's medicine. Japan's traditional medicine, kampo, is similar to and historically derived from Chinese medicine but includes traditional medicines from Japanese folklore. Herbal medicines are the staple of medical treatment in many developing countries and are used for many types of ailments.

European phytomedicines are among the world's best studied medicines, researched in leading European universities and hospitals. Some have been in clinical use under medical supervision for more than 10 years, with tens of millions of documented cases. This form of botanical medicine most closely resembles American medicine. In Europe there have been credible research studies reporting positive effects on a variety of chronic illnesses for herbs such as *Silybum marianum* (milk thistle), *Ginkgo biloba* (ginkgo), *Vaccinium myrtillus* (bilberry extract), and *Ilex guayusa*. Many herbs in China have been studied extensively by methods that are acceptable from the Western perspective; among these herbs are ginseng, fresh ginger rhizome, Chinese foxglove root, baical skullcap root, wild chrysanthemum flower, and licorice root. A number of Ayurvedic herbs also have recently been studied in India under modern scientific conditions, including *Eclipta alba*, Indian gooseberry, neem, turmeric, and trikatu.

Reports of positive effects of herbal preparations in developing countries and Native American Indian herbs are primarily anecdotal. However, since much modern-day medicine is directly or indirectly derived from such folklore sources, it seems illogical to conclude that there are no more significant treatments or cures for major diseases to be found in the world from plant sources.

Diet and Nutrition in the Prevention and Treatment of Chronic Disease

Throughout evolution, human beings adapted to a wide range of naturally occurring foods, but the types of food and the mix of nutrients (in terms of carbohydrates, fats, and proteins) remained relatively constant. Food supplies were often precarious, and the threat of death from starvation was a constant preoccupation for most early humans.

However, about 10,000 years ago the agricultural revolution began making profound dietary changes in many human populations. The ability to produce and store large quantities of dried foods led to preferential cultivation of some foods, such as grains, which constituted new challenges to the human digestive system. Then about 200 years ago, the Industrial Revolution introduced advances in food production, processing, storage, and distribution. Recent technological innovations, along with increased material well-being and lifestyles that have allowed people more freedom in deciding what and when they wish to eat, have led to even further major dietary changes in developed countries. Because changes in the dietary patterns of the more technologically developed countries, such as the United States, have been so dramatic and rapid, the people consuming these affluent diets have had little time to adapt biologically to the types and quantities of food that are available to them today. The longer term adverse health effects of the diet prevailing in these countries—characterized by an excess of energy-dense foods rich in animal fat, partially hydrogenated vegetable oils, and refined carbohydrates but lacking in whole grains, fruits, and vegetables—have become apparent only in recent decades.

Because of the recent, rapid rise in chronic illness related directly or indirectly to diet, the focus of nutrition research has shifted away from eliminating nutritional deficiency to dealing with chronic diseases caused by nutritional excess. Another concern among nutrition researchers is the accumulation of evidence indicating that less-than-adequate intake of some micronutrients over a long period may increase the risks of developing coronary heart disease, cancers, cataracts, and birth defects. In recent decades the data on the relationship between certain dietary habits and nutritional intake have been growing exponentially. Designing interventions based on this wealth of research has become increasingly more difficult and complex.

The Federal Government's approach to dietary intervention, formulated by boards composed of nutrition scientists, generally does not recommend supplementing the typical American diet with vitamins or nutrients beyond the recommended daily allowances (RDAs), nor does it suggest that some foods never be eaten. In contrast, many alternative dietary approaches contend that no amount of manipulation of the typical American diet is enough to promote optimum health or prevent eventual chronic illness. These alternative approaches represent a continuum of philosophies ranging from the concept that supplementing the typical American diet somewhat beyond the RDAs is necessary to promote optimum health, to the idea that supplementation well beyond the RDAs is often required to reverse the effects of long-term deficiencies. Other approaches advocate drastic dietary modification, either eliminating or adding certain types of foods or macronutrients, to treat specific types of conditions such as cancer and cardiovascular disease. Finally, there is the view that certain major staples of the typical American diet, such as meat and dairy products, are basically unhealthy and should be generally avoided.

There is a growing body of data supporting the notion that the RDAs for minerals, such as calcium and magnesium, may be too low and that supplementation may be necessary to prevent the onset of chronic diseases. In addition, the RDAs for a number of vitamins and micronutrients, such as vitamin C, vitamin D, vitamin E, folate, and beta-carotene, may not be adequate to prevent chronic illness. For example, recent studies have found that the RDA for folate may need to be doubled for women as well as men.

Orthomolecular medicine—the therapeutic use of high-dose vitamins to treat chronic disease—promotes improving health and treating disease by using the optimum concentration of substances normally present in the body. Increasing the intake of such nutrients to levels well above those usually associated with preventing overt deficiency disease may have health benefits for some people. There is at least preliminary evidence that orthomolecular remedies may be effective in treating AIDS; bronchial asthma; cancer; cardiovascular disease, heart attacks, and stroke; lymphedema; and mental and neurological disorders.

A variety of alternative diets are offered for treating cancer, cardiovascular disease, and food allergies. Virtually all these interventions focus on eating more fresh and freshly prepared vegetables, fruits, whole grains, and legumes. Allergy to food has become a major area of research. Food intolerance is being studied as a causal or contributing factor in rheumatoid arthritis, and there is evidence that food-elimination diets may help many hyperactive children.

Some alternate dietary lifestyles are believed to offer a greater resistance to illness. These include several variations of the vegetarian diet, such as those consumed by Seventh-Day Adventists and proponents of the macrobiotic diet. Studies have found a significant lowering of risk factors for heart disease and certain forms of cancer in these two groups. Recent studies have also reported that certain cultural eating styles, such as the Asian and Mediterranean diets, appear to lower risk factors for heart disease and certain forms of cancer as well. Although there have been few controlled studies of the benefits of many traditional diets, such as those originally consumed by Native American Indians, diseases such as diabetes and cancer were not a problem for these populations until their diets became more Western, or affluent.

Because dietary and nutritional therapy interventions affect an array of biochemical and physiological processes in the body, evaluating their effectiveness may require equally complex methods. Furthermore, developing a comprehensive health care policy that incorporates diet and nutritional interventions may require taking into account Federal feeding programs and dissemination strategies that might present barriers to the effective propagation of adequate nutritional knowledge.

Part II, CONDUCTING AND DISSEMINATING RESEARCH

Like mainstream medicine, alternative medicine needs reasonable, responsible research and validation of safety and effectiveness. However, several issues must first be addressed: lack of dedicated facilities for alternative medical research, inadequate funding for alternative medical research, lack of training for alternative medical researchers, lack of a centrally located research database, difficulty in designing research, and difficulty obtaining NIH peer review of alternative medical grant applications.

Research Infrastructure: Institutions and Investigators

Although there are pockets of alternative medical research at some U.S. research institutions, including NIH, most has been conducted outside such institutions. A factor that is structured to promote more conventional research over alternative research at most institutions is the peer review process, intended to limit poorer research from being funded or published.

Several alternative medical colleges have research departments and engage in research. Their approach usually differs from that of conventional medical institutes because of a different focus and, more important, less exposure to methodological training. These researchers are more likely to be interested in determining dosages than in investigating whether or how a treatment works. The interest of conventional researchers in dosages and optimal treatment combinations is likely to occur further along in the research process.

However, funding is both limited and precarious for these institutions. Almost without exception, Federal funding has not been available. Limited funding is available from private sources but is inadequate for current needs. Because of the limited funding, at such institutions, infrastructure and faculty have developed only minimally in their research departments. Further, at present there is little communication between these research facilities, other alternative research facilities, and their conventional counterparts. Increased research and communication are likely to benefit the Nation's health care.

Also, some clinical groups need training to become accomplished alternative medical investigators. Some require training in proper and acceptable research methods, and other researchers need exposure to alternative medical practices to be better prepared to evaluate them properly. Indeed, multidisciplinary teams conducting research in alternative medicine may be more successful if they include participants with some level of dual training in conventional medical research methodology and clinical alternative medical practice. Further, alternative medical practitioners have suggested that research in alternative medicine should be performed by individuals and teams trained in as wide as possible an array of relevant research methodologies.

Existing research centers could be enhanced, and new ones could be installed, at alternative medical institutions throughout the United States. Here also, expert faculty from various disciplines would join to evaluate efficacy, safety, clinical effectiveness, cost-effectiveness, and mechanisms of action of alternative medicine through basic as well as clinical research.

Several mainstream medical institutions recently have begun or are developing basic academic medical courses to introduce medical students and physicians in training to the theory, practice, and research of alternative medical therapies. A few other conventional institutions integrate alternative medicine in at least a limited way into the curriculum.

Properly designed, courses such as these will not only provide information on the utility of specific therapeutic approaches but develop a larger framework for understanding the strengths and limitations of more conventional medicine. These courses also will promote recognition of the contributions that theoretical and research models in alternative medicine may make to enlarging conventional research methodology.

Research Databases

A first step in developing a research strategy is to study previously published research literature on the subject and related subjects. Having a central source of information means investigators can go directly to the best and most current research on a topic instead of trying to collect data from disparate sources. Investigators who have access to a comprehensive research database can focus their efforts on the basis of previous research and obtain the information they need to design their own research.

Unfortunately, research into alternative medicine has been hampered because there is currently no easily accessible comprehensive database. Although a great deal of information can be found in the major medical databases on various aspects of alternative medicine, expert searching skills are needed to locate these materials. In addition, much of the little that has been collected on alternative medicine in the major medical databases has not been sufficiently indexed and catalogued. The problem is compounded if there are few journals available for a particular alternative discipline, if the relevant journals are not indexed and catalogued for inclusion in the databases, or if the data were not collected or reported properly. Other potentially valuable information is available only in non-English languages, such as the substantial bodies of literature on traditional Chinese medicine and Ayurvedic medicine.

Research Methodologies

No alternative medical system or method should be recommended for inclusion in the medical health system until it has been adequately tested. Evaluating alternative medical systems is no different from studying conventional systems—appropriate methods must be chosen to evaluate the system. Alternative medical researchers face new challenges as they address factors that lie outside the strictly biological realm. Research design, even for conventional medicine, is difficult and challenging. Researchers in alternative medicine are challenged by the need to apply acceptable research design to procedures or techniques that are hard to quantify.

A review of published conventional research over the years indicates that prospective randomized clinical trials are not always possible or preferred. A 1990 report of the Committee on Technological Innovation in Medicine, Institute of Medicine, supports this tacit reality and discusses methodological options:

> It has also become clear that randomized controlled clinical trials are not necessarily practical or feasible for answering all clinical questions. Therefore, a variety of other methods, such as nonrandomized trials or observational methods, have been adopted to provide complementary information. Traditionally these methods were regarded as weaker than randomized controlled clinical trials for clinical evaluation. Recent methodological advances, such as the use of non-classical statistics and the ability to link large-scale automated data bases for analysis . . . are strengthening these approaches.

The first goal of any research investigation into a medical treatment is to determine whether the treatment makes a clinical or cost difference. The second major concern about designing evaluations is the extent of external validity—the ability to generalize evaluation results to other populations and settings. Whatever methodology or methodologies are used to evaluate an alternative treatment, it may have to take into account a number of factors, including how to measure the perspectives of patients; how to evaluate systematic therapeutic learning, such as with biofeedback; or how to evaluate systems of medicine that adhere to paradigms completely different from those of conventional medicine, such as homeopathy. Other factors, such as disbelief in the treatment by reviewers, also should be taken into account to ensure a truly unbiased evaluation of an alternative therapy.

Peer Review

Peer review is the process in which researchers' peers evaluate the research strengths, weaknesses, and potential publishability or value of their work. Peers are chosen to participate in the evaluation process on the basis of their knowledge of or demonstrated expertise in the area of scientific investigation being considered.

This process is widely used in education, publication, State licensing, research publication, and review of clinical outcomes on a case-by-case basis by physician review organizations mandated by Federal law. While these areas all are relevant to alternative medicine, this report focuses on NIH's evaluation process for research grant and research contract applications.

At NIH, the peer review process is administered by the Division of Research Grants. In the review process, grants are reviewed by a primary and a secondary reviewer in the study section, who present findings to the entire study section. Grants are eventually funded after a second level of review of the application by an advisory council or board of NIH centers and institutes that have funding authority.

The peer review process in alternative medicine is not expected to raise methodological issues substantially different from those encountered in other emerging fields. Alternative medicine challenges established scientists and institutions by proposing models and patterns that differ from what is familiar in conventional medicine. Peer review in alternative medicine will aid reviewers in confronting issues of potential bias stemming from differences in basic assumptions about health and disease that may reflect limitations of current scientific knowledge.

Public Information Activities

As vital as research databases are to the researcher, information libraries are of equal importance to clinician, physician, and patient; without information there is no way a physician or patient can make truly informed choices. An accessible database of alternative medicine information is a vital need for the American public.

Several Institutes at NIH as well as some other Federal agencies include alternative medical practices in some of their information. For example, the National Institute of Neurological Disorders and Stroke includes acupuncture and psychological techniques, the National AIDS Information Clearinghouse provides information on nutrition strategies, the National Institute of Mental Health provides information on biofeedback, and the National Cancer Institute, on chaparral tea and other medicinal herbs. Outside NIH auspices, the Science and Technology Division, Reference Section, of the Library of Congress has reference guides to Acupuncture and Medicinal Plants, among others.

However, a national clearinghouse would provide a clear, concise message for the broader healthcare community, as well as interested members of the lay public, of the benefits of alternative medicine based on a body of scientific information that is current, accurate, and complete. Thus, an OAM-sponsored alternative medicine clearinghouse would provide a gateway for knowledge transfer to several audiences: healthcare practitioners, policymakers, educators, and the public at large.

Information will need to be gathered from a wide range of sources. Furthermore, information will need to be made available to consumers through various means. Electronic access through America OnLine, CompuServe, Genie, and Prodigy will likely be very useful. However, since not all consumers have access to home computers, other means will be required to provide information to the general public. This may be through print information, CD-ROM disks at public libraries, and other community outlets.

Conclusion

Some of the medical systems discussed in this report, such as Ayurvedic medicine and traditional oriental medicine, are centuries old and are still in extensive use in other nations and cultures of the world. Others, such as osteopathy and naturopathy, evolved in the United States in the not-too-distant past but were relegated to the fringes of medicine because the concepts of health and illness they embraced were different from those of conventional biomedicine. Still others, such as some of the mind-body and bioelectromagnetic approaches, are on the frontier of scientific knowledge and understanding.

Many alternative medical practitioners face many barriers before their therapies can become part of mainstream medicine or they can be allowed to peacefully coexist with mainstream medical practitioners. However, consumers are already using their services in rapidly growing numbers. Most people who opt to use alternative therapies do so because they believe conventional medicine has nothing to offer them or because they want to supplement their conventional treatment—or, they want cheaper health care alternatives.

Although biomedicine has revolutionized medicine and the way health and illness are viewed, it is becoming increasingly expensive. This means that significant segments of the population—especially the young, the old, and people with chronic or severe diseases—are being left without adequate health care. Many alternative medical systems, with their emphasis on preventive medicine, may have much to offer in further controlling health care costs. Furthermore, regulations for approving potentially valuable drugs, interventions, and technical devices need to be significantly streamlined in order to bring costs down and offer potentially lifesaving treatments to the public in a timely fashion.

Many of the alternative therapies discussed in this report have already received sufficient clinical evaluations to warrant being included in any serious discussions about developing a comprehensive health care system. Others need to be quickly and thoroughly evaluated to determine their potential for improving the health and the health care of the Nation.

Summary of Part I Recommendations

Mind-Body Interventions

- OAM should develop comprehensive reviews of mind-body literature to document existing work and specify directions for research in the following: clinical applications of mind-body interventions; commonalities and differences among self-regulation strategies; the dynamics of the therapeutic relationship between providers and patients; the influence of social context on health and illness, including the impact of family, work, education, economic status, and culture; the effects of belief, values, and meaning on health and illness; and the influence of nonlocal phenomena on health and illness.

- OAM should fund studies dealing with integrating effective mind-body techniques, giving attention to possible increased cost-effectiveness when these approaches are used integrally rather than singly.

- Studies are needed to investigate in basic terms the nonlocal effects of consciousness. Studies would involve human-machine and human-human interactions and use global or greater degrees of spatial separation. Such research is vital to laying a theoretical foundation for understanding the role of consciousness in health and for progress in the mind-body field.

- OAM/NIH should establish a project to investigate how patient education affects the outcome of research studies. If the findings so justify, develop research designs that inform patients of the nature of the protocol in which they participate and that provide immediate feedback of results.

- OAM/NIH should form a task force on the nature of consciousness, composed of academic representatives from the fields of psychology, neurophysiology, artificial intelligence, physics, medicine, and philosophy. The group's mission would be to formulate a model of consciousness that accounts for manifestations of consciousness that surface in mind-body research.

Bioelectromagnetics Applications in Medicine

- OAM should fund studies to elucidate the physical mechanisms of BEM medical modalities.

- OAM should fund studies that develop assay methods based on EM field interactions in cells for potassium transport, calcium transport, and cytotoxicity. These assays could be applied to studies of such phenomena in cellular systems.

- OAM/NIH should fund studies to develop BEM-based treatments for osteoporosis based on existing work on EM bone repair research. Researchers at the National Aeronautics and Space Administration have expressed interest in collaborative work to develop BEM treatments for weightlessness-induced osteoporosis.

- OAM should fund studies to establish further studies of mechanisms of EM field interactions in cells and tissues, with emphasis on coherent or cooperative states and resonant phenomena in biomolecules and in coherent brain wave states and other long-range interactions in biological systems.

- OAM should fund research into the role of the body's internally generated EM fields and other natural electromagnetic parameters; apply knowledge of such processes to develop novel diagnostic methods and improve understanding of alternative medical treatments such as acupuncture, electroacupuncture, and biofield therapies; and launch exploratory research on the role of the body's energy fields in relation to the role of consciousness states in health and healing.

Alternative Systems of Medical Practice

- OAM/NIH should fund long-term health care utilization and cost-effectiveness studies on individuals who use alternative systems of medicine versus conventional medicine.

- OAM should fund basic research in acupuncture beyond pain management. This research should address the broad range of clinically observed effects of acupuncture treatments.

- OAM/NIH should evaluate a number of specific herbal and natural preparations of systems such as Ayurvedic and naturopathic medicine.

- OAM should establish an initial database with descriptive information about traditional medical practice from medical and nonmedical sources. This database should include a review of scientific data, including quantitative reviews and meta-analyses of studies in selected disciplines.

- OAM should promote and publish consumer-based surveys describing which alternative systems and traditional ethnic medical practices are being used frequently now and for what illnesses.

- OAM/NIH should explore alternative and ethnic medical systems—including historic traditions that may not be replicable in the biomedical model—that recognize the role of body, mind, spirit, and environmental factors in health and disease.

- OAM should fund basic science research to investigate the existence, nature and role of energy (vital force) as an active phenomenon in health and disease.

- OAM should establish collaboration standards for alternative medical practice research to ensure that the research team respects the paradigm under study, that there is joint involvement of alternative or traditional practitioners in biomedical research institutions, and that joint involvement occurs at all stages of research: conception, method design, funding, data collection, evaluation, and publication.

- OAM should support the legislative intent of Congress in creating the Office of Alternative Medicine by focusing on socially and economically critical health conditions and assessing clinical as well as cost outcomes.

- OAM should encourage the addition of alternative systems or ethnomedicine research components to current NIH-sponsored clinical studies.

Manual Healing Methods

- Studies are needed to determine the range of clinical benefits for common physical complaints and problems treated by therapists who use these methods for treating back pain, headache, whiplash, and chronic fatigue syndrome.

- Studies are needed to determine the degree to which a general sense of well-being is enhanced by manual healing methods.

- OAM should work to fund studies to evaluate the effect of structural manipulation on body awareness, motion regulation, range of movement, ability to cope with stress, muscle tone and flexibility, growth and development and aging, autonomic function, electrical patterns in muscles, immune system response, and cardiovascular and respiratory function.

- Studies should be funded to determine the outcomes and the physiological and neurological mechanisms associated with specific manual healing methods.

Pharmacological and Biological Treatments

- OAM should work with the Food and Drug Administration (FDA) to develop a memorandum of understanding so that proposed OAM-approved trials can proceed. FDA and State authorities should consider a moratorium on seizures, raids, import alerts, and licensing actions against physicians, researchers, and health care providers whose work OAM has chosen for evaluation.

Herbal Medicine

- OAM should hold a research organizational conference to facilitate planning in herbal medicine research to help identify state-of-the-art questions in ethnomedical research, existing databases, and research personnel needed to support basic and clinical research needs in this area.

- OAM/NIH should support the training of ethnobotanists, specifically in the field of ethnomedicine, and offer funding opportunities to foster the rebirth of this field at U.S. universities and research institutions. This priority is critical in light of the fact that some traditional knowledge of herbal remedies is in danger of disappearing, as are plant species used in these systems of medicine.

- OAM should work to eliminate the bias against plant medicines by restructuring the requirements for proof of efficacy and concentrating on safety. Eliminate the monosubstance treatment bias by removing the need for extensive chemical analysis of chemically complex natural-product medicines.

- OAM should work to restate the FDA's mandate, taking legislative action if necessary, with respect to herbal products and traditional medications. FDA has limited expertise and resources to evaluate the global herbal medicine inventory. FDA should have a more educational, informational role.

Diet and Nutrition in the Prevention and Treatment of Chronic Disease

- Research is needed to determine how and at what levels antioxidants such as vitamin E, vitamin C, and beta-carotene provide optimal immune enhancement.
- Research is needed into the effects of antioxidants on cancer cells and DNA repair.
- Research is needed into the role of vitamins outside their role as enzyme cofactors. Conduct research in the ability of vitamins and other nutritional supplements to prevent or reverse the effects of free radicals and reactive molecular intermediates.
- Controlled studies are needed in the United States to verify European work on the potential clinical efficacy of minerals such as magnesium and selenium in treating disease. Develop more extensive intervention studies to determine whether adding mineral supplements improves the preventive effects of other dietary interventions such as salt or fat restriction against cardiovascular disease; in particular, do an extended study of magnesium treatment of bronchial asthma.
- Studies are needed on alternative diets, including vegetarian diets, ultra-low-fat diets, high polyunsaturated-fat diets, Mediterranean-type diets, and diets rich in soy foods.
- University-based clinical research needs to be made more available to researchers who investigate diet and nutritional phenomena. Fruitful research efforts would be to screen and summarize pre-World War II data, social science and agricultural data, and world data in foreign databases to develop a bibliography of references that could be added to nationwide databases such as MEDLINE.
- OAM should fund studies that examine widespread popular and folk dietary suggestions for maintaining health or controlling illness. Laboratory testing of the efficacy of ethnic foods used as disease remedies might also provide important strategies.

Summary of Part II Recommendations

Research Infrastructure

- Ultimately, OAM should be upgraded to the Center for Alternative Medicine, similar to the NIH's current National Center for Research Resources. This freestanding unit of NIH would be able to fund as well as investigate systems and processes that fall outside the normal purview of other freestanding NIH units.
- OAM should maintain a working relationship with the FDA to better assist alternative practitioners with the development and regulatory process.
- OAM should investigate areas of mutual interest with NIH and other Public Health Service agencies.
- OAM should help establish research centers at major medical institutions to assess the efficacy, safety, cost-effectiveness, and mechanisms of action of alternative medicine therapies.

Research Databases

- OAM should establish a standing research database committee to work with NLM staff on enhancing the MEDLARS database and MEDLINE. The committee should include alternative researchers and practitioners and include or have access to experts in library research and database management to help develop a program that provides investigators with adequate access to such research data.
- OAM should propose expert alternative medicine investigators or practitioners as candidates for the NLM Literature Selection Technical Review Committee and submit their names to the associate director of library operations, NLM.
- OAM should obtain information on alternative medical practices in China, Japan, India,

Tibet, the former Soviet Union, and industrialized nations throughout Europe.

Research Methodologies

- OAM should sponsor further research methodology conferences to identify or develop methodologies. Conferences that bring alternative practitioners and conventional methodologists together to select and develop methods for alternative medical research are a very high priority.
- OAM should establish an ad hoc review committee to conduct a randomized review of proposed studies. Committee members could be selected from OAM's new mandated advisory council and from among methodologists knowledgeable in alternative practices. The review effort will disclose whether assigners and grant review committees made errors in category and other procedural issues. If a review uncovers problems, the committee should develop guidelines for future peer review committees.
- OAM should continue and expand the program of inviting requests for applications (RFAs) for research grants in needed areas of alternative medicine. The response to the last RFA for exploratory grant applications indicates a tremendous interest and a wealth of promising projects.
- OAM should encourage alternative medical researchers in developing grant proposals by providing a list of resources and potential collaborators and advisers.
- OAM should implement systematic reviews and meta-analyses of existing alternative clinical investigations to objectively summarize existing clinical information, identify methodologic inadequacies in existing alternative medicine research, and document evidence (if any) of an individual therapy's clinical efficacy, toxicity, and (where possible) cost-effectiveness.
- OAM should identify any ongoing NIH-supported studies that could allow for the simultaneous testing of alternative medical therapies as adjuncts or experimental treatments. For example, a controlled trial assessing the efficacy of chemotherapy for a particular malignancy could allow for patients to be randomized to chemotherapy alone or to chemotherapy and an alternative medical practice.

Research Training

- OAM should establish intramural and extramural fellowship training opportunities for both conventional medical researchers and alternative medicine practitioners. Where appropriate, fellowship positions should be added to existing fellowship training programs.
- OAM should develop and maintain lists of current NIH research projects to prevent redundancy and foster joint efforts. Lists of conventional and alternative medical researchers willing to collaborate on research projects and facilitate joint efforts where possible should also be maintained.
- OAM should prepare a list of research methodologists, biostatisticians, and other experienced investigators willing to donate time to help alternative medical researchers.
- OAM should work with directors of medical student education to develop comprehensive programs of undergraduate medical education that explore and critically evaluate the theory, clinical practice, and research implications of alternative medical approaches.
- OAM should develop and offer educational workshops, continuing medical education symposia, and consensus conferences on alternative medical topics.
- OAM should explore opportunities for joint public-private funding to promote research and educational training in alternative medicine.
- OAM should compile lists of research methodologists who are willing to collaborate or serve as resources for alternative investigators and for conventional investigators who want to study alternative practices.
- OAM should foster annual national conferences in each major field of alternative medicine. At these conferences, participants would present current research findings, explore commonalties among alternative therapies, and discuss effective methods of clinical implementation.

- OAM should collaborate with the Foundation for Advanced Education in the Sciences, Inc., to develop continuing education courses in alternative medicine and alternative medical practices.

Peer Review

- OAM should recruit experts within the alternative medical community who are willing to review and give advice on grant applications before they are formally submitted.
- OAM staff should cooperate with staff at the Division of Research Grants (DRG), NIH, to ensure that peer review is conducted with input of those knowledgeable in the field.
- OAM should establish a select committee to continually review the makeup of peer-review panels.
- OAM should encourage DRG to develop a workable and effective NIH appeals process—one that allows due process.

Public Information Activities

- OAM should convene a committee of advisory panel members; OAM staff members; experts on database development; technical, organizational, and legal experts; and others to develop a workable plan to implement the public information clearinghouse mandated by Congress. To coordinate efforts and avoid expensive redundancy, the committee should include a member of the parallel committee that will plan the research database associated with NLM. Since many institutes at NIH have clearinghouses, it is advisable to survey several of them to discover the methods they have found appropriate.
- OAM should develop a consumer-oriented computerized inquiry system devoted to alternative medicine. This system would be similar to health consumer subsections of America OnLine and CompuServe, such as the Cancer Forum.
- OAM should develop hard-copy (i.e., printed) materials for distribution to the public.
- OAM should supply treatment information for herbal medicinals, which (in accordance with current FDA policy) are currently packaged without use instructions. (Including use information on the package is a violation of current FDA rules.) Such a reference document, which is legal, would be of considerable benefit to the public.

Major Contributors

Editorial Review Board

Brian M. Berman, M.D. (Chair)
Director
Laing/UMAB Center for Complementary Medicine
University of Maryland School of Medicine
Baltimore, MD

David B. Larson, M.D., M.P.H. (Cochair/Liaison with Office of Alternative Medicine)
President, National Institute for Healthcare Research
Rockville, MD

Other Board Members

Claire Cassidy, Ph.D.
Research Director
Traditional Acupuncture Institute
Columbia, MD
Director, Paradigms Foundation
Bethesda, MD

Barrie R. Cassileth, Ph.D.
Adjunct Professor of Medicine
University of North Carolina—Chapel Hill
Consulting Professor
Community and Family Medicine
Duke University Medical Center
Chapel Hill, NC

Larry Dossey, M.D.
Author and Consultant
Santa Fe, NM

James S. Gordon, M.D.
Clinical Professor
Departments of Psychiatry and Family Medicine
Georgetown University School of Medicine
Washington, DC

Gar Hildenbrand
Executive Director
Gerson Research Organization
San Diego, CA

Ralph W. Moss, Ph.D.
Editor
The Cancer Chronicles
New York, NY

Richard Pavek
Director
Biofield Research Institute
Sausalito, CA

John C. Reed, M.D., M.P.H.
Director
Pain and Stress Recovery Center
Phoenix, AZ

Beverly Rubik, Ph.D.
Director
Center for Frontier Sciences
Temple University
Philadelphia, PA

NIH Project Officer

Jim Bryant, M.S.
Public Affairs Officer
Office of Alternative Medicine
National Institutes of Health
Bethesda, MD

Science Editors

Managing Editor

James P. Swyers, M.A.
EEI (formerly Editorial Experts, Inc.)
Alexandria, VA

Associate Editor

Linda Silversmith, Ph.D.
EEI (formerly Editorial Experts, Inc.)
Alexandria, VA

Contributing Editors

Harriet Harvey
(Mind-Body Interventions, Pharmacological and Biological Treatments, Diet and Nutrition)
EEI (formerly Editorial Experts, Inc.)
Alexandria, VA

Richard Pavek
(Herbal Medicine, Part II, Appendix F)
Biofield Research Institute
Sausalito, CA

Cheryl Pellerin
(Executive Summary, Herbal Medicine)
EEI (formerly Editorial Experts, Inc.)
Alexandria, VA

Anne T. Phillips, M.L.S.
(Research Databases)
EEI (formerly Editorial Experts, Inc.)
Alexandria, VA

Editorial Assistants

Marc Ciagne (EEI)
Christine Griffin (EEI)

Other Major Contributors[1]

Jeanne Acterberg, Ph.D.
(Mind-Body Interventions)
Professor of Psychology
Saybrook Institute
San Francisco, CA

Michael Balick, Ph.D.
(Herbal Medicine)
Director
The New York Botanical Garden
Bronx, NY

Robert O. Becker, M.D.
(Bioelectromagnetic Applications)
Lowville, NY

Lilian Cheung, D.Sc., R.D.
(Diet and Nutrition)
Director
The Harvard Nutrition and Fitness Project
Harvard School of Public Health
Boston, MA

Effie Chow, Ph.D.
(Alternative Systems of Medical Practice)
President
East West Academy of Healing Arts
San Francisco, CA

James A. Duke, Ph.D.
(Herbal Medicine)
U.S. Department of Agriculture
Beltsville, MD

David Eisenberg, M.D.
(Research Infrastructure)
Instructor of Medicine
Department of Medicine
Harvard Medical School
Beth Israel Hospital
Boston, MA

Robert G. Flower, M.S.
(Bioelectromagnetic Applications)
Applied Science Associates
Alburtis, PA

Elliott Greene, M.A.
(Manual Healing Methods)
President
American Massage Therapy Association
Silver Spring, MD

Carlton F. Hazelwood, Ph.D.
(Bioelectromagnetic Applications, Peer Review)
Professor
Molecular Physiology and Biophysics
Baylor College of Medicine
Houston, TX

Carol Hegedus, M.S., M.A.
(Mind-Body Interventions)
Program Director of Institutional Relations
Fetzer Institute
Kalamazoo, MI

Marian W. Herrmann, M.A.
(Mind-Body Interventions)
Founder
Quanta Center of Learning and Development
Research Investigator
University of Louisville Medical School
Louisville, KY

L. John Hoffer, M.D., Ph.D.
(Diet and Nutrition)
Associate Professor, Faculty of Medicine
McGill University
Associate Director
McGill Nutrition and Food Science Center
Associate Physician
Royal Victoria Hospital
Montreal, Quebec, Canada

Tori Hudson, N.D.
(Alternative Systems of Medical Practice)
Associate Academic Dean
National College of Naturopathic Medicine
Portland, OR

Jennifer Jacobs, M.D.
(Alternative Systems of Medical Practice)
Department of Epidemiology
University of Washington
School of Public Health
Edmonds, WA

---

[1]*This list includes the names of those individuals who made significant writing contributions to the report and/or were consistently involved with the report over the many months required to complete it. Many others at the Chantilly, Virginia, workshop also contributed to the initial discussions and development of broad outlines for various chapters.*

Wayne B. Jonas, M.D.
(Research Methodologies)
Training Director
Medical Research Fellowship
Walter Reed Army Institute of Research
Walter Reed Army Medical Center
Washington, DC

J. Daniel Kanofsky, M.D., M.P.H.
(Diet and Nutrition)
Assistant Professor of Psychiatry and of Epidemiology and Social Medicine
Albert Einstein College of Medicine
Bronx Psychiatric Center
Bronx, NY

Ted Kaptchuk
(Herbal Medicine)
Research Associate
Beth Israel Hospital
Cambridge, MA

Lawrence H. Kushi, Sc.D.
(Diet and Nutrition)
Associate Professor
Division of Epidemiology
University of Minnesota School of Public Health
Minneapolis, MN

Dana Lawrence, D.C.
(Manual Healing Methods)
Professor
National College of Chiropractic
Department of Chiropractic Practice
Lombard, IL

Abraham R. Liboff, Ph.D.
(Bioelectromagnetic Applications)
Professor of Physics
Director of Medical Physics
Oakland University
Rochester, MI

Nancy Lonsdorf, M.D.
(Alternative Systems of Medical Practice)
Medical Director
Maharishi Ayur-Veda Medical Center
Washington, DC

Charles A. Moss, M.D.
(Alternative Systems of Medical Practice)
American Academy of Environmental Medicine
LaJolla, CA

Roger Nelson, Ph.D.
(Mind-Body Interventions)
Research Staff
Princeton Engineering Anomalies Research
Princeton University School of Engineering
Princeton, NJ

Paul Scharff, M.D.
(Alternative Systems of Medical Practice)
Medical Director
Rudolph Steiner Fellowship Foundation
American College of Anthroposophically Extended Medicine
Spring Valley, NY

Mildred Seelig, M.D., M.P.H.
(Diet and Nutrition)
Master of the American College of Nutrition
Editor Emeritus of the *Journal of the American College of Nutrition*
Atlanta, GA
Adjunct Professor of Nutrition
University of North Carolina—Chapel Hill
Chapel Hill, NC

Leanna Standish, N.D., Ph.D.
(Pharmacological and Biological Treatments)
Director of Research
Bastyr College of Natural Health Sciences
Seattle, WA

John Upledger, D.O.
(Manual Healing Methods)
Medical Director
The Upledger Institute
Palm Beach Gardens, FL

Jan Walleczek, Ph.D.
(Bioelectromagnetic Applications)
Staff Scientist
Veterans Affairs Medical Center
Loma Linda, CA

Walter C. Willett, M.D., Dr.P.H.
(Diet and Nutrition)
Professor of Epidemiology and Nutrition
Harvard School of Public Health
Boston, MA

This report was produced by EEI (formerly Editorial Experts, Inc.) under contract NIH-263-89-C-0016.

Introduction

by Larry Dossey, M.D. and James P. Swyers, M.A.

> The Constitution of this Republic should make special provision for Medical Freedom as well as Religious Freedom.... To restrict the art of healing to one class of men and deny equal privileges to others will constitute the Bastille of medical science. All such laws are un-American and despotic. They are fragments of monarchy and have no place in a Republic.
>
> —Benjamin Rush
> Surgeon General of the Continental Army of the United States
> Signer of the Declaration of Independence

History of Medicine in the United States

Medicine in the United States has evolved from an eclectic mix of Native American, African, Eastern, and European botanical traditions. In colonial and postcolonial America, there were dozens of competing medical philosophies, each claiming to have the "divine right" to practice medicine. By the early 1800s, medical practitioners included homeopaths, naturopaths, botanics, and Thomsonians. Competition was fierce, and the practice of medicine was essentially wide open (Hogan, 1979).

However, in the mid-1800s, the medical system we now refer to as biomedicine[1] began to dominate the scene. Biomedicine was shaped by two important sets of observations made in the early 1800s: (1) specific organic entities—bacteria—were responsible for producing particular disease states and characteristic pathological damage; and (2) certain substances—antitoxins and vaccines—could improve an individual's ability to ward off the effects of these and other pathogens. Armed with this knowledge, investigators and clinicians began to conquer a myriad of devastating infectious diseases and to perfect surgical procedures. As their conquests mounted, biomedical scientists came to believe that once they found the offending pathogen, metabolic error, or chemical imbalance, all afflictions—including many mental illnesses—would eventually yield to the appropriate vaccine, antibiotic, or chemical compound (Gordon, 1980). This philosophy eventually led them to extend their purview beyond the bounds of physical and even mental disease to conditions that previously had been viewed in religious, moral, economic, or political terms. For example, births and deaths, which traditionally had taken place at home, were moved to the hospital.

During the late 1800s, the American Medical Association (AMA), which was first organized in 1847, sponsored and lobbied for enactment of State licensing laws. By 1900, every State had enacted such a law. The result was a quick decline in competition from other schools of medical practice (Starr, 1982). The ability of biomedicine to eliminate competition was further strengthened with the passage of the Pure Food and Drug Act of 1906 and the first court trial under this act in 1908 (McGinnis, 1991). In 1910, the fate of competing forms of medicine was

[1]*This is the more accurate technical term for the style of medical practice in which practitioners hold either an M.D. (medical doctor) or D.O. (doctor of osteopathy) degree. Other terms for this system include* allopathy, Western medicine, regular medicine, conventional medicine, mainstream medicine, *and* cosmopolitan medicine. *All of these terms have some applicability, but none is as accurate as* biomedicine. Allopathy, *the most specific of these terms, denotes a tendency to choose therapies that oppose symptoms* (allo = *opposite) and enables parallels with terms such as osteopathy, homeopathy, and naturopathy. The other terms* (mainstream, conventional, *etc.) are less accurate but are better known and thus will be used throughout this text interchangeably with* biomedicine.

sealed with the release of a report by Abraham Flexner, a U.S. educator and founder of the Institute for Advanced Study in Princeton, NJ. Flexner's report, *Medical Education in the United States and Canada,* was funded by the Carnegie Foundation and was instrumental in upgrading medical education. However, it also enabled medical schools with a greater orientation toward biomedicine research to receive preferential treatment from the large philanthropic foundations that were then awarding money for medical education. Indirectly, this development led to the demise of the more financially strapped alternative medical schools (King, 1984).

Although the Flexner Report is properly credited with closing many substandard medical teaching establishments, an unfortunate side effect was a complete stifling of all competing schools of thought regarding the origins of illness and the appropriateness of therapies (Coulter, 1973). This effect occurred even though Flexner had no firsthand knowledge of medicine or medical science, or of the scientific method and its potential inadequacies (King, 1984). Indeed, in the years after his report was published, Flexner became increasingly disenchanted with the rigidity of the educational standards that had become identified with his name (Starr, 1982).

With the loss of their medical schools, all but a few alternative medical systems and practices vanished into obscurity. In 1907 there were approximately 160 medical schools in the United States; by 1914, 4 years after the Flexner Report, that number had declined to around 100 (King, 1984). Thus, by the early part of this century, biomedicine had become the standard, or convention, for every facet of health and illness. As a result, for the next half century it overshadowed "less scientific" paradigms, and those who adopted and practiced it accumulated great power and prestige. Rival healing professions and perspectives gradually disappeared, were relegated to "fringe" status, or were swallowed up by the biomedical paradigm. Some alternative medicines degenerated into the stereotypical "snake oil" proprietary medicines, further eroding the credibility of legitimate alternative medicine practitioners.

Several decades ago, however, consumer confidence in conventional medicine began to show some signs of waning. Reports emerged on the side effects and inadequacies of widely used drugs, and new strains of bacteria suddenly appeared that were resistant to the first "magic bullet" antibiotics. The use of new, more powerful antibiotics eventually resulted in microbes that could thwart them, too. Meanwhile, cures for arthritis, allergies, hypertension, cancer, depression, cardiovascular disease, digestive problems, and other chronic conditions—which had replaced infectious disease as the major killers and cripplers—eluded the best minds of biomedicine. Also, the civil rights, consumer's, and women's movements raised serious questions about the availability and equity of the allocation of health care resources under this system (Gordon, 1980).

As a result, many Americans began to look outside conventional medicine for relief. Indeed, according to a recent survey conducted by Dr. David Eisenberg of the Harvard School of Medicine and Ronald Kessler of the Survey Research Center, so-called alternative therapies appear to be as popular as ever (Eisenberg et al., 1993). This survey found that in 1990 an estimated 61 million Americans used an alternative therapy and 22 million saw a provider of alternative therapies for a principal medical condition.

More intriguing, Americans appear to have made more total visits to practitioners of alternative medicine than to conventional primary care physicians—425 million visits versus 388 million—even though most of these visits to alternative practitioners were paid out of pocket (i.e., were not covered by medical insurance). Americans spent an estimated $13.7 billion on alternative therapies in 1990, of which $10.3 billion was paid out of pocket. This is almost as much as the out-of-pocket expenditure for all hospital care in the United States that year ($12.8 billion), and it is nearly half the amount spent out of pocket for all physicians' services in the United States ($23.5 billion). Thus, alternative medicine appears to represent a significant portion of Americans' health care expenditures. Furthermore, as the Eisenberg and Kessler survey showed, the majority of people seeking alternative medical therapies are those with chronic illnesses who believe that conventional medicine has few, if any, effective treatments for their conditions.

Distinction Between Alternative and Conventional Medicine

In a narrow sense, alternative medical practices today are often defined as those that are not widely practiced in hospitals or taught in conventional U.S. medical school curriculums (Eisenberg et al., 1993). However, "alternative" medicine can refer to any one of a number of practices, techniques, and systems that may challenge the commonly assumed viewpoints or bureaucratic priorities of our dominant professionalized system of health care.

Besides wide differences in the philosophical underpinnings and the types of therapies offered by mainstream and alternative medicine, there are also major differences in how therapies are administered and how the practitioners and patients interact. For example, conventional medicine practitioners tend to give their patients standardized treatments (typically drugs or surgery or both) and medical advice on the basis of whether the patient fits into one of a number of broadly defined symptomatic categories. Furthermore, the educational theory most familiar to conventional physicians and the one they most frequently use when interacting with their patients is "physician centered." In this model, the physician is the authoritative expert and the patient is a receptive participant (Brunton, 1984). This type of communication has been found to be lacking in addressing patient needs; it encourages passivity in patients, which may undermine the patient's commitment and determination to carry out the recommended treatment regimen (McCann and Blossom, 1990).

In comparison, because alternative medical practitioners often see each patient as unique, they tend to individualize treatment to the extreme and to create elaborate procedures for identifying individual suitability and sensitivity to the interventions. They also frequently use multiple treatment modalities and judge effectiveness by using multiple or unusual outcomes, many of them subjective and patient derived (Jonas, 1993). Furthermore, many alternative systems of medicine are converging toward a client-centered relationship, where emphasis is placed on the patient's responsibility in the healing process. Patient- centered exchanges have been found to maximize the collaboration between the physician and patient, thus enhancing the benefits of a therapy. Indeed, Rosenberg (1971) showed that patients who feel they have some control over their treatment have better outcomes.

Unifying Threads Among the Alternative Medical Systems

Because the term *alternative medicine* is used to describe such a wide variety of medical systems and therapies, they cannot easily be categorized. Despite this diversity, most alternative systems of medicine do hold some common beliefs. First, there is the overarching belief that humans have built-in recuperative powers, such as when a cut heals into a scar. Most alternative medicine adherents believe that this phenomenon, referred to as *vis medicatrix naturae* (the healing power of nature), can be speeded up, sometimes to an astonishing degree, by the proper stimuli (Inglis, 1965). Thus, alternative medical practitioners typically focus on therapies designed to stimulate the patient's constitution to fight on its own behalf, on the assumption that this emphasis on enhancing the natural healing process is the most appropriate foundation of any medical therapy.

In addition, several other unifying threads are common to most alternative medical systems. These include emphasis on the

- *Integration of individuals in the "stream of life,"* that is, one's relationships and place in society, one's sense of value and self-esteem, and the various meanings and values one perceives in life (Dossey, 1991).
- *Importance of religious and spiritual values to health.* These factors are largely ignored or considered of secondary importance in contemporary medical science (Larson and Larson, 1991; Larson et al., 1992; Levin and Schiller, 1987).
- *Attribution of a causal, independent role to the various "manifestations of consciousness."* One's thoughts, attitudes, feelings, emotions, values, and perceived meanings are capable of directly affecting one's physical function. This causal view of the mind has been called "downward causation" by Nobel laureate Roger Sperry; it contrasts with the idea of "upward causation," which is currently favored in medical science. Upward causation views all mental activity as a derivative of the biochemical and physiological processes of the brain; essentially, the mind is equated with the brain, and thus the mind is regarded as a "brain in disguise." Almost all alternative medical systems maintain that consciousness may manifest itself "through" or "via" the

brain, but they do not equate the two (Sperry, 1987, 1991).

- *Maintaining the Hippocratic injunction: first do no harm.* In general, many alternative practitioners use the least harmful therapies first. In addition, most alternative therapies tend to avoid suppressing symptoms because the symptoms are understood to be a manifestation of a more profound underlying imbalance—in physiology, attitude, and lifestyle—that must be addressed. Therefore, most alternative medical practitioners tend to rely primarily on diet, exercise, relaxation techniques, and lifestyle and changes in attitude to bring about changes in health.

- *Use of whole substances.* Alternative practitioners understand that pharmacological agents, which may be extracted or synthesized from plants, may be more potent and fast acting. However, whole foods and herbs are believed to produce fewer adverse side effects.

In addition, the following concepts often are used by alternative systems of medicine and their practitioners and are important in understanding the rationale for such treatments:

- *Holism.* Holism is the principle that all aspects of the person—physical, emotional, mental, and psychosocial health; diet; lifestyle; and so on—are interrelated and must be considered in treatment, not just the specific disease or specific body part that is affected. The holistic practitioner looks equally at the relationship among these aspects of the total person and at the presenting disorder. Closely associated with the principle of holism is the principle of balance.

- *Balance and imbalance.* Balance refers to harmony among organs in the body and among body systems, in a person's diet, and in relationships to other individuals, society, and the environment. Balance or imbalance in any of these systems is understood to holistically affect other systems as well. Thus people who are out of balance with society find their organs affected because of the societal imbalance. The quality of imbalance is expressed in similar but slightly different ways in different alternative medical systems—too hot or too cold, too *yin* (weak, quiet) or too *yang* (strong, loud), too high or too low, too wet or too dry, too sweet or too salty. To achieve balance, energy must be equalized between the imbalanced portions. People who use this term often do not use the concept of "disease"[2] or use it in a much modified form.

- *Energy* refers to the force necessary to achieve balance; the part of the system that is deficient needs to acquire energy while the part that has excess needs to release energy. Thus (in traditional Chinese medicine, for example) when an organ is imbalanced, it is either too yang or too yin. Therefore, *qi* (the Chinese term for energy) must be transferred from the yang organ to the yin organ to restore balance and reestablish harmony among the organs; the harmony achieved extends holistically into all aspects (mental, physical, and psychosocial) of the person with beneficial effect. In practice, the holistic practitioner is likely to boost the vis medicatrix naturae by, for example, stimulating the immune system, balancing organ function by moving energy from the excessive organ to the deficient organ, altering diet to include more (or less) hot (or cold) foods, and prescribing more (or less) specific exercise or other lifestyle changes.

- *Healing and curing.* Because of the focus on the total person, many alternative practitioners often measure their treatment success, or lack of it, on healing the total person—bringing all aspects of the person into better balance, rather than just focusing on curing a given disease or disorder. In this view, where total outcome is more important than specific result, it is possible for the person to be *healed*

[2]Disease *is a technical concept, especially developed in biomedicine, that refers to a limited, well-defined condition such as a specific infection (measles) or deficiency (beri-beri). It has expanded to take in many less well-defined conditions for which the "cause" is complex, such as duodenal ulcer, stroke, or breast cancer. Some conditions, especially psychosocial conditions such as alcoholism and depression, which straddle the line between moral failing and disease, are becoming "medicalized," or pushed away from the moral failing category and into the disease category. In contrast,* illness *and* sickness *are social terms that emphasize sensations of unwellness and discomfort and imply a change in relationship toward family and work. Sociologically speaking, people take on the "sick role" at the time when they claim sickness and those around them accept the claim. People can have a disease and not know it, in which case they are not ill or sick because they have not recognized their condition of frailty and have not sought the sick role. Or a person can feel ill or sick and seek the sick role but be denied it, at least by medical specialists, if they "can find no wrong." When both sickness and disease overlap, everyone involved in the communication agrees that "something is wrong with this person."*

without the disease being *cured*, although the intent is always to do both.

Interface Between Alternative and Conventional Medicine

In some areas, the distinction between what is alternative and what is conventional is not always so clear-cut, because there is a constant progression of therapies from the "fringe" into the mainstream. For example, manipulative therapies such as chiropractic were considered fringe therapies 20 years ago but now are gaining increasing acceptance in mainstream medicine in the United States (Cherkin et al., 1989). In a recent survey of conventional physicians in Britain, 75 percent said that some alternative practices had become conventional between 1982 and 1987. Fifty-four percent said that musculoskeletal manipulation had become conventional, 47 percent reported the same for hypnosis, and 45 percent said that acupuncture had become conventional for certain problems (Reilly and Taylor, 1991).

This increasing acceptance of some forms of alternative medicine is demonstrated by the fact that in the past few decades, a small but growing number of M.D.s in America have organized and taken courses in manipulative medicine to better serve their patients (Gevitz, 1993). In addition, an estimated 3,000 conventionally trained physicians—M.D.s and D.O.s (doctors of osteopathy)—have been trained to incorporate acupuncture as a treatment modality in their medical practices through courses such as those affiliated with the University of California, Los Angeles, School of Medicine; the New York University School of Medicine and Dentistry; and St. Louis University Medical School (Lytle, 1993).

Furthermore, a number of tenets of naturopathy, especially those linking particular foods to the incidence of certain diseases such as cancer, are beginning to gain more credence in mainstream science. Many recent case control and cohort studies indicate associations between high intake of red meat and increased risk of some forms of cancer (Willett, 1990); other studies have focused on the anticancer protective effects of a vegetarian diet (Rao and Janezic, 1992). Such associations have led to increased interest among researchers worldwide in investigating the role that micronutrients and other substances in fruits and vegetables may play in preventing or inhibiting serious disease (Lee, 1993). (See the "Diet and Nutrition" chapter for more information on the latest research regarding these issues.)

Given that what is considered alternative today may be the accepted treatment for a particular condition in a decade or two, the following question arises: Could any of today's fringe therapies have a significant, immediate impact on the pressing and costly medical problems facing the Nation if they were more widely available?

Barriers to Progress on Alternative Medicine Research

Barriers to a fair, unbiased, scientific evaluation of alternative therapies can be categorized as structural barriers (problems caused by classification, definition, cultural, or language barriers), regulatory and economic barriers (the legal and cost implications of compliance or noncompliance with Federal and State regulations), and belief barriers (obstacles caused by ideology, misconceptions, myths, etc.).

Structural Barriers

As mentioned previously, a basic problem in investigating alternative therapies is that a clear definition of alternative medicine is almost impossible to devise. Alternative therapies are often referred to by a diverse group of sometimes derogatory pseudonyms, including "unconventional," "unorthodox," "integrated," "nonmainstream," "traditional," "nontraditional," "natural," "unscientific," "holistic," "wholistic," and many others, making classification difficult (Jonas, 1993). Other questions arise: Is the use of megavitamins, food supplements, or nutritional regimens to treat disease considered medicine, or is it a lifestyle change, or both? Can having one's aching back massaged be considered a medical therapy? How should spiritual healing and prayer—some of the oldest, most widely applied, and least studied unconventional approaches—be classified?

Because the line between conventional and alternative is imprecise and frequently changing, an approach to evaluation must be devised that is useful for comparing all types of therapy. The unfamiliar diagnostic outcome categories in many alternative approaches may require two sets of classification criteria (Wiegart et al., 1991). Traditional acupuncture, for example, classifies patients according to excesses or deficiencies in vital energy, or *chi,* in contrast to Western diagnostic classifications that are based on pathological or symptom complexes (coronary artery disease, depression, etc.). Scientists rarely understand and may oversimplify these alternative medicine concepts and thus may design methodologically correct research on the basis of incorrect classifications, resulting in unusable data (Bensoussan, 1991; Patel, 1991).

In addition, reprints of original research in alternative medicine are difficult to locate. Many alternative medicine research studies, especially those conducted in other countries, are not published in scientifically reviewed literature, and much of what does exist is not in English. For example, more than 600 research articles or abstracts have been published on the medical effects of *qigong* (a Chinese term for a form of energy), but few have been translated from Chinese (Sancier et al., 1993). The retrieval of information on alternative medicine from online databases is often inadequate, because these databases do not routinely collect articles from alternative medicine journals (Bareta et al., 1990; Dickerson, 1990; Easterbrook et al., 1991) or because the ones they do collect are not accessible by standard search languages (see the "Research Databases" chapter).

Many alternative medicine practitioners are primarily clinicians rather than researchers, and medical practice is their primary priority. Therefore, case series and anecdotal reports are often their only evidence that a practice is effective. Even so, the quality of the research presented by alternative medical practitioners is not always poor, and the fact that an article is published in an alternative medical journal does not mean the study is inferior. For example, a meta-analysis of 107 published controlled trials of homeopathic treatments to assess their methodological quality found that while many of the trials were of "low" methodological quality, there appeared to be an overall positive effect from the homeopathic treatment regardless of the quality of the trial. The authors of the study noted that while no definitive conclusions about the effectiveness of homeopathic treatments could be drawn, the meta-analysis supported a legitimate case for the further evaluation of homeopathy (Kleijnen et al., 1991).

Therefore, one cannot assume that practices unfamiliar to conventional physicians and researchers are necessarily backed by poor-quality research. Surprisingly, adequate methods for judging the quality of research in individual alternative medicine studies, both published and unpublished, still remain an underdeveloped research area. Scientists who conduct reviews of the literature on alternative medicine must be comprehensive, systematic, and explicit (Fuchs and Garber, 1990; Larson et al., 1986; Sachett et al., 1991).

Finally, many conventional physicians remain virtually unaware that alternative approaches exist, even though their patients are seeing them and alternative medical practitioners simultaneously for the same condition. The Eisenberg-Kessler survey (Eisenberg et al., 1993) found that 70 percent of patients seeking alternative practices did not reveal to their conventional physicians that they had done so. Patients' unwillingness to reveal this information to their conventional physicians may be largely due to the physician-centered model discussed above. Recently, an increasing number of members of the conventional medical community have called for physicians to move toward a patient-centered model for educating and interacting with patients. The impetus for this is a realization that the majority of patients want to participate in their clinical decisionmaking and are more likely to adhere to a prescribed therapy using this approach (Brody and Larson, 1992; Brunton, 1984; Titus et al., 1980).

Regulatory and Economic Barriers

Today there are literally hundreds of treatments that are considered alternative, or outside the range of conventional medical treatment modalities. These treatments include various forms of behavioral, psychological, and spiritual interventions, as well as a host of herbal, pharmacological, nutritional, and mechanical therapies. Promoters of these therapies include trained physicians and other allied health care practitioners as well as laypersons.

The U.S. Food and Drug Administration (FDA) is the Federal agency most responsible for protecting consumers against unsafe and ineffective medicines and health products in the marketplace. Armed with broad regulatory powers delegated to the agency by the Food, Drug, and

Cosmetic Act (FDCA), FDA oversees distribution of the Nation's food supply, oversees development and marketing of new drugs and medical devices, and generally supervises the promotion of these items to ensure that consumers are not harmed or defrauded.

Under the FDCA, new drugs require extensive laboratory and animal testing before their sponsors can petition FDA for an investigational new drug (IND) application for limited testing in humans. IND applications must state in detail how the clinical trials will be conducted (e.g., how subjects will be selected and how many will be involved with the studies), where the studies will be done and by whom, and how the product's safety and effectiveness will be evaluated.

Clinical trials are generally done in three phases. Phase I studies are designed to determine the safety of the product using small numbers of healthy subjects. Phase II studies are concerned more with the effectiveness of the product, usually employ up to several hundred volunteers diagnosed with the particular disease or condition under investigation, and may take 2 years or more to complete. Phase III studies, which may require several hundred to several thousand subjects and take 4 years or more to complete, are then designed to elaborate the correct dosage and frequency of administration of the product (Evers, 1988).

The entire drug approval process is time-consuming and extremely expensive, forcing treatment sponsors to spend millions of dollars each year to comply with FDA's safety and efficacy regulations. For example, a manufacturer must submit more than 100,000 pages of supporting documentation in connection with a single new drug application (Hect, 1983). It can take up to 10 years and cost hundreds of millions of dollars to obtain FDA approval of a new drug (Evers, 1988; also see the "Herbal Medicine" chapter). These astronomical costs are beyond the reach of all but a few corporations and can be recouped only by exercising the legal 17-year monopolies conferred by the U.S. patent laws. With a patent, drug companies can and do charge whatever the market will bear.

Thus, the current Federal mechanisms of regulating medical research do not favor the evaluation of many forms of alternative treatment. Because the costs of developing, evaluating, and marketing new drugs are so prohibitive, pharmaceutical companies are not likely to invest time and effort in therapies, such as nutritional or behavioral approaches, that cannot be patented and are therefore unlikely to offer the opportunity to recover their investment and provide a return to stockholders. This means that many alternative therapies are likely to be casualties of the formal research process.

Although foods are exempt from such extensive premarketing clearance, the FDA often regulates foods as if they were drugs whenever any health claims are associated with a product, even though the same product may also qualify as a food or as a cosmetic. A recent controversy surrounding the advertising campaign of a popular breakfast cereal demonstrates how overzealous FDA can be at times. FDA disapproved of the manufacturer's claims that its cereal would help prevent colon cancer, even though the company had prepared the advertisement in cooperation with the National Cancer Institute. FDA launched a probe into the matter, which it later had to abandon (Evers, 1988).

FDA has long attempted to regulate vitamins and minerals as drugs. The AMA supports this view and has urged Congress to grant FDA such authority (U.S. Congress, 1984). To date, Congress has not chosen to extend FDA's drug jurisdiction to encompass vitamins and minerals, except in cases where therapeutic claims are made for products.

Although the FDCA is the most comprehensive law designed to prevent interstate marketing of unapproved drugs, several other Federal statutes also are applicable to promotion or sale. The Federal Trade Commission (FTC) often uses the term *false advertisement* under the Federal Trade Commission Act to prevent the manufacturers of alternative therapies from promoting their products or services. Courts have generally held that the FTC does not have to show that an advertiser lacked good faith or intended to deceive, nor must it show that actual deception occurred. Rather, it has to show only that the potential to deceive might be there.

The FTC frequently seeks to hinder what it considers false advertising dealing with disease prevention or cure. For example, in 1983 the FTC sought to prohibit the manufacturer of a dietary supplement—which contained vitamins A, C, and E; selenium; beta-carotene; and dehydrated vegetables—from advertising its product as reducing the risk of certain cancers. The manufacturer's claims were based on the findings of a report entitled *Diet, Nutrition, and Cancer*, published by the National Research Council (1982). The FTC successfully argued that the manufacturer's representations went well beyond the report's conclusions and thus were false, misleading, and deceptive because they conveyed the impression that simply consuming daily portions of the product would prevent cancer. Accordingly, an injunction was issued prohibiting such advertisements (Evers, 1988).

In addition to FDA and FTC restrictions and regulations, the Federal Government routinely uses numerous other statutes to curtail the promotion of alternative treatments and practices. Statutes such as the mail fraud and wire fraud statutes and the "smuggling statute" are among the many laws that provide criminal penalties for those who promote unapproved products through the mail or on the radio or attempt to import them from overseas. Penalties can be fines of up to $10,000 or 5 years' imprisonment or both.

Another major barrier to the investigation and acceptance of alternative medicine is the existence in all States of medical practice acts that limit the practice of healing arts to holders of medical licenses. The history of medical licensure illustrates not only the enormous power bestowed on professional groups by regulation, but also the ways licensing has been used to eliminate or curtail the activities of alternative medical practitioners, regardless of whether their methods have been proved harmful. For example, throughout this century the medical professional organizations have used a variety of weapons to harass osteopathic and chiropractic physicians. Indeed, conventional medical organizations have historically prohibited their members from even consulting with "sectarian" practitioners such as homeopaths and chiropractors (see below). Medical organizations establish such prohibitions for reasons that have to do as much with ideology as with economics. The ideological reasons are discussed below.

Belief Barriers

Conventional physicians in general adhere to a number of beliefs and misconceptions about themselves and the type of medicine they practice that prevent them from viewing anything labeled "alternative" in a positive light or taking it seriously. The following are some of the ideological grounds for conventional physicians' skepticism of alternative systems of medicine and their therapies.

- *Confidence in high technology.* High-tech diagnostic and therapeutic procedures in modern medicine are often enormously attractive to the physician. However, confidence in these instruments and procedures often exceeds the evidence for their effectiveness (Grimes, 1993). As a result, many alternative therapies, which are often relatively "low tech," may be considered ineffective.

- *Safety in the status quo.* Once in place, established therapies often tend to prevail over new or alternative treatments. How much and what kind of evidence is necessary for implementing an alternative therapy? This question has not been fully answered even for conventional therapies. For example, acceptance of a new drug therapy usually requires repeated, double-blind, placebo-controlled, randomized clinical trials, whereas implementation of new surgical techniques may at times be done without any controlled trials at all (Eddy, 1990).

- *The "one true" medical profession.* A longstanding belief held by many conventional medical practitioners is that there should be only one representative voice for the whole of medicine (Gevitz, 1989). That is, only the members of their profession, holders of a certain degree from approved institutions, are the bona fide, rightful, and exclusive representatives of medicine, and they should be allowed to control all aspects of medical practice (Inglis, 1965). For example, in the 1960s the AMA decided to contain and eliminate chiropractic as a profession. To do so, in 1963 the AMA formed its Committee on Quackery, which worked aggressively—both overtly and covertly—to find ways to cut off chiropractors from their base of patients. One of the AMA's principal means of achieving this goal was to make it unethical for a medical physician to associate with an "unscientific practitioner." Then, in 1966, the AMA's House of Delegates passed a resolution calling chiropractic an "unscientific cult." To complete the circle, the AMA's Judicial Council issued an opinion holding that it was unethical for a physician to associate professionally with chiropractors (Gevitz, 1989).

Although the AMA gradually relaxed some of its taboos regarding chiropractors, these relaxed positions were generally not communicated to AMA members (Gevitz, 1989). However, in the August 1987 *Wilk et al. v. the American Medical Association* decision, a Federal judge found that the AMA, the American College of Radiology, and the American College of Surgeons had conspired to intentionally harm the chiropractic profession and were thus guilty of violating the Sherman Antitrust Act (Special Communication, 1988). Under the court's ruling, the AMA was ordered to cease and desist its hampering of chiropractors and to send a copy of the injunction to each of its members.

- *Stereotypes.* One stereotype of alternative medicine that is widely propagated is that it attracts people with "weak" minds (i.e., the uneducated and the poor) who easily succumb to the "sideshow" lures of "snake oil" salespeople, who are not qualified to give medical advice or to practice medicine. However, recent studies of cancer patients indicate that, much to the contrary, well-educated persons with higher incomes are more likely to use alternative treatments, primarily because they want to take charge of their health (Lerner and Kennedy, 1992; McGinnis, 1991). Furthermore, more than 60 percent of practitioners of alternative treatments for cancer hold an M.D., a Ph.D., or both from an accredited medical school or graduate school (Cassileth et al., 1984). In addition, the term *quack,* as a blanket indictment of all those who practice alternative forms of medicine, is often used more as an insult than as an objective assessment of someone's skills and intentions. According to Dr. David J. Hufford, professor of behavioral science at the Pennsylvania State College of Medicine, the term *quack* generally means "one who pretends to have medical knowledge but does not; that is, it implies the element of fraud." Hufford contends that most alternative healers do not pretend to have medical knowledge but possess some other sort of knowledge that they and their clients believe is relevant to health. "Certainly the use of caution to protect oneself and one's family from unscrupulous and incompetent health care pretenders should be part of everyone's concern. But this is not limited to alternative medicine," he maintains (Hufford, 1990).

The barriers facing many aspects of alternative medicine today are typical of the barriers that have faced novel scientific ideas throughout the centuries. At the root of this conflict is the fact that alternative and mainstream medical scientists often have two diametrically opposed views, not just on which drugs and vaccines are appropriate or most effective for a particular condition, but on the nature of life itself.

The 20th-century scientific philosopher Thomas Kuhn put this age-old conflict into perspective by stating that scientific doctrines rest not just on facts, but more fundamentally on paradigms (i.e., broad views of how those facts should be organized).[3] Differences in views among groups of people are a reflection of the different scientific paradigms they adhere to. According to Kuhn, because unusual scientific discoveries often require more than incremental adjustments to the dominant scientific paradigm, the hapless innovator who stumbles upon some new set of facts that run counter to the dominant paradigm often finds it necessary to elaborate a whole new paradigm to accommodate them. When this happens, the innovator often becomes a scientific outcast, for, as Kuhn wrote, "to desert the paradigm is to cease practicing the science it defines" (Kuhn, 1970). For example, Louis Pasteur, the father of microbiology, was thrown out of the Academy of Medicine for suggesting that microbes that could not be seen by the naked eye were responsible for causing food to spoil and that spontaneous generation (life arising from nonliving matter) was an impossibility (Kostychev, 1978).

---

[3]*A paradigm is an overarching cosmological conceptual scheme; an explanatory model explains a limited set of events or observations from within a paradigm and using the guidance of a paradigm. Alternative words for paradigm include* worldview, framework, *and* weltanschauung, *all of which suggest the largeness of the concept. A paradigm tells whole societies in whole historical periods how to think about such "big issues" as goodness, success, holiness, love, and evil. Much of a paradigm is out of awareness—that is, people act on it without realizing that they have other choices. In contrast, an explanatory model is the way one discipline, denomination, or health care system explains itself—the details of its assumptions, logic, and rationale—and much of this is within the awareness of its practitioners, and is therefore open to argument, criticism, and change.*

Thus, bridging the gap between the different paradigms of the conventional medical and alternative medical communities is and always has been a formidable challenge. However, as the public turns increasingly to alternative medical practitioners for treatment, pressure is mounting on the mainstream scientific and medical communities as well as on Federal and State scientific and regulatory bodies to speed up the investigation and evaluation of "novel" approaches. The public is demanding a streamlined evaluation process not only to provide it with more health care options, but also to provide definitive answers about the safety and efficacy of alternative therapies that are being offered.

Role of the Office of Alternative Medicine

In response to this increasing public pressure, in 1992 Congress established the Office of Alternative Medicine (OAM) in the Office of the Director of the National Institutes of Health (NIH). OAM's mandate is to facilitate the evaluation of alternative medical treatments that might offer promise for addressing a number of serious health problems that afflict the Nation. OAM also was mandated to establish an information clearinghouse to exchange information with the public about alternative medicine. In addition, OAM was charged with supporting research training in topics related to alternative medicine that are not typically included in the training curriculums of mainstream physicians and other health professionals.

OAM has been guided through its early stages by an ad hoc advisory panel of alternative medical practitioners and mainstream medical researchers who have an interest in alternative medicine. With its recent formal charter as an NIH advisory council status, this panel will play an increasing role in helping OAM to fulfill its mandate.

OAM's mandate is not to be an advocate of any particular alternative medicine treatment, but rather to advocate the fair scientific evaluation of alternative therapies that are found to have *potential* for improving the health and well-being of a significant number of people. In doing so, OAM has positioned itself as an intermediary between the alternative medical community and the Federal research and regulatory communities, in order to help reduce the barriers that may keep promising alternative therapies from coming to light.

Organization of This Report

Traditionally, alternative medical disciplines often have been divided into four categories on the basis of the type of treatment or treatments offered by their practitioners. The psychological and spiritual category (often referred to as mind-body) includes practitioners who use psychological techniques such as mental imaging, hypnosis, and art therapy. The diet and nutrition category includes those who recommend dietary supplementation with vitamins or minerals and prescribe specific diets, such as a vegetarian or macrobiotic diet, for specific conditions. The drug and biological category comprises specialists in the use of assorted chemicals, drugs, serums, and vaccines (e.g., treatments to enhance the immune system) and the injection of live cells from fetuses and animals. The fourth category, involving treatment with physical forces and devices, includes chiropractors, massage and touch therapists, acupuncturists, and practitioners of various electrotherapies.

This report deviates from this scheme in several ways. For example, although it includes the above-mentioned categories—mind-body, diet and nutrition, biologics and pharmacologics (i.e., drugs), and manual healing (i.e., massage, chiropractic, etc.)—it also includes a separate section on bioelectromagnetic therapies instead of grouping them with massage and chiropractic. In addition, there is a chapter on alternative systems of medicine (i.e., homeopathy, traditional Asian medicine, etc.) as well as a chapter on herbal medicine. Part II deals with issues that are germane to all areas of alternative medicine, including research methodology issues, peer review, research training, database establishment, and so on.

Each chapter presents an overview of the discipline (i.e., historical background as well as how the system or therapy is used today), the research base, future research opportunities, barriers to research, and key issues. Many sections also contain specific recommendations relating to priorities for research and evaluation activities as well as specific illnesses or groups of patients that may benefit from such therapies.

This report is by no means all-inclusive; a number of alternative medical systems and therapies are not discussed here. For instance, midwifery is not discussed, even though in many States midwifery is considered outside the mainstream of medicine and midwives are legally prevented from practicing. Midwifery and a number of other important alternative medicine disciplines were left out because of limited time and resources rather than because of a conscious decision to overlook them. The present plan is for this report to be updated so that later editions will be more accurate and more comprehensive.

Neither is this a consensus document. Contributors to this report do not necessarily agree with all of its content and recommendations. It covers such an array of topics and required input from such a diverse group of experts and disciplines that reaching consensus even within a particular area of expertise, such as diet and nutrition, would have been virtually impossible without a prohibitively lengthy and costly peer review process. Because much of the research on alternative medicine, by definition, has been conducted outside the mainstream of medicine, it is not possible to verify all of the individual claims of efficacy made in this report. Rather, the report is a good-faith effort to point out research directions to OAM and other Federal agencies where there is at least some evidence to suggest that further inquiry is warranted.

Claire Cassidy, Ph.D., James S. Gordon, M.D., Ralph W. Moss, Ph.D., and Richard Pavek contributed to this section.

References

Bareta, J., D. Larson, J. Lyons, and J. Zorc. 1990. A comparison of manual and MEDLARS reviews of the literature on consultation-liaison psychiatry. Am. J. Psychiatry 147:1040.

Bensoussan, A. 1991. Contemporary acupuncture research: the difficulties of research across scientific paradigms. Am. J. Acupunc. 19(4):357–365.

Brody, D., and D. Larson. 1992. The role of primary care physicians in managing depression. J. Gen. Intern. Med. 7:243–247.

Brunton, S.A. 1984. Physicians as patient teachers. In Personal Health Maintenance (Special Issue). West. J. Med. 141:855–860.

Cassileth, B.R., E.J. Lusk, T.B. Strouse, and B.J. Bodenheimer. 1984. Contemporary unorthodox treatments in cancer medicine: a study of patients, treatments, and practitioners. Ann. Intern. Med. 101:105–112.

Cherkin, D., F.A. MacCornack, and A.O. Berg. 1989. Family physicians' views of chiropractors: hostile or hospitable? Am. J. Public Health 79(5):636–637.

Coulter, H. 1973. Divided Legacy: The Conflict Between Homeopathy and the American Medical Association. North Atlantic Books, Richmond, Calif.

Dickerson, K. 1990. The existence of publication bias and risk factors for its occurrence. JAMA 263:1385.

Dossey, L. 1991. Meaning and Medicine. Bantam, New York.

Easterbrook, P.J., J.A. Berlin, R. Gopolan, and D.R. Matthews. 1991. Publication bias in clinical research. Lancet 337:867.

Eddy, D.M. 1990. Should we change the rules for evaluating medical technologies? In A.C. Geligns, ed. Modern Methods of Clinical Investigation. National Academy Press, Washington, D.C.

Eisenberg, D., R. Kessler, C. Foster, F.E. Norlock, D.R. Calkins, and T.L. Delbanco. 1993. Unconventional medicine in the U.S.: prevalence, costs, and patterns of use. N. Engl. J. Med. 328(4):245–252.

Evers, M.S. 1988. Unconventional Cancer Treatments: Legal Constraints on the Availability of Unorthodox Cancer Treatments. Congress of the United States, Office of Technology Assessment.

Fuchs, V.R., and A.M. Garber. 1990. The new technology assessment. N. Engl. J. Med. 323:673.

Gevitz, N. 1989. The chiropractors and the AMA: reflections on the history of the consultation clause. Perspect. Biol. Med. 32:281–299.

Gevitz, N. 1993. The scope and challenge of unconventional medicine. Advances, The Journal of Mind-Body Health 9(3):4–11.

Gordon, J.S. 1980. The paradigm of holistic medicine. In A. Hastings, ed. Health for the Whole Person. Westview Press, Boulder, Colo.

Grimes, D.A. 1993. Technology follies: the uncritical acceptance of medical innovation. JAMA 269:3030–3033.

Hect. 1983. Slashing away at red tape in the new drug approval process. FDA Consumer February:10–11.

Hogan, D. 1979. The Regulation of Psychotherapists, Vol. 1. Ballinger, Cambridge, Mass.

Hufford, D.J. 1990. Unconventional Cancer Treatments. Congress of the United States, Office of Technology Assessment.

Inglis, B. 1965. The Case for Unorthodox Medicine. G.P. Putnam's Sons, New York.

Jonas, W.B. 1993. Evaluating unconventional medical practices. Journal of NIH Research 5:64–67.

King, L.S. 1984. The Flexner Report of 1910. JAMA 251(8):1079–1086.

Kleijnen, J., P. Knipschild, and G. ter Riet. 1991. Clinical trials of homeopathy. BMJ 302(6772): 316–323.

Kostychev, S.P. 1978. Pasteur, his life and achievements. Oxford and IBH Pub. Co., New Delhi.

Kuhn, T.S. 1970. The structure of scientific revolutions. In International Encyclopedia of Unified Science, Vol. 2. University of Chicago Press, Chicago.

Larson, D.B., and S.S. Larson. 1991. Religious commitment and health: valuing the relationship. Second Opinion: Health, Faith, and Ethics 17(1):26–40.

Larson, D.B., K.A. Sherrill, J.S. Lyons, F.C. Craigie Jr., et al. 1992. Associations between dimensions of religious commitment and mental health reported in the American Journal of Psychiatry and Archives of General Psychiatry: 1978–1989. Am. J. Psychiatry 149(4):557–559.

Larson, D., et al. 1986. Systematic analysis of research on religious variables in four major psychiatric journals, 1978–1982. Am. J. Psychiatry 143(3):329–334.

Lee, H.P. 1993. Diet and cancer: a short review. Ann. Acad. Med. Singapore 22(3):355–359.

Lerner, I.J., and B.J. Kennedy. 1992. The prevalence of questionable methods of cancer treatments in the United States. CA Cancer J. Clin. 42:181–191.

Levin, J.S., and P.L. Schiller. 1987. Is there a religious factor in health? Journal of Religion and Health 26:9–36.

Lytle, C.D. 1993. An Overview of Acupuncture. Center for Devices and Radiological Health, U.S. Department of Health and Human Services, Public Health Service, Food and Drug Administration.

McCann, D.P., and H.J. Blossom. 1990. The physician as a patient educator: from theory to practice. Western J. Med. 153:44–49.

McGinnis, L.S. 1991. Alternative therapies, 1990: an overview. Cancer 67:1788–1792.

National Research Council. Assembly of Life Sciences. Committee on Diet, Nutrition, and Cancer. 1982. Diet, Nutrition, and Cancer. National Academy Press, Washington, D.C.

Patel, M.S. 1991. Problems in the evaluation of alternative medicine. Soc. Sci. Med. 25:669.

Rao, A.V., and S.A. Janezic. 1992. The role of dietary phytosterols in colon carcinogenesis. Nutr. Cancer 18(1):43–52.

Reilly, D.T., and M.A. Taylor. 1991. Developing Integrated Medicine: Report of the Research Council on Complementary Medicine (RCCM) Research Fellowship in Complementary Medicine. Department of Medicine, University of Glasgow.

Rosenberg, S. 1971. Patient education leads to better care for heart patients. HSMHA Health Rep. 86:793–802.

Sachett, D.L., R.B. Haynes, G.H. Guyatt, and P. Tugwell, eds. 1991. Clinical Epidemiology: A Basic Science for Clinical Medicine. Little, Brown & Co., Boston.

Sancier, K.M., W. Croft, W. Lee, and R. Burke. 1993. Permuted Title/Keyword Index of Qigong. The Qigong Institute, San Francisco.

Special Communication. 1988. JAMA 259(1):81–82.

Sperry, R.W. 1987. Structure and significance of the consciousness revolution. Journal of Mind and Behavior 8:37–66.

Sperry, R.W. 1991. Search for beliefs to live by consistent with science. Zygon 26(2):237–258.

Starr, P. 1982. The Social Transformation of American Medicine. Basic Books, Inc., New York.

Titus, E., J. Low, R. Clark, et al. 1980. Patient Education as Adult Education: A Workshop—Patient Education in a Primary Care Setting. Proceedings of the 4th National Conference, Memphis, Tenn.

U.S. Congress, House of Representatives, Select Committee on Aging, Subcommittee on Health and Long-Term Care. 1984. Quackery: A $10 Billion Scandal (hearing May 31, 1984). U.S. Government Printing Office, Washington D.C.

Wiegart, F.C., C.W. Kramers, and R. van Wijk. 1991. Clinical research in complementary medicine: the importance of patient selection. Comp. Med. Research 5:110.

Willett, W.C. 1990. Epidemiologic studies of diet and cancer. Med. Oncol. Tumor Pharmacother. 7(2–3):93–97.

Part I
Fields of Practice

Mind-Body Interventions

PANEL MEMBERS AND CONTRIBUTING AUTHORS

Jeanne Achterberg, Ph.D.—Cochair
Larry Dossey, M.D.—Cochair
James S. Gordon, M.D.—Cochair
Carol Hegedus, M.S., M.A.
Marian W. Herrmann, M.A.
Roger Nelson, Ph.D.

Introduction

Most traditional medical systems appreciate and make use of the extraordinary interconnectedness of the mind and the body and power of each to affect the other. In contrast, modern Western medicine has regarded these connections as of secondary importance.

The separation between mind and body was established during the 17th century. Originally it permitted medical science the freedom to explore and experiment on the body while preserving for the church the domain of the mind. In the succeeding three centuries, the medicine that evolved from this focus on the body and its processes has yielded extraordinary discoveries about the nature and treatment of disease states.

However, this narrow focus has also tended to obscure the importance of the interactions between mind and body and to overshadow the possible importance of the mind in producing and alleviating disease. The focus of medical research has been on the biology of the body and of the brain, which is part of the body. Concern with the mind has been left to non-biologically oriented psychiatrists, other mental health professionals, philosophers, and theologians. Psychosomatic medicine, the discipline that has addressed mind-body connections, is a subspecialty within the specialty of psychiatry.

During the past 30 years, there has been a powerful scientific movement to explore the mind's capacity to affect the body and to rediscover the ways in which it permeates and is affected by all of the body's functions. This movement has received its impetus from several sources. It has been spurred by the rise in incidence of chronic illnesses—including heart disease, cancer, depression, arthritis, and asthma—which appear to be related to environmental and emotional stresses. The prevalence, destructiveness, and cost of these illnesses have set the stage for the exploration of therapies that can help individuals appreciate the sources of their stress and reduce that stress by quieting the mind and using it to mobilize the body to heal itself.

During the same time, medical researchers have discovered other cultures' healing systems, such as meditation, yoga, and tai chi, which are grounded in an understanding of the power of mind and body to affect one another; developed techniques such as biofeedback and visual imagery, which are capable of facilitating the mind's capacity to affect the body; and examined some of the specific links between mental processes and autonomic, immune, and nervous system functioning—most dramatically illustrated by the growth of a new discipline, psychoneuroimmunology.

The clinical aspect of the enterprise that explores, appreciates, and makes use of mind-body interactions has come to be called mind-body medicine. The techniques that its practitioners use are mind-body interventions. The chapter discusses the evidence that supports the mind-body approach, describes some of these techniques, and summarizes the results of some of the most effective interventions.

This approach is not only producing dramatic results in specific arenas, it is forming the basis for a new perspective on medicine and healing. From this perspective it is becoming clear that every interaction between doctors and patients—

between those who give help and those who receive it—may affect the mind and in turn the body of the patient. From this perspective all of medicine, indeed all of health care, is grounded in the mind-body approach. And all interventions, alternative or conventional, can be enhanced by it.

Meaning of *Mind-Body*

Any discussion of mind-body interventions brings the old questions back to life: What are mind and consciousness?[1] How and where do they originate? How are they related to the physical body? In approaching the field of mind-body interventions, it is important that the mind not be viewed as if it were dualistically isolated from the body, as if it were doing something *to* the body. Mind-body relations are always mutual and bidirectional—the body affects the mind and is affected by it. Mind and body are so integrally related that, in practice, it makes little sense to refer to therapies as solely "mental" or "physical." For example, activities that appear overwhelmingly "physical," such as aerobic exercise, yoga, and dance, can have healthful effects not only on the body but also on such "mental" problems as depression and anxiety; and "mental" approaches such as imagery and meditation can benefit physical problems such as hypertension and hypercholesterolemia as well as have salutary psychological effects. Even the use of drugs and surgery has its psychological side. The use of these methods often requires placebo-controlled, double-blind studies to estimate and factor out the physical effects of patients' beliefs and expectations.

When the term *mind-body* is used in this report, therefore, there is no implication that an object or thing—the mind—is somehow acting on a separate entity—the body. Rather, "mind-body" could perhaps best be regarded as an overall *process* that is not easily dissected into separate and distinct components or parts. This point of view, which was put forward a century ago by William James, the father of American psychology, has recently been reaffirmed by brain researchers Francis Crick and Christof Koch (1992).

Timeless Factors in Healing

Throughout history the value of "human" factors in healing has been recognized. These factors include closeness, caring, compassion, and empathy between therapist and patient. Though these factors are theoretically acknowledged by contemporary medicine, they are largely ignored in current practice, partly because they are hard to define and measure and cannot be easily taught. In many mind-body interventions, however, their relevance is obvious. A research agenda for the future should include an investigation of the impact of these qualities on healing—not only on alternative, mind-body interventions but on orthodox therapies as well.

Healing and Curing

Mind-body interventions frequently lead patients to new ways of experiencing and expressing their illness. For example, although healing usually denotes an objective improvement in health, patients commonly state that they feel "healed" but not "cured"—that is, they experience a profound sense of psychological or spiritual well-being and wholeness although the actual disease remains. Distinctions between curing (the actual eradication of a disease) and healing (a sense of wholeness and completeness) have little place in contemporary medical practice but are important to patients. A place should be made for these distinctions. Acknowledging that "healing without curing" is both permissible and honorable requires the recognition of spiritual elements in illness.[2] It also requires honoring the wishes of individuals in deciding what is best in the course of their disease process. Sometimes, zealous attempts to cure may have disastrous effects on patients' quality of life for the years they have left.

---

[1]*In this report,* mind *and* consciousness *are used interchangeably, and the following definition is accepted: "Our use of the term* consciousness *is intended to subsume all categories of human experience, including those commonly termed 'conscious,' 'subconscious,' 'superconscious,' or 'unconscious,' without presumption of specific psychological or physiological mechanisms" (Jahn and Dunne, 1987).*

[2]*"Spiritual elements are those capacities that enable a human being to rise above or transcend any experience at hand. They are characterized by the capacity to seek meaning and purpose, to have faith, to love, to forgive, to pray, to meditate, to worship, and to see beyond present circumstances" (Clifford Kuhn, quoted in Aldridge, D. 1993. Is there evidence for spiritual healing?* Advances *9:4–85). "The spiritual dimension . . . is that aspect of the person concerned with meaning and the search for absolute reality that underlies the world of the senses and the mind and, as such, is distinct from adherence to a religious system" (J. Hiatt. 1986. Spirituality, medicine, and healing.* Southern Medical Journal *79:736–743.*

Evidence of Mind-Body Effects in Contemporary Medical Science

Social Isolation

Biological scientists have long been aware of the importance of social relationships on health. As the evolutionary biologist George Gaylord Simpson observed, "No animal or plant lives alone or is self-sustaining. All live in communities including other members of their own species and also a number, usually a large variety, of other sorts of animals and plants. *The quest to be alone is indeed a futile one, never successfully followed in the history of life*" (emphasis added) (Simpson, 1953, p. 53).

This observation is nowhere truer than in the human domain, where perceptions of social isolation and aloneness may set in motion mind-body events of life-or-death importance. This point has been demonstrated in research on many dimensions of human experience, among them the following:

Bereavement. The idea that a person can die from being separated suddenly from a loved one is rooted in history and spans all cultures—the "broken heart" syndrome. In the United States, 700,000 people aged 50 or older lose their spouses annually. Of these, 35,000 die during the first year after the spouse's death. Researcher Steven Schleifer of Mount Sinai Hospital, New York, calculates that 20 percent, or 7,000, of these deaths are directly caused by the loss of the spouse. The physiological processes responsible for increased mortality during bereavement have been the subject of extensive investigations and include profound alterations in cardiovascular and immunological responses. In study after study, the mortality of the surviving spouse during the first year of bereavement has been found to be 2 to 12 times that of married people the same age (Dimsdale, 1977; Engel, 1971; Holmes and Rahe, 1967; Lown et al., 1980; Lynch, 1977; Schleifer et al., 1983; Stoddard and Henry, 1985). These studies have far-reaching therapeutic implications as well. Individual and group support can—and have been shown to—help mitigate the devastating effects of loss.

Poor education and illiteracy. A more general and pervasive form of isolation results from poor education and illiteracy, which are in turn associated with increased incidence of disease and death. As Thomas B. Graboys of Harvard Medical School has stated, poor education is "an Orwellian recipe in which the estranged worker, besieged from above and below, mixes internal rage and incessant frustration into a fatal brew" (Graboys, 1984).

Many believe that the common factor in poor education, poor health, and higher mortality is simply that the poorly educated take worse care of themselves. However, research shows that smoking, exercise, diet, and accessibility to health care, while important, do not explain the poorer health and earlier death of these people; the influence of social isolation and poor education is more powerful. Moreover, poor education appears to be only a stand-in or proxy for stress and loneliness—that is, low education actually does its damage through the stress and social isolation to which it leads (Berkman and Syme, 1982; House et al., 1982, 1988; Ruberman et al., 1984; Sagan, 1987).

The underlying pathophysiological processes by which social isolation may bring about poor health have been illuminated by studies of primates in the wild. Low-ranking baboons, whose entire life is spent in constant danger with little control, demonstrate high circulating levels of hydrocortisone, which remain elevated even when the stressful event has passed. In addition, chronic psychological stress and isolation have been associated with decreased concentrations of high-density lipoproteins, which protect against heart disease, and weaker immune systems with fewer circulating disease-fighting lymphocytes (Sapolsky, 1990).

Work Status

Attitude toward work and work status may also be intimately related to health and well-being. Several lines of evidence point to these correlations:

- When researcher Peter L. Schnall and his colleagues examined the relationship between "job strain," blood pressure, and the mass of the heart's left ventricle, they found—after adjusting for age, race, body-mass index, type A behavior, alcohol intake, smoking, the nature of the work site, sodium excretion, education, and the physical demand level of the job—that job strain was significantly related to hypertension. They concluded that "job strain may be a risk factor for both hypertension and structural changes of the heart in working men" (Schnall et al., 1990; Williams, 1990).

- Epidemiologist C. David Jenkins demonstrated in 1971 that most people in the United States who experience their first heart attack when they are under the age of 50 have *no* major risk factors. Although Jenkins's findings must be tempered by the more recent redefinition of what constitutes "normal" cholesterol and blood pressure, the point remains: a purely physical approach may be inadequate for understanding the origins of coronary artery disease in our culture (Jenkins, 1971).

- In a 1973 survey in Massachusetts, a special Department of Health, Education, and Welfare task force reported that the best predictor for heart attack was none of the classic risk factors, but the level of one's job dissatisfaction (*Work in America: Report of a Special Task Force to the Secretary of Health, Education, and Welfare*, 1973). It is possible that this finding may be related to the observation that heart attacks in the United States, as well as in other Western industrialized nations, cluster on Monday mornings from 8 to 9 a.m., the beginning of the work week (Kolata, 1986; Muller et al., 1987; Rabkin et al., 1980; Thompson et al., 1992).

- Robert A. Karasek and colleagues have shown that the job characteristics of high demand and low decision latitude have predictive value for myocardial infarction. Occupational groups embodying these personality traits—waiters in busy restaurants, assembly line workers, and gas station attendants, for example—are at increased risk for heart attack. Their hypothesis is that increasing job demands are harmful when environmental constraints prevent optimal coping or when coping does not increase possibilities for personal and professional growth and development (Bergrugge, 1982; Bruhn et al., 1974; Karasek et al., 1982, 1988; Palmore, 1969; Sales and House, 1971; Syme, 1991).

- Psychologist Suzanne C. Kobasa and colleagues have identified job qualities that offer protection against cardiovascular morbidity and mortality, even in psychologically stressful job settings. They refer to the "three Cs": (1) control—a sense of personal decisionmaking; (2) challenge—the sense of personal growth and wisdom; becoming a better person; and (3) commitment to life on and off the job—to work, community, family, and self. Persons experiencing these qualities are said to possess "hardiness" and are relatively immune to job-induced illness or death (Kobasa et al., 1982).

Perceived Meaning and Health

Perceived meaning—how one perceives an event or issue, what something symbolizes or represents in one's mind—has direct consequences to health.[3] The annals of medicine are replete with anecdotes illustrating the power of perceived meaning—for example, accounts of sudden death after receiving bad news. Moreover, perceived meanings affect not just health, they also influence the types of therapies that are chosen. For example, if "body" means "machine," as it has tended to for people since the Industrial Revolution, illness is likely to be seen as a breakdown or malfunction, and the tendency is to prefer mechanically oriented approaches to treating illness.

Therapies, therefore, are likely to be designed to repair the machine when it malfunctions—surgery, drugs, irradiation, and so on. Or, if illness symbolizes an attack from the outside by "invading" pathogens or foreign substances, as it does to many people, people are apt to look for magic bullets in the form of antibiotics or other substances to protect them from these threats. Society may even declare counterattacks, such as the "wars" on acquired immunodeficiency syndrome (AIDS), heart disease, cancer, high blood pressure, or cholesterol. Perceived meanings, therefore, can be translated into the body as potent influences, and they can strongly influence the design of medical interventions.

More recently, careful studies have indicated the pivotal role of perceived meaning in health. Sociologists Ellen Idler of Rutgers University and Stanislav Kasl of the Department of Epidemiology and Public Health at Yale Medical School studied the impact of people's opinions on their health—what their health *meant* to them. The study involved more than 2,800 men and women, and the findings were consistent with the results of five other large studies involving more than 23,000

[3] *For a review of the impact of perceived meaning on health, see Dossey, 1991.*

people. All these studies lead to the same conclusion: One's own opinion about his or her state of health is a better predictor than objective factors, such as physical symptoms, extensive exams, and laboratory tests, or behaviors such as cigarette smoking. For instance, people who smoked were twice as likely to die during the next 12 years as people who did not, whereas those who said their health was "poor" were seven times more likely to die than those who said their health was "excellent" (Idler and Kasl, 1991).

Placebo Response

Dorland's Illustrated Medical Dictionary, twenty-fifth edition, defines the word *placebo* (in Latin, "I will please") as an inactive substance or preparation given to satisfy the patient's symbolic need for drug therapy and used in controlled studies to determine the efficacy of medicinal substances. It is also a procedure with no intrinsic therapeutic value, performed for such purposes. Although the placebo response is perhaps the most widely known example of mind-body interaction in contemporary scientific medicine,[4] it is at the same time one of the most undervalued and neglected assets in today's medical practice (Benson and Epstein, 1975). Even the definition from the medical dictionary suggests the term's uselessness apart from its narrow role in testing drugs. However, throughout most of medical history—in the centuries before antibiotics and other "wonder drugs"—the placebo effect was the central treatment physicians offered their patients (Benson and Epstein, 1975). Doctors hoped that their reassuring attention and their belief in their treatments would mobilize powers within their patients to fight their illnesses.

Today the placebo response is considered primarily a way of testing new drugs: if patients who have been given a placebo improve as much as those who took the new medication, the drug is dismissed as ineffective and with it the placebo. "Since a beneficial effect is the desired result," say cardiologist Herbert Benson and psychiatrist Mark Epstein, "should not the placebo effect be further investigated so that we might better explain its worthwhile consequences?" (Benson and Epstein, 1975).

The placebo response relies heavily on the interrelationship between doctor and patient. Patients bring with them to the doctor's office their attitudes, expectations, hopes, and fears. Doctors, in turn, have their own biases, attitudes, expectations, and methods of communication, which have a profound effect on patients. Doctors who believe in the efficacy of their treatment communicate that enthusiasm to their patients; those who have strong expectations of specific effects and are self-confident and attentive are the most successful at eliciting a positive placebo response (Wheatley, 1967). It is the interrelationship between the doctor and patient and the congruence of their expectations that bring about a positive placebo response. If the congruence is lacking, a favorable response rarely occurs (Hankoff et al., 1960).

The placebo response says a great deal about the importance of the doctor-patient relationship and the need to pay greater attention to it—and to provide further medical training on how that relationship can be heightened. It is particularly important in this highly technological era of medicine, when doctor-patient contacts are diminishing.

Although the literature of mind-body interaction documenting the placebo response is too vast to be reviewed here, several additional mind-body issues raised by this research deserve emphasis:

- The placebo response is almost ubiquitous. Studies show that in virtually any disease, roughly one-third of all symptoms improve when patients are given a placebo treatment without drugs (Goleman and Gurin, 1993).
- Placebo responses can be extraordinarily dramatic and offer valuable insights into the extent of the "powers of the mind" (Levoy, 1989).
- The *nocebo* response, a toxic or negative placebo event, raises serious questions about what is meant by "the natural course" or "the inherent biology" of any particular disease and suggests the great degree to which attitudes and expectations can affect one's state of health and the course of an illness.
- Nocebo effects can also be dramatic, are very common, and should be more widely acknowledged. Even anaphylactoid reactions (Wolf

[4] *T.J. Silber, for example, writing in the* Journal of the American Medical Association *in 1979, found 1,500 articles on the subject of placebos in English, German, and Spanish.*

and Pinsky, 1954) and addictions to placebos (Rhein, 1980)—reactions not commonly thought to be "mental" in origin—have been reported, along with a variety of other noxious reactions. In one controlled study by the British Stomach Cancer Group, 30 percent of the control (placebo-treated) group lost their hair, and 56 percent of the same group had "drug-related" nausea or vomiting (Fielding et al., 1983).

Spirituality, Religion, and Health

"Spirituality" is, generally speaking, one's inward sense of something greater than the individual self or the meaning one perceives that transcends the immediate circumstances. "Religion" may be described as the outward, concrete expression of such feelings.

The therapeutic potential of spirituality and religion have generally been neglected in the teaching and practice of medicine. However, epidemiologists Jeffrey S. Levin and Harold Y. Vanderpool have assembled what they term an "epidemiology of religion"—a large body of empirical findings "lying forgotten at the margins of medical research . . . specifically . . . nearly 250 published studies dating back over 150 years which [present] the results of epidemiologic, sociomedical, and biomedical investigations into the effects of religion. Nearly all of these investigations were large-scale studies" (Levin, 1989; Levin and Schiller, 1987; Levin and Vanderpool, 1991; Vanderpool and Levin, 1990).

Reviewing this immense database, Schiller and Levin found significant associations with variables such as religious attendance and subjective religiosity for a wide assortment of health outcomes, including cardiovascular disease, hypertension and stroke, uterine and other cancers, colitis and enteritis, general mortality, and overall health status (Schiller and Levin, 1988). These data are so consistent that Levin and Vanderpool suggest that infrequent religious attendance or observance should be regarded as a consistent risk factor for morbidity and mortality of various types (Levin and Vanderpool, 1987).

These findings are consistent with those of David B. Larson and Susan S. Larson, who surveyed 12 years of issues of the *American Journal of Psychiatry* and the *Archives of General Psychiatry*. They found that 92 percent of the studies that measured participation in religious ceremony, social support, prayer, and relationship with God showed benefit for mental health, whereas 4 percent were neutral, and 4 percent showed harm (Larson and Larson, 1991). Craigie and colleagues, in a 1990 review of 10 years of issues of the *Journal of Family Practice*, reported similar findings: 83 percent of studies showed benefit for physical health, 17 percent were neutral, and 0 percent showed harm (Craigie et al., 1990).

Matthews, Larson, and Barry made a major contribution in bringing together the research in this field—a two-volume report that compiles hundreds of studies, titled *The Faith Factor: An Annotated Bibliography of Clinical Research on Spiritual Subjects* (Matthews et al., 1993). Because research indicates that religious and spiritual meanings are correlated with increased physical and mental health and a lower incidence of a variety of diseases, and because religious and spiritual issues also affect profoundly how physicians regard death and treat the elderly, the quarantine against bringing up these matters in the doctor-patient relationship must be lifted. Becoming sensitive to these delicate issues does not require physicians to advocate any particular religious point of view. It does imply, however, that they should honor the salutary effects of spiritual meanings in their patients' lives, and inquire about spiritual and religious issues as assiduously as any *physical* factor.[5]

Spontaneous Remission of Cancer

The belief that life-threatening diseases such as cancer may disappear suddenly and completely is universal. This idea is usually coupled with the conviction that radical healing is somehow connected with one's state of mind.

Opinions vary as to how often cancer regresses spontaneously, leaving the person healthy. In their 1966 book on spontaneous regression of cancer, Everson and Cole collected 176 case reports from various countries around the world and concluded that spontaneous regression oc-

[5]*Larson and Larson assembled a teaching module that physicians could fruitfully follow in dealing with these delicate issues with patients without appearing to advocate any particular religious tradition or point of view (Larson and Larson, 1991). In the study, physicians who were not religious seemed to achieve better results with the inquiry than physicians who were.*

curs in one of 100,000 cases of cancer. Other authorities believe the incidence may be much higher. Everson and Cole found that almost any therapy to induce remission seems to work *some* of the time. Regression of cancer follows such diverse measures as intercessory prayer, conversion to Christian Science, mud packs, vitamin therapy, and force-feeding. They found that spontaneous regression occurs after both insulin and electroshock treatments. Since almost any treatment seems to work occasionally but not consistently, many have concluded that these measures are equally worthless and that spontaneous regression of cancer is purely a random event (Everson and Cole, 1966).

This point of view is a historical oddity. Prior to the 20th century, both physicians and patients believed the mind was a major factor in the development and course of cancer. In the years since Everson and Cole's review, this perspective has been recovered and reexamined. Many investigators—including psychologist Lawrence LeShan (1977) of New York and psychiatrist Steven Greer (1985) of King's College Hospital, London—have produced studies that suggest that emotions, attitudes, and personality traits may affect the onset of cancer as well as its course and outcome.

The Institute of Noetic Sciences has just published the most comprehensive investigation of spontaneous remission ever done—*Spontaneous Remission: An Annotated Bibliography* (O'Regan and Hirshberg, 1993).[6] This 15-year project was the work of biochemist Caryle Hirshberg and researcher Brendan O'Regan, who combed 3,500 references from more than 800 journals in 20 languages. The report deals not only with cancer but also with the spontaneous remission of a wide spectrum of diseases. It is the largest database of medically reported cases of spontaneous remission in the world. Key findings are as follows:

- Remission is a widely documented phenomenon, almost certainly more common than generally believed.
- Remission is an extremely promising area of research. Studying the psychobiological processes involved may provide important clues to understanding the body's self-regulatory processes and the breakdowns that precede the onset of many diseases.
- Data on remissions can have an important influence on how patients are treated and handled when diagnosed with a terminal illness. Restoring hope may help instill a "fighting spirit," an important factor in recovery from illness.

This interest in the possible role of the mind in the causation and course of cancer has been significantly stimulated by the discovery of the complex interactions among the mind and the neurological and immune systems, the subject of the rapidly expanding discipline of psychoneuroimmunology.

The relationship between psychological strategies and the regression of cancer is immensely complex and cannot be fully reviewed here. Two salient points should be made, however, that contradict popular belief and illustrate the complexity of these events: (1) Although an aggressive, fighting stance is generally advocated in stimulating spontaneous regression of cancer, University of California-Los Angeles psychologist Shelley E. Taylor has shown that (a) psychological denial following the diagnosis of breast cancer and (b) openly facing the disease and its implications are associated with near-equal survival statistics (Taylor, 1989). (2) Sometimes a mode of psychological acceptance, not aggressiveness, toward the diagnosis seems to set the stage for spontaneous remission. This point is particularly obvious in a series of spontaneous cancer remissions reported from Japan by Y. Ikemi and colleagues (Ikemi et al., 1975).

The profound differences in the psychological stances taken by people who survive cancer suggest that not only is there extreme variation *between* cultures, there are profound differences in the psychology of cancer survivors *within* cultures as well. Because the causal mechanisms involved are not known, and in view of the sheer variety of the psychological states that are apparently involved in spontaneous regression of cancer, physicians are currently unjustified in recommending uniformly that patients with cancer adopt a specific psychological stance in hopes of getting well. Still, spontaneous remission of cancer is a fact. Far more knowledge is needed

[6]*This publication can be obtained from the Institute of Noetic Sciences, Box 909, Sausalito, CA 94966-0909.*

about when and why it happens and what can be done to promote it.

Specific Therapies

The Panel on Mind-Body Interventions has selected the following therapies in an attempt to illustrate the diversity of this field and to illustrate some of the scientific work that has been done. The panel has not attempted to be exhaustive in this review, nor does it believe an exhaustive approach is possible in this document. Space does not allow discussion of many alternative therapies in which mind-body interactions are obviously prominent, such as anthroposophically extended medicine (see the "Alternative Systems of Medical Practice" chapter), Christian Science, and many others. Even though the sampling of specific therapies is necessarily restricted, the panel hopes this limited discussion will contribute to the development of a larger dialog in which all perspective mind-body interventions can eventually be considered.

Psychotherapy

It may be an error to focus on psychotherapy as an adjunctive therapy. Only from a perspective that views doctors as mechanics does psychotherapy become simply a technique. In fact, psychotherapy is the medium and basis of all care. It influences to some degree the efficacy of all health interventions, even those thought to be purely physical in nature.

Derived from Greek words meaning "healing of the soul," *psychotherapy* means treatment of emotional and mental health, which is in turn closely interwoven with physical health. Psychotherapy encompasses a wide range of specific treatments, including combining medication with discussion, listening to the patient's concerns, and using more active behavioral and emotive approaches. It also should be understood more generally as the matrix of interaction in which all the helping professions operate.

The number of health care professionals in the United States with some level of training in psychiatric and psychological counseling is immense. Currently, the American Psychiatric Association registers approximately 37,000 members; the American Psychological Association, 54,562 (approximately 60 percent clinical and 40 percent research and academic). The Department of Labor estimates that there are between 380,000 and 400,000 social workers; the American Medical Association lists 615,000 physicians, and the American Nurses Association lists 2,000,000 nurses. All of these people, as well as alternative health care practitioners, make conscious or unconscious use of psychotherapeutic interventions in their contacts with patients.

Conventional psychotherapy is conducted primarily by means of psychological methods such as suggestion, persuasion, psychoanalysis, and reeducation. It can be divided into the following six general categories. All of the following therapies can be undertaken either individually or in groups.

1. *Psychodynamic therapy* is derived from psychoanalysis. Current emotional reactions are related to past experiences, usually those of early childhood. It is generally directed toward changing fundamental personality patterns.
2. *Behavior therapy* emphasizes making specific behavior changes, such as learning not to be afraid of public speaking.
3. *Cognitive therapy* facilitates changing specific behaviors but focuses on habitual thoughts that affect behavior.
4. *Systems therapy* emphasizes relationship patterns and may involve all family members in therapy sessions.
5. *Supportive therapy* concentrates on helping people in major emotional crises, and treatment may include drug therapy.
6. *Body-oriented therapy* hypothesizes that emotions are encoded in and may be expressed as tension and restriction in any part of the physical body. Therapy uses breathing techniques, movement, and manual pressure and probing to help people release emotions that are believed to have been located in their tissues.

Any and all of these approaches may be used, but if a patient has a physical illness, the therapist focuses on short-term treatment dealing with any emotional state directly related to the physical condition. For example, depression and anxiety are common effects of any serious illness and may make it worse. Psychotherapy helps patients acknowledge the presence of these emotions and diminish their effects, thus enhancing recovery.

According to a study by James J. Strain (1993), an average of "one of every five people in the United States has a psychological disorder every six months—most commonly anxiety, depression, substance abuse, or acute confusion." At present, approximately three-fifths of patients with psychological problems are seen only by primary care physicians, many of whom are not well trained in psychotherapy and do not have adequate time to spend with each patient. Thus, despite the enormous need for psychological care, most people with medical illnesses do not receive screening or treatment for their psychiatric symptoms.

Clinical applications. Studies have shown that psychotherapy has had beneficial effects with medical crises and somatic illness.

Medical crises. Research indicates that psychotherapeutic treatment can hasten a recovery from a medical crisis and is in some cases the best treatment for it. According to Strain, brief psychotherapy reduced the hospital stay of elderly patients with broken hips by an average of 2 days. These patients had fewer rehospitalizations and spent fewer days in rehabilitation (Strain, 1993). Other studies show that psychotherapy is most effective when begun soon after a patient is admitted to a hospital. Currently, however, most psychological problems associated with physical illnesses remain undiagnosed or are not identified until near the end of a hospital stay.

In-hospital psychotherapy helps people cope with fears about their medical state by providing them with a supportive atmosphere in which to verbalize feelings. This atmosphere may give them a sense that their concerns are understood. It may also, by altering mood and attitude, be a significant factor in improving outcome. At the University of Minnesota, 100 patients preparing to go through bone marrow transplant for leukemia were examined for depression. Of the 13 patients diagnosed with major depression, all but one died in the following year; but all of the other 87 patients were still alive 2 years later.

Somatic illness. Somatic illnesses, in which physical symptoms appear to have no medical cause, are often improved markedly with psychotherapy. The emotional mechanism triggering somatic illness is presumed to be a problem that is not acceptable to the person and is transformed into a physical ailment. Studies measuring rates of return visits to a health maintenance organization after receiving a brief interval of psychotherapy are very positive. Another study demonstrated a reduction in visits following group support and psychotherapeutic treatment. A physician who recognizes this condition can save time and money and alleviate the physical suffering of the patient.

Cost-effectiveness. Psychotherapy has been shown to speed patients' recovery time from illness. Faster recovery in turn leads to smaller medical bills and fewer return visits to medical practitioners. In a study by Nicholas Cummings (Cummings and Bragman, 1988), patients who frequently visited medical clinics were offered short-term psychotherapy, and "these patients showed significant declines in their visits to doctors, days spent in the hospital, emergency room visits, diagnostic procedures, and drug prescriptions." The overall health care costs decreased by 10 to 20 percent in the years following brief psychotherapy.

A more specific example of cost-effectiveness was demonstrated in a study by Margaret Caudill and colleagues (1991), in which 10 group sessions of 90 minutes of psychotherapy and relaxation techniques significantly reduced the severity of pain. In a study of clinic use by chronic pain patients, patients who participated in the outpatient behavioral medicine program used 36 percent fewer clinic visits than those who did not. Cost savings were estimated at more than $100 per patient per year (Caudill et al., 1991).

Support groups. Social, cultural, and environmental contexts, which have a powerful impact on bringing about both psychological and physiological change, should be more fully investigated. The literature on support groups demonstrates that in a wide variety of physical illnesses, such as heart disease, cancer, asthma, and strokes, a support group can have a powerful positive effect.

Consider the potential role of group support and psychological counseling in cancer and heart disease, the two major causes of death in the United States. One recent, well-publicized example of this ubiquitous effect is David Spiegel's study on women with metastatic breast cancer.

Women who took part in a support group lived an average of 18 months longer (a doubling of the survival time following diagnosis) than those who did not participate. In addition, all the long-term survivors belonged to the therapy group (Spiegel et al., 1989).

In a well-known study of patients with established coronary artery disease, group support, and psychological counseling were combined with diet and exercise. Symptoms such as angina pectoris rapidly diminished or disappeared altogether, and after 1 year the coronary artery obstructions were demonstrated to be smaller. This strongly suggests that coronary artery disease, the Nation's most deadly and expensive health care problem, is reversible through a complementary, noninvasive, diet and behavioral modification approach that emphasizes group psychotherapy (Ornish, 1990). (See the "Diet and Nutrition" chapter for more details on this approach.)

Support groups have two other major benefits: (1) they help members form bonds with one another, an experience that may empower members for the rest of their lives; and (2) they are inexpensive or even free (e.g., Alcoholics Anonymous).

Research needs and opportunities. Future opportunities for research on the interconnectedness of mind and body include the following:

- Studies should be directed toward devising methods for integrating psychotherapy into all aspects of health care and evaluating its efficacy in all treatments.
- Researchers should try to understand better how small shifts in behavior, thoughts, and attitudes can help change a person's entire physical and psychological state.
- Whether behavioral intervention can delay or prevent the onset of illness should be assessed.
- How support groups work should be explored. What types of groups are best? Leaderless or directed groups? Participants with single or mixed diagnoses? With time-limited or open-ended sessions? What type of personality is most likely to find them useful? Are they harmful to certain types of individuals? If so, what types?
- The role of psychotherapy in treating serious illness should be emphasized. Unfortunately, many people, including health care professionals and academicians, consider psychotherapeutic intervention in physical illness a luxury or frill. However, the studies cited above suggest that psychological intervention works best when used early and may actually make the difference between life and death in certain illnesses.
- Research should be undertaken on just how the body records and expresses emotions and on the possible effectiveness of body-oriented therapies in releasing physical tensions and resolving emotional problems.
- Mental health researchers should direct more attention to certain anomalous and unexplained mind-body events that have long existed on the periphery of medicine and that are generally ignored. Examples include the falling off of warts with suggestion; psychological profiles of extremely long-lived people; and the spontaneous and unanticipated remission of "fatal" cancer. If explained, these events could yield major gains in understanding the mind and its relationship to the body and could yield valuable new approaches to health.
- Mental health departments in teaching institutions should be bolder in entertaining novel explanations of mind and consciousness and the relationship between mind and brain. Currently, almost all academic institutions teach models of consciousness that largely equate mind and consciousness with the physical brain. This perspective is incomplete; it entirely ignores the considerable data implying that a nonlocal concept of consciousness may be a more encompassing explanation for the manifestations of consciousness. (See Dossey, 1989, 1992; Jahn, 1981; and Josephson and Ramachandran, 1980.) For patients, a physically based view of illness is restrictive, expensive, and often harmful. As long as mind is equated with brain, the routine tendency to employ physical interventions such as drugs for mental disturbances will continue to overshadow other methods that conceivably might be safer, more effective, and less costly.
- Mental health professionals should explore other areas of science—areas usually considered "off base" and "irrelevant"—for perspec-

tives that might be enriching. Quantum mechanics, dissipative structure theory, chaos theory, and nonlinear dynamics are only a few areas of science that have great potential relevance for understanding the mind and consciousness.[7]

- The concept of what constitutes appropriate areas for psychiatric intervention should be enlarged. Impressive evidence exists that "disorders of meaning" (a person's sense that his or her life lacks meaning) are epidemic in society and that these disorders can have life-and-death consequences. Mental health professionals should deal more effectively with issues involving meanings and values, which are usually shunted aside by medical professionals. Some of these problems are spiritual and require a reexamination of the traditional distinctions psychiatrists have made between psychiatry and religion, and between "science" and "spirit."[8]
- The cost-effectiveness of psychiatric intervention in physical illness deserves to be better known and should be more widely publicized. In an era of continued escalation of health care costs, these interventions offer a very real opportunity to improve health and limit costs simultaneously.

Meditation

Meditation is a self-directed practice for relaxing the body and calming the mind. The meditator makes a concentrated effort to focus on a single thought—peace, for instance; or a physical experience, such as breathing; or a sound (repeating a word or mantra, such as "one" or a Sanskrit word such as "kirim"). The aim is to still the mind's "busyness"—its inclination to mull over the thousand demands and details of daily life.

Most meditative techniques have come to the West from Eastern religious practices—particularly those of India, China, and Japan—but they can be found in all cultures of the world. Christian contemplation—saying the rosary or repeating the "Hail Mary"—brings similar effects and can be said to be akin to meditation. Michael Murphy, the cofounder of Esalen Institute, claims that the concentration used in Western sports is itself a form of meditation. While most meditators in the United States practice sedentary meditation, there are also many moving meditations, such as the Chinese martial art tai chi, the Japanese martial art aikido, and walking meditation in Zen Buddhism. Yoga can also be said to be a meditation.

Until recently, the primary purpose of meditation has been religious, although its health benefits have long been recognized. During the past 15 years, it has been explored as a way of reducing stress on both mind and body. Cardiologists, in particular, often recommend it as a way of reducing high blood pressure.

There are many forms of meditation—with many different names—ranging in complexity from strict, regulated practices to general recommendations, but all appear to produce similar physical and psychological changes (Benson, 1975; Chopra, 1991; Goleman, 1977; Mahesh Yogi, 1963).

If practiced regularly, meditation develops habitual, unconscious microbehaviors that produce widespread positive effects on physical and psychological functioning. Meditating even for 15 minutes twice a day seems to bring beneficial results.

While many individuals and groups have examined the effects of meditation, two major meditation programs have extensive bodies of research: transcendental meditation and the relaxation response.

Transcendental meditation. Transcendental meditation (TM) was developed by the Indian leader Maharishi Mahesh Yogi, who eliminated from yoga certain elements he considered nonessential. In the 1960s he left India and came to the United States, bringing with him this reformed yoga, which he felt could be grasped and practiced more easily by westerners. His new method did not require the often difficult physical or mental exercises required by yoga and could be

---

[7]As an example of the cross-fertilization that might occur between the disciplines of psychiatry and modern physics, see Zohar, 1990. See also Jahn, 1981; and Josephson and Ramachandran, 1980.

[8]See Ravindra, 1991. Ravindra is both an academic physicist and a theologian at Dalhousie University. See also the "Spirituality, Religion, and Health" section of this chapter.

easily taught in one training session. TM was soon embraced by some celebrities of that day, such as the Beatles, and can now probably claim well over 2 million practitioners.

TM is simple. To prevent distracting thoughts a student is given a mantra (a word or sound) to repeat silently over and over again while sitting in a comfortable position. Students are instructed to be passive and, if thoughts other than the mantra come to mind, to notice them and return to the mantra. A TM student is asked to practice for 20 minutes in the morning and again in the evening.

In 1968, Harvard cardiologist Herbert Benson was asked by TM practitioners to test them on their ability to lower their own blood pressures. At first, Benson refused this suggestion as "too far out" but later was persuaded to do so. Benson's studies and an independent investigation at the University of California at Los Angeles were followed by much additional research on TM at Maharishi International University in Fairfield, IA, and at other research centers. Published results from these studies report that the use of TM is discretely associated with

- reduced health care use;
- increased longevity and quality of life;
- reduction of chronic pain (Kabat-Zinn et al., 1986);
- reduced anxiety;
- reduction of high blood pressure (Cooper and Aygen, 1978);
- reduction of serum cholesterol level (Cooper and Aygen, 1978);
- reduction of substance abuse (Sharma et al., 1991);
- longitudinal increase in intelligence-related measures (Cranson et al., 1991);
- treatment of posttraumatic stress syndrome in Vietnam veterans (Brooks and Scarano, 1985);
- blood pressure reduction in African-American persons (Schneider et al., 1992); and
- lowered blood cortisol levels initially brought on by stress (MacLean et al., 1992).

Relaxation response. Convinced that meditation was a possible treatment for high blood pressure, Benson later pursued his investigation at the Mind-Body Medical Institute at Harvard Medical School. He identified what he calls "the relaxation response," a constellation of psychological and physiological effects that appear common to many practices: meditation, prayer, progressive relaxation, autogenic training, and the presuggestion phase of hypnosis and yoga (Benson, 1975). He published his method in a book of the same name.

Over a period of 25 years, Benson and colleagues have developed a large body of research. During this time, meditation in general and the relaxation response specifically have slowly moved from alternative to mainstream medicine, although they are still overlooked by many conventional doctors. Benson's research has demonstrated a wide range of effects from meditation (or the relaxation response) on bodily functions: oxygen consumption and carbon dioxide and lactate production, adrenocorticotropic hormone excretion, blood elements such as platelets and lymphocytes, cell membranes, norepinephrine receptors, brain wave activity, and utilization of medical resources.

In addition, one study by Benson's group indicated that chronic pain patients who meditated had a net reduction in general health care costs, suggesting that this approach is cost-effective (Caudill et al., 1991).[9]

Although the positive effects of meditation clearly outnumber and outweigh the negative effects, the latter have also been studied (Blackmore, 1991). Potential adverse effects include adverse psychological feelings (e.g., feelings of negativity, disorientation) in a small percentage of meditators after meditation retreats; and elicitation of acute episodes of psychosis by intensive meditation in schizophrenics.

---

[9] *Although TM and the relaxation response have been most intensively studied, other investigators (including Jon Kabat-Zinn, Ilan Kutz, and Joan Borysenko) have demonstrated the effectiveness of South Asian vipassana, or mindfulness meditation, in the reduction of chronic pain and as an adjunct to psychotherapy (Kabat-Zinn et al., 1985; Kutz et al., 1985).*

Despite the breadth and clarity of the research[10] indicating that meditation is a useful, low-cost intervention, it continues to be regarded as unconventional and is still ignored by most medical professionals. The report of the National Research Council (NRC) on meditation, which drew heavily on a negative review by Holmes (1984), emphasized concerns about weak experimental designs, failure to discriminate meditation from other sources of effects, and conceptual issues such as the lack of an underlying mechanism. A critique of the NRC report by Orme-Johnson and Alexander responded to these criticisms using quantitative reviews which they claimed provided strong arguments for taking a deeper look at meditation (Orme-Johnson and Alexander, 1992). The Mind-Body panel's critique of the NRC report is in appendix B of this report.

Current clinical use. In September 1987, science writer Daniel Goleman reported in the *New York Times Magazine* that some 400 universities offered some level of training in behavioral medicine, including meditation, and "thousands of hospitals, clinics, and individual practitioners offer the treatments." Harvard Medical School's Mind-Body Medical Institute has several thousand patient visits per year in its clinical arm and maintains an active research program as well as training programs for doctors, nurses, social workers, and psychologists, in conjunction with the school's continuing education program (Benson and Stuart, 1992). Other hospitals want clinics of this kind, and dissemination is proceeding. The first affiliate is at Mercy Hospital in Chicago. Others sites being negotiated are Morristown, NJ; Columbus, OH; Charlottesville, VA; and Houston, TX. Many other independent clinics employ meditation techniques, such as the Cambridge Hospital behavioral medicine program and the University of Massachusetts Medical School program.

Meditation and healing. In addition to being used by individuals, meditation is also an important part of the unconventional healing approaches used by mental, spiritual, and psychic healers. Almost all healers consider some form of meditation or quiet prayer fundamental to their practice. (Mental healing is discussed in the "Prayer and Mental Healing" section.) Indeed, the state of focused attention and exclusive concern that some doctors demonstrate in orthodox medicine can be thought of as a form of meditation. In addition, meditation is often practiced by some physicians for their own benefit, even though they do not use it in treating their patients.

Cost-effectiveness and potential economic impact. Insurance statistics for a group of 2,000 meditators compared with 600,000 nonmeditators show that the use of medical care was 30 percent to 87 percent less for meditators in all but one of 18 categories (childbirth) (McSherry, 1990; Orme-Johnson, 1987). In another study at the Harvard Community Health Plan, patients who attended a 6-week behavioral medicine group that included meditation made significantly fewer visits to physicians during the 6 months that followed; the savings were estimated at $171 per patient.

If the definition of meditation is expanded to include more or less formal religious practices that emphasize quiet prayer, the number of people using some form of meditation becomes enormous and the potential health benefits correspondingly large. In the United States, TM has been taught to well over a million people, and it is estimated that most continue the practice regularly. Benson's Mind-Body Medical Institute currently has 7,000 patient visits per year and has trained thousands of health professionals in applying the relaxation response.

Theory and rationale. How and why does meditation work? There are several related theories about the underlying mechanism. Ken

[10]*The most comprehensive review of meditation research is a set of five volumes compiled by Maharishi International University (Orme-Johnson and Farrow, 1977) (a sixth is in preparation), containing more than 500 original research, review, and theoretical papers by some 360 researchers at 200 universities and a meta-analysis. Comparing various techniques for reducing trait anxiety, researchers found the largest overall effect was produced by TM (Eppley et al., 1989). Murphy and Donovan surveyed more than 600 studies of physiological and psychological effects of meditation (Murphy, 1992; Murphy and Donovan, 1989). Schneider addressed the search for an optimal behavioral treatment for hypertension (Schneider et al., 1992). Walsh and Vaughan provide a compact and readable summary of the state of the art in meditation research as a chapter in a new book (Walsh and Vaughan, in press).*

Walton, director of the Neurochemistry Laboratory, Maharishi International University, states:

> The frequently striking results of [studies of TM] have not been widely discussed in the medical literature, purportedly because "there is no reasonable mechanism" which could explain such a spectrum of health effects from a simple mental technology. . . . Only in the last year has the stress connection emerged with the degree of clarity it now has. The . . . bottom line is the proposed vicious circle linking chronic stress, serotonin metabolism, and hippocampal regulation of the hypothalamic-pituitary-adrenocortical (HPA) axis (Nelson, 1992).

Similarly, Everly and Benson have proposed that meditation is effective in a wide variety of disorders that may be called "disorders of arousal," in which the limbic system of the brain has become overstimulated. Relaxation and meditation training serve to "retune" the nervous system by damping the production of adrenergic catecholamines, which stimulate limbic activity. Everly and Benson (1989) suggest also that excessive limbic activity may inhibit immune function—a possibility that may account for the association of chronic stress and increased susceptibility to infection.

Research needs and opportunities. The following points may be made about research needs in the area of meditation:

- More than 30 years of research, as well as the experiences of a large and growing number of individuals and health care providers, suggest that meditation and similar forms of relaxation can lead to better health, higher quality of life, and lowered health care costs. This research should be collected and critically evaluated, and its results should be widely disseminated to health professionals.
- Some of the research needs to be replicated and the physiological and biochemical dimensions more fully investigated to facilitate education, application, and acceptance into mainstream medicine.
- Research is needed into the commonalities and differences of meditation and other forms of self-regulation such as hypnosis, relaxation, and guided imagery.
- The nature and purpose of meditation need to be made more explicit by its advocates. In most traditions, meditation was originally considered primarily a technique for changing consciousness and achieving spiritual understanding; improvements in health were considered only byproducts. Today, meditation seems to be popularly regarded as utilitarian, as simply as a tool for improving physical health. Future research should compare the health benefits that result when meditation is undertaken for explicit health reasons versus for its own sake.
- Most meditation research has involved young or middle-aged Americans who have practiced meditation for several months to several years. Understanding would be enhanced by more studies of advanced, expert meditators who have spent a lifetime of meditation in a variety of traditions and cultures. This approach would be more likely to shed light on the maximal health benefits possible from meditation.
- Many different schools of meditation exist, advocating a variety of techniques. Prospective studies should investigate whether any particular school offers special health benefits.
- To ameliorate the objections of many Christian religious groups to meditation, cross-disciplinary dialog and communication should be encouraged that would examine (1) the commonalities between Christian prayer and contemplation and Eastern meditation, and (2) the extraordinary similarities in the esoteric mystical traditions of East and West.

Most important, meditation techniques offer the potential of learning how to live in an increasingly complex and stressful society while helping to preserve health in the process. Given their low cost and demonstrated health benefits, these simple mental technologies may be some of the best candidates among the alternative therapies for widespread inclusion in medical practice and for investment of medical resources.

Imagery

Imagery is both a mental process (as in imagining) and a wide variety of procedures used in therapy to encourage changes in attitudes, behavior, or physiological reactions. As a mental process, it is often defined as "any thought representing a sensory quality" (Horowitz, 1983). It includes, as well as the visual, all the senses—aural, tactile, olfactory, proprioceptive, and kinesthetic. *Imagery* is often used synonymously with *visualization*; this use is misleading, because the latter refers only to *seeing* something in the mind's eye, whereas imagery can mean imagining through any sense, as through hearing or smell.

Imagery is a common ingredient in many behavioral therapies not specifically labeled imagery. Since it often involves directed concentration, it can also be thought of as a form of meditation (see the "Meditation" section). Imagery can be taught either individually or in groups, and the therapist often uses it to affect a particular result, such as quitting smoking or bolstering the immune system to attack cancer cells.

Practices that have a component of imagery are almost ubiquitous. They include, among many others, biofeedback, desensitization and counterconditioning, psychosynthesis, neurolinguistic programming, gestalt therapy, rational emotive therapy, and hypnosis (see the "Hypnosis" section). Any therapy that relies on imagery or fantasy to motivate, communicate, solve problems, or evoke heightened awareness and sensitivity could be described as a form of imagery. Forms of meditation that involve repeating a sound or mantra (e.g., TM) or focusing attention on an object that has no concurrent external referent (such as a whale in the ocean) could also be developed as aspects of imagery. Likewise, relaxation techniques that involve instruction (e.g., "Your hands are heavy"), such as autogenic training, have an imagery component.

Whether imagery differs from hypnosis in terms of purpose and state of consciousness is currently debated. Hypnotherapists, particularly those who train clients in methods of self-hypnosis, are often indistinguishable from practitioners of imagery. What has been agreed on is that there is a correlation between the ability to image and the capacity to enter into an altered state of consciousness, including the hypnotic state (Barber, 1984; Hilgard, 1974; Lynn and Rhue, 1987).

Numerous studies indicate that mental imagery can bring about significant physiological and biochemical changes. These findings, which have encouraged the development of imagery as a health care tool, include its capacity to affect the following: oxygen supply in tissues (Olness and Conroy, 1985); cardiovascular changes (Barber, 1969); vascular or thermal change (Green and Green, 1977); the pupil and the cochlear reflex (Luria, 1968); heart rate and galvanic skin response (Jordan and Lenington, 1979); salivation (Barber et al., 1964; White, 1978); gastrointestinal activity (Barber, 1978); increase in breast size (Barber, 1984); the Mantoux reaction (Black et al., 1963); and blood glucose levels (Stevens, 1983). Several hundred studies using biofeedback, which Green and Green (1977) refer to as an "imagery trainer," expand the list considerably, running the gamut from effects on the firing of single motorneurons (Basmajian, 1963) to brain wave alterations (Brown, 1977).

Some of these findings are from well-controlled studies, but the vast majority represent reports of single cases or small studies that have not been replicated. Nevertheless, the overriding conclusion is that there is a relationship between imagery of bodily change and actual bodily change. Without question, imagery calls for further and more precise investigation.

Clinical applications. Procedures for imagery fall into at least three major categories: (1) evaluation or diagnostic imagery, (2) mental rehearsal, and (3) therapeutic intervention.

Techniques used in evaluation or diagnostic imagery involve asking the person to describe his or her condition in sensory terms. The therapist gathers information regarding the disease, the effect of treatment, and any natural inner healing resources the person might be sensing. The patient is asked, literally, "How do you feel?" In psychotherapy settings, dreams or fantasies might be used in this way, as a means to gaining insight or control over a situation.

Evaluation imagery is usually done early in a therapy session and serves as a format for designing both mental rehearsal and therapeutic intervention strategies. It also is an indicator of the person's understanding of the mechanisms of health and disease and provides opportunity for patient education.[11]

---

[11] *Many evaluation formats appear in the nursing literature. For a comprehensive presentation of this information as it relates to nursing practice and assessment, see Dossey et al., 1992, and Zahourek, 1988. General health evaluation tools, as well as those specific to certain diseases, have been published by Achterberg and Lawlis (1980, 1984).*

Mental rehearsal is an imagery technique used before medical techniques, usually in an attempt to relieve anxiety, pain, and side effects, which are exacerbated by heightened emotional reactions. Surgery or a difficult treatment is rehearsed before the event so that the patient is prepared and is rid of any unrealistic fantasies.

Typically, a relaxation strategy is taught, then the treatment and recovery period are described in sensory terms as the patient is taken on a guided imagery "trip." Care is taken to be factual without using emotion-laden or fear-provoking words, and the medical procedure is reframed in a positive way whenever possible. The patient is taught coping techniques such as distraction, mental dissociation, muscle relaxation, and abdominal breathing.

Published results with mental rehearsals (or sensory education) are almost uniformly positive and often dramatic. Effects include reduced pain and anxiety; decreased length of hospital stay; the use of fewer pain medicines, barbiturates, tranquilizers, and other medications; and reduced treatment side effects. Mental rehearsal is a cornerstone of certain natural childbirth practices. It has also been tested in burn debridement (Kenner and Achterberg, 1983) and as a preparation for spinal surgery (Lawlis et al., 1985), cholecystectomy, pelvic examination, cast removal, and endoscopy (Johnson et al., 1978). In each of these instances, rehearsal through imagery has been found to diminish pain and discomfort and to reduce side effects.

Imagery as a therapeutic intervention is based on the idea that the images have either a direct or an indirect effect on health. Therefore, either the patients are shown how to use their own flow of images about the healing process or, alternatively, they are guided through a series of images that are intended to soothe and distract them, reduce any sympathetic nervous system arousal, or generally enhance their relaxation. The practitioner may also use "end state" types of imagery, having patients imaging themselves in a state of perfect health, well-being, or successfully achieved goals.

A major and serious criticism of imagery literature (as well as hypnosis literature) is that clinic protocols are seldom provided. Therefore, it is impossible to know what type of therapeutic strategy was used, and of course it cannot be replicated. Some practitioners even regard their protocols as trade secrets and refuse to divulge them.

Whether imagery is merely an antidote to feelings of helplessness or whether the image itself has the capacity to induce the desired physical effect is still unclear. Existing research suggests both conclusions are justified, depending on the situation in question.

Imagery has been successfully tested as a strategy for alleviating nausea and vomiting associated with chemotherapy in cancer patients (Frank, 1985; Scott et al., 1986), to relieve stress (Donovan, 1980), and to facilitate weight gain in cancer patients (Dixon, 1984). It has been successfully used and tested for pain control in a variety of settings; as adjunctive therapy for several diseases, including diabetes (Stevens, 1983); and with geriatric patients to enhance immunity (Kiecolt-Glaser et al., 1985).

Imagery is usually combined with other behavioral approaches. It is best known in the treatment of cancer as a means to help patients mobilize their immune systems (Borysenko, 1987; Siegel, 1986; Simonton et al., 1978), but it also is used as part of a multidisciplinary approach to cardiac rehabilitation (Ornish, 1990; Ornish et al., 1983) and in many settings that specialize in treating chronic pain.

In a survey of alternative techniques used by cancer patients (Cassileth et al., 1984), imagery was cited as the fourth most frequently used. And 46 percent of the respondents listed "self" as practitioner, indicating that imagery is often used as a self-help tool.

Imagery assessment tools. The measurement of imagery as a mental process is fraught with the same problems faced in measuring any other so-called hypothetical construct, including learning, motivation, and perception. So far, psychology has risen to the occasion and developed reliable and meaningful measurement strategies.

A number of instruments with varying purposes, degrees of validity, and reliability are currently in use for measuring imagery. Sheikh and Jordan (1983) have reviewed the imagery test used for psychological diagnosis. Imagery of cancer, diabetes, and spinal pain have been specifically analyzed by Achterberg and Lawlis, using a protocol to elicit sensory information on healing mechanisms, treatment, and the disease itself (Achterberg and Lawlis, 1984). These tests have been found to be accurate predictors of treatment outcome in a number of clinics and rehabilitation facilities.

Research accomplishments. Recent studies suggest a direct impact or correlation between imagery (both as a mental process and a set of procedures) and immunology. These findings include the following:

- Correlations between various types of leukocytes and components of cancer patients' images of their disease, treatment, and immune system (Achterberg and Lawlis, 1984).
- Increased phagocytic activity following biofeedback-assisted relaxation (Peavey et al., 1985).
- Enhanced natural killer cell function following a relaxation and imagery training procedure with geriatric patients (Kiecolt-Glaser et al., 1985) and in adult cancer patients with metastatic disease (Gruber et al., 1988).
- Changes in lymphocyte reactivity following hypnotic procedures (Hall, 1982–83) and instruction in relaxation and imagery in adult cancer patients with metastatic disease.
- Altered neutrophil adherence or margination, as well as white blood cell count, following an imagery procedure (Schneider et al., 1983).
- Increased secretory immunoglobulin A (IgA) (significantly higher than control group) following training in location, activity, and morphology of IgA and 6 weeks of daily imaging.
- The specificity of imagery training was suggested by a study on training patients in cell-specific imagery of either T lymphocytes or neutrophils. The effects of training, which were assessed after 6 weeks, were statistically associated with the type of imagery procedure employed (Achterberg and Rider, 1989).

Research issues. Although this early research is very promising, further investigations are badly needed. Longitudinal studies are virtually nonexistent. Consequently, the major question remains: Will the physiological-biochemical changes noted in imagery studies have an ultimate impact on health or on the course of the disease?

Distinguishing clinical from statistical significance is critical. Relying on statistical significance alone may obscure much valuable information, such as the few outstanding cases in which the methods were remarkably successful.

For complex clinical research, innovative research paradigms and statistical treatments are needed. Traditional research methodology is based on the idea of a univariate, linear model, which is rare (if not completely absent) in the real world. The spirit of discovery is not served by clinging to models that obscure much of the richness of the human condition. Furthermore, there are a number of complex variables that need to be accounted for in developing a research design. The following are examples:

- The randomized control group design is often impossible, impractical, and unnecessary. Its general efficacy and the ethics of its application are now being seriously challenged (Rider et al., 1990). Other designs should be considered.
- Participant and therapist-researcher motivation and belief are critical and significant variables to consider in this type of behavioral research and should serve as factors in group selection and measurement.
- Studies should be designed to maximize the possibility of good outcome on health and well-being.
- Research into the relationship between imagery and biological parameters—particularly those related to immunology—is hindered by the state of the art in that area. For instance, normative data are often absent, and reliability of assay procedures is questionable. Clinical significance of any changes may or may not be known. The specific impact of diet, season, environment, age, mood, or even the time of day on many of the immune assays is not well studied.

Research needs and opportunities. Existing data suggest at least two major research directions:

1. The impact of imagery as part of a multimodal treatment with conditions such as cancer, AIDS, or autoimmune disorders. The research should include repeat immunologic testing and followup. Specific studies could be embedded within the overall design; for example, studies on the effect of imagery specifically

designed to enhance medical treatment, the relationship between imagery and outcome of disease, types of patients who respond to imagery, and so on.

2. Replication and expansion of earlier intriguing—but small or poorly controlled—studies that indicated a direct effect of imagery on biologic function.

Hypnosis

Hypnosis, derived from the Greek word *hypnos* (sleep), and hypnotic suggestion have been a part of healing since ancient times. The induction of trance states and the use of therapeutic suggestion were a central feature of the early Greek healing temples, and variations of these techniques were practiced throughout the ancient world.

Modern hypnosis began in the 18th century with Franz Anton Mesmer, who used what he called "magnetic healing" to treat a variety of psychological and psychophysiological disorders, such as hysterical blindness, paralysis, headaches, and joint pains. Since then, the fortunes of hypnosis have ebbed and flowed. The famous Austrian neurologist Sigmund Freud at first found hypnosis extremely effective in treating hysteria and then, troubled by the sudden emergence of powerful emotions in his patients and his own difficulty with its use, abandoned it.

In the past 50 years, however, hypnosis has experienced a resurgence, first with physicians and dentists and more recently with psychologists and other mental health professionals. Today it is widely used for addictions, such as smoking and drug use, for pain control, and for phobias, such as the fear of flying.

Hypnosis is a state of attentive and focused concentration in which people can be relatively unaware of, but not completely blind to, their surroundings. If something demands attention—such as a fire in the wastebasket—hypnotized people easily rouse themselves to react to the situation. In this state of concentration, people are highly responsive to suggestion. But, contrary to popular folklore, people cannot be hypnotized involuntarily or follow suggestions against their wishes. They must be *willing* to concentrate their thoughts and to follow the suggestions offered. In the end, all hypnotherapy is self-hypnosis. Some people—usually those with a vivid fantasy life—are better hypnotic subjects than others.

Hypnosis has three major components: absorption (in the words or images presented by the hypnotherapist); dissociation (from one's ordinary critical faculties); and responsiveness. A hypnotherapist either leads a client through relaxation, mental images, and suggestions or teaches clients to do this for themselves. Many hypnotherapists provide guided audiotapes for their clients so they can practice the therapy at home. The images presented are specifically tailored to the particular client's problems and may employ one or all of the senses.

Physiologically, hypnosis resembles other forms of deep relaxation: a generalized decrease in sympathetic nervous system activity, a decrease in oxygen consumption and carbon dioxide eliminations, a lowering of blood pressure and heart rate, and an increase in certain kinds of brain wave activity (Spiegel et al., 1989).

The most prominent organization of clinical professionals in the field is the American Society for Clinical Hypnosis, which numbers approximately 3,000 members (M.D.s and Ph.D.s). In addition, there are probably thousands of others who use hypnotherapy as part of their practice (e.g., R.N.s, M.S.W.s, marriage and family counselors, and lay therapists).

Clinical applications. One of the most dramatic uses of hypnosis is the treatment of congenital ichthyosis (fish skin disease), a genetic skin disorder that covers the surface of the skin with grotesque hard, wartlike, layered crust. Dermatologists thought ichthyosis was incurable until an anesthesiologist, Arthur Mason, in the mid-1950s used hypnosis by chance to effectively treat a patient he thought had warts. After Mason used hypnosis on the patient (a 16-year-old boy), the boy's scales fell off, and within 10 days, normal pink skin replaced it. Since that time, hypnosis has been used to treat ichthyosis—not always resulting in complete cure but often resulting in dramatic improvement (Goldberg, 1985).

Hypnosis is, however, most frequently used in more common ailments, either independently or in concert with other treatment. The following are a few examples:

- *Pain management.* Pain increases with heightened fear and anxiety. Because hypnotherapy helps a person gain control over fear and anxiety, pain is also reduced. Hypnotic suggestion (one may suggest that a part of the body become numb) can be used instead of or together with an anesthetic. Twelve controlled studies have demonstrated that hypnosis is a superior way to reduce migraine attacks in children and teenagers. In one experiment, schoolchildren were randomly assigned a placebo or propranolol, a blood-pressure lowering agent, or taught self-hypnosis; only the children using self-hypnosis had a significant drop in severity and frequency of headaches (Olness et al., 1989). Another pain study of patients who were chronically ill reports a 113-percent increase in pain tolerance among highly hypnotizable subjects versus a control group who did not receive hypnosis (Debenedittis et al., 1989).

- *Dentistry.* Some people have learned how to tolerate dental work with hypnotherapy as the only anesthetic. Even when an anesthetic is used, hypnotherapy can also be employed to reduce fear and anxiety, control bleeding and salivation, and reduce postoperative discomfort.

- *Pregnancy and delivery.* Women who have hypnosis prior to delivery have shorter labors and more comfortable deliveries. Women have also used self-hypnosis to control pain during delivery (Rossi, 1986).

- *Anxiety.* Hypnosis can be used to establish a new reaction to specific anxiety-causing activities such as stage fright, plane flights, and other phobias.

- *Immune system function.* Hypnotherapy can have a positive effect on the immune system. One study has shown that hypnosis can raise immunoglobulin levels of healthy children (Olness et al., 1989). Another study reported that self-hypnosis led to an increase in white blood cell activity (Hall, 1982–83).

Other studies in the past 40 years have shown that hypnosis can affect a wide variety of physical responses, including reduction of bleeding in hemophiliacs (Lucas, 1965), reduction in severity of attacks of hay fever and asthma (Mason and Black, 1958), increased breast size (Honiotest, 1977; LeCron, 1969; Staib and Logan, 1977; Willard, 1977; Williams, 1973), the cure of warts (Ahser, 1956; Sinclair-Geiben and Chalmers, 1959; Surman et al., 1973; Ullman and Dudek, 1960), the production of skin blisters and bruises (Bellis, 1966; Johnson and Barber, 1976), and control of reaction to allergens such as poison ivy and certain foods (Ikemi, 1967; Ikemi and Nakagawa, 1962; Platonov, 1959).

No one knows exactly how such bodily changes are brought about by hypnosis, but they clearly occur because of the connections between mind and body. It is also clear that suggestions have the capacity to affect all systems and organs of the body in a variety of ways.

To flow naturally in and out of hypnotic states is common; it happens to people watching television, for instance. We are also likely to move into a trance state in situations of extreme stress. When a person in a position of power yells, the yelling may have effects that become as strong as posthypnotic suggestions. When physicians or other health care providers make predictions about an illness, they may have a similar effect. It is particularly important that physicians understand this state and the potential power of the positive and negative suggestions they use with their patients.

Research needs and opportunities. The following needs exist in the area of hypnosis:

- Because of the profound influence of hypnosis, an understanding of how to apply it in all therapeutic settings is needed. Future study must be directed toward influencing and maximizing the beneficial capacity of trance states occurring in doctors' offices and on operating tables as well as minimizing the destructive effects of negative or offhand remarks made in these places. And of course, further research is needed on explicit, hypnotic treatment for specific illnesses.

- The cases in which hypnosis has resulted in dramatic improvements of severely disfiguring genetic diseases such as ichthyosis deserves further scientific attention. They raise fundamental questions about the extent and limits of the mind's powers and suggest that such limits may be very wide indeed.

- Hypnosis is often reserved as a "backup" therapy to be used when conventional treatments fail. However, the examples above show the broad spectrum of its usefulness and suggest that in some conditions hypnosis may be appropriately considered as a first-line therapy instead of a last resort.

Biofeedback

Originating in the late 1960s, biofeedback is a treatment method that uses monitoring instruments to feed back to patients physiological information of which they are normally unaware. By watching the monitoring device, patients can learn by trial and error to adjust their thinking and other mental processes in order to control bodily processes heretofore thought to be involuntary, such as blood pressure, temperature, gastrointestinal functioning, and brain wave activity.

Biofeedback can be used to treat a wide variety of conditions and diseases ranging from stress, alcohol and other addictions, sleep disorders, epilepsy, respiratory problems, and fecal and urinary incontinence to muscle spasms, partial paralysis or muscle dysfunction caused by injury, migraine headaches, hypertension, and a variety of vascular disorders. More applications are being developed yearly.

In a normal session, electrodes are attached to the area being monitored (the involved muscles for muscle therapy, the head for brain wave activity); these electrodes feed the information to a small monitoring box that registers the results by a sound tone that varies in pitch or on a visual meter that varies in brightness as the function being monitored decreases or increases. A biofeedback therapist leads the patient in mental exercises to help the patient reach the desired result (e.g., muscle relaxation or contraction, or more alpha and theta brain waves). Through trial and error, patients gradually train themselves to control the inner mechanism involved. Training for some disorders requires 8 to 10 sessions. Patients with long-term or severe disorders may require longer therapy. Obviously, the aim of the treatment is to teach patients to regulate their own inner mental and bodily processes without help from the machine. In its simplest form, biofeedback therapy always involves a therapist, a patient, and a monitoring device capable of providing accurate physiological information.

A major reason why many patients like biofeedback training is that, like behavioral approaches in general, it puts them in charge, giving them a sense of mastery and self-reliance over their illnesses and health. Such an attitude may play a crucial role in the lower health care costs seen in patients after learning biofeedback skills.

Background. In 1961, experimental psychologist Neal Miller proposed that the autonomic, or visceral, nervous system was entirely trainable. Miller's suggestion ran contrary to prevailing orthodoxy, which held that all autonomic responses—heart rate, blood pressure, regional blood flow, gastrointestinal activity, and so on—were beyond voluntary control. In a remarkable series of experiments he showed that instrumental learning and control of such processes were indeed possible. One result of his work was the creation of biofeedback therapy.

In the succeeding three decades, Miller's work has been expanded by scores of researchers. Approximately 3,000 articles and 100 books have been published to date describing biofeedback and its applications. There are currently about 10,000 practitioners in the United States. Two organizations certify biofeedback professionals and paraprofessionals, and more than 2,000 individuals have received national certification.

Biofeedback does not belong to any particular field of health care but is used in many disciplines, including internal medicine, dentistry, physical therapy and rehabilitation, psychology and psychiatry, pain management, and more.

The most common forms of biofeedback involve the measurement of muscle tension (electromyographic, or EMG, feedback), skin temperature (thermal feedback), electrical conductance or resistance of the skin (electrodermal feedback), brain waves (electroencephalographic, or EEG, feedback), and respiration. More recently, increasingly sophisticated measurement devices have expanded biofeedback possibilities. Sensors can now measure and feed back the activity of the internal and external rectal sphincters (for the treatment of fecal incontinence), the activity of the detrusor muscle of the urinary bladder (for the treatment of urinary incontinence), esophageal motility, and stomach acidity (pH). Currently there are approximately 150 applications for biofeedback. Medical awareness of biofeedback is increasing, and referrals to biofeedback clinics continue to climb. Some treatments are already widely accepted. The American Medical Association, for example, has endorsed EMG biofeedback training for treating muscle contraction headaches.

Research accomplishments and clinical applications. Substantial research exists demonstrating the effectiveness of biofeedback in a number of conditions, including bronchial asthma, drug and alcohol abuse, anxiety, tension and migraine headaches, cardiac arrhythmias, essential hypertension, Raynaud's disease/syndrome, fecal and urinary incontinence, irritable bowel (spastic colon) syndrome, muscle reeducation (strengthening weak muscles, relaxing overactive ones), hyperactivity and attention deficit disorder, epilepsy, menopausal hot flashes, chronic pain syndromes, and anticipatory nausea and vomiting associated with chemotherapy (Basmajian, 1989).

Like all other forms of therapy, biofeedback is more useful for some clinical problems than for others. For example, biofeedback is the preferred treatment in Raynaud's disease/syndrome (a painful and potentially dangerous spasm of the small arteries) and certain types of fecal and urinary incontinence. However, it is one of several preferred treatments for muscle contraction (tension) headaches, migraine headaches, irritable bowel (spastic colon) syndrome, hypertension, asthma, and a variety of neuromuscular disorders, especially during rehabilitation. EEG biofeedback therapy is one of several preferred treatments for certain patients with epilepsy or attention deficit disorder.

Cost-effectiveness. Biofeedback-assisted relaxation training has been shown to be associated with decrease in medical care costs to patients, decrease in number of claims and costs to insurers in claims payments, reduction of medication and physician usage, reduction in hospital stays and rehospitalization, reduction of mortality and morbidity, and enhanced quality of life (Schneider, 1987).

Efforts are being made to further increase the cost-effectiveness of biofeedback therapy through the use of group and classroom instruction, reduced therapist contact, and home-based training. No studies have yet been made that discuss cost-benefit issues for the nonrelaxation-based biofeedback therapies, such as neuromuscular education and seizure reduction training.

Research needs and opportunities. The following are some of the research questions about biofeedback that need answering:

- What is actually learned during biofeedback? An awareness of some internal response or an awareness of associations between stimuli and responses?
- What variables influence learning in the biofeedback setting? How do they exert their effects? For example, what are the effects of the quality and quantity of reinforcements used to promote learning?
- What is the full range of bodily responses that can be modified by instrumental training procedures? Are the influences of biofeedback large enough to make a clinical difference? Or, are they laboratory curiosities?
- Which physiological responses are best to modify with respect to a specific disorder? For example, is lowering of blood pressure best achieved by feedback of blood pressure, or is feedback of muscle tension or skin temperature more effective?
- To what extent does transfer of training take place from the laboratory to real life? Can an individual self-regulate a physiological response at home as well as in a clinic? How long does the learning last?
- How do motivation and expectancy relate to the successful learning of biofeedback skills? What criteria predict who will be a successful biofeedback subject?
- How does biofeedback compare with other approaches (e.g. meditation, relaxation, suggestion, hypnosis) in altering physiological processes?
- How can biofeedback's effects be separated from other treatment variables such as the therapist's attention, verbal exchanges, suggestion, patient expectation, the clinical atmosphere, or participation in a self-help program?
- In which situations can biofeedback-assisted learning be used in lieu of pharmacological or surgical therapies, and in which situations as an adjunct to these approaches?
- For what conditions might group instruction in biofeedback skills be as effective as individ-

ual teaching? How can subjects be identified as more suitable for group teaching or individual instruction?

- How can biofeedback teaching procedures be more widely applied to the medical problems of children? Might the widespread teaching of biofeedback skills to children emphasizing self-care and self-responsibility at a young age counteract the widespread dependence and reliance on the medical system demonstrated by adults?
- What innovations in chip and microprocessor technology are needed to open up new areas of experimental and clinical research in biofeedback? How might miniaturization provide opportunities for patients to wear portable devices in real-life situations, thus expanding biofeedback learning?

Progress in this field, as in many other alternative and orthodox therapies, will entail three general steps or phases:

1. Pilot studies to determine whether there are any promising effects worthy of investigation and to detect any negative side effects or practical difficulties. These may be anecdotal case reports, systematic case studies, or uncontrolled single-group studies.
2. Controlled comparisons with the best available other techniques or with placebo treatments, using larger groups of patients, double-blind procedures, and adequate followup.
3. Broad clinical trials on large patient populations under ordinary conditions, to determine the effectiveness of the treatment in conditions other than unusually favorable ones with especially talented therapists.

Most clinical research in biofeedback has been done in Phase I, although some studies have appeared in Phase II. Phase III studies are needed and can be expected if funding becomes available.

Yoga

In India, where it has been practiced for thousands of years, yoga is a way of life that includes ethical precepts, dietary prescriptions, and physical exercise. Its practitioners have long known that their discipline has the capacity to alter mental and bodily responses normally thought to be far beyond a person's ability to modulate. During the past 80 years, health professionals in India and the West have begun to investigate the therapeutic potential of yoga. To date, thousands of research studies have shown that with the practice of yoga a person can indeed learn to control such physiological parameters as blood pressure, heart rate, respiratory function, metabolic rate, skin resistance, brain waves, body temperature, and many other bodily functions (see also the "Ayurvedic Medicine" section in the "Alternative Systems of Medical Practice" chapter).

As the practice of yoga has gradually moved into the West, it has been used most often as part of an integral program of health enhancement as well as for the treatment of chronic diseases. A prime example of the latter application is Dr. Dean Ornish's use of yoga in conjunction with dietary changes, moderate aerobic exercise, meditation, and group support to reverse coronary artery disease (Ornish, 1990) (see the "Diet and Nutrition" chapter).

For the most part, the West has adopted three aspects of entirely different yoga practices: the postures (or asanas) of hatha yoga, the breathing techniques of pranayama yoga, and meditation. Studies of meditation were discussed previously in this section. Here, the focus is on the therapeutic utility of programs that combine hatha yoga and pranayama yoga.

A typical yoga session as practiced in the United States lasts 20 minutes to an hour. Some people practice daily at home, while others practice one to three times a week in a class. A session usually begins with gentle postures to relax tension in the muscles and joints, then moves to more difficult postures. Every movement should be made gently and slowly, and practitioners are urged not to stretch beyond what is comfortable for them. Rather, practice should be "easeful." Emphasis is placed on breathing slowly from deep in the abdomen. Specific pranayama breathing exercises also are an important part of the practice. Guided (or self-guided) relaxation, meditation, and sometimes visualization follow the asanas. The session frequently ends with chanting, such as a repeating *Om shanti* ("Let there be peace"), to bring the body and mind into a deeper state of relaxation.

The physical and psychological benefits of yoga reportedly include massage of muscles and internal organs; increased blood circulation; rebalancing of the sympathetic and parasympathetic nervous systems; increase in brain endorphins, enkephalins, and serotonin; deeper breathing; increased lymph circulation; countering of the effects of gravity on the body; increasing nutrient supply to the tissues; and augmenting alpha and theta brain wave activity, which reflects a greater degree of relaxation.

Research. Since it began in the 1920s, scientific research on yoga has been enormous. Some 1,600 studies are listed by Monroe and colleagues (1989), and many more have been undertaken since that bibliography was published in 1989. Following are a few examples of those studies:

- Rats who were placed in headstands for an hour a day and then subjected to a variety of shocks adapted more rapidly to stressful situations than the control group (Udupa, 1978).
- Human beings doing postures such as the shoulder stand daily became more "stress hardy" (Gaertner et al., 1965).
- People practicing yogic meditation showed a 200-percent increase in skin resistance (less stress) within 10 minutes after beginning to meditate. The anxiety level remained altered (reduced) for long periods after the meditation training session ended (Benson, 1972).
- With the practice of yoga, the heart works more efficiently (Ornish et al., 1983), and the respiratory rate decreases (Bakker, 1976).
- Blood pressure is lowered, accumulated carbon dioxide diminishes, and the brain waves reflect a more relaxed state (Anand and Chhina, 1961; Blacknell et. al., 1975; Fenwick et al., 1977).
- EEG synchronicity, a unique change in brain waves found only in deep meditation, reflects improved communication between the right and left brain with regular yoga practice (Banquet, 1972).
- Physical fitness (as measured by the Fleishman Battery of Physical Fitness) is improved (Therrien, 1968).
- With yoga training in conjunction with dietary changes, cholesterol levels have been shown to drop an average of 14 points in 3 weeks (Ornish et al., 1983).
- Yoga brings increased chest expansion, better breath-holding abilities, and increased vital capacity and tidal volume (Maris and Maris, 1979; Shivarpita, 1981).
- Blood sugar levels improve and diabetes is better controlled after regular yoga practice (Monroe and Fitzgerald, 1986).
- Yoga, because of its psychological benefits, has been used successfully for drug treatment among prisoners, to help people stop smoking (Benson, 1969), and to improve job satisfaction (Maris and Maris, 1979).
- Yoga can be used successfully as an adjunctive therapy for asthma (Gore, 1982), high blood pressure (Blacknell et al., 1975), drug addiction (Benson, 1969), heart disease (Ornish et al., 1983), migraine headaches (Benson et al., 1977), and cancer (Frank, 1975).
- Yoga has been used successfully with arthritis and the arthritic symptoms of lupus (Coudron and Coudron, 1987).

Research needs and opportunities. Although many possibilities to further research can be considered, two areas are of primary importance—surgery and cancer. Yoga should be studied as a form of pain relief for surgical patients. Use of yoga both before and after surgery should be studied and evaluated in terms of the number of days of recuperation and the level of pain experienced. Studies also should be done with cancer patients who practice 1 hour of yoga a day for a year together with specific, ongoing lifestyle changes: a low-fat, high-fiber diet and weekly group support meetings.

Dance Therapy

Because dance is a direct expression of the mind and body, it is an intimate and powerful medium for therapy. Throughout the world, people have always danced to celebrate major events, to bond communities, to share sentiments, and to heal the sick and the alienated.

Applications. The use of dance as a medical therapy in the United States began in 1942 through the pioneering efforts of Marian Chace. Psychiatrists in Washington, DC, found that their patients were deriving therapeutic benefits from attending Chace's dance classes. As a result,

Chace was asked to work on the back wards of St. Elizabeth's Hospital with patients who had been considered too disturbed to participate in group activities. At about the same time, Trudi Schoop, a dancer and mime, volunteered to work with patients at Camarillo State Hospital in California. A group approach for nonverbal and noncommunicative patients was needed, and dance/movement therapy (DMT) met that need.

In 1956, dance therapists from across the country founded the American Dance Therapy Association, which has now grown to more than 1,100 members.[12] It publishes a journal, the *American Journal of Dance Therapy*; fosters research; monitors standards for professional practice; and develops guidelines for graduate education. It also maintains a registry for therapists: the certification registered dance therapist (D.T.R.) is granted to individuals with a master's degree and 700 hours of supervised clinical internship; the certification "Academy of Dance Therapists Registered" (A.D.T.R.) is awarded after therapists have completed 3,640 hours of supervised clinical work, which qualifies an individual to teach, supervise, and engage in private practice.

Dance/movement therapists are employed in a wide range of facilities, work with diverse populations, and address the needs of a broad spectrum of specific disorders and disabilities. Typically, dance/movement therapists work with individuals who have social, emotional, cognitive, or physical problems. Evolving specializations include using DMT as a disease prevention and health promotion service with healthy people and as a method of reducing the stress of caregivers and of patients with cancer, AIDS, and Alzheimer's disease.

Therapy goals vary according to the population served: for the emotionally disturbed, goals are to express feelings, gain insight, and develop attachments; for the physically disabled, to increase movement and self-esteem, have fun, and heighten creativity; for the elderly, to maintain a healthy body, enhance vitality, develop relationships, and express fear and grief; and for the mentally retarded, to motivate learning, increase body awareness, and develop social skills.

The underlying assumption in DMT is that visible movement behavior is analogous to personality. Thus, the process of changing how one moves (e.g., from fragmented to integrated or graceful) can effect total functioning. Specific aspects in DMT—such as music, rhythm, and synchronous movement—promote the healing processes by altering mood states, reawakening stored memories and feelings, organizing thoughts and actions, reducing isolation, and establishing rapport. Dancing in a group creates the emotional intensity necessary for behavioral change, and physical activity increases the endorphin level, inducing a state of well-being. Total body movement stimulates functioning of body systems (circulatory, respiratory, skeletal, and neuromuscular). Activating muscles and joints reduces body tension and body armoring. Unspeakable events, expressed in dance, can then be verbalized.

DMT has been demonstrated to be clinically effective in developing body image, improving self-concept, increasing self-esteem, facilitating attention, ameliorating depression, decreasing fears and anxieties, expressing anger, decreasing isolation, increasing communication skills, fostering solidarity, decreasing bodily tension, reducing chronic pain, enhancing circulatory and respiratory functions, reducing suicidal ideas, increasing feelings of well-being, promoting healing, and increasing verbalization (Fisher and Stark, 1992).

Research needs and opportunities. Although the efficacy of DMT has been demonstrated since the 1940s through extensive clinical practice, the following kinds of research should be done:

- Experimental studies to establish cause-effect relationships between specific approaches and patient outcomes. For example, what is the effect of daily DMT on depressed teenagers and drug abusers? What are the effects of psychotropic drugs on the ability of patients to respond to DMT? What are the effects of DMT on the ability of autistic children to communicate (Holtz, 1990)?
- Regression studies to isolate the independent and interactive effect of DMT. In many settings DMT is but one of several treatment modalities. Studies addressing the question of how much of the variation in patient change is

[12] *The American Dance Therapy Association is located at 2000 Century Plaza, Suite 108, Columbia, MD 21044-3363, telephone 410-997-4040.*

accounted for by DMT alone and by DMT in combination with other therapies would yield useful information (Holtz, 1990).

- Studies about how specific elements of dance—such as exuberance, vitality, social contact, and bonding—promote healing, longevity, and health-enhancement. Can the effects of these different components be dissected and quantified?
- If dance is engaged in for a specific purpose, is its therapeutic effect diminished? That is, to what extent does the effect of dance depend on spontaneity?
- Studies indicate that DMT is an aid to recovery after illness. However, few studies exist on the use of dance therapy for prevention of illness. Studies could be done to evaluate the adjunctive use of dance in blood pressure control or in reduction of blood lipids.

Music Therapy

Throughout history, music has been used to facilitate healing. Aristotle believed the flute in particular was powerful. Pythagoras taught his students to change emotions of worry, fear, sorrow, and anger through the daily practice of singing and playing a musical instrument. The first accounts of the influence of music on breathing, blood pressure, digestion, and muscular activity were documented during the Renaissance (Munro and Mount, 1978).

Music, more than the spoken word, "lends itself as a therapy because it meets with little or no intellectual resistance, and does not need to appeal to logic to initiate its action . . . [and] is more subtle and primitive, and therefore its appeal is wider and greater" (Altshuler, 1948). This wide appeal, as well as the considerable research base, suggests music may be used more and more both by itself and in conjunction with other treatments to ameliorate certain illnesses.

Music therapy began as a profession in the 1940s, when the Veterans Administration Hospital incorporated music into rehabilitation programs for disabled soldiers returning from World War II. The National Association for Music Therapy, Inc. (NAMT), was established in the United States in 1950. At the same time, degree programs were developing to educate and train professional music therapists. Since then, the organization has established curricular programs in music therapy, which include both clinical practice and internships at sites in a wide variety of medical and community settings; organized an impressive scientific database for the profession; developed standards of practice and a code of ethics; and fostered the development of a theoretical rationale for music's beneficial effect on the mind and body.

There are more than 5,000 registered music therapists (R.M.T.s) in the United States, and more than 80 undergraduate and graduate degree programs. In addition, there are 165 clinical internship training sites. A baccalaureate degree in music therapy requires course work in music therapy; psychology; music; biological, social, and behavioral sciences; disabling conditions; and general studies. It includes field work in community facilities or on-campus clinics serving individuals with special needs. After graduation, a student must serve a 6-month internship in an approved facility to be eligible to take the exams to become a board-certified therapist.

Two refereed journals are sponsored by NAMT: the *Journal of Music Therapy* and *Music Therapy Perspectives.* Three published indexes in music therapy exist with more than 6,000 citations of periodical articles published between 1960 and 1980 (Eagle, 1976, 1978; Eagle and Minter, 1984). An electronic database of medical music therapy (Computer-Assisted Information Retrieval Service System, CAIRSS) has been established with citations from more than 1,000 journals including empirical studies, case reports, and program reviews.

Music therapy is used in psychiatric hospitals, rehabilitation facilities, general hospitals, outpatient clinics, day care treatment centers, residences for people with developmental disabilities, community mental health centers, drug and alcohol programs, senior centers, nursing homes, hospice programs, correctional facilities, halfway houses, schools, and private practice.

Music therapy is used to address physical, psychological, cognitive, and social needs of individuals with disabilities and illnesses. After assessing the strengths and needs of each client, a qualified music therapist provides the appropriate treatment, which can include creating music, singing, moving to music, or just listening to it.

Music therapy can be used to meet medical goals in many areas, including the following:

- *Physical and emotional stimulation for those with chronic pain or impaired movement.* Music evokes a wide range of emotional responses. It can be a sedative to promote relaxation, or it can be a stimulant to promote movement to other physical activity (Coyle, 1987; Kerkvliet, 1990; Zimmerman et al., 1989).

- *Communication for those with autism or communication disorders.* Music is a unique form of communication. Using music with people who are nonverbal or who have difficulty communicating facilitates their social interaction and may increase their functioning (Grimm and Pefley, 1990; Street and Cappella, 1989).

- *Emotional expression for those with mental health problems.* Music can be used to express a wide variety of emotions, ranging from anger and frustration to affection and tenderness. These feelings often take the form of vocalizations that may or may not employ words (Jochims, 1990; Schmettermayer, 1983).

- *Associations with music for those with Alzheimer's disease and other dementias.* Selecting music from an individual's past may evoke memories of times, places, and persons. These memories can contribute additional information to the treatment of the individual (Clair and Bernstein, 1990; Gibbons, 1988; Hanser, 1990).

Research accomplishments. Thousands of specific research studies have been undertaken in the clinical uses of music in medical and dental treatment, and many others are currently in process. Among those clinical uses are the following:

- *As an analgesic.* As early as 1914, Kane investigated using a phonograph in the operating room for calming patients prior to anesthesia. Music as an analgesic for dental procedures was one of the earliest and most thoroughly investigated areas. It also has been used successfully during childbirth and with obstetric patients. A 1985 study using music as an anxiolytic showed suppressed stress hormone levels in orthopedic, gynecologic, and urologic surgery patients (Bonny and McCarron, 1984; Frandsen, 1989).

- *As a relaxant and anxiety reducer for infants and children.* Many studies have dealt with music's effect on hospitalized infants and pediatric patients. Lullabies in the neonatal nursery increased the weight gain and movements of newborns; music activities reduced fear, distress, and anxiety in hospitalized infants, toddlers, and their families and promoted "wellness" attributes in very ill children (Aldridge, 1993; Armatas, 1964; Atterbury, 1974; Chetta, 1981; Crago, 1980; Daub and Kirschner-Hermanns, 1988; Fagen, 1982; Kamin et al., 1982; Locsin, 1981; MacClelland, 1979; Mullooly et al., 1988; Oyama et al., 1983; Sanderson, 1986; Tanioka et al., 1985).

- *With burn patients.* Burn patients experienced alleviation of aesthetic sterility and distraction from constant pain.

- *With terminally ill individuals.* Cancer patients, using music therapy, increased their ability to discuss their feelings and talk about the trauma of the disease (Fagen, 1982; Frampton, 1986; Gilbert, 1977; Walter, 1983).

- *With persons with cerebral palsy.* As early as 1950, music therapy together with physical therapy was shown to reduce the neurological problems of children with cerebral palsy.

- *With individuals who have had strokes or have Parkinson's disease.* Federal funding from the Administration on Aging is currently being used for research into the effects of music therapy and physical therapy on people with strokes or Parkinson's disease.

- *With persons who have sensory impairments or AIDS.* Many studies have explored the applications of music therapy to individuals who have sensory impairments (visual and hearing), mental retardation, or AIDS.

- *With elderly persons.* In 1991 the U.S. Senate Special Committee on Aging convened a hearing on the therapeutic benefits of music for elderly persons, which included neurologist Dr. Oliver Sacks, singer Theodore Bikel, rock musician Mickey Hart, music therapists, and clients. The hearing record documents in detail the benefits of music therapy to the elderly (Special Committee on Aging, 1991). After the hearing, Senator Harry Reid (D–NV) introduced the Music Therapy for Older Americans Act, which was later folded into the Older

Americans Act Amendments of 1992. This act lists music therapy as both a supportive and a preventive health service. The new Title IV initiative creates research and demonstration projects and education and training initiatives, for which Congress appropriated nearly $1 million. In 1993, six nationwide music therapy projects were funded (Renner, 1986).

- *With persons with brain injuries.* In 1993, the Office of Alternative Medicine awarded one of its first 30 grants "to investigate any beneficial effects of a specific music therapy intervention on empirical measures of self-perception, empathy, social perception, depression, and emotional expression in persons with brain injuries." This research is now under way (Lehmann and Kirchner, 1986; Lucia, 1987).

Research needs and opportunities. In areas where it has not been done, systematic review and meta-analysis should be performed to assess the quality and outcomes of the research. In addition, further research is needed in the following areas:

- Neurological functioning, communication skills, and physical rehabilitation.
- Perception of pain, need for medication, and length of hospital stay.
- Cognitive, emotional, and social functioning in those with cognitive impairments.
- Emotional and social well-being of caregivers and families of those with disabilities.
- Clinical depression and other mental disorders.
- Disease prevention and health promotion of persons with disabilities.

Art Therapy

Art therapy is a means for patients to reconcile emotional conflicts, foster self-awareness, and express unspoken and frequently unconscious concerns about their disease. In addition to its use in treatment, it can be used to assess individuals, couples, families, and groups. It is particularly valuable with children, who often cannot talk about their most pressing and painful concerns.

The connection between art and mental health began to be recognized with the advent of mental institutions in the late 1800s and the early 1900s. Prinzhorn's book *Artistry of the Mentally Ill*, published in 1922, with stunning art made by institutionalized adults, helped ignite inquiries into the spontaneous graphic outpouring of disturbed patients. In addition to the interest in the artistic or diagnostic value of the patients' productions, there was the realization that the production of art was valuable in rehabilitating a patient's mental health.

In the 1940s, Margaret Naumberg blended ideas about psychoanalytic interpretive techniques and art to develop art as a tool to help release "the unconscious by means of spontaneous art expression . . . and on the encouragement of free association. . . . The images produced . . . constitute symbolic speech" (Naumberg, 1958). A decade later, Edith Kramer began her own exploration into the use of art. She focused her approach on the artmaking process itself. In her brand of therapy, a therapist is able to bring "unconscious material closer to the surface by providing an area of symbolic experience wherein changes may be tried out, gains deepened and cemented. The art therapist must be at once artist, therapist, and teacher . . ." (Kramer, 1958). Then, in 1958, Hana Kwiatkowska translated what she knew as an artist into the field of family work and introduced specific evaluation and treatment techniques at the National Institute of Mental Health.

Art therapy was formalized in the founding of the American Art Therapy Association in 1969.[13] Along with the Art Therapy Credentials Board, the 4,000-member organization sets standards for the profession, strives to educate the public about the field, has a code of ethics and a system of approving educational programs and registering art therapists, and will soon certify art therapists. Registered art therapists (A.T.R.s) must have graduate degree training and a strong foundation in the studio arts as well as in therapy techniques and must complete a supervised internship with work experience. Currently, 2,250

[13] *References documenting work in art therapy in addition to those cited in this report can be obtained from the American Art Therapy Association, Inc., 1202 Allanson Road, Mundelein, IL 60060, telephone 708-949-6064, fax 708-566-4580.*

art therapists are registered by the association. They practice in psychiatric centers, drug and alcohol rehabilitation programs, prisons, day care treatment programs, schools for the mentally retarded, residences for the developmentally delayed, geriatric centers, and hospices. Two journals are available: *Journal of Art Therapy* and *Art Therapy Journal.*

Art therapy differs from regular art classes such as painting, sculpture, and drawing, in that the therapist is trained both in diagnosis and in helping patients with specific health problems. In their art, for instance, patients may focus on parts of their bodies that unconsciously concern them but which they have never mentioned to their physicians or nurses. Such revelation can lead to further investigation and additional diagnosis. In helping patients express their feelings about a disease—such as cancer, for instance—therapists may lead them to draw images of themselves with cancer. These images may reveal a great deal about their feelings about their cancer, its severity, and its effect on their health and well-being.

Research accomplishments. Research on art therapy has been conducted in clinical, educational, physiological, forensic, and sociological arenas. Studies on art therapy have been conducted in many areas.

- Burn recovery in adolescent and young patients (Appleton, 1990).
- Eating disorders.
- Emotional impairment in young children (Bowker, 1990).
- Reading performance (Catchings, 1981).
- Chemical addiction (Chickerneo, 1993).
- As a prognostic aid in childhood cancer.
- As an aid in assessing ego development and psychological defensiveness in young children (Kaplan, 1986; Levick, 1983).
- Childhood bereavement (Zambelli et al., 1989).
- As a modifier of locus of control in behavior-disordered students.
- Sexual abuse in adolescents.
- Deafness, aphasia, autism, emotional disturbance, physical handicap, and brain injury in children (Silver, 1966).

Research needs and opportunities. Among the areas for further research are the following:

- Test the effect of art therapy on anxiety levels of patients subjected to invasive medical procedures.
- Determine whether art therapy enhances recovery and diminishes hospital stays for hospitalized patients.
- Examine whether art enhances relaxation art in guided imagery and relaxation training.
- Develop specific art interventions for children with communication problems and test the impact on their academic and social performance.
- Determine whether clients' choice of art materials and quality of art affects their psychophysical state.
- Assess group therapy as a tool to improve corporate working relationships.
- Assess self-portraits as a prognostic indicator for clients with eating disorders.
- Examine use of art therapy with juvenile offenders to assess moral development and modify impact of peer pressure.
- Investigate art therapy as an avenue to pain control.
- Test whether art therapy increases acceptance of physical and psychological changes in the elderly.
- Assess the utility of art therapy as a coping technique with survivors of natural disasters.

Prayer and Mental Healing

The use of prayer in healing began in human prehistory and continues to this day. Contemporary surveys reveal that most Americans pray and that they pray frequently, and almost always when they or their loved ones are ill.

The terms *mental healing* and *spiritual healing* are frequently used interchangeably. What does "spiritual" mean in this context? For many healers, spiritual healing is an integral part of their personal religion (e.g., healing comes from Jesus, Mary, a particular saint, God, and so on). Yet this cannot be the whole story, because spiritual and prayer-based healing is universal. It cannot be attributed to any particular religious point of view; it occurs in nontheistic traditions such as Buddhism just as it does in the theistic traditions of the West and in animistic societies as well. What is the unifying principle in mental-spiritual healing that seemingly transcends personal religious views? Is mental-spiritual healing a direct effect of mind or consciousness? Are personal religious interpretations irrelevant? What is the most fundamental, basic requirement for mental-spiritual healing, without which it cannot occur?

Techniques vary widely from culture to culture and are too diverse to be reviewed here. Overall patterns can nonetheless be discerned among mental-spiritual healers practicing in the United States.

One of the most thorough and innovative evaluations of this field is by psychologist Lawrence LeShan, a pioneer in investigating the relationship between psychological states and cancer (LeShan, 1966). LeShan found that mental-spiritual healing methods are of two main types. In type 1 healing, which LeShan considered the most important and prevalent kind, the healer enters a prayerful, altered state of consciousness in which he views himself and the patient as a single entity. There need be no physical contact and there is no attempt to "do anything" or "give something" to the person in need, only the desire to unite and "become one" with him or her and with the Universe, God, or Cosmos.

Type 1 healers uniformly emphasize the importance of empathy, love, and caring in this process. When healing takes place, it does so in the context of an enveloping sense of unity, compassion, and love. These healers state that this type of healing is a natural process that does not violate the laws of innate bodily function but rather speeds up ordinary healing—a very rapid self-repair or self-recuperation.

LeShan's type 2 healers, on the other hand, do touch the patient and describe some "flow of energy" through their hands to the patient's area of pathology. Feelings of heat are common in both healer and patient. In this mode, unlike type 1, the healer *tries* to heal. Some type 2 healers see themselves as originators of this healing power; others describe themselves as transmitters of it.

Type 1 healers do not have to be close to the patient to facilitate healing; for them, the degree of spatial separation from the person in need is irrelevant. Type 2 healers work on site in the presence of the patient.

These healing techniques are offered only as generalities. Some healers use both methodologies, even in the same healing session, and other healing methods could be described.

Rationale. How does this type of healing occur? There is no explanation within contemporary medical science, particularly for type 1, nonlocal healing.

The absence of an underlying "mechanism" is the greatest impediment to progress in this field, if such a word is even applicable. The lack of an explanation for these events prompts many people to dismiss them without investigating the evidence: since they *cannot* occur, they *do not* occur. Proponents of this foregone conclusion regard any "evidence" for mental healing as illusory, nothing more than artifacts of poor experimentation or data processing, or chance results of complex random processes.

The absence of a known mechanism, however, does not necessarily mean that mental healing does not or cannot occur, or that the research supporting it is necessarily flawed. Until the turn of this century, scientists had no explanation for a very common event: sunshine. An understanding of why the sun shines had to await the development of modern nuclear physics. Of course, the ignorance of scientists did not annul sunlight. Likewise, although the evidence is not so immediate, mental healing may be valid in the absence of a validating theory.

What might a future model of the mind that permits mental-spiritual healing look like? Such a model will almost certainly be *nonlocal*.

The idea prevalent in contemporary science is that the mind and consciousness are entirely local phenomena—that is, they are localized to the brain and body and confined to the present moment. From this point of view, distant healing cannot occur in principle, since the mind cannot stray outside the "here and now" to cause a remote event. Studies in distant mental influence and mental healing, however, challenge these assumptions. Dozens of laboratory experiments suggest that the mind can bring about changes in faraway physical bodies, even when the distant person or organism is shielded from all known sensory and electromagnetic influences. They imply that mind and consciousness may not always be localized or confined to points in space, such as brains or bodies, or in time, such as the present moment (Braud, 1992; Braud and Schlitz, 1991; Jahn and Dunne, 1987).

For medicine, the implications of a nonlocal concept of the mind may be profound. Among them are the following:

- Nonlocal models of the mind may be helpful in understanding the actual dynamics of healing. They may help explain instances in which a cure appears suddenly, radically, and unexpectedly; or when healing appears to be influenced by events occurring at a distance from the patient and outside his or her awareness.

- Nonlocal manifestations of consciousness may complicate traditional experimental designs and require innovative research methods because they suggest, among other things, that the mental state or expectation of the experimenter may influence the experiment's outcome, even under "blind" conditions (Solfvin, 1984).

At the same time, however, nonlocal manifestations suggest unmistakable *spiritual* qualities of the psyche, including the possibility that a nonlocal consciousness might survive the death of the *local* brain. The temporal barrier may also be violated: information apparently may be received by a distant person, at global distances, *before* it is mentally transmitted by the sender (Radin and Nelson, 1989). These events, replicated by careful observers under laboratory conditions, suggest that there is some aspect of the psyche that is unconfinable to points in space or to points in time. In sum, these events point toward a nonlocal model of consciousness, which at the very least allows for the possibility of distant healing information exchange and perhaps distant healing influences.

A nonlocal model of consciousness implies that at some level of the psyche there are no fundamental spatiotemporal separations between individual minds. If so, at some level and in some sense there may be unity and oneness of all minds—what Nobel physicist Erwin Schroedinger called the One Mind.[14]

In a nonlocal model of consciousness, therefore, distance is not fundamental but is completely overcome—in which case the mind of the healer and the patient are not genuinely separate but in some sense united. "Distant" healing thus becomes a misnomer, and because of the unification of consciousness, the patient may be said to be healing himself or herself.

Offering nonlocality as the bedrock of mental healing merely shifts the question: instead of asking how mental healing occurs, now one must ask how nonlocality happens. Currently no one knows, not even the physicists whose many experiments have established it as a solid part of modern physics. The saying comes to mind, "Physicists never really understand a new theory, they just get used to it." Perhaps the same may be said of physicians and their attempts to understand mental healing. Nonlocal mental models imply "action at a distance," which has been an abhorrent concept to most scientists since Galileo. But that situation may be changing. Physicists have repeatedly documented that nonlocal phenomena occur in the subatomic, quantum domain, wherein information can seemingly be "transferred" between distant sites by processes that are "immediate, unmitigated, and unmediated."[15] Whether *quantum* nonlocality is a possible explanation or rationale for *biological* or *mental* nonlocality is a question for future research. Nobel prize-winning physicist Brian D. Josephson of Cambridge University has suggested that nonlocal events occur in the biological world as well as the quantum domain. He proposes that human ways of knowing, particularly the human capacity to perceive patterns and

[14]*For a discussion of Schroedinger's views on the nonlocal, unitary nature of human consciousness, see L. Dossey, "Erwin Schroedinger," in* Recovering the Soul *(Dossey, 1989, pp. 125–139). Nonlocality, furthermore, implies infinitude in space and time, because a limited nonlocality is a contradiction in terms. A nonlocal model of the mind, therefore, suggests that some component of the psyche is omnipresent, eternal, and immortal. For elaboration, see* Recovering the Soul.

[15]*For a review of the current status of nonlocality in contemporary physics, see physicist Nick Herbert's* Quantum Reality *(Herbert, 1987).*

meaning, make possible "direct interconnections between spatially separated objects." Josephson suggests that these interconnections permit the operation of "psi functioning" between humans, currently held by biomedical science as impossible (Josephson and Pallikara-Viras, 1991). In any case, the fact that nonlocal events are now studied by physicists in the microworld suggests a greater permissiveness and freedom to examine phenomena in the biological and mental domains—such as mental healing—that may possibly be analogous.

Research accomplishments and major reviews. Anecdotal accounts of the power of prayer in "mental," "spiritual," "psychic," "distant," or "absent" healing are both legendary and legion. Countless books on these subjects are available, but this literature contains little scientific value.

Scientific attempts to assess the effects of prayer and spiritual practices on health began in the 19th century with Sir Francis Galton's treatise entitled "Statistical Inquiries into the Efficacy of Prayer" (Galton, 1872). Galton assessed the longevity of people frequently prayed for, such as clergy, monarchs, and heads of state. He concluded that there was no demonstrable effect of prayer on longevity. Judged by modern research standards, Galton's study contains many flaws, but he succeeded in advancing the idea that healing methods involving prayer and similar spiritual practices could be subjected to empirical scrutiny.

Since Galton's time, a sizable body of scientific evidence has accumulated in the field of spiritual healing showing positive results. This information is little known to the scientific community. Psychologist William G. Braud, a leading researcher in this field, summarizes this research in a recent review:

> There exist many published reports of experiments in which persons were able to influence a variety of cellular and other biological systems through mental means. The target systems for these investigations have included bacteria, yeast, fungi, mobile algae, plants, protozoa, larvae, insects, chicks, mice, rats, gerbils, cats, and dogs, as well as cellular preparations (blood cells, neurons, cancer cells) and enzyme activities. In human "target persons," eye movements, muscular movements, electrodermal activity, plethysmographic activity, respiration, and brain rhythms have been affected through direct mental influence (Braud, 1992; Braud and Schlitz, 1991).

These studies in general assess the ability of humans to affect physiological functions of a variety of living systems at a distance, including studies in which the "receiver" or "target" is unaware that such an effort is being made. The fact that these studies commonly involve nonhuman targets is important; lower organisms are presumably not subject to suggestion and placebo effects, a frequent criticism when human subjects are involved.

Many of these studies do not describe the psychological strategy of the influencer as actual "prayer," in which one directs entreaties to a Supreme Being, a Universal Power, or God. But almost all of them involve a state of prayerful*ness*—a feeling of genuine caring, compassion, love, or empathy with the target system, or a feeling that the influencer is one with the target.

In addition to the review by Braud, two other major reviews of this field have been published in the past decade by researchers Jerry Solfvin and Daniel J. Benor (Benor, 1990, 1993; Solfvin, 1984). These reviews examine the results of more than 130 controlled studies of distant mental effects, approximately half of which show statistically significant results. *The Future of the Body: Explorations Into the Further Evolution of Human Nature,* a scholarly, encyclopedic work by Michael Murphy, cofounder of the Esalen Institute, reviews the major research accomplishments in the field of mental healing and related fields and is a valuable guide (Murphy, 1992). The potential relevance of this area for medical practice has been examined by Larry Dossey (1993).

Experiments in distant hypnosis deserve intense scientific scrutiny. In such studies a subject is hypnotized remotely, is unaware when the hypnosis is taking place, and has no sensory contact with the hypnotist. Several such experiments were performed in France in the late 1800s by Janet and Gilbert and were repeated with greater refinement in 260 laboratory experiments in 1933 and 1934 by Vasiliev and colleagues in Leningrad (Vasiliev, 1976). These studies offer tantalizing suggestions that the human mind may display nonlocal characteristics (see the next section). For reasons to be discussed there, exploring this possibility scientifically should be given high priority.

Extent of the nonlocal perspective. The nonlocal manifestations of consciousness are not limited to prayer. Consciousness appears to manifest nonlocally in secular laboratory settings as freely as in a church, implying that prayer is only one of the possible avenues for the expression of these events. If nonlocal mental events are indeed ubiquitous, they may pervade all healing endeavors to some degree, even those that appear overwhelmingly mechanical, such as pharmacological and surgical therapies. Therefore it is unclear whether any therapy can be considered totally mechanical or "objective" (Braud, 1992). Nonlocal mental events may affect all therapies to some degree, and the nonlocal perspective may have to be considered when *any* therapy is assessed.

Research needs and opportunities. In addition to demonstrating whether there is a distant healing effect of the mind, future research should examine the following questions:

- How robust, reliable, and dependable is the mental healing effect?
- What qualities in the praying person and the recipient facilitate and retard distant healing effects?
- How can talented or potential healers be identified?[16]
- Is healing a "gift," or can individuals be trained to heal?[17]
- Do some prayers work better than others in mental-spiritual healing?[18]
- Why does the ability to heal fluctuate? Why is it not constant? Are mental healers like talented athletes, who can be either "hot" or "cold"? Since healing abilities seem to fluctuate, how can experimental protocols allow for this variation? Is it justifiable to apply the same experimental designs to healers as to penicillin, which presumably does not have an "off" day?
- How can mental healing be integrated with orthodox medical approaches, particularly in hospital environments? Can medical and surgical approaches be used simultaneously with mental healing, or are these methods incompatible?
- Can mental healing be tested in the same way as a new drug or surgical procedure? Is the randomized, prospective, double-blind methodology equally appropriate for physically and for mentally-spiritually based therapies?
- How can the public be protected from fraudulent or misguided mental "healers"? Is it possible to establish a requirement akin to board certification for healers in an attempt to ensure efficacy and protect consumers from worthless "healers" and predatory quacks?[19]
- What about more general ethical considerations? Is a mental healer justified in attempting to heal people without their knowledge and consent?
- Is it possible to *harm* distant organisms and *aid* them through distant mental influences?[20]

---

[16]*Efforts to identify potential spiritual healers and encourage or accelerate their development are being made by the National Federation of Spiritual Healers of America, Inc., P.O. Box 2022, Mt. Pleasant, SC 29465.*

[17]*An exemplary training program for spiritual healers is the Consciousness Research and Training Project, Inc., 315 East 68th Street, Box 9G, New York, NY 10021-5692. The director is Joyce Goodrich, Ph.D. This organization developed from the research of psychologist Lawrence LeShan, a pioneer in the scientific study of spiritual healing, and it advocates his general philosophy in this area.*

[18]*This question has also been investigated extensively by Spindrift, Inc., of Lansdale, PA (see next footnote). These researchers have repeatedly demonstrated in quantitative experiments that although both approaches work, an open-ended "Thy will be done" prayer strategy is more effective than a specific, goal-directed request in bringing about healing. These results may depend, however, on innate personality characteristics of the praying person, a possibility that Spindrift has not addressed.*

[19]*Spindrift researchers have developed a laboratory test they believe can prove which healers are talented and which are not. They have shown that healers differ widely in their abilities. Spindrift's suggestion that all so-called healers "take the test" evoked bitter criticism and hostility from the Christian Science Church ("It is heresy to bring God into the laboratory!"). See L. Dossey, "How Should We Pray? The Spindrift Experiments," in* Recovering the Soul *(New York: Bantam, 1989), 55–62.*

[20]*This possibility is suggested by many anthropological accounts such as the "death prayer," used at a distance by Kahuna shamans of Hawaii. These phenomena are unlike hexing and voodoo, which are local in nature, mediated through sensory exchanges between perpetrator and recipient.*

There are two related but separate directions of research in the field of nonlocal therapy: (1) the need to develop actual healing methods, and (2) the need to shed light on the fundamental nature of human consciousness. The first goal obviously requires the use of some type of living organisms as the recipient, but the second need not. In fact, the effects of consciousness can be studied in certain laboratory settings that offer greater precision and control than is offered by the usual experiments that involve living organisms as recipients. An example is the sophisticated studies in remote human-machine interactions that have been done for a decade at the Princeton Engineering Anomalies Research laboratory by Robert G. Jahn, former dean of engineering of Princeton University, and his colleagues (Jahn and Dunne, 1987).

Conclusions. Appallingly little is known about the origins of consciousness and how it relates to the physical brain. Although hypotheses purporting to explain consciousness abound, there simply is no consensus among expert neuroscientists, psychologists, artificial intelligence researchers, and philosophers as to its nature. Perhaps the lack of knowledge is not surprising; in medical research, scientists usually consign consciousness to last-place status and opt for "practical" research areas—the development of new drugs, surgical therapies, vaccines, and so forth.

Research in this area is analogous to basic investigations in other exotic areas of science such as particle physics, which have no immediate, bottom-line value. There is a need to know more about the basic, fundamental nature of consciousness—its spatial and temporal characteristics and its precise relationship with matter, including the brain. Without this basic understanding, progress in all forms of therapy, alternative and traditional, will be hampered, because the effects of consciousness are to some degree involved in all of them.

Summary

The mind-body interventions described in this chapter are part of a neglected dimension in health care. They offer what people are hungry for—a medicine that addresses more than the body. In addition to preventing or curing illnesses, these therapies by and large provide people with the chance to be involved in their own care, to make vital decisions about their own health, to be touched at deep emotional levels, and to be changed psychologically in the process.

There is nothing inherent in many alternative medical therapies that necessarily sets them apart from the way contemporary drugs and surgery are used. Because they are, after all, *things*, it is possible to use diets, herbs, homeopathic remedies, and most other alternative treatments with the same impersonal, remote objectivity that prompts people today to say, "My doctor doesn't care about *me*!" It is possible to convert any alternative technique into the "new penicillin" or the "latest surgery"—something given or done *to* a body without regard for the person involved. The mind-body approach outlined here is potentially a corrective to this tendency, a reminder of the importance of human connection and the power of patients acting on their own behalf.

But caring and compassion are not enough, and "putting the patient back into health care" is not sufficient. Alternative therapies, including the mind-body approaches that have been described, must be proved to work, must be safe, and must be cost-effective. While more work needs to be done, evidence also is already substantial that many of these mind-body therapies, if appropriately selected and wisely applied, meet these demands.

Recommendations

To further the development of alternative medical practices and mind-body interventions, the Panel on Mind-Body Interventions recommends the following:

- Development of educational materials, models, and programs in each of the mind-body areas discussed in this chapter, and dissemination to faculty and students in medical and other schools of health education.

- Development of comprehensive reviews of the literature in the various areas of the mind-body field. Such reviews would document the enormous body of work already done and specify directions for future research, thus facilitating the most efficient use of resources. Five areas should receive focus in a comprehensive review:

1. The theoretical foundations, research accomplishments, and clinical applications of mind-body interventions as well as the commonalities and differences among various self-regulation strategies.

2. The dynamics of the therapeutic relationship between providers and patients. What qualities, for example, allow therapists and patients to work well together? What factors distinguish "technicians" from "healers"? How do beliefs and attitudes of both patients and physicians affect health care and treatment outcomes?

3. The influence of social context on health and illness, including the impact of family, work, education, economic status, and culture.

4. The effects of belief, values, and meaning on health and illness.

5. The influence of nonlocal phenomena on health and illness.

- Development of a clearinghouse for information dealing with mind-body approaches to health and illness, including the publication of a journal on mind-body medicine.

- Evaluation of the legal, regulatory, and economic barriers to the integration of the mind-body perspective and techniques into the health care system.

- Institution of studies dealing with integration of mind-body techniques already shown to be effective (e.g., biofeedback plus hypnosis plus imagery), with attention to possible increases in cost-effectiveness when these approaches are used integrally rather than singly.

- Comparison of the long- and short-term effects of various self-regulation strategies.

- Basic investigations of the nonlocal effects of consciousness. These studies would involve human-machine as well as human-human interactions and would employ degrees of spatial separation of global or greater distances. Such research is vital in laying a theoretical foundation for understanding the role of consciousness in health in general and for progress in the mind-body field.

- Research addressing mind-body factors in chronic illness in poor and minority communities.

- Development of stress reduction techniques and nonpharmacological health education programs in elementary and secondary schools. Such programs would emphasize the role of self-responsibility in young children as well as the impact of attitudes, beliefs, and emotions in health.

- Development of drug rehabilitation and recidivism-reduction programs that emphasize mind-body techniques.

- A project to investigate how patient education affects the outcome of research studies. If the findings so justify, research designs should be developed that inform patients fully of the nature of the protocol in which they are participating and that provide immediate feedback of results.

- Funding and support of small pilot programs in the mind-body field.

- A study of the psychosocial characteristics of people who experience spontaneous remissions of cancer and chronic disease.

- Development of research methods that include subjective ways of knowing and "state-specific" observations.

- The beginning of a systematic study of what it means to be healthy.

- A task force on the nature of consciousness to be formed within the Office of Alternative Medicine. This task force would be composed of representatives from various disciplines whose work deals with the nature of consciousness, including psychologists, neurophysiologists, artificial intelligence experts, physicists, physicians, and philosophers. The mission of this group would be to formulate a model of consciousness that, as completely as possible, would account for the manifestations of consciousness that surface in mind-body research. Such a model would be of significant value in legitimizing the area of mind-body interventions and in stimulating progress in this field.

References

Achterberg, J., and G.F. Lawlis. 1980. Bridges of the Bodymind: Behavioral Approaches to Health Care. Institute for Personality and Ability Testing, Champaign, Ill.

Achterberg, J., and G.F. Lawlis. 1984. Imagery and Disease: Diagnostic Tools? Institute for Personality and Ability Testing, Champaign, Ill.

Achterberg, J., and M.S. Rider. 1989. The effect of music-mediated imagery on neutrophils and lymphocytes. Biofeedback Self Regul. 14:247–257.

Ahser, R. 1956. Respectable hypnosis. BMJ 1:309–313.

Aldridge, K. 1993. The use of music to relieve pre-operational anxiety in children attending day surgery. Australian Journal of Music Therapy 4:19–35.

Altshuler, I. 1948. A psychiatrist's experience with music as a therapeutic agent. In D. Schullian and M. Schoen, eds. Music as Medicine. Henry Schuman, New York.

Anand, B.K., and G.S. Chhina. 1961. Investigation on yogis claiming to stop their heartbeats. Indian J. Med. Res. 49:90–94.

Appleton, V.B. 1990. Transition from trauma: art therapy with adolescent and young adult burn patients. DAI 51:2282–2283.

Armatas, C. 1964. A study of the effect of music on postoperative patients in the recovery room. Unpublished master's thesis, University of Kansas.

Atterbury, R. 1974. Auditory pre-sedation for oral surgery patients. Audioanalgesia 38(6):12–14.

Bakker, R. 1976. Decreased respiratory rate during the TM technique: a replication. In T. Orme-Johnson and J. Farrow, eds. Scientific Research in Transcendental Meditation Programme. Maharishi European Research University Press, Geneva, Switzerland: vol. 1, pp. 140–141.

Banquet, J.P. 1972. EEG and meditation. JAMA 224:791–799.

Barber, T.X. 1969. Hypnosis: A Scientific Approach. Van Nostrand, New York.

Barber, T.X. 1978. Hypnosis, suggestion, and psychosomatic phenomena. Am. J. Clin. Hypn. 21:12–27.

Barber, T.X. 1984. Changing "unchangeable" bodily processes by (hypnotic) suggestions: a new look at hypnosis, imaging and the mind-body problem. Advances 1(2):7–40.

Barber, T.X., H.M. Chauncey, and R.A. Winer. 1964. The effect of hypnotic and non-hypnotic suggestion on parotid gland response to gustatory stimuli. Psychosom. Med. 26:374–380.

Basmajian, J.V. 1963. Control of individual motor units. Science 141:440–441.

Basmajian, J.V., ed. 1989. Biofeedback: Principles and Practice for Clinicians. Williams and Wilkins, Baltimore.

Bellis, J.M. 1966. Hypnotic pseudo-sunburn. Am. J. Clin. Hypn. 8:310–312.

Benor, D. 1993. Healing Research. (4 vols.) Helix Verlag, Munich.

Benor, D.J. 1990. Survey of spiritual healing research. Complementary Medical Research 4:9–33.

Benson, H. 1969. Yoga and drug abuse (letter). N. Engl. J. Med. 281:1133.

Benson, H. 1972. The physiology of meditation. Sci. Am. 226:84–90.

Benson, H. 1975. The Relaxation Response. Morrow, New York.

Benson, H., and M. Epstein. 1975. The placebo effect: a neglected asset in the care of patients. JAMA 232:1225–1227.

Benson, H., J. B. Kotch, and K.D. Crassweller. 1977. Relaxation response: bridge between psychiatry and medicine. Med. Clin. North Am. 61:929–938.

Benson, H., and E. Stuart. 1992. The Wellness Book: The Comprehensive Guide to Maintaining Health and Treating Stress-Related Illness. Birch Lane Press, New York.

Bergrugge, L.M. 1982. Work satisfaction and physical health. J. Community Health 7:262–283.

Berkman, L. and S. Syme. 1982. Social networks, host resistance, and mortality: a nine-year follow-up study of Alameda County residents. Am. J. Epidemiol. 109:186–204.

Black, S., J.H. Humphrey, and J.S. Niven. 1963. Inhibition of mantoux reaction by direct suggestion under hypnosis. BMJ 6:1649–1652.

Blackmore, S. 1991. Is meditation good for you? New Scientist (July 6):30–33.

Blacknell, B., J.B. Harrison, S.S. Bloomfield, H.G. Magenheim, S. Nidich, and P. Gartside. 1975. Effects of transcendental meditation on blood pressure: a controlled pilot experiment (abstract). Psychosom. Med. 37:86.

Bonny, H., and N. McCarron. 1984. Music as an adjunct to anaesthesia in operative procedures. J. Am. Assoc. Nurse Anesth. (February):55–57.

Borysenko, J. 1987. Minding the Body, Mending the Mind. Bantam, New York.

Bowker, C.A. 1990. A comparison of particular aspects of artistic expression in normal and emotionally impaired elementary-age boys. DAI 51:1.

Braud, W.G. 1992. Human interconnectedness: research indications. ReVision 14:140–148.

Braud, W.G., and M. Schlitz. 1991. Consciousness interactions with remote biological systems: anomalous intentionality effects. Subtle Energies 2.

Brooks, J.S., and T. Scarano. 1985. Transcendental meditation in the treatment of post-Vietnam adjustment. Journal of Counseling and Development 65:212–215.

Brown, B. 1977. Stress and the Art of Biofeedback. Harper and Row, New York.

Bruhn, J.G., A. Paredes, C.A. Adsett, and S. Wolf. 1974. Psychological predictors of sudden death in MI. J. Psychosom. Res. 18:187–191.

Cassileth, B.R., E.J. Lusk, T.B. Strouse, and B. Bodenheimer. 1984. Contemporary unorthodox treatments in cancer medicine: a study of patients, treatments, and practitioners. Ann. Intern. Med. 101:105–112.

Catchings, Y.P. 1981. A study of the effect of an integrated art and reading program on the reading performance of fifth-grade children. DAI 42:6.

Caudill, M., R. Schnable, P. Zuttermeister, H. Benson, and R. Friedman. 1991. Decreased clinic use by chronic pain patients: response to behavioral medicine intervention. Journal of Chronic Pain 7:305–310.

Chetta, H. 1981. The effect of music and desensitization on preoperative anxiety in children." J. of Music Ther. 18:74–87.

Chickerneo, N. 1993. New images, ancient paradigm: a study of the contribution of art to spirituality in addiction recovery. DAI 51:3781.

Chopra, D. 1991. Creating Health: How to Wake Up the Body's Intelligence. Houghton-Mifflin, New York.

Clair, A.A., and B. Bernstein. 1990. A comparison of singing, vibrotactile, and nonvibrotactile instrumental playing responses in severely regressed persons with dementia of the Alzheimer's type. J. Music Ther. 27:119–125.

Computer-Assisted Information Retrieval Service System (CAIRSS), the bibliographic database of music research literature.

Cooper, M., and M. Aygen. 1978. Effect of meditation on blood cholesterol and blood pressure. Journal of the Israel Medical Association 95:1–2.

Coudron, L., and O. Coudron. 1987. Le Yoga et les troubles du système osteo-articulaire. Annals de IIIe Colloque Yoga Santé (May).

Coyle, N. 1987. A model of continuity of care for cancer patients with chronic pain. Med. Clin. North Am. 71:259–270.

Crago, B. 1980. Reducing the stress of hospitalization for open heart surgery. Unpublished doctoral dissertation, University of Massachusetts.

Craigie, F.C., Jr., D.B. Larson, and I.Y. Liu. 1990. References to religion in The Journal of Family Practice: dimensions and valence of spirituality. J. Fam. Pract. 30:477–480.

Cranson, R.W., et al. 1991. Transcendental meditation and improved performance on intelligence-related measures: a longitudinal study. Personality and Individual Differences 12:1105–1116.

Crick, F. and C. Koch. 1992. The problem of consciousness. Sci. Am. 267:153–159.

Cummings, N.A., and J.I. Bragman, J.I. 1988. Triaging the "somatizer" out of the medical system into the psychological system. In E.M. Stern and V.F. Stern, eds. Psychotherapy and the Somatizing Patient (pp. 109–112). Hayward Press, New York.

Daub, D., and R. Kirschner-Hermanns. 1988. Reduction of preoperative anxiety: a study comparing music, Thalamonal, and no premedication. Anaesthetist 37:594–597.

Debenedittis, G., A.A. Panerai,and M.A. Villamira. 1989. Effects of hypnotic analgesia and hypnotizability on experimental ischemic pain. Int. J. Clin. Exp. Hypn. 37:55–69.

Dimsdale, J.E. 1977. Emotional causes of sudden death. Am. J. Psychiatry 134:1361–1366.

Dixon, J. 1984. Effect of nursing interventions on nutritional and performance status in cancer patients. Nurs. Res. 33:330–335.

Donovan, M. 1980. Relaxation with guided imagery: a useful technique. Cancer Nurs. 3:27–32.

Dossey, B.M., C.E. Guzzetta, and C.V. Kenner. 1992. Critical care nursing: body-mind-spirit (3rd ed.) J.B. Lippincott, Philadelphia.

Dossey, L. 1989. Recovering the Soul. Bantam, New York.

Dossey, L. 1991. Meaning and Medicine. Bantam, New York.

Dossey, L. 1992. Era III medicine: the next frontier. ReVision 14(3):128–139.

Dossey, L. 1993. Healing Words: The Power of Prayer and the Practice of Medicine. Harper San Francisco, San Francisco.

Eagle, C.T., Jr. 1976. Music Therapy Index, Vol. 1. National Association for Music Therapy. Lawrence, Kan.

Eagle, C.T., Jr. 1978. Music Psychology Index, Vol. 2. Institute for Therapeutics Research, Denton, Tex.

Eagle, C.T., Jr., and J.J. Minter. 1984. Music Psychology Index, Vol. 3. Orynx Press, Phoenix, Ariz.

Engel, G.L. 1971. Sudden and rapid death during psychological stress: folklore or folk wisdom? Ann. Intern. Med. 74:771–782.

Eppley, K.R., A.I. Abrams, and J. Shear. 1989. Differential effects of relaxation technique on trait anxiety: a meta-analysis. J. Clin. Psychol. 45:957–974.

Everly, G.S., Jr., and H. Benson. 1989. Disorders of arousal and the relaxation response: speculations on the nature and treatment of stress-related diseases. Int. J. Psychosom. 36:15–21.

Everson, T.C., and W.H. Cole. 1966. Spontaneous Regression of Cancer. Saunders, Philadelphia.

Fagen, T.S. 1982. Music therapy in the treatment of anxiety and fear in terminal pediatric patients. Music Therapy. 2:13–23.

Fenwick, P.B., S. Donaldson, L. Gillis, et al. 1977. Metabolic and EEG changes during TM: an explanation. Biol. Psychol. 5:101–118.

Fielding, J.W.L., S.L. Fagg, B.G. Jones, et al. 1983. An interim report of a prospective, randomized, controlled study of adjuvant chemotherapy in operable gastric cancer: British stomach cancer group. World J. Surg. 7:390–399.

Fisher, A.C., and A. Stark. 1992. Dance/Movement Therapy Abstracts: Doctoral Dissertations, Masters' Theses, and Special Projects Through 1990. Marian Chace Memorial Fund of the American Dance Therapy Association, Columbia, Md.

Frampton, D. 1986. Restoring creativity to the dying patient. BMJ 293:1593–1595.

Frandsen, J. 1989. Nursing approaches in local anaesthesia for ophthalmic surgery. J. Ophthalmic Nurs. Technol. 8:135–138.

Frank, J. 1985. The effects of music therapy and guided visual imagery on chemotherapy induced nausea and vomiting. Oncol. Nurs. Forum 12:47–52.

Frank, J.D. 1975. The faith that heals. Johns Hopkins Med. J. 137:127–131.

Gaertner, H., et al. 1965. Influence of Sirsasana headstand postures of thirty minutes duration on blood composition and circulation. Acta Physiol. Pol. 16:44.

Galton, F. 1872. Statistical inquiries into the efficacy of prayer. Fortnightly Review 12:125–135.

Gibbons, A.C. 1988. A review of the literature for music development/education and music therapy with the elderly. Music Therapy Perspectives 5:33–40.

Gilbert, J. 1977. Music therapy perspectives on death and dying. J. Music Ther. 14:165–171.

Goldberg, B. 1985. Hypnosis and the immune response. Int. J. Psychosom. 32(3): 34–36.

Goleman, D.J. 1977. The Varieties of the Meditative Experience. Irvington Publishers, New York.

Goleman, D.J. and J. Gurin. 1993. Mind Body Medicine. Consumer Reports Books, Yonkers, N.Y.

Gore, M.M. 1982. Effect of yogic treatment on some pulmonary functions in asthmatics. Yoga Mimamsa 20:51–58.

Graboys, T.B. 1984. Stress and the aching heart. N. Engl. J. Med. 311:594–595.

Green, E., and A. Green. 1977. Beyond Biofeedback. Delta, New York.

Greer, S. 1985. Cancer: psychiatric aspects. In G.K. Granville, ed. Recent Advances in Clinical Psychiatry. Churchill Livingstone, Edinburgh.

Grimm, D. and P. Pefley. 1990. Opening doors for the child "inside." Pediatr. Nurs. 16:368–369.

Gruber, B.L., N.R. Hall, S.P. Hersh, and P. Dubois. 1988. Immune system and psychological changes in metastatic cancer patients using relaxation and guided imagery: a pilot study. Scandinavian Journal of Behavior Therapy 17:25–46.

Hall, H. 1982–83. Hypnosis and the immune system. Journal of Clinical Hypnosis 25:92–93.

Hankoff, L.D., D. Englehardt, N. Freedman, D. Mann, and R. Margolis. 1960. The doctor-patient relationship in a psychopharmacological treatment setting. J. Nerv. Ment. Dis. 131(6):540–546.

Hanser, S.B. 1990. A music therapy strategy for depressed older adults in the community. Journal of Applied Gerontology 9:283–298.

Herbert, N. 1987. Quantum Reality. Anchor/Doubleday, Garden City, N.Y.

Hilgard, J.R. 1974. Imaginative involvement: some characteristics of highly hypnotizable and non-hypnotizable subjects. Int. J. Clin. Exp. Hypn. 22:138–156.

Holmes, D.S. 1984. Meditation and somatic arousal reduction: a review of the experimental evidence. Am. Psychol. 39:1–10.

Holmes, T.H., and R.H. Rahe. 1967. The Social Readjustment Rating Scale. J. Psychosom. Res. 11:213–218.

Holtz, G. 1990. Suggested research—my top 10. American Journal of Dance Therapy 12.

Honiotest, G.J. 1977. Hypnosis and breast enlargement—a pilot study. Journal of International Society for Professional Hypnosis 6:8–12.

Horowitz, M. 1983. Image Formation. Jason Aronson, Inc., New York.

House, J., K.R. Landis, and D. Umberson. 1988. Social relationships and health. Science 241:540–545.

House, J., C. Robbins, and H. Metzner. 1982. The association of social relationships and activities with mortality: prospective evidence from the Tecumseh study. Am. J. Epidemiol. 116:123–140.

Idler, E. L., and S. Kasl. 1991. Health perceptions and survival: do global evaluations of health status really predict mortality? J. Gerontol. 46:S55–S65.

Ikemi, Y. 1967. Psychological desensitization in allergic disorders. In J. Lassner, ed. Hypnosis and Psychosomatic Medicine (pp. 160–165). Springer-Verlag, New York.

Ikemi, Y., and S. Nakagawa. 1962. A psychosomatic study of contagious dermatitis. Kyushu J. Med. Sci. 13:335–350.

Ikemi, Y., S. Nakagawa, T. Nakagawa, and M. Sugita. 1975. Psychosomatic consideration of cancer patients who have made a narrow escape from death. Dynamic Psychiatry 31:77–92.

Jahn, R.G., ed. 1981. The Role of Consciousness in the Physical World. AAAS Selected Symposium 57. Westview, Boulder, Colo.

Jahn, R.G., and B.J. Dunne. 1987. Precognitive Remote Perception. In Margins of Reality: The Role of Consciousness in the Physical World (pp. 149–191). Harcourt Brace Jovanovich, New York.

Jenkins, C.D. 1971. Psychological and social precursors of coronary artery disease. N. Engl. J. Med. 284:417–418.

Jochims, S. 1990. Coping with illness in the early phase of severe neurologic diseases: a contribution of music therapy to psychological management in steroid neurologic disease pictures. Psychother. Psychosom. Med. Psychol. 40:115–122.

Johnson, J., V.H. Rice, S.S. Fuller, and M.P. Endress. 1978. Sensory information, instruction in a coping strategy and recovery from surgery. Res. Nurs. Health 1:4–17.

Johnson, R.F.Q., and T.X. Barber. 1976. Hypnotic suggestions for blister formation: subjective and physiological effects. Am. J. Clin. Hypn. 18:172–181.

Jordan, C.S., and K.T. Lenington. 1979. Psychological correlates of eidetic imagery and induced anxiety. Journal of Mental Imagery. 3:31–42.

Josephson, B.D., and F. Pallikara-Viras. 1991. Biological utilization of quantum nonlocality. Foundations of Physics. 21:197–207.

Josephson, B.D., and V.S. Ramachandran, eds. 1980. Consciousness and the Physical World. Pergamon Press, New York.

Kabat-Zinn, J., L. Lipworth, and R. Burney. 1985. The clinical use of mindfulness meditation for the self-regulation of chronic pain. J. Behav. Med. 8:163:190.

Kabat-Zinn, J., L. Lipworth, et al. 1986. Four-year follow-up of a meditation-based program for the self-regulation of chronic pain. Clin. J. Pain 2:150–173.

Kamin, A., H. Kamin, R. Spintge, and R. Droh. 1982. Endocrine effect of anxiolytic music and psychological counseling before surgery. In R. Droh and R. Spintge, ed. Angst, Schmerz, Musik in der Anasthesie (pp. 163–166). Editiones Roche, Basel, Switzerland..

Kaplan, F.F. 1986. Level of ego development as reflected in patient drawings. DAI 46:2166.

Karasek, R.A., T.G. Theorell, J. Schwartz, C. Pieper, and L. Alfredsson. 1982. Job, psychosocial factors and coronary heart disease. Adv. Cardiol. 29:62–67.

Karasek, R.A., T. Theorell, J.E. Schwartz, et al. 1988. Job characteristics in relation to the prevalence of myocardial infarction in the U.S. Health Examination Survey (HES) and the Health and Nutrition Examination Survey (HANES). Am. J. Public Health 78(8):910–918.

Kenner, C., and J. Achterberg. 1983. Non-pharmacologic pain relief for burn patients. Presented at the Annual Meeting of the American Burn Association, New Orleans.

Kerkvliet, G. 1990. Music therapy may help control pain. J. Natl. Cancer Inst. 82:350–352.

Kiecolt-Glaser, J.K., R. Glaser, D. Williger, et al. 1985. Psychosocial enhancement of immunocompetence in a geriatric population. Health Psychol. 4:25–41.

Kobasa, S.C., S.R. Maddi, and S. Kahn. 1982. Hardiness and health: a prospective study. J. Pers. Soc. Psychol. 42:168–177.

Kolata, G. 1986. Heart attacks at 9:00 a.m. Science 233:417–418.

Kramer, E. 1958. Art Therapy in a Children's Community. Schocken Books, New York.

Kutz, I., J.Z. Borysenko, and H. Benson. 1985. Meditation and psychotherapy: a rationale for the integration of dynamic psychotherapy, the relaxation response, and mindfulness meditation. Am. J. Psychiatry 142:1–8.

Larson, D.B., and S.S. Larson. 1991. Religious commitment and health: valuing the relationship. Second Opinion: Health, Faith, and Ethics 17:26–40.

Lawlis, G.F., D. Selby, G. Hinnant, and C. McCoy. 1985. Reduction of postoperative pain parameters by presurgical relaxation instructions for spinal pain patients. Spine 10(7):649–651.

LeCron, L.M. 1969. Breast development through hypnotic suggestion. J. Am. Soc. Psychosom. Dent. Med. 16:58–61.

Lehmann, W., and D. Kirchner. 1986. Initial experiences in the combined treatment of aphasia patients following cerebrovascular insult by speech therapists and music therapists. Zeitschrift für Alzenforschung 41:123–128.

LeShan, L. 1966. The Medium, the Mystic, and the Physicist. Viking, New York.

LeShan, L.L. 1977. You can fight for your life: emotional factors in the causation of cancer. M. Evans, New York.

Levick, M.F. 1983. Resistance: developmental image of ego defenses, manifestations of adaptive and maladaptive defenses in children's drawings. DAI 43:10.

Levin, J.S. 1989. Religious factors in aging, adjustment, and health: a theoretical overview. In W.M. Clements, ed. Religion, Aging and Health: A Global Perspective. Compiled by the World Health Organization. Haworth Press, New York.

Levin, J.S., and P.L. Schiller. 1987. Is there a religious factor in health? Journal of Religion and Health 26:9–36.

Levin, J.S., and H.Y. Vanderpool. 1987. Is frequent religious attendance really conducive to better health?: toward an epidemiology of religion. Soc. Sc. Med. 24:589–600.

Levin, J.S., and H.Y. Vanderpool. 1991. Religious factors in physical health and the prevention of illness. Prev. Hum. Serv. 9:41–64.

Levoy, G. 1989. Inexplicable recoveries from incurable diseases. Longevity (October):37–42.

Locsin, R. 1981. The effect of music on the pain of selected post-operative patients. J. Adv. Nurs. 6:19–25.

Lown, B., R.A. DeSilva, P. Reich, and B.J. Murawski. 1980. Psychophysiological factors in sudden cardiac death. Am. J. Psychiatry 137:1325–1335.

Lucas, O.N. 1965. Dental extractions in the hemophiliac: control of the emotional factors by hypnosis. Am. J. Clin. Hypn. 7:301–307.

Lucia, C.M. 1987. Toward developing a model of music therapy intervention in the rehabilitation of head trauma patients. Music Therapy Perspectives 4:34–39.

Luria, A.R. 1968. The Mind of a Mnemonist. Basic Books, New York.

Lynch, J.J. 1977. The Broken Heart: The Medical Consequences of Loneliness. Basic Books, New York.

Lynn, S.J., and J.W. Rhue. 1987. Hypnosis, imagination, and fantasy. J. Mental Imagery. 11:101–113.

MacClelland, D.C. 1979. Music in the operating room. AORN J. 29:252–260.

MacLean, C.R.K., K.G. Walton, et al. 1992. Altered cortisol response to stress after four months' practice of the transcendental meditation program. Presented at the 18th Annual Meeting of the Society for Neuroscience, Anaheim, Calif., October 30.

Mahesh Yogi, M. 1963. Transcendental Meditation. New American Library, New York.

Maris, L., and M. Maris. 1979. Mechanics of stress release: the TM program and occupational stress. Police Stress 1:29–36.

Mason, A.A., and S. Black. 1958. Allergic skin responses abolished under treatment of asthma and hay fever by hypnosis. Lancet 1:877–880.

Matthews, D.A., D.B. Larson, and C.P. Barry. 1993. The Faith Factor: An Annotated Bibliography of Clinical Research on Spiritual Subjects. National Institute for Healthcare Research, Rockville, Md.

McSherry, E. 1990. Medical economics. In D. Wedding, ed. Medicine and Behavior (pp. 463–484). Mosby and Co., St. Louis.

Monroe, R.E., and L. Fitzgerald. 1986. Follow-up survey on yoga and diabetes. Yoga Biomedical Bulletin 1:4, 61.

Monroe, R., A.K. Ghosh, and D. Kalish. 1989. Yoga Research Bibliography, Scientific Studies on Yoga and Meditation. Yoga Biomedical Trust, Cambridge, England.

Muller, J.E., P.L. Ludmer, S.N. Willich, and G.H. Tofler. 1987. Circadian variation in the frequency of sudden death. Circulation 75:131–138.

Mullooly, V., R. Levin, and H. Feldman. 1988. Music for postoperative pain and anxiety. J. N.Y. State Nurses Assoc. 19:4–7.

Munro, S., and B. Mount. 1978. Music therapy in palliative care. Can. Med. Assoc. J. 119:1029–1034.

Murphy, M. 1992. The Future of the Body: Explorations Into the Further Evolution of Human Nature. Jeremy P. Tarcher, Los Angeles. pp. 257–283.

Murphy, M., and S. Donovan. 1989. The Physical and Psychological Effects of Meditation: A Review of Contemporary Meditation Research With a Comprehensive Bibliography, 1931–1988. Esalen Institute of Exceptional Functioning, San Rafael, Calif.

Naumberg, M. 1958. Art therapy: its scope and function. In E.F. Hammer, ed. The Clinical Application of Projective Drawings (pp. 511–517). Charles C. Thomas, Springfield, Ill.

Nelson, R. 1992. Personal communication. NIH Mind-Body Interventions Panel.

Olness, K., and M. Conroy. 1985. A pilot study of voluntary control of transcutaneous PO by children. Int. J. Clin. Exp. Hypn. 33:1.

Olness, K., T. Culbert, and D. Uden. 1989. Self-regulation of salivary immunoglobulin A by children. Pediatrics 83:66–71.

O'Regan, B., and C. Hirshberg. 1993. Spontaneous Remission: An Annotated Bibliography. Institute of Noetic Sciences, Sausalito, Calif.

Orme-Johnson, D.W. 1987. Medical care utilization and the transcendental meditation program. Psychosom. Med. 49:493–507.

Orme-Johnson, D.W., and C.N. Alexander. 1992. Critique of the National Research Council's report on meditation. (Manuscript available from the first author, Maharishi International University, Fairfield, Iowa.)

Orme-Johnson, D.W., and F.T. Farrow, eds. 1977. Scientific Research on the Transcendental Meditation Program: College Papers, Vol. 1–5. MERU Press, Los Angeles.

Ornish, D. 1990. Can lifestyle changes reverse coronary artery disease? Lancet 336:129.

Ornish, D., L.W. Scherwitz, R.D. Doody, et al. 1983. Effects of stress management training and dietary changes in treating ischemic heart disease. JAMA 249:54–59.

Oyama, T., Y. Sato, M. Kudo, R. Spintge, and R. Droh. 1983. Effect of anxiolytic music on endocrine function in surgical patients. In R. Droh and R. Spintge, eds. Angst, schmerz, musik in der anasthesie (pp. 147–152). Editiones Roche, Basel, Switzerland.

Palmore, E. 1969. Predicting longevity: a follow-up controlling for age. Gerontologist 9:247–250.

Peavey, B., G.F. Lawlis, and P. Goven. 1985. Biofeedback-assisted relaxation: effects on phagocytic capacity. Biofeedback Self Regul. 10:33–47.

Platonov, K. 1959. The Word as a Psychological and Therapeutic Factor. Foreign Language Publishing House, Moscow.

Rabkin, S.W., F.A.L. Mathewson, and R.B. Tate. 1980. Chronobiology of cardiac sudden death in men. JAMA 244:1357–1358.

Radin, D.L., and R.D. Nelson. 1989. Consciousness-related effects in random physical systems. Foundations of Physics 19:1499–1514.

Ravindra, R., ed. 1991. Science and Spirit. Paragon House, New York.

Renner, M. 1986. Means for the activation of the elderly: music for fun. Krankenpfl. Soins Infirm. 79:85–86.

Rhein, R.W., Jr. 1980. Placebo: deception or potent therapy? Med. World News (Feb. 4):39–47.

Rider, M.S., J. Achterberg, G.F. Lawlis, A. Goven, R. Toledo, and J.R. Butler. 1990. Effect of immune system imagery on secretory IgA. Biofeedback Self Regul. 15:317–333.

Rossi, E.L. 1986. The Psychobiology of Mind-Body Healing: New Concepts of Therapeutic Hypnosis. W.W. Norton, New York.

Ruberman, W.E., E. Weinblatt, J.D. Goldberg, and B.S. Chaudhary. 1984. Psychosocial influences on mortality after myocardial infarction. N. Engl. J. Med. 311:552–559.

Sagan, L.A. 1987. The Health of Nations: True Causes of Sickness and Well-Being. Basic Books, New York.

Sales, S.M., and J. House. 1971. Job dissatisfaction as a possible risk factor in coronary artery disease. J. Chronic Dis. 23:861–873.

Sanderson, S. 1986. The effect of music on reducing preoperative anxiety and postoperative anxiety and pain in the recovery room. Unpublished master's thesis. Florida State University.

Sapolsky, R.M. 1990. Stress in the wild. Sci. Am. (January):116–123.

Schiller, P.L., and J.S. Levin. 1988. Is there a religious factor in health care utilization?: a review. Soc. Sci. Med. 27:1369–1379.

Schleifer, S.J., S.E. Keller, M. Camerino, J.C. Thornton, and M. Stein. 1983. Suppression of lymphocyte stimulation following bereavement. JAMA 250:374–377.

Schmettermayer, R. 1983. Possibilities for inclusion of group music therapeutic methods in the treatment of psychotic patients. Psychiatr. Neurol. Med. Psychol. (Leipz.) 35:49–53.

Schnall, P.L., C. Pieper, J.E. Schwartz, et al. 1990. The relationship between "job strain," workplace diastolic blood pressure, and left ventricular mass index: results of a case-control study. JAMA 263:1929–1935.

Schneider, C.J. 1987. Cost-effectiveness of biofeedback and behavioral medicine treatments: a review of the literature. Biofeedback Self Regul. 12(2):71–92.

Schneider, J., C.S. Smith, and S. Whitcher. 1983. The relationship of mental imagery to neutrophil function. Uncirculated manuscript, Michigan State University. (For an abridged version, see Achterberg and Lawlis, 1984.)

Schneider, R.H., C.N. Alexander, and R.K. Wallace. 1992. In search of an optimal behavioral treatment for hypertension: a review and focus on transcendental meditation. In E.H. Johnson, W.D. Gentry, and S. Julius, eds. Personality, Elevated Blood Pressure, and Essential Hypertension. Hemisphere, Washington, D.C.

Scott, D.W., D.C. Donohue, R.C. Mastrovito, and T.B. Hakus. 1986. Comparative trial of clinical relaxation and an antiemetic drug regimen in reducing chemotherapy-related nausea and vomiting. Cancer Nurs. 9:178–188.

Sharma, H.M., B.D. Triguna, and D. Chopra. 1991. Maharishi Ayur-Veda: modern insights into ancient medicine. JAMA 265:2633–2634, 2637.

Sheikh, A.A., and C.S. Jordan. 1983. Clinical uses of mental imagery. In A.A. Sheikh, ed. Imagery: Current Theory, Research, and Application. John Wiley, New York.

Shivarpita, J.H. 1981. The effects of Hatha Yoga postures and breathing. Research Bulletin of Himalayan International Institute 3:4–10.

Siegel, B. 1986. Love, Medicine and Miracles. Harper and Row, New York.

Silver, R. 1966. The role of art in the conceptual thinking, adjustment, and aptitude of deaf and aphasic children. DAI 27:5.

Simonton, O.C., S. Simonton, and J. Creighton. 1978. Getting Well Again. J.P. Tarcher, Los Angeles.

Simpson, G.G. 1953. Life of the Past. Yale University Press, New Haven.

Sinclair-Geiben, A.H.C., and D. Chalmers. 1959. Evaluation of treatment of warts by hypnosis. Lancet, 2:480–482.

Solfvin, J. 1984. Mental Healing. In S. Krippner, ed. Advances in Parapsychological Research vol. 4, McFarland and Company, Jefferson, N.C.

Special Committee on Aging, U.S. Senate. 1991. Forever Young: Music and Aging. Pub. No. 102-9, U.S. Government Printing Office, Washington, D.C.

Spiegel, D., J.R. Bloom, H.C. Kraemer, and E. Gottheil. 1989. Effect of psychosocial treatment on survival of patients with metastatic breast cancer. Lancet 2(8668):888–891.

Staib, A.R., and D.R. Logan. 1977. Hypnotic stimulation of breast growth. Am. J. Clin. Hypn. 19:201–208.

Stevens, L. 1983. An intervention study of imagery with diabetes mellitus. Doctoral dissertation, University of North Texas.

Stoddard, J.B., and J.P. Henry. 1985. Affectional bonding and the impact of bereavement. Advances 2:19–28.

Strain, J.J. 1993. Psychotherapy and medical conditions. In D. Galman and J. Guin, eds. Mind-Body Medicines. Consumer Reports Books, New York.

Street, R.J., and J. Cappella. 1989. Social and linguistic factors influencing adaptation in children's speech. J. Psycholinguist. Res. 18:497–519.

Surman, O.S., S.K. Gottlieb, T.P. Hackett, and E.L. Silverberg. 1973. Hypnosis in the treatment of warts. Arch. Gen. Psychiatry 28:439–441.

Syme, S.L. 1991. Control and health: a personal perspective. Advances 7:16–27.

Tanioka, F., T. Takazawa, S. Kamata, M. Kudo, A. Matsuki, and T. Oyama. 1985. Hormonal effect of anxiolytic music in patients during surgical operations under epidural anaesthesia. In R. Droh and R. Spintge, eds. Music in Medicine (pp. 285–290). Editiones Roche, Basel, Switzerland.

Taylor, S.E. 1989. Positive Illusions: Creative Self-Deception and the Healthy Mind. Basic Books, Inc., New York.

Therrien, R. 1968. Influence of a 5BX and a Hatha Yoga training programme of selected fitness measures. Completed Research in HPER 11:125.

Thompson, D.R., J.E.F. Pohl, and T.W. Sutton. 1992. Acute myocardial infarction and day of the week. Am. J. Cardiol. 69:266–257.

Udupa, K.N. 1978. Disorders of Stress and Their Management by Yoga. Benares Hindu University, Benares, India.

Ullman, M., and S. Dudek. 1960. On the psyche and warts: II. hypnotic suggestion and warts. Psychosom. Med. 22:68–76.

Vanderpool, H.Y., and J.S. Levin. 1990. Religion and medicine: how are they related? Journal of Religion and Health 29:9–20.

Vasiliev, L.L. 1976. Experiments in Distant Influence. Dutton, New York.

Walsh, R., and F. Vaughan. In press. Paths Beyond Ego: The Transpersonal Vision. J.P. Tarcher, Los Angeles.

Walter, B. 1983. A little music: why the dying aren't allowed to die. Nurs. Life 3:52–57.

Wheatley, D. 1967. Influence of doctors' and patients' attitudes in the treatment of neurotic illness. Lancet 2(526):1133–1135.

White, K.D. 1978. Salivation: the significance of imagery in its voluntary control. Psychophysiology 15(3):196–203.

Willard, R.D. 1977. Breast enlargement through visual imagery and hypnosis. Am. J. Clin. Hypn. 19:195–200.

Williams, J.E. 1973. Stimulation of breast growth by hypnosis. J. Sex Res. 10:316–326.

Williams, R.B. 1990. Editorial: the role of the brain in physical disease: folklore, normal science, or paradigm shift? JAMA 263:1971–1972.

Wolf, S., and R.A. Pinsky. 1954. Effects of placebo administration and occurrence of toxic reactions. JAMA 15:339–341.

Work in America: Report of a Special Task Force to the Secretary of Health, Education, and Welfare. 1973. MIT Press, Cambridge, Mass.

Zahourek, R., ed. 1988. Relaxation and Imagery. Philadelphia: W.B. Saunders, Philadelphia.

Zambelli, G.C. , E.J. Clark, and M. Heegard. 1989. Art therapy for bereaved children. In H. Wadeson, J. Durkin, and D. Perach, eds. Advances in Art Therapy (pp. 60–80). John Wiley and Sons, New York.

Zimmerman, L., B. Pozehl, K. Duncan, and R. Schmitz. 1989. Effects of music in patients who had chronic cancer pain. West. J. Nurs. Res. 11:298–309.

Zohar, D. 1990. The Quantum Self: Human Nature and Consciousness Defined by the New Physics. William Morrow, New York.

Bioelectromagnetics Applications in Medicine

PANEL MEMBERS AND CONTRIBUTING AUTHORS

Beverly Rubik, Ph.D.—Chair
Robert O. Becker, M.D.
Robert G. Flower, M.S.
Carlton F. Hazlewood, Ph.D.
Abraham R. Liboff, Ph.D.
Jan Walleczek, Ph.D.

Overview

Bioelectromagnetics (BEM) is the emerging science that studies how living organisms interact with electromagnetic (EM) fields. Electrical phenomena are found in all living organisms. Moreover, electrical currents exist in the body that are capable of producing magnetic fields that extend outside the body. Consequently, they can be influenced by external magnetic and EM fields as well. Changes in the body's natural fields may produce physical and behavioral changes. To understand how these field effects may occur, it is first useful to discuss some basic phenomena associated with EM fields.

In its simplest form, a magnetic field is a field of magnetic force extending out from a permanent magnet. Magnetic fields are produced by moving electrical currents. For example, when an electrical current flows in a wire, the movement of the electrons through the wire produces a magnetic field in the space around the wire (fig. 1). If the current is a direct current (DC), it flows in one direction and the magnetic field is steady. If the electrical current in the wire is pulsing, or fluctuating—such as in alternating current (AC), which means the current flow is switching directions—the magnetic field also fluctuates. The strength of the magnetic field depends on the amount of current flowing in the wire; the more current, the stronger the magnetic field. An EM field contains both an electrical field and a magnetic field. In the case of a fluctuating magnetic or EM field, the field is characterized by its rate, or frequency, of fluctuation (e.g., one fluctuation per second is equal to 1 hertz [Hz], the unit of frequency).

A field fluctuating in this fashion theoretically extends out in space to infinity, decreasing in strength with distance and ultimately becoming lost in the jumble of other EM and magnetic fields that fill space. Since it is fluctuating at a certain frequency, it also has a wave motion (fig. 2). The wave moves outward at the speed of light (roughly 186,000 miles per second). As a result, it has a wavelength (i.e., the distance between crests of the wave) that is inversely related to its frequency. For example, a 1-Hz frequency has a wavelength of millions of miles, whereas a 1-million-Hz, or 1-megahertz (MHz), frequency has a wavelength of several hundred feet, and a 100-MHz frequency has a wavelength of about 6 feet.

All of the known frequencies of EM waves or fields are represented in the EM spectrum, ranging from DC (zero frequency) to the highest frequencies, such as gamma and cosmic rays. The EM spectrum includes x rays, visible light, microwaves, and television and radio frequencies, among many others. Moreover, all EM fields are force fields that carry energy through space and are capable of producing an effect at a distance. These fields have characteristics of both waves and particles. Depending on what types of experiments one does to investigate light, radio waves, or any other part of the EM spectrum, one will find either waves or particles called *photons*.

A photon is a tiny packet of energy that has no measurable mass. The greater the energy of the photon, the greater the frequency associated with its waveform. The human eye detects only

Figure 1. An electrical current in a wire produces a magnetic field in the space around the wire.

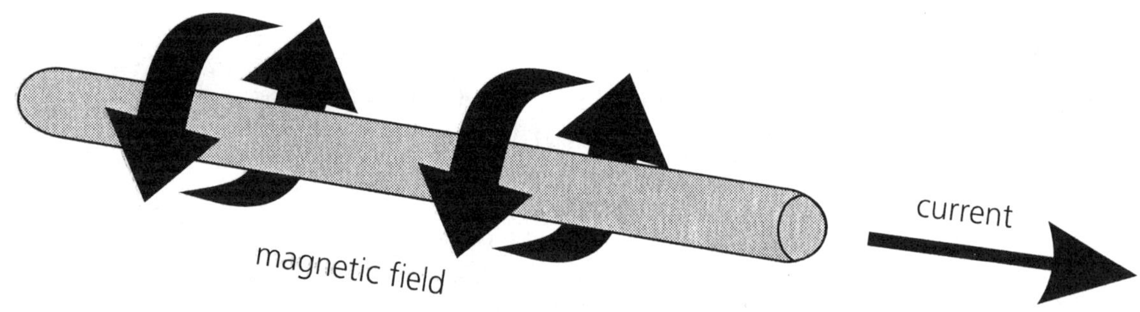

Figure 2. Electromagnetic theory showing a wave in which the electric field is perpendicular to the magnetic field and also to the direction of propagation.

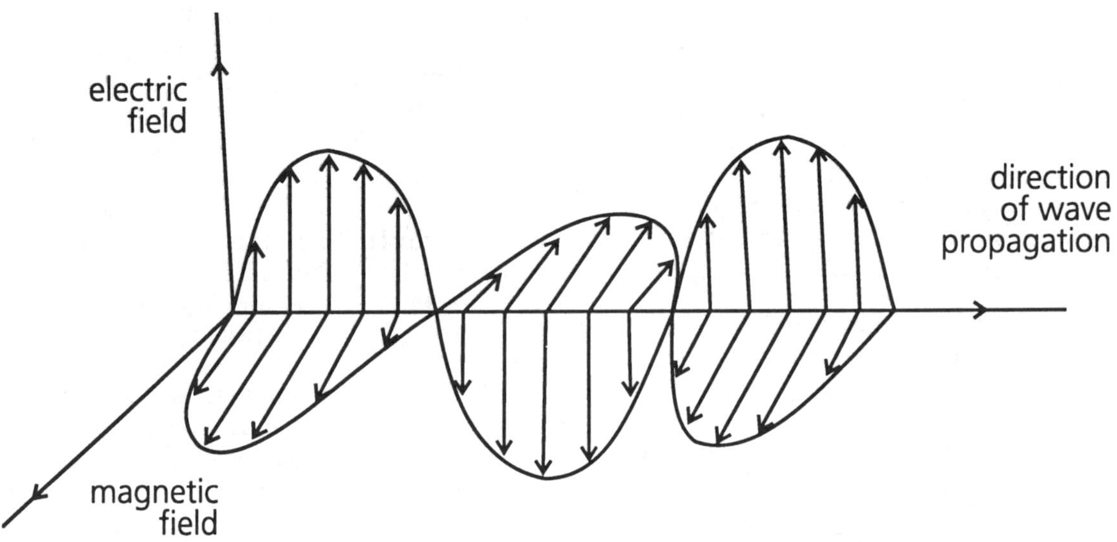

a narrow band of frequencies within the EM spectrum, that of light. One photon gives up its energy to the retina in the back of the eye, which converts it into an electrical signal in the nervous system that produces the sensation of light.

Table 1 shows the usual classification of EM fields in terms of their frequency of oscillation, ranging from DC through extremely low frequency (ELF), low frequency, radio frequency (RF), microwave and radar, infrared, visible light, ultraviolet, x rays, and gamma rays. For oscillating fields, the higher the frequency, the greater the energy.

Endogenous fields (those produced within the body) are to be distinguished from *exogenous* fields (those produced by sources outside the body). Exogenous EM fields can be classified as either natural, such as the earth's geomagnetic field, or artificial (e.g., power lines, transformers, appliances, radio transmitters, and medical de-

Table 1. Electromagnetic Spectrum

Frequency range (Hz)*	Classification	Biological effect
0	Direct current	Nonionizing
0 – 300	Extremely low frequency	Nonionizing
$300 - 10^4$	Low frequency	Nonionizing
$10^4 - 10^9$	Radio frequency	Nonionizing
$10^9 - 10^{12}$	Microwave and radar bands	Nonionizing
$10^{12} - 4 \times 10^{14}$	Infrared band	Nonionizing
$4 \times 10^{14} - 7 \times 10^{14}$	Visible light	Weakly ionizing
$7 \times 10^{14} - 10^{18}$	Ultraviolet band	Weakly ionizing
$10^{18} - 10^{20}$	X rays	Strongly ionizing
Over 10^{20}	Gamma rays	Strongly ionizing

* Division of the EM spectrum into frequency bands is based on conventional but arbitrary usage in various disciplines.

vices). The term *electropollution* refers to artificial EM fields that may be associated with health risks.

In radiation biophysics, an EM field is classified as *ionizing* if its energy is high enough to dislodge electrons from an atom or molecule. High-energy, high-frequency forms of EM radiation, such as gamma rays and x rays, are *strongly* ionizing in biological matter. For this reason, prolonged exposure to such rays is harmful. Radiation in the middle portion of the frequency and energy spectrum—such as visible, especially ultraviolet, light—is *weakly* ionizing (i.e., it can be ionizing or not, depending on the target molecules).

Although it has long been known that exposure to strongly ionizing EM radiation can cause extreme damage in biological tissues, only recently have epidemiological studies and other evidence implicated long-term exposure to nonionizing, exogenous EM fields, such as those emitted by power lines, in increased health hazards. These hazards may include an increased risk in children of developing leukemia (Bierbaum and Peters, 1991; Nair et al., 1989; Wilson et al., 1990a).

However, it also has been discovered that oscillating nonionizing EM fields in the ELF range can have vigorous biological effects that may be beneficial and thus nonharmful (Becker and Marino, 1982; Brighton and Pollack, 1991). This discovery is a cornerstone in the foundation of BEM research and application.

Specific changes in the field configuration and exposure pattern of low-level EM fields can produce highly specific biological responses. More intriguing, some specific frequencies have highly specific effects on tissues in the body, just as drugs have their specific effects on target tissues. The actual mechanism by which EM fields produce biological effects is under intense study. Evidence suggests that the cell membrane may be one of the primary locations where applied EM fields act on the cell. EM forces at the membrane's outer surface could modify ligand-receptor interactions (e.g., the binding of messenger chemicals such as hormones and growth factors to specialized cell membrane molecules called receptors), which in turn would alter the state of large membrane molecules that play a role in controlling the cell's internal processes (Tenforde and Kaune, 1987). Experiments to establish the full details of a mechanistic chain of events such as this, however, are just beginning.

Another line of study focuses on the endogenous EM fields. At the level of body tissues and organs, electrical activity is known to exhibit macroscopic patterns that contain medically useful information. For example, the diagnostic procedures of electroencephalography (EEG) and electrocardiography are based on detection of endogenous EM fields produced in the central nervous system and heart muscle, respectively. Taking the observations in these two systems a step further, current BEM research is exploring the possibility that weak EM fields associated with nerve activity in other tissues and organs might also carry information of diagnostic value. New technologies for constructing extremely sensitive EM transducers (e.g., magnetometers and electrometers) and for signal processing recently have made this line of research feasible.

Recent BEM research has uncovered a form of endogenous EM radiation in the visible region of the spectrum that is emitted by most living organisms, ranging from plant seeds to humans (Chwirot et al., 1987, Mathew and Rumar, in press, Popp et al., 1984, 1988, 1992). Some evidence indicates that this extremely low-level light, known as biophoton emission, may be important in bioregulation, membrane transport, and gene expression. It is possible that the effects (both beneficial and harmful) of exogenous fields may be mediated by alterations in endogenous fields. Thus, externally applied EM fields from medical devices may act to correct abnormalities in endogenous EM fields characteristic of disease states. Furthermore, the energy of the biophotons and processes involving their emission as well as other endogenous fields of the body may prove to be involved in energetic therapies, such as healer interactions.

At the cutting edge of BEM research lies the question of how endogenous body EM fields may change as a result of changes in consciousness. The recent formation and rapid growth of a new society, the International Society for the Study of Subtle Energies and Energy Medicine, is indicative of the growing interest in this field.[1]

Figure 3 illustrates several types of EM fields of interest in BEM research.

Medical Applications of Bioelectromagnetics

Medical research applications of BEM began almost simultaneously with Michael Faraday's discovery of electromagnetic induction in the late 1700s. Immediately thereafter came the famous experiments of the 18th-century physician and physicist Luigi Galvani, who showed with frog legs that there was a connection between electricity and muscle contraction. This was followed by the work of Alessandro Volta, the Italian physicist whose investigation into electricity led him to correctly interpret Galvani's experiments with muscle, showing that the metal electrodes and not the tissue generated the current. From this early work came a plethora of devices for the diagnosis and treatment of disease, using first static electricity, then electrical currents, and, later, frequencies from different regions of the EM spectrum. Like other treatment methods, certain devices were seen as unconventional at first, only to become widely accepted later. For example, many of the medical devices that make up the core of modern, scientifically based medicine, such as x-ray devices, at one time were considered highly experimental.

Most of today's medical EM devices use relatively large levels of electrical, magnetic, or EM energy. The main topic of this chapter, however, is the use of the nonionizing portion of the EM spectrum, particularly at low levels, which is the focus of BEM research.

Nonionizing BEM medical applications may be classified according to whether they are *thermal* (heat producing in biologic tissue) or *nonthermal*. Thermal applications of nonionizing radiation (i.e., application of heat) include RF hyperthermia, laser and RF surgery, and RF diathermy.

The most important BEM modalities in alternative medicine are the nonthermal applications of nonionizing radiation. The term *nonthermal* is used with two different meanings in the medical and scientific literature. *Biologically* (or medically) nonthermal means that it "causes no significant gross tissue heating"; this is the most common usage. *Physically* (or scientifically) nonthermal means "below the thermal noise limit at physiological temperatures." The energy level of thermal noise is much lower than that

[1]*A more detailed introduction to the field of BEM and an overview of research progress is available in the following monographs and conference proceedings: Adey, 1992; Adey and Lawrence, 1984; Becker and Marino, 1982; Blank, 1993; Blank and Findl, 1987; Brighton and Pollack, 1991; Brighton et al., 1979; Liboff and Rinaldi, 1974; Marino, 1988; O'Connor et al., 1990; O'Connor and Lovely, 1988; Popp et al., 1992; and Ramel and Norden, 1991.*

Figure 3. Examples of natural and created EM fields, exogenous and endogenous.

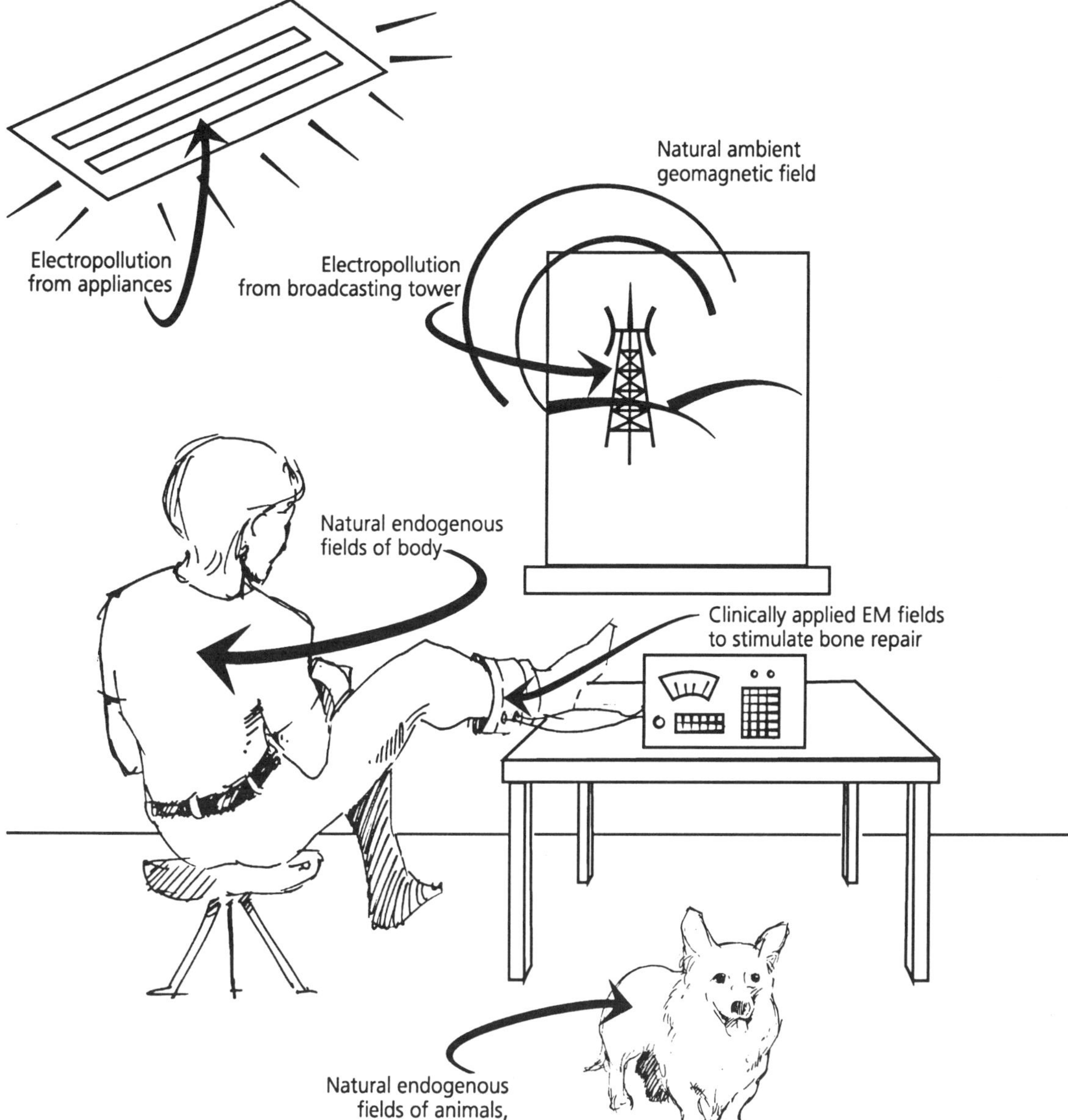

required to cause heating of tissue; thus, any physically nonthermal application is automatically biologically nonthermal.

All of the nonthermal applications of nonionizing radiation are nonthermal in the biological sense. That is, they cause no significant heating of tissue. Some of the newer, unconventional BEM applications are also physically nonthermal. A variety of alternative medical practices developed outside the United States employ nonionizing EM fields at nonthermal intensities. For instance, microwave resonance therapy, which is used primarily in Russia, employs low-intensity (either continuous or pulse-modulated), sinusoidal microwave radiation to treat a variety of conditions, including arthritis, ulcers, esophagitis, hypertension, chronic pain, cerebral palsy, neurological disorders, and side effects of cancer chemotherapy (Devyatkov et al., 1991). Thousands of people in Russia also have been treated by specific frequencies of extremely low-level microwaves applied at certain acupuncture points.

The mechanism of action of microwave resonance therapy is thought to involve modifications in cell membrane transport or production of chemical mediators or both. Although a sizable body of Russian-language literature on this technique already exists, no independent validation studies have been conducted in the West. However, if such treatments prove to be effective, current views on the role of information and thermal noise (i.e., order and disorder) in living systems, which hold that biological information is stored in molecular structures, may need revision. It may be that such information is stored at the level of the whole organism in the endogenous EM field, which may be used informationally in biological regulation and cellular communication (i.e., not due to energy content or power intensity). If exogenous, extremely low-level nonionizing fields with energy contents well below the thermal noise limit produce biological effects, they may be acting on the body in such a way that they alter the body's own field. That is to say, biological information would be altered by the exogenous EM fields.

The eight major new (or "unconventional") applications of nonthermal, nonionizing EM fields are as follows:

1. Bone repair.
2. Nerve stimulation.
3. Wound healing.
4. Treatment of osteoarthritis.
5. Electroacupuncture.
6. Tissue regeneration.
7. Immune system stimulation.
8. Neuroendocrine modulations.

These applications of BEM and the evidence for their efficacy are discussed in the following section.

Research Base

Applications 1 through 5 above have been clinically tested and are in limited clinical use. On the basis of existing animal and cellular studies, applications 6 through 8 offer the potential for developing new clinical treatments, but clinical trials have not yet been conducted.

Bone Repair

Three types of applied EM fields are known to promote healing of nonunion bone fractures (i.e., those that fail to heal spontaneously):

- Pulsed EM fields (PEMFs) and sinusoidal EM fields (AC fields).
- DC fields.
- Combined AC–DC magnetic fields tuned to ion-resonant frequencies (these are extremely low-intensity, physically nonthermal fields) (Weinstein et al., 1990).

Approval of the U.S. Food and Drug Administration (FDA) has been obtained on PEMF and DC applications and is pending for the AC–DC application. In PEMF and AC applications, the repetition frequencies used are in the ELF range (Bassett, 1989). In DC applications, magnetic field intensities range from 100 microgauss to 100 gauss (G), and electric currents range from less than 0.1 microampere to milliamperes (Baranowski and Black, 1987).[2] FDA approval of these therapies covers only their use to promote healing of nonunion bone fractures, not to accelerate routine healing of uncomplicated fractures.

Efficacy of EM bone repair treatment has been confirmed in double-blind clinical trials (Barker et al., 1984; Sharrard, 1990). A conservative estimate is that as of 1985 more than 100,000 people had been treated with such devices (Bassett et al., 1974, 1982; Brighton et al., 1979, 1981; Goldenberg and Hansen, 1972; Hinsenkamp et al., 1985).

Stimulation and Measurement of Nerve Activity

These applications fall into the following seven categories:

---

[2]*Gauss is a unit of magnetic flux density. For comparison, a typical magnet used to hold papers vertically on a refrigerator is 200 G.*

1. *Transcutaneous electrical nerve stimulation (TENS).* In this medical application, two electrodes are applied to the skin via wires attached to a portable electrical generating device, which may be clipped to the patient's belt (Hagfors and Hyme, 1975). Perhaps more than 100 types of FDA-approved devices in this category are currently available and used in physical therapy for pain relief. All of them operate on the same basis.
2. *Transcranial electrostimulation (TCES).* These devices are similar to the TENS units. They apply extremely low currents (below the nerve excitation threshold) to the brain via two electrodes applied to the head and are used for behavioral/psychological modification (e.g., to reduce symptoms of depression, anxiety, and insomnia) (Shealy et al., 1992). A recent meta-analysis covering at least 12 clinical trials selected from more than 100 published reports found that TCES can alleviate anxiety disorders (Klawansky et al., 1992). With support from the National Institutes of Health (NIH), TCES is under evaluation for alleviation of drug dependence.
3. *Neuromagnetic stimulation.* In this application, which has both diagnostic and therapeutic uses, a magnetic pulse is applied noninvasively to a part of the patient's body to stimulate nerve activity. In diagnostic use, a pulse is applied to the cerebral cortex, and the patient's physiological responses are monitored to obtain a dynamic picture of the brain-body interface (Hallett and Cohen, 1989). As a treatment modality, it is being used in lieu of electroshock therapy to treat certain types of affective disorder (e.g., major depression) and seizures (Anninos and Tsagas, 1991). Neuromagnetic stimulation also is used in nerve conduction studies for conditions such as carpal tunnel syndrome.
4. *Electromyography.* This diagnostic application detects electrical potentials associated with muscle contraction. Specific electrical patterns have been associated with certain abnormal states (e.g., denervated muscle). This method, along with electromyographic biofeedback, is being used to treat carpal tunnel syndrome and other movement disorders.
5. *Electroencephalography.* This neurodiagnostic application detects brainwaves. Coupled with EEG biofeedback it is used to treat a variety of conditions, such as learning disabilities, attention deficit and hyperactivity disorders, chronic alcoholism, and stroke.
6. *Electroretinography.* This diagnostic application monitors electrical potentials across the retina to assess eye movements. This is one of the few methods available for noninvasive monitoring of rapid eye movement sleep.
7. *Low-energy emission therapy.* This application uses an antenna positioned in the patient's mouth to administer amplitude-modulated EM fields. It has been shown to affect the central nervous system, and pilot clinical studies show efficacy in treating insomnia (Hajdukovic et al., 1992) and hypertension (Pasche et al., 1989).

Soft-tissue Wound Healing

The following studies have demonstrated accelerated healing of soft-tissue wounds using DC, PEMF, and electrochemical modalities:

- When wound healing is abnormal (retarded or arrested), electric or magnetic field applications may trigger healing to occur. A review of several reports indicates that fields may be useful in this regard (Lee et al., 1993; Vodovnik and Karba, 1992).
- PEMFs have been used clinically to treat venous skin ulcers. Results of several double-blind studies showed that PEMF stimulation promotes cell activation and cell proliferation through an effect on the cell membrane, particularly on endothelial cells (Ieran et al., 1990; Stiller et al., 1992).
- ELF and RF fields are applied to accelerate wound healing. Since skin wounds have unique electrical potentials and currents, stimulation of these electrical factors by a variety of exogenous EM fields can aid in the healing process by causing dedifferentiation (i.e., conversion to a more primitive form) of the nearby cells followed by accelerated cell proliferation (O'Connor et al., 1990).
- An electrochemical treatment that provides scarless regenerative wound healing uses electricity solely to introduce active metallic ions, such as silver, into the tissue. The electric field plays no role itself (Becker, 1987, 1990, 1992).
- PEMF increases the rate of formation of epithelial (skin) cells in partially healed wounds (Mertz et al., 1988).

- AC EM fields promote the repair of injured vascular networks (Herbst et al., 1988).
- EM devices have been patented for treating atherosclerotic lesions (i.e., small blood clots that build up on the walls of arteries and cause cardiovascular disease) and to control tissue growth (Gordon, 1986; Liboff et al., 1992b).

Osteoarthritis

In a recent clinical trial using a double-blind, randomized protocol with placebo control, osteoarthritis (primarily of the knee) treated noninvasively by pulsed 30-Hz, 60-G PEMFs showed the treatment group improved substantially more than the placebo group (Trock et al., 1993). It is believed that applied magnetic fields act to suppress inflammatory responses at the cell membrane level (O'Connor et al., 1990).

Electroacupuncture

Electrical stimulation via acupuncture needles is often used as an enhancement or replacement for manual needling. Clinical benefits have been demonstrated for the use of electrical stimulation (electrostimulation) in combination with acupuncture as well as for electrostimulation applied directly to acupuncture points.

As an enhancement of acupuncture, a small-scale study showed electrostimulation with acupuncture to be beneficial in the treatment of post-operative pain (Christensen and Noreng, 1989). Other controlled studies have shown good success in using electrostimulation with acupuncture in the treatment of chemotherapy-induced sickness in cancer patients (Dundee and Ghaly, 1989). In addition, electrical stimulation with acupuncture was recently shown to be beneficial in the treatment of renal colic (Lee et al., 1992).

As a replacement for acupuncture, electrostimulation applied in a controlled study to acupuncture points by a TENS unit was effective in inducing uterine contractions in post-term pregnant women (Dunn and Rogers, 1989). Further, research with rats has shown that electrostimulation at such points can enhance peripheral motor nerve regeneration (McDevitt et al., 1987) and sensory nerve sprouting (Pomeranz et al., 1984).

Regeneration

Animal research in this area indicates that the body's endogenous EM fields are involved in growth processes and that modifications of these fields can lead to modest regeneration of severed limbs (Becker, 1987; Becker and Spadero, 1972; Smith, 1967). Russian research and clinical applications, along with studies now under way in the United States, indicate that low-intensity microwaves apparently stimulate bone marrow stem cell division and may be useful in enhancing the effects of chemotherapy by maintaining the formation and development, or hematopoiesis, of various types of blood cells (Devyatkov et al., 1991).

The following studies are also relevant to the use of BEM for regeneration:

- PEMF applications to promote peripheral nerve regeneration (Orgel et al., 1992; Sisken, 1992).
- The "diapulse" method of using pulsed, high-frequency EM fields for human wrist nerve regeneration (Wilson et al., 1974).
- DC applications to promote rat spinal cord regeneration (Fehlings et al., 1992; Hurlbert and Tator, 1992).
- Swedish work showing that BEM promotes rat sciatic nerve regeneration (Kanje and Rusovan, 1992; Rusovan and Kanje, 1991, 1992; Rusovan et al., 1992).

Immune System

During the past two decades, the effects of EM exposure on the immune system and its components have been extensively studied. While early studies indicated that long-term exposure to EM fields might negatively affect the immune system, there is promising new research showing that applied EM fields may be able to beneficially modulate immune responses. For example, studies with human lymphocytes show that exogenous EM or magnetic fields can produce changes in calcium transport (Walleczek, 1992) and cause mediation of the mitogenic response (i.e., the stimulation of the division of cellular nuclei; certain types of immune cells begin to divide and reproduce rapidly in response to certain stimuli, or mitogens). This finding has led to research investigating the possible augmentation by applied EM fields of a type of immune cell population called natural killer cells, which are important in helping the body fight against cancer and viruses (Cadossi et al., 1988a, 1988b; Cossarizza et al., 1989a, 1989b, 1989c).

Potential Neuroendocrine Modulations

Low-level PEMFs have typically been shown to suppress levels of melatonin, which is secreted by the pineal gland and is believed to regulate the body's inner clock (Lerchl et al., 1990; Wilson et al., 1990b). Melatonin, as a hormone, is oncostatic (i.e., it stops cancer growth). Thus, if melatonin can be suppressed by certain magnetic fields, it also may be possible to employ magnetic fields with different characteristics to stimulate melatonin secretion for the treatment of cancer. Other applications may include use of EM fields to affect melatonin secretion to normalize circadian rhythms in people with jet lag and sleep cycle disturbances.

Table 2 provides an overview of selected citations to the refereed literature for these applications.

Future Research Opportunities

Although to date there is an extensive base of literature on the use of BEM for medical applications, the overall research strategy into this phenomenon has been quite fragmented. Because of BEM's potential for the treatment of a wide range of conditions, an integrated research program is needed that includes both basic and clinical research in BEM. These two approaches should be pursued vigorously and simultaneously along parallel tracks.

Basic research is needed to refine or develop new BEM technologies with the aim of establishing the fundamental knowledge about the body's endogenous EM fields and how they interact with clinically applied EM fields. A basic understanding of the BEM of the human body might provide insight into the scientific bioenergetic or bioinformational principles by which other areas of alternative medicine, such as homeopathy, acupuncture, and energetic therapies, may function. Furthermore, fundamental knowledge of BEM principles in the human body, in conjunction with psychophysiological states, might help facilitate understanding of mind-body regulation.

Clinical research, including preclinical assessments, is also essential, with the aim of bringing the most promising BEM treatments and diagnostics from limited use into widespread use as quickly as possible. Although a number of BEM devices show promise as new diagnostics or therapeutics, they must be tested on humans to show exactly when they are effective and when they are not. Moreover, measures of clinical effectiveness and safety are required for FDA approval of BEM medical devices. Ultimately, knowledge about the safety of new BEM medical devices can be ascertained only from the appropriate clinical trials.

Basic

The current status of basic research in BEM may be summarized as follows:

- Nonionizing, nonthermal exogenous EM fields exert measurable bioeffects in living organisms. In general, the organism's response to applied EM fields is highly frequency specific and the dose-response curve is nonlinear (i.e., application of an additional amount of the EM field does not elicit a response of equal magnitude; the response eventually diminishes no matter how additional EM stimuli are applied). Extremely weak EM fields may, at the proper frequency and site of application, produce large effects that are either clinically beneficial or harmful.
- The cell membrane has been proposed as the primary site of transduction of EM field bioeffects. Relevant mechanisms may include changes in cell-membrane binding and transport processes, displacement or deformation of polarized molecules, modifications in the conformation of biological water (i.e., water that comprises organisms), and others.
- The physical mechanisms by which EM fields may act on biomolecules are far too complex to discuss here. However, the following references propose such physical mechanisms: Grundler et al., in press; Liboff, 1985, 1991; and Liboff et al., 1991.
- Endogenous nonthermal EM fields ranging from DC to the visible spectral region may be intimately involved in regulating physiological and biochemical processes.

Consequently, the following pressing needs should be addressed in developing a basic BEM research program:

Table 2. Selected Literature Citations on Biomedical Effects of Nonthermal EM Fields

	Frequency range of EM fields				
Location or type of bioeffect	**DC**	**ELF, including sinusoidal, pulsed, and mixed**	**RF and microwave**	**IR, visible, and UV light**	**Review articles and monographs**
Bone and cartilage, including treatments for bone repair and osteoporosis	Brighton et al., 1981; Baranowsi & Black, 1987; Papatheofanis, 1989	Bassett et al., 1982; Barker et al., 1984; Brighton et al., 1985; Hinsenkamp et al., 1985; Huraki et al., 1987; Bassett, 1989; Madroñero, 1990; Sharrard, 1990; Grande et al., 1991; Magee et al., 1991; Pollack et al., 1991; Skerry et al., 1991; Ryaby et al., 1992			Brighton et al., 1979
Soft tissue, including wound healing, regeneratrion, and vascular-tissue effects	Becker, 1987; Becker, 1990; Becker, 1992; Vodovnik & Karba, 1992	Gordon, 1986; Herbst et al., 1988; Mertz et al., 1988; Yen-Patton et al., 1988; Albertini et al., 1990; Ieran et al., 1990; Im & Hoopes, 1991; Kraus, 1992; Liboff et al., 1992b; Stiller et al., 1992; Vodovnik & Karba, 1992	Devyatkov et al., 1991		Vodovnik & Karba, 1992
Neural tissue, including nerve growth and regeneration		Wilson et al., 1974; Rusovan & Kanje, 1991; Subramanian et al., 1991; Horton et al., 1992; Rusovan & Kanje, 1992; Rusovan et al., 1992			

Table 2. Selected Literature Citations on Biomedical Effects of Nonthermal EM Fields (cont.)

Location or type of bioeffect	Frequency range of EM fields				
	DC	ELF, including sinusoidal, pulsed, and mixed	RF and microwave	IR, visible, and UV light	Review articles and monographs
Neural stimulation effects, including TENS and TCES		Hagfors & Hyme, 1975; Hallett & Cohen, 1989; Anninos & Tsagas, 1991; Klawansky et al., 1992			
Psychophysiological and behavioral effects			Pasche et al., 1989; Devyatkov et al., 1991; Hajdukovic et al., 1992	Thomas et al., 1986	O'Connor & Lovely, 1988
Electroacupuncture	McDevitt et al., 1987	Pomeranz et al., 1984; Christensen & Noreng, 1989; Dundee & Ghaly, 1989; Lee et al., 1992			
Neuroendocrine effects, including melatonin modifications	Feinendegen & Muhlensiepen, 1987	Lerchl et al., 1990; Wilson et al., 1990a, 1990b			O'Connor & Lovely, 1988
Immune system effects		Cadossi et al., 1988a; Cadossi et al., 1988b; Cossarizza et al., 1989a; Cossarizza et al., 1989b; Rosenthal & Obe, 1989; Phillips & McChesney, 1991; Walleczek, 1992			
Arthritis treatments		Grande et al., 1991; Trock et al., 1993	Devyatkov et al., 1991		

Table 2. Selected Literature Citations on Biomedical Effects of Nonthermal EM Fields (cont.)

Location or type of bioeffect	Frequency range of EM fields: DC	ELF, including sinusoidal, pulsed, and mixed	RF and microwave	IR, visible, and UV light	Review articles and monographs
Cellular and subcellular effects, including effects on cell membrane, genetic system, and tumors	Easterly, 1982; Liburdy & Tenforde, 1986; Foxall et al., 1991; Miklavčič et al., 1991; Short et al., 1992	Cohen et al., 1986; Takahashi et al., 1987; Adey, 1992; Marron et al., 1988; Onuma & Hui, 1988; Brayman & Miller, 1989; Cossarizza et al., 1989a, 1989b; De Loecker et al., 1989; Goodman et al., 1989; Rodemann et al., 1989; Brayman & Miller, 1990; Lerchl et al., 1990; Omote et al., 1990; Greene et al., 1991; Liboff et al., 1991	Guy, 1987; Chen & Ghandi, 1989; Brown & Chattpadhyay, 1991; Devyatkov et al., 1991		Adey & Lawrence, 1984; Marino, 1988; Blank & Findl, 1987; Ramel & Norden, 1991; Grundler et al., in press
Endogenous EM fields, including biophotons		Mathew & Rumar, in press	Mathew & Rumar, in press	Popp et al., 1984; Chwirot et al., 1987; Chwirot, 1988; Popp et al., 1988	Wijk & Schamhart, 1988; Popp et al., 1992

Note: Reports listed in table 2 are selected from refereed medical and scientific journals, multiauthor monographs, conference proceedings, and patents. See References for identification of sources. This is a representative selection from a large body of relevant sources and is not meant to be exhaustive or definitive.

- Standardized protocols for measuring dosages for therapeutically applied EM fields should be established and followed uniformly in BEM research. Protocols are needed for characterizing (i.e., defining and measuring) EM field sources (both exogenous and endogenous) and EM parameters of biological subjects. Such variables must be characterized in greater detail than is commonly practiced in clinical research. Artifacts caused by ambient EM fields in the laboratory environment (e.g., from power lines and laboratory equipment) must be avoided.

- In general, a balanced, strategic approach to basic research—including studies in humans, animals, and cells along with theoretical modeling and close collaboration with other investigators in alternative medicine—will produce the most valuable results in the long run.

- Many independent parameters characterize nonthermal nonionizing EM fields, including pulsed vs. nonpulsed and sinusoidal vs. other waveforms; frequency; phase; intensity (as a function of spatial position); voltage; and current. If multiple fields are combined, these parameters must be specified for each component. Additional parameters necessary for characterizing the medical application of EM fields include the site of application and the time course of exposure. All of these can be experimentally varied, producing an enormous range of possibilities. To date, there has been little systematic research to explore the potential biological effects of this vast array of applied field parameter characteristics.

Clinical

Clinical trials of BEM-based treatments for the following conditions may yield useful results relatively soon: arthritis, psychophysiological states (including drug dependence and epilepsy), wound healing and regeneration, intractable pain, Parkinson's disease, spinal cord injury, closed head injury, cerebral palsy (spasticity reduction), learning disabilities, headache, degenerative conditions associated with aging, cancer, and acquired immunodeficiency syndrome (AIDS).

EM fields may be applied clinically as the primary therapy or as adjuvant therapy along with other treatments in the conditions listed above. Effectiveness can be measured via the following clinical markers:

- In arthritis, the usual clinical criteria, including decrease of pain, less swelling, and thus a greater potential for mobility.

- In psychophysiological problems, relief from symptoms of drug withdrawal and alleviation of depressive anxiety and its symptoms.

- In epilepsy, return to greater normality in EEG, more normal sleep patterns, and reduction in required drug dosages.

- In wound healing and regeneration, repair of soft tissue and reduction of collagenous tissue in scar formation; regrowth via blastemal (primitive cell) formation and increase in tensile strength of surgical wounds; alleviation of decubitus chronic ulcers (bedsores); increased angiogenesis (regrowth of vascular tissue such as blood vessels); and healing of recalcitrant (i.e., unresponsive to treatment) chronic venous ulcers.

For instance, a short-term, double-blind clinical trial of magnetic field therapy could be based on the protocol of Trock et al. (1993) for osteoarthritis of the knee or elbow. This protocol is as follows:

- A suitable patient population is divided into treatment and control groups. Individual assignments are coded and remain unknown to patients, clinicians, and operators until treatment and assessment are complete.

- Pretreatment clinical markers are assessed by clinicians or by patients themselves or both.

- Treatments consist of 3 to 5 half-hour sessions each week for a total of 18 treatments over 5–6 weeks.

- During treatment, each patient inserts the affected limb into the opening of a Helmholtz coil (a solenoid about 12 inches in diameter and 6 inches long) and rests while appropriate currents are applied to the coil via a preset program.

- The treatment is noninvasive and painless; the patient feels nothing; there is no measurable transfer of heat to the patient.

- The control group follows the same procedure except that, unknown to operator and patient, a "dummy" apparatus (altered internally so that no current flows in the coil) is used.

- Patients' posttreatment clinical markers are assessed.
- Appropriate data reduction (scoring of assessments, decoding of the treatment and control groups, and statistical analysis) is performed.

Clinical trials of BEM-based treatments for a variety of other conditions could follow a similar general outline.

Key Issues

Certain key issues or controversies surrounding BEM have inhibited progress in this field. These issues fall into several distinct areas: medical controversy, scientific controversy, barriers, and other issues.

Medical Controversy

A number of uncharacterized "black box" medical treatment and diagnostic devices—some legal and some illegal—have been associated with EM medical treatment. Whether they operate on the basis of BEM principles is unknown. Among these devices are the following: radionics devices, Lakhovsky multiple-wave oscillator, Priore's machine, Rife's inert gas discharge tubes, violet ray tubes, Reich's orgone energy devices, EAV machines, and biocircuit devices. There are at least six alternative explanations for how these and other such devices operate: (1) They are ineffectual and are based on erroneous application of physical principles. (2) They may be operating on BEM principles, but they are uncharacterized. (3) They may operate on acoustic principles (sound or ultrasound waves) rather than BEM. (4) In the case of diagnostic devices, they may work by focusing the intuitive capacity of the practitioner. (5) In the case of long-distance applications, they may operate by means of nonlocal properties of consciousness of patient and practitioner. (6) They may be operating on the energy of some domain that is uncharacterized at present.

A recent survey (Eisenberg et al., 1993) showed that about 1 percent of the U.S. population used energy healing techniques that included a variety of EM devices. Indeed, more of the respondents in this 1990 survey used energy healing techniques than used homeopathy and acupuncture in the treatment of either serious or chronic disease. In addition to the use of devices by practitioners, a plethora of consumer medical products that use magnetic energy are purported to promote relaxation or to treat a variety of illnesses. For example, for the bed there are mattress pads impregnated with magnets; there are magnets to attach to the site of an athletic injury; and there are small pelletlike magnets to place over specific points on the body. Most of these so-called therapeutic magnets, also called biomagnets, come from Japan. However, no known published journal articles demonstrating effectiveness via clinical trials exist.

Some of the medical modalities discussed in this report, although presently accepted medically or legally in the United States, have not necessarily passed the most recent requirements of safety or effectiveness. FDA approval of a significant number of BEM-based devices, primarily those used in bone repair and neurostimulation, was "grandfathered." That is, medical devices sold in the United States prior to the Medical Device Law of the late 1970s automatically received FDA approval for use in the same manner and for the same medical conditions for which they were used prior to the law's enactment. Grandfathering by the FDA applies not only to BEM devices but to all devices covered by the Medical Device Law. However, neither the safety nor the effectiveness of grandfathered devices is established (i.e., they are approved on the basis of a "presumption" by the FDA, but they usually remain incompletely studied). Reexamination of devices in use, whether grandfathered or not, may be warranted.

There are three possible ways of resolving controversies associated with BEM and its application: (1) elucidating the fundamental principles underlying the device, or at least the historical basis for the development of the device; (2) conducting properly designed case control studies and clinical trials to validate effects that have been reported or claimed for BEM-based treatments; and (3) increasing the medical community's awareness of well-documented, controlled clinical trials that indicate the effectiveness of specific BEM applications (see table 2).

Scientific Controversy

Some physicists claim that low-intensity, nonionizing EM fields have no bioeffects other than resistive (joule) heating of tissue. One such argument is based on a physical model in which the only EM field parameter considered relevant to biological systems is power density (Adair, 1991). The argument asserts that measurable nonthermal bioeffects of EM fields are "impossible" because they contradict known physical laws or would require a "new physics" to explain them.

However, numerous independent experiments reported in the refereed-journal research literature conclusively establish that nonthermal bioeffects of low-intensity EM fields do indeed exist. Moreover, the experimental results lend support to certain new approaches in theoretical modeling of the interactions between EM fields and biological matter. Most researchers now feel that BEM bioeffects will become comprehensible not by forsaking physics but rather by developing more sophisticated, detailed models based on known physical laws, in which additional parameters (e.g., frequency, intensity, waveform, and field directionality) are taken into account.

Barriers

The following barriers to BEM research exist:

- Members of NIH review panels in medical applications might not be adequately knowledgeable about alternative medical practices or BEM. This is the most serious barrier.
- Funding in BEM research is weighted heavily toward the study of hazards of EM fields; there is little funding for potential beneficial medical applications or the study of basic mechanisms of EM interactions with life processes. Also, the bulk of EM field research is administered by the Department of Defense and the Department of Energy, agencies with missions unrelated to medical research. The small amount of BEM work funded by NIH thus far has addressed mostly the hazards of EM fields. In late 1993 the National Institute of Environmental Health Sciences issued requests for grant application in the areas of (1) cellular effects of low-frequency EM fields and (2) effects of 60-Hz EM fields in vivo. The latter project is concerned solely with safety in power line and appliance exposures. However, the former apparently does not rule out the investigation of possible beneficial effects from low-frequency fields, although the focus is clearly on assessing previously reported effects of 60-Hz EM fields on cellular processes.
- Regulatory barriers to making new BEM devices available to practitioners are formidable. The approval process is slow and exorbitantly expensive even for conventional medical devices.
- Barriers in education include the following: (1) basic education in biological science is weak in physics, (2) undergraduate- and graduate-level programs in BEM are virtually nonexistent, and (3) multidisciplinary training is lacking in medicine and biology.
- The mainstream scientific and medical communities are basically conservative and respond to emerging disciplines, such as BEM, with reactions ranging from ignorance and apathy to open hostility. Consequently, accomplished senior researchers may not be aware of the opportunities for fruitful work in (or in collaboration with others in) BEM, while junior researchers may be reluctant to enter a field perceived by some as detrimental to career advancement.

Other Issues

Other key issues that need to be considered in developing a comprehensive research and development agenda for BEM include the following:

- Separate studies prepared for the Office of Technology Assessment, the National Institute of Occupational Safety and Health, and the Environmental Protection Agency have recommended independently that research on fundamental mechanisms of EM field interactions in humans receive high priority (Bierbaum and Peters, 1991; Nair et al., 1989; U.S. EPA, 1991). Moreover, a 1985 report prepared by scientists at the Centers for Devices and Radiological Health recommended that future research on EM field interactions with living systems "be directed at exploring beneficial medical applications of EMR (electromagnetic radiation) modulation of immune responses" (Budd and Czerski, 1985).
- Elucidation of the physical mechanisms of BEM medical modalities is the single most powerful key to developing efficient and optimal clinical intervention. Even a relatively small advance beyond present knowledge of fundamental mechanisms would be of considerable practical value. In addition, progress in the development of a mechanistic explanation of the effects of alternative medicine could

increase its acceptability in the eyes of mainstream medicine and science.

- BEM potentially offers a powerful new approach to understanding the neuroendocrine and immunological bases of certain major medical problems (e.g., wound healing, cancer, and AIDS). However, substantial funding and time are required to perform the basic research needed in developing this approach.

- BEM may provide a comprehensive biophysical framework grounded in fundamental science, through which many alternative medical practices can be studied. BEM offers a promising starting point for scientifically exploring various traditional alternative medical systems (Becker and Marino, 1982).

Basic Research Priorities

The most fruitful topics for future basic research investigations of BEM may include the following:

- Developing assay methods based on EM field interactions in cells (e.g., for potassium transport, calcium transport, and cytotoxicity). These assays could then be applied to existing studies of such phenomena in cellular systems.

- Developing BEM-based treatments for osteoporosis, on basis of the large body of existing work on EM bone repair and other research (e.g., Brighton et al., 1985; Cruess and Bassett, 1983; Liboff et al., 1992a; Madroñero, 1990; Magee et al., 1991; Skerry et al., 1991). NASA researchers have already expressed interest in collaborative work to develop BEM treatments for weightlessness-induced osteoporosis.

- Measuring neurobiochemical changes in the blood in response to microcurrent skin stimulation in animals or humans with different frequencies, waveforms, and carrier waves. Such measurements should be made for preclinical evaluation of neurostimulation devices.

- Furthering studies of mechanisms of EM field interactions in cells and tissues with emphasis on coherent or cooperative states and resonant phenomena in biomolecules; and on coherent brainwave states and other long-range interactions in biological systems.

- Studying the role of water as a mediator in biological interactions with emphasis on the quantum EM aspects of its conformation (i.e., "structure," as implied in some forms of homeopathy). The response of biologic water to EM fields should be studied experimentally. A novel informational capacity of water in relation to EM bioeffects may provide insights into homeopathy and healer interactions (i.e., "laying on of hands").

- Studying in detail the role of the body's internally generated (endogenous) EM fields and the body's other natural electromagnetic parameters (see the "Manual Healing Methods" chapter). Knowledge of such processes should be applied to develop novel diagnostic methods and to understand alternative medical treatments such as acupuncture, electroacupuncture, and biofield therapies. Furthermore, exploratory research on the role of the body's energy fields in relation to the role of states of consciousness in health and healing should be launched.

- Establishing a knowledge base (an intelligent database) to provide convenient access to all significant BEM work in both basic and clinical research.

- Performing systematic reviews as well as meta-analytic reviews of existing BEM studies to identify the frequency and quality of research concerning BEM as well as most promising clinical end points for BEM treatments in humans.

Summary

Just as exposure to high-energy radiation has unquestioned hazards, radiation has long been a key weapon in the fight against many types of cancers. Likewise, although there are indications that some EM fields may be hazardous, there is now increasing evidence that there are beneficial bioeffects of certain low-intensity nonthermal EM fields.

In clinical practice, BEM applications offer the possibility of more economical and more effective diagnostics and new noninvasive therapies for medical problems, including those considered intractable or recalcitrant to conventional treatments. The sizable body of recent work cited in this chapter has established the feasibility of treatments based on BEM, although the mainstream medical community is largely unaware of this work.

In biomedical research, BEM can provide a better understanding of fundamental mechanisms of communication and regulation at levels ranging from intracellular to organismic. Improved knowledge of fundamental mechanisms of EM field interactions could lead directly to major advances in diagnostic and treatment methods.

In the study of other alternative medical modalities, BEM offers a unified conceptual framework that may help explain how certain diagnostic and therapeutic techniques (e.g., acupuncture, homeopathy, certain types of ethnomedicine, and healer effects) may produce results that are difficult to understand from a more conventional viewpoint. These areas of alternative medicine are currently based entirely on empirical (i.e., experimentation and observation rather than theory) and phenomenological (i.e., the classification and description of any fact, circumstance, or experience without any attempt at explanation) approaches. Thus, their future development could be accelerated as a scientific understanding if their mechanisms of action are ascertained.

References

Adair, R.K. 1991. Constraints on biological effects of weak extremely low-frequency electromagnetic fields. Physical Review 43:1039–1048.

Adey, W.R. 1992. Collective properties of cell membranes. In B. Norden and C. Ramel, eds. Interaction Mechanisms of Low-level Electromagnetic Fields in Living Systems. Symposium, Royal Swedish Academy of Sciences, Stockholm (pp. 47–77). Oxford University Press, New York.

Adey, W.R., and A.F. Lawrence, eds. 1984. Nonlinear Electrodynamics in Biological Systems (conference proceedings). Plenum Press, New York.

Albertini, A., P. Zucchini, G. Nocra, R. Carossi, and A. Pierangeli. 1990. Effect of PEMF on irreversible ischemic injury following coronary artery occlusion in rats. Transactions of Bioelectrical Repair and Growth Society 10:20.

Anninos, P.A., and N. Tsagas. 1991. Magnetic stimulation in the treatment of partial seizures. Int. J. Neurosci. 60:141–171.

Baranowski, T.J., and J. Black. 1987. Stimulation of osteogenesis. In M. Blank and E. Findl, eds. Mechanistic Approaches to Interactions of Electric and Electromagnetic Fields With Living Systems (pp. 399–416). Plenum Press, New York.

Barker, A.T., R.A. Dixon, W.J.W. Sharrard, and M.L. Sutcliffe. 1984. Pulsed magnetic field therapy for tibial nonunion: interim results of a double-blind trial. Lancet. 1 (8384):994–996.

Bassett, C.A.L. 1989. Fundamental and practical aspects of therapeutic uses of pulsed electromagnetic fields (PEMFs). CRC Critical Reviews in Biomedical Engineering 17:451–529.

Bassett, C.A.L., S.N. Mitchell, and S.R. Gaston. 1982. Pulsing electromagnetic field treatment in ununited fractures and failed arthrodoses. JAMA 247:623–628.

Bassett, C.A.L., R.D. Pawluk, and A.A. Pilla. 1974. Augmentation of bone repair by inductively coupled electromagnetic fields. Science 184:575–577.

Becker, R.O. 1987. The effect of electrically generated silver ions on human cells. Proceedings of 1st International Conference on Gold and Silver in Medicine, Bethesda, Md., May 13–14, pp. 227–243.

Becker, R.O. 1990. A technique for producing regenerative healing in humans. Frontier Perspectives 1(2):1–2.

Becker, R.O. 1992. Effect of anodally generated silver ions on fibrosarcoma cells. Electro- and Magnetobiology 11:57–65.

Becker, R.O., and A.A. Marino. 1982. Electromagnetism and Life. State University of New York Press, Albany, New York.

Becker, R.O., and J.A. Spadero. 1972. Electrical stimulation of partial limb regeneration in mammals. Bull. N.Y. Acad. Med. 48:627–641.

Bierbaum, P.J., and J.M. Peters, eds. 1991. Proceedings of the Scientific Workshop on the Health Effects of Electric and Magnetic Fields on Workers. Cincinnati, Ohio, January 30–31. National Institute of Occupational Safety and Health (NIOSH) Report No. 91-111. NTIS Order No. PB-91-173-351/A13. National Technical Information Service, Springfield, Va.

Blank, M., ed. 1993. Electricity and Magnetism in Biology and Medicine. Proceedings of the 1st World Congress for Electricity and Magnetism in Biology and Medicine, Orlando, Fla., June 14–19, 1992. San Francisco Press, Inc., San Francisco.

Blank, M., and E. Findl, eds. 1987. Mechanistic Approaches to Interactions of Electric and Electromagnetic Fields With Living Systems. Plenum Press, New York.

Brayman, A., and M. Miller. 1989. Proportionality of 60-Hz electric field bioeffect severity to average induced transmembrane potential magnitude in a root model system. Radiat. Res. 117:207–213.

Brayman, A., and M. Miller. 1990. 60-Hz electric field exposure inhibits net apparent H-ion excretion from excised roots of Zea mays L. Radiat. Res. 123:22–31.

Brighton, C.T., J. Black, Z.B. Friedenberg, J.L. Esterhai, L. Day, and J.F. Connally. 1981. A multicenter study of the treatment of nonunion with constant direct current. J. Bone Joint Surg. (Br.) 63A:2–12.

Brighton, C.T., J. Black, and S.R. Pollack, eds. 1979. Electrical Properties of Bone and Cartilage: Experimental Effects and Clinical Applications. Grune and Stratton, Inc., New York.

Brighton, C.T., M.J. Katz, S.R. Goll, C.E. Nichols, and S.R. Pollack. 1985. Prevention and treatment of sciatic denervation disuse osteoporosis in the rat tibia with capacitively coupled electrical stimulation. Bone 6:87–97.

Brighton, C.T., and S.R. Pollack, eds. 1991. Electromagnetics in Medicine and Biology. San Francisco Press, Inc., San Francisco.

Brown, H.D., and S.K. Chattpadhyay. 1991. EM-field effect upon properties of NADPH-cytochrome P-450 reductase with model substrates. Cancer Biochem. Biophys. 12(3):211–215.

Budd, R.A., and P. Czerski. 1985. Modulation of mammalian immunity by electromagnetic radiation. J. Microw. Power Electromagn. Energy 20:217–231.

Cadossi, R., G. Emilia, and G. Torelli. 1988a. Lymphocytes and pulsing magnetic fields. In A.A. Marino, ed. Modern Bioelectricity. Marcel Dekker, Inc., New York.

Cadossi, R., R. Iverson, V.R. Hentz, P. Zucchini, G. Emilia, and G. Torelli. 1988b. Effect of low-frequency low-energy pulsing electromagnetic fields on mice undergoing bone marrow transplantation. International Journal of Immunopathology and Pharmacology 1:57–62.

Chen, J., and O.P. Gandhi. 1989. RF currents in an anatomically based model of a human for plane-wave exposures (20–100 MHz). Health Phys. 57(1):89–98.

Christensen, P.A., and M. Noreng. 1989. Electroacupuncture and postoperative pain. Br. J. Anaesth. 62:258–262.

Chwirot, W.B. 1988. Ultraweak photon emission and anther meiotic cycle in Larix europaea (experimental investigation of Nagl and Popp's electromagnetic model of differentiation). Experientia 44:594–599.

Chwirot, W.B., R.S. Dygdala, and S. Chwirot. 1987. Quasi-monochromatic-light-induced photon emission from microsporocytes of larch shows oscillating decay behavior predicted by the electromagnetic model of differentiation. Cytobios 47:137–146.

Cohen, M.M., A. Kunska, J.A. Astemborsky, and D. McCulloch. 1986. The effect of low-level 60-Hz electromagnetic fields on human lymphoid cells. Circ. Res. 172:177–184.

Cossarizza, A., D. Monti, F. Bersani, et al. 1989a. Extremely low-frequency pulsed electromagnetic fields increase cell proliferation in lymphocytes from young and aged subjects. Biochem. Biophys. Res. Commun. 160:692–698.

Cossarizza, A., D. Monti, F. Bersani, et al. 1989b. Extremely low-frequency pulsed electromagnetic fields increase interleukin-2 (IL-2) utilization and IL-2 receptor expression in mitogen-stimulated human lymphocytes from old subjects. FEBS Lett. 248:141–144.

Cossarizza, A., D. Monti, P. Sola, et al. 1989c. DNA repair after irradiation in lymphocytes exposed to low-frequency pulsed electromagnetic fields. Radiat. Res. 118:161–168.

Cruess, R.L., and C.A.L. Bassett. 1983. The effect of pulsing electromagnetic fields on bone metabolism in experimental disuse osteoporosis. Clin. Orthop. 173:245–250.

De Loecker, W., P.H. Delport, and N. Cheng. 1989. Effects of pulsed electromagnetic fields on rat skin metabolism. Biochim. Biophys. Acta 982:9–14.

Devyatkov, N.D., Y.V. Gulyaev, et al. 1991. Digest of Papers. International Symposium on Millimeter Waves of Non-Thermal Intensity in Medicine. Cosponsored by Research and Development Association "ISTOK" and Research Institute of U.S.S.R. Ministry of Electronic Industry ("ORION"). Moscow, October 3–6. (In Russian.)

Dundee, J.W., and R.G. Ghaly. 1989. Acupuncture prophylaxis of cancer chemotherapy-induced sickness. J. R. Soc. Med. 82:268–271.

Dunn, P.A., and D. Rogers. 1989. Transcutaneous electrical nerve stimulation at acupuncture points in the induction of uterine contractions. Obstet. Gynecol. 73:286–290.

Easterly, C. 1982. Cardiovascular risk from exposure to static magnetic fields. American Industrial Hygiene Association Journal 43:533–539.

Eisenberg, D.M., R.C. Kessler, C. Foster, et al. 1993. Unconventional medicine in the United States: prevalence, costs, and patterns of use. N. Engl. J. Med. 328:246–252.

Fehlings, M.G., R.J. Hurlbert, and C.H. Tator. 1992. An examination of direct current fields for the treatment of spinal cord injury. Paper presented at the 1st World Congress for Electricity and Magnetism in Biology and Medicine, Orlando, Fla., June 14–19.

Feinendegen, L.E. and H. Muhlensiepen. 1987. In vivo enzyme control through a strong stationary magnetic field: The case of thymidine kinase in mouse bone marrow cells. Int. J. Radiat. Biol. 52(3):469–479.

Foxall, P.J.D., G.H. Neild, F.D. Thompson, and J.K. Nicholson. 1991. High-resolution NMR spectroscopy of fluid from polycystic kidneys suggests reversed polarity of cyst epithelial cells. Journal of the American Society of Nephrology 2(3):252.

Goldenberg, D.M., and H.J. Hansen. 1972. Electric enhancement of bone healing. Science 175:1118–1120.

Goodman, R., L. Wei, J. Xu, and A. Henderson. 1989. Exposures of human cells to low-frequency electromagnetic fields results in quantitative changes in transcripts. Biochim. Biophys. Acta 1009:216–220.

Gordon, R.T. 1986. Process for the Treatment of Atherosclerotic Lesions. U.S. Patent No. 4,622,953, November 18.

Grande, D.A., F.P. Magee, A.M. Weinstein, and B.R. McLeod. 1991. The effect of low-energy combined AC and DC magnetic fields on articular cartilage metabolism. In C.T. Brighton and S.R. Pollack, eds. Electromagnetics in Medicine and Biology. San Francisco Press, Inc., San Francisco.

Greene, J.J., W.J. Skowronski, J.M. Mullins, and R.M. Nardone. 1991. Delineation of electric and magnetic field effects of extremely low frequency electromagnetic radiation on transcription. Biomedical and Biophysical Research Communications 174(2):742–749.

Grundler, W., F. Kaiser, F. Keilmann, and J. Walleczek. In press. Mechanisms of electromagnetic interaction with cellular systems. Naturwissenschaften. From a workshop sponsored by the Deutsche Forschungsgemeinschaft (DFG) at the Max-Planck-Institut für Festkörperforschung, Stuttgart, Germany, September 11–12.

Guy, A.W. 1987. Dosimetry association with exposure to non-ionizing radiation: very low frequency to microwaves. Health Phys. 53(6):569–584.

Hagfors, N.R., and A.C. Hyme. 1975. Method and structure of preventing and treating ileus, and reducing acute pain by electrical pulse stimulation. U.S. Patent No. 3,911,930, October 14.

Hajdukovic, R., M. Mitler, B. Pasche, and M. Erman. 1992. Effects of low-energy emission therapy (LEET) on sleep structure (abstract). Sleep Research 21:206.

Hallett, M., and L.G. Cohen. 1989. Magnetism: a new method for stimulation of nerve and brain. JAMA 262 (4):538–541.

Herbst, E., B.F. Sisken, and H.Z. Wang. 1988. Assessment of vascular network in rat skin flaps subjected to sinusoidal EMFs using image analysis techniques. Transactions of the 8th Annual Meeting of the Bioelectrical Repair and Growth Society. Washington, D.C., October 9–12.

Hinsenkamp, M., J. Ryaby, and F. Burny. 1985. Treatment of nonunion by pulsing electromagnetic fields: European multicenter study of 308 cases. Reconstr. Surg. Traumatol. 19:147–151.

Horton, P., J.T. Ryaby, F.P. Magee, and A.M. Weinstein. 1992. Stimulation of specific neuronal differentiation proteins in PC12 cells by combined AC/DC magnetic fields. Presented at the 1st World Congress for Electricity and Magnetism in Biology and Medicine, Orlando, Fla., June 14–19.

Huraki, Y., N. Endo, M. Takigawa, A. Asada, H. Takahashe, and F. Suzuki. 1987. Enhanced responsiveness to parathyroid hormone and induction of functional differentiation of cultured rabbit costal chondrocytes by a pulsed electromagnetic field. Biochim. Biophys. Acta 931:94–110.

Hurlbert, R.J., and C.H. Tator. 1992. Effect of disc vs. cuff electrode configuration on tolerance of the rat spinal cord to DC stimulation. Paper presented at the 1st World Congress for Electricity and Magnetism in Biology and Medicine, Orlando, Fla., June 14–19.

Ieran, M., S. Zaffuto, M. Bagnacani, M. Annovi, A. Moratti, and R. Cadossi. 1990. Effect of low-frequency pulsing electromagnetic fields on skin ulcers of venous origin in humans: a double-blind study. J. Orthop. Res. 8:276–282.

Im, M.J., and J.E. Hoopes. 1991. Effects of electrical stimulation on ischemia/reperfusion injury in rat skin. In C.T. Brighton and S.R. Pollack, eds. Electromagnetics in Medicine and Biology. San Francisco Press, Inc., San Francisco.

Kanje, M., and A. Rusovan. 1992. Reversal of the stimulation of magnetic field exposure on regeneration of the rat sciatic nerve by a Ca^{2+} antagonist. Paper presented at the 1st World Congress for Electricity and Magnetism in Biology and Medicine, Orlando, Fla., June 14–19.

Klawansky, S., A. Yueng, C. Berkey, N. Shah, C. Zachery, and T.C. Chalmers. 1992. Meta-analysis of randomized control trials of the efficacy of cranial electrostimulation in treating psychological and physiological conditions. Report of the Technology Assessment Group, Department of Health Policy and Management, Harvard University School of Public Health, August 28.

Kraus, W. 1992. The treatment of pathological bone lesion with nonthermal, extremely low frequency electromagnetic fields. Bioelectrochemistry and Bioenergetics 27:321–339.

Lee, R.C., D.J. Canaday, and H. Doong. 1993. A review of the biophysical basis for the clinical application of electric fields in soft tissue repair. J. Burn Care Rehabil. 14:319–335.

Lee, Y.H., W.C. Lee, M.T. Chen, et al. 1992. Acupuncture in the treatment of renal colic. J. Urol. 147:16–18.

Lerchl, A., K.O. Nonaka, K.A. Stokkan, and R.J. Reiter. 1990. Marked rapid alterations in nocturnal pineal serotonin metabolism in mice and rats exposed to weak intermittent magnetic fields. Biochem. Biophys. Res. Commun. 169:102–108.

Liboff, A.R. 1985. Geomagnetic cyclotron resonance in living cells. J. of Biol. Phys. 13:99–104.

Liboff, A.R. 1991. The cyclotron resonance hypothesis: experimental evidence and theoretical constraints. In C. Ramel and B. Norden, eds. Interaction Mechanisms of Low-Level Electromagnetic Fields With Living Systems. Oxford University Press, London, pp. 130–147.

Liboff, A.R., B.R. McLeod, and S.D. Smith. 1991. Resonance transport in membranes. In C.T. Brighton and S.R. Pollack, eds. Electromagnetics in Medicine and Biology. San Francisco Press, Inc., San Francisco.

Liboff, A.R., B.R. McLeod, and S.D. Smith. 1992a. Techniques for Controlling Osteoporosis Using Noninvasive Magnetic Fields. U.S. Patent No. 5,100,373, March 31.

Liboff, A.R., B.R. McLeod, and S.D. Smith. 1992b. Method and Apparatus for Controlling Tissue Growth with an Applied Fluctuating Magnetic Field, U.S. Patent No. 5,123,898, June 23.

Liboff, A.R., R.A. Rinaldi, eds. 1974. Electrically mediated growth mechanisms in living systems. Ann. N.Y. Acad. Sci. 238(October 11).

Liburdy, R.P., and T.S. Tenforde. 1986. Magnetic field-induced drug permeability in liposome vesicles. Radiat. Res. 108:102–111.

Madroñero, A. 1990. Influence of magnetic fields on calcium salts crystal formation: an explanation of the "pulsed electromagnetic field" technique for bone healing. J. Biomed. Eng. 12:410–412.

Magee, F.P., A.M. Weinstein, R.J. Fitzsimmons, D.J. Baylink, and B.R. McLeod. 1991. The use of low-energy combined AC and DC magnetic fields in the prevention of osteopenia. In C.T. Brighton and S.R. Pollack, eds. Electromagnetics in Medicine and Biology. San Francisco Press, Inc., San Francisco.

Marino, A.A., ed. 1988. Modern Bioelectricity. Marcel Dekker, Inc., New York.

Marron, M.T., E.M. Goodman, P.T. Sharpe, and B. Greenebaum. 1988. Low-frequency electric and magnetic fields have different effects on the cell surface. FEBS Lett. 230(1–2):13–16.

Mathew, R., and S. Rumar. The non-exponential decay pattern of the weak luminescence from seedlings in Cicer arietinum L. stimulated by pulsating electric fields. Experientia. In press.

McDevitt, L., P. Fortner, and B. Pomeranz. 1987. Application of weak electrical field to the hindpaw enhances sciatic motor-nerve regeneration in the adult rat. Brain Res. 416:308–314.

Mertz, P.M., S.C. Davis, and W.H. Eaglstein. 1988. Pulsed electrical stimulation increases the rate of epithelialization in partial thickness wounds. Transactions of the 8th Annual Meeting of the Bioelectrical Repair and Growth Society, Washington, D.C., October 9–12.

Miklavčič, D., S. Reberšek, G. Serša, et al. 1991. Nonthermal antitumor effect of electrical direct current on murine fibrosarcoma SA-1 tumor model. In C.T. Brighton and S.R. Pollack, eds. Electromagnetics in Medicine and Biology. San Francisco Press, Inc., San Francisco.

Nair, I., M.G. Morgan, and H.K. Florig. 1989. Biological Effects of Power Frequency Electric and Magnetic Fields (Background Paper). Office of Technology Assessment, Report No. OTA-BP-E-53. U.S. Government Printing Office, Washington, D.C.

O'Connor, M.E., R.H.C. Bentall, and J.C. Monahan, eds. 1990. Emerging Electromagnetic Medicine conference proceedings. Springer-Verlag, New York.

O'Connor, M.E., and R.H. Lovely, eds. 1988. Electromagnetic Fields and Neurobehavioral Function. Alan R. Liss, Inc., New York.

Omote, Y., M. Hosokawa, M. Komatsumoto, et al. 1990. Treatment of experimental tumors with a combination of a pulsing magnetic field and an antitumor drug. Jpn. J. Cancer Res. 81:956–961.

Onuma, E., and S. Hui. 1988. Electric field-directed cell shape changes, displacement, and cytoskeletal reorganization are calcium dependent. J. Cell Biol. 106:2067–2075.

Orgel, M.G., R.J. Zienowicz, B.A. Thomas, and W.H. Kurtz, 1992. Peripheral nerve transection injury: the role of electromagnetic field therapy. Paper presented at the 1st World Congress for Electricity and Magnetism in Biology and Medicine, Orlando, Fla., June 14–19.

Papatheofanis, F.J., and B.J. Papatheofanis. 1989. Acid and alkaline phosphase activity in bone following intense magnetic field irradiation of short duration. Int. J. Radiat. Biol. 55(6):1033–1035.

Pasche, B., T.P. Lebet, A. Barbault, C. Rossel, and N. Kuster. 1989. Electroencephalographic changes and blood pressure lowering effect of low energy emission therapy (abstract). Bioelectromagnetics Society Proceedings, F-3-5.

Phillips, J.L., and L. McChesney. 1991. Effect of 72-Hz pulsed magnetic field exposure on macromolecular synthesis in CCRF-CEM cells. Cancer Biochem. Biophys. 12:1–7.

Pollack, S.R., C.T. Brighton, D. Plenkowski, and N.J. Griffith. 1991. Electromagnetic Method and Apparatus for Healing Living Tissue. U.S. Patent No. 5,014,699, May 14.

Pomeranz, B., M. Mullen, and H. Markus. 1984. Effect of applied electrical fields on sprouting of intact saphenous nerve in adult rat. Brain Res. 303:331–336.

Popp, F.A., A.A. Gurwitsch, H. Inaba, et al. 1988. Biophoton emission (multiauthor review). Experientia 44:543–600.

Popp, F.A., K.H. Li, and Q. Gu, eds. 1992. Recent Advances in Biophoton Research and Its Applications. World Scientific Publishing Co., Singapore and New York.

Popp, F.A., W. Nagl, K.H. Li, et al. 1984. Biophoton emission: new evidence for coherence and DNA as source. Cell Biophys. 6:33–52.

Ramel, C., and B. Norden, eds. 1991. Interaction Mechanisms of Low-Level Electromagnetic Fields With Living Systems. Oxford University Press, London.

Rodemann, H.P., K. Bayreuther, and G. Pfleiderer. 1989. The differentiation of normal and transformed human fibroblasts in vitro is influenced by electromagnetic fields. Exp. Cell Res. 182:610–621.

Rosenthal, M., and G. Obe. 1989. Effects of 50-Hz electromagnetic fields on proliferation and on chromosomal alterations in human peripheral lymphocytes untreated or pretreated with chemical mutagens. Mutat. Res. 210:329–335.

Rusovan, A., and M. Kanje. 1991. Stimulation of regeneration of the rat sciatic nerve by 50-Hz sinusoidal magnetic fields. Exp. Neurol. 112:312–316.

Rusovan, A., and M. Kanje. 1992. D600, a Ca^{2+} antagonist, prevents stimulation of nerve regeneration by magnetic fields. NeuroReport 3:813–814.

Rusovan, A., M. Kanje, and K.H. Mild. 1992. The stimulatory effect of magnetic fields on regeneration of the rat sciatic nerve is frequency dependent. Exp. Neurol. 117:81–84.

Ryaby, J.T., D.A. Grande, F.P. Magee, and A.M. Weinstein. 1992. The effect of combined AC/DC magnetic fields on resting articular cartilage metabolism. Presented at the 1st World Congress for Electricity and Magnetism in Biology and Medicine, Orlando, Fla., June 14–19.

Sharrard, W.J.W. 1990. A double-blind trial of pulsed electromagnetic fields for delayed union of tibial fractures. J. Bone Joint Surg. (Br.) 72B:347–355.

Shealy, N., R. Cady, D. Veehoff, et al. 1992. Neuro-chemistry of depression. American Journal of Pain Management 2:31–36.

Short, W.O., L. Goodwill, C.W. Taylor, et al. 1992. Alteration of human tumor cell adhesion by high-strength static magnetic fields. Invest. Radiol. 27:836–840.

Sisken, B.F. 1992. Nerve regeneration: implications for clinical applications of electrical stimulation. Paper presented at the 1st World Congress for Electricity and Magnetism in Biology and Medicine, Orlando, Fla., June 14–19.

Skerry, T.M., M.J. Pead, M.J., and L.E. Lanyon. 1991. Modulation of bone loss during disuse by pulsed electromagnetic fields. J. Orthop. Res. 9:600–608.

Smith, S.D. 1967. Induction of partial limb regeneration in Arana pipicus by galvanic stimulation. Anat. Rec. 158:89–97.

Stiller, M.J., G.H. Pak, J.L. Shupack, S. Thaler, C. Kenny, and L. Jondreau. 1992. A portable pulsed electromagnetic field (PEMF) device to enhance healing of recalcitrant venous ulcers: a double-blind placebo-controlled clinical trial. Br. J. Dermatol. 127:147–154.

Subramanian, M., C.H. Sutton, B. Greenebaum, and B.F. Sisken. 1991. Interaction of electromagnetic fields and nerve growth factor on nerve regeneration in vitro. In C.T. Brighton and S.R. Pollack, eds. Electromagnetics in Medicine and Biology. San Francisco Press, Inc., San Francisco.

Takahashi, K., I. Kaneko, and E. Fukada. 1987. Influence of pulsing electromagnetic field on the frequency of sister-chromatid exchanges in cultural mammalian cells. Experientia 43:331–332.

Tenforde, T.S., and W.T. Kaune. 1987. Interaction of extremely low frequency electric and magnetic fields with humans. Health Phys. 53:585–606.

Thomas, J.R., J. Schrot, and A.R. Liboff. 1986. Low-intensity magnetic fields alter operant behavior in rats. Bioelectromagnetics 7:349.

Trock, D.H., A.J. Bollet, R.H. Dyer, Jr., L.P. Fielding, W.K. Miner, and R. Markoll. 1993. A double-blind trial of the clinical effects of pulsed electromagnetic fields in osteoarthritis. J. Rheumatol. 20:456–460.

U.S. Environmental Protection Agency. 1991. Evaluation of the Potential Carcinogenicity of Electromagnetic Fields. Report #EPA/600/6-90/05B. Unreleased preliminary draft (March).

Vodovnik, L., and R. Karba. 1992. Treatment of chronic wounds by means of electric and electromagnetic fields. Part 1: literature review. Med. Biol. Eng. and Comput. (May):257–266.

Walleczek, J. 1992. Electromagnetic field effects on cells of the immune system: the role of calcium signalling. FASEB Lett. 6:3177–3185.

Weinstein, A.M., B.R. McLeod, S.D. Smith, and A.R. Liboff. 1990. Ion resonance-tuned electromagnetic fields increase healing rate in ostectomized rabbits. Abstracts of 36th Annual Meeting of Orthopedic Research, February 5–8, 1990, New Orleans.

Wijk, R.V., and D.H.J. Schamhart. 1988. Regulatory aspects of low-intensity photon emission. Experientia 44:586–593.

Wilson, B.W., R.G. Stevens, and L.E. Anderson, eds. 1990a. Extremely Low Frequency Electromagnetic Fields: The Question of Cancer. Battelle Press, Columbus, Ohio.

Wilson, B.W., C.W. Wright, J.E. Morris, et al. 1990b. Evidence for an effect of ELF electromagnetic fields on human pineal gland function. J. Pineal Res. 9:259–269.

Wilson, D.H., P. Jagdeesh, P.P. Newman, and D.G.F. Harriman. 1974. The effects of pulsed electromagnetic energy on peripheral nerve regeneration. Ann. N.Y. Acad. Sci. 238:575–585.

Yen-Patton, G.P.A., W.F. Patton, D.M. Beer, and B.S. Jacobson. 1988. Endothelial cell response to pulsed electromagnetic fields: stimulation of growth rate and angiogenesis in vitro. J. Cell. Physiol. 134:37–46.

Alternative Systems of Medical Practice

PANEL MEMBERS

Jennifer Jacobs, M.D.—Cochair
John C. Reed, M.D.—Cochair

Michael Balick, Ph.D.
Steven Birch
Gerald Bodeker, Ed.D.
Carola Burroughs
Carlo Calabrese, N.D., M.P.H.
Edward Chapman, M.D.
Deepak Chopra, M.D.
Effie Chow, Ph.D.
Patricia Culliton, M.A., Dipl.Ac.
Robert Duggan
Peter Hindebergh, M.D.
Tori Hudson, N.D.
Ted Kaptchuk
Fredi Kronenberg, Ph.D.
Nancy Lonsdorf, M.D.
Robert S. McCaleb
Kevin McNamee, D.C., L.Ac.
Paul Ortega

CONTRIBUTING AUTHORS

John C. Reed, M.D., Lead Author

Background
Claire Cassidy, Ph.D.
John C. Reed, M.D.
Traditional Oriental Medicine
Effie Chow, Ph.D.
Steven Birch
John C. Reed, M.D.
Acupuncture
John C. Reed, M.D.
Ayurvedic Medicine
Nancy Lonsdorf, M.D.
Homeopathic Medicine
Jennifer Jacobs, M.D.
Brian Berman, M.D.
Anthroposophically Extended Medicine
Paul Scharff, M.D.
Naturopathic Medicine
Tori Hudson, N.D.
Environmental Medicine
Charles Moss, M.D.
Community-Based Health Care Practices
Claire Cassidy, Ph.D.
Rayna Green, Ph.D.
Clara Sue Kidwell, Ph.D.
Pat Locke

Background

In the United States many people think of mainstream biomedicine as the world's standard health care system, assuming it is used by most people most of the time.[1] Actually, careful estimates reveal that worldwide only 10 to 30 percent of human health care is delivered

[1]*The term* health care system *is used two ways. In one sense, a health care system encompasses all the health care available to a nation of people. According to this meaning, in the United States all people are immersed in the health care system to the extent that they are connected to the health-protective infrastructure (e.g., clean water, sewer systems, vaccinations) and use any form of specialist health care, including both community-based and professionalized health care practitioners. In the second sense, a health care system is all the components that together make up the practice of any particular form of medical care, such as osteopathy, acupuncture, psychotherapy, biomedicine, or hands-on healing. Each such system provides explanations for the cause and cure of illness; identifies and trains specialists; provides locales, equipment, and* materia medica *for practice; and arranges for social and legal mandates for practice. All health care provided by specialists (that is, apart from household and popular remedies) is delivered from within a health care system. However, the complexity and extension of health care systems vary widely, from the relatively experiential and localized practices of community-based traditional healers to the extensive, complex, and intensely professionalized practices of cosmopolitan doctors.*

by the conventional, biomedically oriented health care system. The remaining 70 to 90 percent of health care sought out by people includes everything from self-care according to folk principles to care rendered in an organized health care system based on an alternative tradition of practice (Dean, 1981; Hufford, 1992).

Such strikingly high usage of alternative health care systems also is reflected in a number of recent surveys. For example, a nationwide telephone survey of 1,539 people, conducted in 1990, indicated that up to one in three Americans used alternative therapies (Eisenberg et al., 1993). Another telephone survey conducted in 1992 in the States of Maryland and Pennsylvania reported that someone in 33 percent of 1,165 households consulted chiropractors, 25 percent, massage therapists; and 16 percent, spiritual healers (Kirby, 1992). One biomedical clinic survey of 660 cancer patients showed that 54 percent used alternative medical care along with conventional care, and 8 percent used strictly alternative care (Cassileth et al., 1984). In addition, a survey of 628 cancer patients found the utilization rate of folk treatments for cancer to be 70 percent (Hufford, 1992). Finally, an acupuncture clinic survey of 180 general-care patients showed that 70 percent sought other alternative professional or community-based health care in addition to biomedical and acupuncture care (Cassidy, 1994).

Given the immense political and economic investment this country has made in its "mainstream" medicine, these statistics are quite surprising. However, to better understand why alternative systems of medicine not only survive but thrive, it is worthwhile to first examine how people typically go about choosing their health care.

Studies show that most people go through a "hierarchy of resort" when seeking health care assistance (Romanuicci-Ross, 1969). That is, when ill, they usually begin by trying simple home remedies, often consulting friends and family about what to do. Only if the condition persists and worsens do people typically seek help from health care specialists.

The hierarchy of health care specialists includes the *popular, community-based, and professionalized* (Hufford, 1988; Kleinman, 1980). All are similar in that they aim to help people stay or get well and use manipulation (from laying on of hands to surgery), chemical substances (foods and drugs), or psychospiritual approaches (e.g., talking, suggesting, praying, drumming) as therapeutic techniques. They differ, however, in factors such as how much training they require of practitioners, how intensely they scrutinize and theorize about their own methods, how widely their practice is spread, and to whom they primarily aim their care.

Popular health care is what most people practice and receive at home, such as drinking hot honey and lemonade to relieve a sore throat. People get information about popular health care primarily from family or friends; it can be centuries old or relatively new to that family or social circle. People also learn about popular medicine from magazines, television, and other informal sources. In the United States, popular medicine often uses the words but not necessarily the underlying thinking of biomedicine.

Community-based health care refers to the nonprofessionalized yet specialized health care practices of both rural and urban people. The term *community-based* is used to avoid the stereotypes associated with the terms *folk* and *tribal*. Information in such systems is commonly passed on orally (through workshops, apprenticeships, and so on) and through informal and popular media sources. Some community-based practices have ancient roots (such as rootwork among African-Americans, powwowing among European-Americans, *curanderismo* among Hispanic-Americans, and religious pilgrimage and psychic healing traditions), while others have developed relatively recently, such as the various 12-step programs (e.g., Alcoholics Anonymous), popular weight loss programs, and various health and natural foods dietary practices. In contrast to popular and professionalized systems, these community-based systems characteristically focus on community health care or on the individual as part of the community. They also usually fuse concepts of medicine and religion or spirituality in such a way that all care is explained as being influenced by a "higher power."

Professionalized health care is characteristically urban and complexly organized. It is the most intellectualized and formalized type of health care. Certain of these have been called the "Great Tradition" medical care systems. Examples of such professionalized health care systems include conventional Western biomedicine, Asian-

Indian Ayurveda, traditional oriental medicine, and traditional Persian medicine (Unani), all of which have evolved over time within major urban cultures. Other systems such as chiropractic medicine, osteopathic medicine, anthroposophically extended medicine, environmental medicine, and homeopathic medicine have been the result of the formalization and expansion of the teachings of a specific creative founder within the Western rational and intellectual culture. Each of these major formal systems of medical practice has the following general characteristics: (1) a theory of health and disease; (2) an educational scheme to teach its concepts; (3) a delivery system involving practitioners who usually practice in offices, clinics, or hospitals; (4) a material support system to produce its medicines and therapeutic devices; (5) a legal and economic mandate to regulate its practice; (6) a set of cultural expectations on the role of the medical system; and (7) a means to confer "professional" status on the approved providers.

Two major types of illnesses are recognized in most of these systems, though one or the other is usually emphasized: the *naturalistic* illness (which results from an accident, infection, intoxication, malformation, aging, environmental stress, etc.) and the *personalistic* illness (which is the result of malfunction in relationships between people). A third category of illness is increasingly proposed: the *energetic* illness, which is the result of abnormalities in the flow of subtle energies.

Studies show that people are quite astute at knowing what sorts of conditions to take to what sorts of practitioners. The practitioners at the top of the hierarchy, those that are the most "socially foreign" (i.e., hard to reach from the point of view of the patient), are consulted last and usually only when the condition is unresponsive, very serious, or chronically debilitating. For example, rural Mexicans go to the *curandero* or *curandera* for "folk" illnesses, to the nun or nurse for mild biomedical conditions, and to the biomedical physician for the most serious conditions (Young, 1981). Likewise, in urban America many people consult a registered nurse, pharmacist, or health food salesperson before taking their concerns to the medical doctor. One-third of the users of unconventional therapy are estimated to use it for "nonserious" conditions, health promotion, or disease prevention. However, in the case of more serious health problems, the medical doctor is not the most socially foreign type of practitioner in the United States, because M.D.s and D.O.s (doctors of osteopathy) are abundant. People consulting alternative practitioners for an identified health problem are much more likely to have first consulted a medical doctor (Eisenberg et al., 1993). This point suggests that many of the alternative practitioners are rendering care to people with conditions either unresponsive to or unsatisfactorily treated by standard biomedical care.

Of the types of health care listed above, only the professionalized practitioners have received much, if any, scientific study regarding the causes of illness and the explanations and results of treatment. Indeed, community-based practices have been virtually ignored by conventional medicine on the assumption that these superstitious ways are dying out. On the other hand, popular and community-based systems have been studied primarily by social scientists, historians, and folklorists. These researchers, though not primarily concerned with clinical results or health outcomes, have provided most of the clinical material currently available. Health educators have made use of such studies in designing culturally sensitive outreach programs (see the "Diet and Nutrition" chapter).

In recent years, the professionalized biomedical health care system has initiated a number of programs in an attempt to influence popular health practices on the basis of sound epidemiological concerns, addressing such issues as smoking and health, diet and cardiovascular disease, sexual behavior and human immunodeficiency virus (HIV), and healthy childbirth practices. The comparative clinical effectiveness of indigenous community-based health care practices remains, however, a fruitful field for further research.

The remainder of this chapter comprises three major sections, the first of which describes several examples of professionalized alternative health care systems. The following section focuses on community-based practices. Except for the epidemiological issues addressed in the "Diet and Nutrition" chapter, *popular* practices are not discussed in this document, because the emphasis is on health care delivered by the community of alternative medicine practitioners rather than by laypeople. The last major section addresses the barriers, key issues, and overall priorities for research in alternative systems of medical practice.

Professionalized Health Systems

This section includes discussions of representative health systems whose practitioner base and standards of practice are such that outcomes research may lead to generalizable conclusions applicable to the improvement of the Nation's health care delivery system. These systems are

- traditional oriental medicine,
- acupuncture,
- Ayurvedic medicine,
- homeopathic medicine,
- anthroposophically extended medicine,
- naturopathic medicine, and
- environmental medicine.

Traditional oriental medicine and Ayurvedic medicine are professionalized health systems that are enjoying popularity beyond the ethnic Asian community and are building practitioner bases, educational systems, and popular awareness in North America. Likewise, acupuncture, both as a treatment method and as a formal professional medical system, has an established formal educational base, extensive legal sanction for a variety of practitioners, and a broad base of public support and acceptance in the United States.

Homeopathic medicine has maintained a sound educational base for both professional practitioner training and popular self-help support and has the only officially established "alternative" drug production system regulated by the Food and Drug Administration (FDA). Naturopathy has a base in two formally accredited naturopathic medical schools in the United States and legal recognition of practitioners in a number of States. Anthroposophically extended medicine, while limited in availability in the United States, has a track record of thoughtful research and drug development in Europe that exemplifies the possibilities for "scientific alternatives" in our own health care system. Environmental medicine is a modern specialty area within biomedicine that has developed in ecological theory of health and disease.

Discussion of these professionalized systems is intended as an overview only. The serious student or researcher will find an extensive global database for future research. Each of the following subsections ends with a discussion of current research issues and recommendations for future research.

Traditional Oriental Medicine

Overview. Traditional oriental medicine is a sophisticated set of many systematic techniques and methods. Many of these methods are widely known in the United States, including acupuncture, herbal medicines, acupressure, qigong, and oriental massage techniques. Traditional oriental medicine is rooted in Chinese culture and has spread, with variations, throughout other Asian countries, particularly Japan, Korea, and Vietnam. As a professionalized health system, it has a range of applications from health promotion to the treatment of illness.

The fundamental concepts of oriental medicine are embedded in the philosophical and metaphysical worldviews of Taoism, Confucianism, and Buddhism, which began evolving and spreading throughout East Asia 2,500 years ago. Whereas the religions and philosophies of the Western world developed around the theme of separation of mind, body, and spirit, the Eastern philosophies undergirding oriental medicine consider the whole person and nature to be systematically interrelated.

Chinese medicine developed concurrently with Chinese culture out of its shamanic, tribal origins in the pre-Christian era. By the beginning of the Han Dynasty (200 B.C.E.) the Chinese had acquired and documented formidable medical experience. The first mention of the Shen Nung pharmacopoeia dates from the first century A.D. (Unschuld, 1986). Anatomic dissections and surgeries were practiced during the earlier eras, although in later centuries the Confucian belief in the sacredness of the human body prevented further developments in surgery and anatomic research. The early Chinese State distinguished various sorts of doctors, including medical physicians, surgeons, dietitians, veterinary surgeons, and community-based health officers. By the close of the Han era (220 A.D.), the Chinese had a clear idea of preventive medicine and first aid, knew pathology and dietetics, and had devised breathing practices to promote longevity. After Buddhist influences were assimilated, particularly a tolerance for judging medical practices by their results and not by their theories, the characteristic qualities and components of Chinese medicine had developed by 500 A.D. These qualities and components were expanded during periods of cultural intellectual growth that paralleled the Middle Ages and the Renaissance in Western Europe (Unschuld, 1985).

During the colonial periods of encounter with Western culture, the systems of oriental medicine became fragmented. As Western medical science followed the spread of Western social and political power throughout East Asia, some traditional methods were relegated to folk and quasi-religious practitioners. However, since 1949, traditional Chinese medicine has enjoyed a Government-sponsored renaissance in the People's Republic of China (PRC) (Hiller and Jewel, 1983; Unschuld, 1992). Today, both traditional- and Western-oriented medical training, research, and institutional practice are available throughout mainland China (Quinn, 1972). In addition, traditional practices survive in various degrees in other East Asian countries (Sonoda, 1988).

The most striking characteristic of oriental medicine is its emphasis on diagnosing disturbances of qi (pronounced "chee"), or vital energy, in health and disease (Unschuld, 1985; Wiseman et al., 1985). There are many aspects of healthy balance and function in oriental medicine, and these aspects are described qualitatively or metaphorically as "disharmonies" among forms of vital energy. The concept of yin and yang harmony is a basic description of the interaction between the active and passive, stimulating and nurturing, masculine and feminine, and "heavenly" and "earthly" qualities that characterize living things. Imbalances of yin and yang can manifest within the functions of internal organs in their generation of metabolic energy, can propagate along energetically active channels represented on the body as the acupuncture meridians, and can undergo transformations of expression according to the system of "five phases." Each phase of energy has a characteristic quality of material expression represented by the elemental natures of fire, earth, metal, water, and wood. The Chinese systematically incorporated into their theories new discoveries of environmental and infectious influences on healthy qi and incorporated the emotional, psychological, and personality aspects of illness into the five-phase system.

Diagnosis in oriental medicine involves the classical procedures of observation, listening, questioning, and palpation, including feeling the quality of the pulses and the sensitivity of various body parts. The well-trained physician is taught to use all procedures together in evaluating the patient and to search for details of habit, lifestyle, nutritional indulgence, and specific mediating circumstances. Physical and emotional aspects of health are assumed to be interrelated; for example, fullness of the lungs is said to produce dreams of sorrow and weeping. A range of traditional therapies is prescribed to correct physical symptoms, restore energetic balance, and redirect and normalize the patient's qi.

The professionalization of oriental medicine has taken diverse paths in both East Asia and the United States. Currently, the model in the PRC, which was established after the 1949 revolution, involves the organized training of practitioners in schools of traditional Chinese medicine. The curriculum of these schools includes acupuncture, oriental massage, herbal medicine, and pharmacology, though the theoretical style of making a diagnosis and designing a treatment plan is the one traditionally associated with herbal medicine (Flaws, 1993). The graduates of these colleges are generally certified in one of the four specialty areas at a training level roughly equivalent to that of the Western bachelor's degree (Flaws, 1993). In contrast, in Japan there is a distinct profession of acupuncture, and the herbs used in traditional herbal medicine products (*kampo*) are prescribed by medically trained physicians or pharmacists (Birch, 1993).

In the United States the professional practitioner base for oriental medicine is organized around acupuncture and oriental massage. There are about 6,500 acupuncturist practitioners in the United States. The American Oriental Body Work Therapy Association has approximately 1,600 members representing practitioners of tuina, shiatsu, and related techniques (Flaws, 1993). Many American schools of acupuncture are evolving into "colleges of oriental medicine" by adding courses in oriental massage, herbal medicine, and dietary interventions. They are also offering diplomas and master's or doctor's degrees in oriental medicine. Although graduates of these programs are exposed to herbal medicine pharmacology, only the States of California and Nevada include a specific section evaluating knowledge of herbal medicine in the state acupuncturist licensing examination. The legal sanctioning of oriental medical practice is most extensive in New Mexico, where the acupuncturists have established an exclusive profession of oriental medicine. Their legal scope of practice is currently similar to that of primary care M.D.s and D.O.s, and their State statute restricts other licensed New Mexico health professionals' ability to advertise or bill for oriental medicine or acupuncture services (New Mexico Association of Acupuncture and Oriental Medicine, 1993).

As with any new profession in the United States, the issues of appropriate formal training, State-by-State legal scope of practice, official title and privileges of practitioners, and professional monopoly on health practices are currently controversial, even among the community of oriental medicine advocates. Furthermore, the position of oriental medicine practices and practitioners within the broader U.S. health care system continues to be a subject of heated political, economic, and intellectual debate (Birch, 1993; Flaws, 1993; National Council Against Health Fraud, 1991; New Mexico Association of Acupuncture and Oriental Medicine, 1993).

The treatment modalities most associated with traditional oriental medicine and used regularly by practitioners include acupuncture, moxibustion, acupressure, remedial massage, cupping, qigong, herbal medicine, and nutritional and dietary interventions. These are discussed below. Acupressure, massage, and qigong are also discussed in the "Manual Healing Methods" chapter.

Acupuncture. It is important to remember that acupuncture was but one branch among several therapies. It involves the direct manipulation of the network of energetic meridians, which are believed to connect not only with the surface or structural body parts but also to influence the deeper internal organs. The needle is inserted at appropriately chosen energetic points to disperse or activate the qi by a variety of technical manipulations. Western-style research showing that acupuncture could relieve pain and cause surgical analgesia through the release of pain-inhibiting chemicals (endorphins) in the nervous system led to the first theories of how acupuncture might work in terms of a biomedical science model (Han, 1987). This model does not, however, account for the many different ways acupuncture is used clinically to improve or correct ailing body functions. Because acupuncture has attracted major interest in the United States, an expanded section on acupuncture is included in this chapter.

Moxibustion. Moxibustion using *Artemisia vulgaris* (a plant of the composite, or daisy, family) evolved in early times in northern China. In this cold, mountainous region, the effect of heating the body on the energetically active points was a logical development. Moxibustion is thought to have preceded the use of needles. The crushed leaves, or moxa, of *vulgaris* may be used in loose or cigar form. In theory, the burning from the moxa releases a radiant heat that penetrates deeply and is used to affect the balance and flow of qi.

Acupressure. The energy points and channels can be treated with direct physical pressure by the fingertips or hands of the therapist. Simple points may be used for first aid or symptomatic relief or entire systems of manual therapy (e.g., shiatsu, jin shin jyutsu) may be used to effect the overall well-being of the body.

Remedial massage. The techniques of remedial massage (an-mo and tuina) are described in medical texts of the Han period. Later, in the Tang dynasty, massage was taught in special institutes. An-mo tonifies the system using pressing and rubbing hand motions, while tuina soothes and sedates using thrusting and rolling hand motions. Both systems employ a complex series of hand movements called the eight *kua* on specific body areas to produce the desired effects.

Cupping. Cupping is a technique of applying suction over selected points or zones in the body. A vacuum is created by warming the air in a jar of bamboo or glass and overturning it onto the body to disperse areas of local congestion. This therapy is used in the treatment of arthritis, bronchitis, and sprains, among other ailments.

Qigong. Qigong is the art and science of using breath, movement, and meditation to cleanse, strengthen, and circulate the vital life energy and blood.[2] Three basic principles are observed in the performance of the exercises: relaxation and repose; association of breathing with attention; and the interaction of movement and rest. Tai chi and other practices of oriental physical culture emphasize maintaining internal and external balance while encountering one's environment. Certain of the qigong exercises, particularly the *gou lin* form, have been used for immune stimulation and self-help in cancer patients (Sancier, 1991, 1993). These personal practices are the "internal" qigong type. Certain qigong "masters" are considered to be "energetic healers," who via "external" qigong use some of their own energy to strengthen the vitality of others who have ailments.

Herbal medicine. There is a complex series of practices regarding the preparation and administering of herbs in Chinese medicine (Unschuld, 1986). The traditional *materia medica* in China included approximately 3,200 herbs and 300 mineral and animal extracts (Bensky and Gamble, 1986). Herbal prescriptions cover the entire range of medical ailments, including pain, hormone disturbances, breathing disorders, infections, and chronic debilitating illnesses. Medications are classified according to their energetic qualities (e.g., heating, cooling, moisturizing, drying) and prescribed for their action on corresponding organ dysfunction, energy disorders, disturbed internal energy, blockage of the meridians, or seasonal physical demands. One unique aspect of traditional prescribing is the use of complex mixtures containing many ingredients. Such prescriptions are systemically compounded to have several effects: to principally affect the disease or disharmony, to balance out any potential side effects of the principal therapy, and to direct the therapy to a specific area or a physical process in the body. (See the "Herbal Medicine" chapter for details on specific Chinese herbs and how they are used).

Nutrition and dietetics. Dietary interventions are also individualized on the basis of the physical characteristics of both the patient's constitution and the patient's illness disturbance. Foods are characterized according to their energetic qualities (e.g., tonifying, dispersing, heating, cooling, moistening, drying). Emphasis is given to eating in harmony with seasonal shifts and life activities.

Research base. Although extensive research has been done in China through the institutions of traditional Chinese medicine, much of this clinical research has been empirical, that is, reports of observed results of various treatments. Many of these reports have been difficult to translate into Western languages and into the standard formulas or analysis typical for Western biomedical research. Because of the interest in applying acupuncture for pain and for chronic conditions, much research has focused on these two areas. However, clinical practice experience in the Asian countries suggests there is a role for complementary use of traditional therapies with a myriad of modern Western "scientific" medical interventions (Sun, 1988; Unschuld, 1992; Wong et al., 1991).

Only in the past quarter-century have biomedical scientists in China been characterizing and identifying the active agents in much of the traditional medical formulary (Hsu et al., 1982, 1985). However, extensive research has been published detailing the pharmacology and toxicity of many traditional oriental herbs (Bensky and Gamble, 1986; Hsu et al., 1982, 1985; Ng et al., 1991). How many clinical trials of traditional oriental herbal medicine have been conducted and what extent and validity the findings have are unclear. Few references to published studies appear in the databases available in the West. Although some individual studies appear quite promising, only preliminary conclusions can be drawn about the field until more complete literature searches are conducted. (See the "Herbal Medicine" chapter for a more complete

[2]*The word* qi *is principally used in relation to the biofield flux, the material of the biofield. The former phonetic spelling is* ch'i; *both are pronounced "chee"; originally also used as a root word similar to the use of the word* energy. *It was used with modifiers to describe hormones, nutrition factors, etc., such as the following.* Ching qi: *(meridian qi)—the qi that flows through the twelve meridians.* Fa qi—*external qi (wei qi) used in healing.* Jing qi—*essence (sexual essence—ancient usage, hormones in current usage).* Ku qi—*caloric energy from plants.* Qi density—*relative quantity of qi.* Ren qi—*internal qi that fills the spaces between the meridians in the body.* Wei qi—*external portion of the body's qi (aura).* Receiving hand—*hand with a polarity that receives the flow (qi). Sending hand—hand with a polarity that sends the flow (qi).* Flows—*movement of qi through the body or movement of qi from one of the practitioner's hands to the other through the patient's body.*

discussion of the status of herbal medicine research in China.)

Tsutani conducted an extensive search to find the number of clinical trials of herbal medicine in China (Tsutani, 1993). Of 148 studies retrieved from computerized databases, 39 were double blind, used random allocation, or were randomized controlled clinical trials. He conducted a combined computerized and manual search of the Japanese literature and retrieved references to 59 controlled studies on the use of kampo (Japanese traditional herbal medicine). An additional unpublished search by Birch of computer-indexed herbal medicine studies published in the period 1978–92 located 23 studies in English and 44 in other languages (Chinese 37, Japanese 5, German 1, French 1). In general, the methodological quality of these studies was poor, and they had multiple study design problems, including poor experimental design, lack of randomization, unclear entry criteria and end points, and lack of consideration of the traditional uses of the herbs (Birch, 1993).

Research in the medical effects of qigong has been a subject of interest in the PRC in recent years and was the topic of six international conferences between 1986 and 1991. Patients who practice internal qigong exercises combining meditation and gentle body movement were shown to have better results in therapy for hypertension, cancer, and coronary artery disease (Sancier, 1991, 1993). Qigong exercise also was shown to affect the blood chemistry of individuals practicing it. In addition, studies on external qigong have included measurements of the effect of qi emitted by master practitioners on cell cultures, germination rate of seeds, and electroencephalographic measurements of human recipients (Sancier and Hu, 1991).

Measurements of emissions from external qigong practitioners suggested that infrasonic energy was present in frequency ranges from 8 to 12.5 hertz (lower than the human ear can hear) and in intensities measurably different than background-noise level (Sancier and Hu, 1991). These suggestive findings parallel certain studies done in the West on mind-body interactions and nonlocal or "energetic" healing. (See the "Manual Healing Methods" and "Mind-Body Interventions" chapters.) Unfortunately, these Chinese studies are available only in abstract or conference proceedings formats in English. It is not known whether the complete papers are published in the Chinese literature with supporting data that would allow a methodological evaluation of the quality of the studies.

Future research opportunities. Although many diseases may be helped by the modalities of traditional oriental medicine, documenting its benefit in conditions of greatest concern to the United States should have research priority: cancer, acquired immune deficiency syndrome (AIDS), cardiovascular diseases, neuromuscular disabilities, chronic fatigue syndrome, psychosomatic problems, alcohol and drug addictions, and chronic pain.

Clinical research into the nondrug modalities of traditional oriental medicine includes opportunities for investigating manual healing therapies, bioelectricity and magnetic physical interventions, and the use of body-mind interactions for health purposes. Issues and criteria for such future research are discussed in other chapters of this report.

The use of traditional oriental herbal medicines and formulas in China and Japan has been studied for therapeutic value in the following areas: chronic hepatitis; rheumatoid arthritis; hypertension; atopic eczema; various immunologic disorders, including AIDS; and certain cancers (Hirayama et al., 1989; Sheehan and Atherton, 1992; Smith, 1987; Sun, 1988; Tao et al., 1989; Wong et al., 1991; Xu et al., 1989; Zhao et al., 1993). It would be useful to repeat these studies in the United States using high-quality research criteria. Research into the application of traditional oriental products could be roughly organized in three levels: first, publication of appropriate safety studies; second, pharmacological studies characterizing the contents, action, and components of single herbs and herbal formulas; and third, controlled clinical trials for specified conditions. The expense of this research endeavor can be lessened if World Health Organization proposals (see the "Herbal Medicine" chapter and app. C) allowing the documentation of traditional use are adopted by U.S. regulatory authorities (McCaleb, 1993). Given the large-scale use of over-the-counter herbal products as "food supplements" in the U.S. market, studies involving postmarketing surveillance of the use, clinical results, and complications of currently available products also would be appropriate (Ng et al., 1991).

Examples of creative basic research would include viewing the pH balance of body fluids as a representation of yin-yang balance, noting changes in organ and tissue receptor sites following treatment with herbal preparations, and investigating various neurological responses to massage and acupressure interventions. There is a major opportunity for cataloging and translating research done in China, Japan, and Korea in order to stimulate further development of the field in the United States.

Outcomes research can also address the application of traditional oriental medicine as a system. Such research would involve comparing (a) the overall health improvement and cost of care of a population working with a program of mixed interventions prescribed by practitioners of traditional oriental medicines with (b) the health indices of a control group using conventional care.

Acupuncture

Overview. Acupuncture involves stimulating specific anatomic points in the body for therapeutic purposes. Puncturing the skin with a needle is the usual method of application, but practitioners may also use heat, pressure, friction, suction, or impulses of electromagnetic energy to stimulate the points. Acupuncture was an evolving part of the medical practices of the Chinese people and is described in two surviving historical texts: the well-known medical treatise *Huang Ti Nei Ching Su Wên (The Yellow Emperor's Classic of Internal Medicine),* and *Shi Ji (Book of History),* both dating to the period 200–100 B.C.E.

Over the centuries, acupuncture spread throughout the medical practices of the Asiatic peoples around the Pacific Rim. However, it has been practiced as a medical art in Western Europe for several hundred years, having been brought home by the traders, diplomats, and missionary priests who encountered it during their travels in the Orient. By the late 19th century, acupuncture was known and used on the east coast of the United States. Sir William Osler's American medical textbook, which was first published in 1892 and was updated periodically through 1947, recommended acupuncture for treating lumbago or lower back pain (Lytle, 1993). Acupuncture also reached the United States on the west coast as an ethnic practice among Asian immigrants in the 19th and 20th centuries.

George Soulie de Morant, a French diplomat in China at the turn of the century, became an accomplished acupuncturist. On his return to France he began systematically introducing the full range of acupuncture to the French and European medical community. He published significant texts in 1934, 1939, 1941, and 1955 that represent a landmark effort to expand Western biomedical explanations of the physiology of health and disease to include the classical and empirical observations of Chinese acupuncture. His influence did much to establish acupuncture as an accepted clinical art in Europe (Zmiewski, 1994).

In the past 40 years acupuncture has become a well-known and reasonably available treatment in both developed and developing countries. Since the reopening of relations between the United States and the PRC, acupuncture has attracted increased attention from the American public and governmental agencies (Chen, 1973). With the emergence of traditional Chinese medicine as an organized system of practice in the PRC, formal training programs in acupuncture and oriental medicine have expanded throughout the world. Schools and training programs of acupuncture in the United States incorporate varying degrees of traditional Chinese medicine as well as European acupuncture approaches and elements of the traditional and modern practice traditions from Japan, Korea, and Vietnam.

Because the traditional view of health and illness in oriental medicine is related to a proper balance of qi, or energy, in the body, acupuncture is used to regulate or correct the flow of qi to restore health. Acupuncture treatment points are chosen on the basis of diagnosis of a medical problem by history and physical exam using one or more models of how the body operates in health and disease. The model, or "tradition," that is used to guide treatment may vary according to the cultural background and education of the practitioner as well as the nature of the patient's problem. Acupuncture prescriptions can be simple or sophisticated. A series of 10 or more treatments is usually prescribed for a chronic illness or physical rehabilitation. On the other hand, one to four treatments may suffice for minor injuries, a self-limited illness, or a seasonal "tune up."

Modern theories of acupuncture are based on laboratory research conducted in the past 40 years. Acupuncture points have been found to have certain electrical properties, and stimulation of these points has been shown to alter the chemical neurotransmitters in the body. Many of the therapeutic effects of acupuncture can be clearly related to the mechanism of neurotransmitter release via peripheral nerve stimulation. This mechanism is associated with changes in the balance of the natural physiological chemicals in the body, which can be used for a therapeutic effect (Pomeranz, 1986). Other therapeutic effects may be related to mechanical stimulation or alteration of the natural electrical currents or electromagnetic fields in the body.

Although the physiological effects of acupuncture stimulation in experimental animals have been well documented, the use of acupuncture treatments for clinical illness in humans has remained controversial within much of the mainstream medical community in the United States. Some controversy comes from the "foreignness" of traditional Chinese interpretations of medical illness, and some may be due to an unfamiliarity with the existing global research base. In 1973 the commissioner of the FDA announced that devices used in acupuncture, including the specialized needles, electrical stimulators, and associated paraphernalia, would be considered investigational on the basis of the perception at that time that "the safety and effectiveness of acupuncture devices [had] not yet been established by adequate scientific studies to support the many and varied uses for which such devices are being promoted including uses for analgesia and anesthesia" (Lytle, 1993). This designation is still official FDA policy.

In the subsequent 20 years, however, acupuncture has become an increasingly established health care practice in the United States. Furthermore, there are currently more than 40 schools and colleges of acupuncture and oriental medicine in the United States, 20 of which are either approved or in candidacy status with the National Accreditation Commission for Schools and Colleges of Acupuncture and Oriental Medicine. There are licensure or registration statutes in 28 States for the practitioner graduates of these programs. There are an estimated 6,500 acupuncturist practitioners in the United States, of whom 3,300 have taken the examination of the National Commission for the Certification of Acupuncturists. In addition to these practitioners, naturopathic and chiropractic physicians also can legally incorporate acupuncture in their practice in a limited number of States.

Besides the "alternative" medical practitioners who are trained in acupuncture, an estimated 3,000 conventionally trained physicians (M.D.s and D.O.s) have taken courses to incorporate acupuncture as a treatment modality in their medical practices. Such courses have been affiliated with the UCLA School of Medicine, the New York University School of Medicine and Dentistry, and St. Louis University Medical School (Helms, 1993). Proficiency certification examination for physician acupuncturists has been offered for a number of years in Canada by the Acupuncture Foundation of Canada, and similar examinations are currently in development in the United States, Australia, and New Zealand (Williams, 1994). The gradual acceptance of acupuncture therapeutics based on clinical practice experience in American medicine is reflected by the incorporation of descriptions of this discipline into most current textbooks of physical medicine and pain management (Chapman and Gunn, 1990; Lee and Liao, 1990). Moreover, a recent review estimated that patient visits for acupuncture to physician and nonphysician practitioners are occurring at a rate of 9 to 12 million per year in the United States (Lytle, 1993). Thus, the continued FDA "experimental" designation, which is echoed by the reference committee of the American Medical Association (AMA), is considered by many to be obsolete in the face of the large-scale use of acupuncture by legally sanctioned practitioners in the United States as well as in many other countries' health care systems.

Research base. Acupuncture is one of the most thoroughly researched and documented of the so-called alternative medical practices. A series of controlled studies on the treatment of a variety of conditions has shown compelling, though not statistically conclusive, evidence for the efficacy of acupuncture. These conditions are osteoarthritis (Dickens and Lewith, 1989), chemotherapy-induced nausea (J. Dundee et al., 1989), asthma (Fung and Chow, 1986), back pain (Gunn and Milbrandt, 1980), painful menstrual cycles (Helms, 1987), bladder instability (Phillip et al., 1988), and migraine headaches (Vincent, 1990).

Moreover, in spite of the unenviable challenge of serving as the "alternative" therapy of "last resort," acupuncture studies have shown positive results in managing chronic pain (Patel et al., 1989) and drug addiction (Bullock et al., 1989; Smith, 1988), two areas where conventional Western medicine has generally failed. Indeed, the criminal justice systems in New York City and Portland, OR, have mandated acupuncture as part of their detoxification and probation programs for drug abusers.

In addition, basic science research in animal models suggests that neurological pathways are the mechanism by which acupuncture relieves pain (Pomeranz, 1986). There also is work showing acupuncture effects in treating veterinary medical problems, such as bacteria-induced diarrhea in pigs (Hwang and Jenkins, 1988). A broad range of applications in human medicine also has been explored.

The risk and safety issues in acupuncture also have been thoroughly investigated (Lytle, 1993). In a recent review of 3,255 acupuncture citations in the world scientific literature, the conditions of study in 365 Western and 344 Chinese clinical research papers were tabulated (American Foundation of Medical Acupuncture, 1993). The number of studies per topic was as follows: surgical applications, 77; pain (chronic and acute pain of all types), 222; neurological disorders, 62; organic illness (e.g., heart, lungs), 200; women's reproductive disorders, 43; mental illness, 29; addiction therapy, 54; and acupuncture treatment complications, 11. The diversity of clinical applications and supporting basic physiology studies points to acupuncture having a therapeutic effect that exceeds a purely placebo or culturally dependent action.

Acupuncture research involves tailoring the study design and question to one of several levels of clinical investigation. At the most basic level, one can study the effect of stimulating a specific acupuncture point on a specific physiological response. For example, Dundee and colleagues conducted a series of investigations involving more than 500 patients for a 5-year period, evaluating the effect on nausea of stimulating the acupuncture point PC-6 (*neiguan*). These studies involved manual needling, electrical stimulation on the needle, acupressure, and noninvasive electrical stimulation. Control groups included patients with no treatment as well as patients who were needled at a sham point (a point unrelated to the accepted treatment meridian). The patients being investigated were undergoing minor gynecologic operations under general anesthesia. Results of the active acupuncture treatments showed better response than was shown by controls or by those who received sham acupuncture treatments. Indeed, needle acupuncture gave slightly better results than the then-standard antinausea drugs (R. Dundee et al., 1989).

Moreover, the effect of acupuncture in the treatment of specific clinical conditions has been measured. For example, Helms (1987) studied 43 women suffering from dysmenorrhea (painful menstrual periods); the patients were divided into four groups: real acupuncture, sham acupuncture, standard controls (no intervention), and visitation controls (visits to the treating physician). The patients were free to take their previously used pain medications during the 3-month treatment period and a followup period. Ninety-one percent of the real acupuncture treatment group showed improvement, whereas only 36 percent of the sham acupuncture group showed improvement. Only 18 percent of the standard control group and 10 percent of the visitation control group showed improvement. In addition, there was a 41-percent decrease in use of pain medication in the real acupuncture group, versus no change in the others (Helms, 1987). Furthermore, the improvement noted in the real acupuncture treatment group persisted beyond the end of the active treatment period.

Although acupuncture effects on pain problems can be considered purely subjective phenomena, acupuncture treatments also can be studied in terms of their effect on altering patient behavior and use of medical care. Bullock et al. (1989) studied 80 severe alcoholics through the Hennipen County, MN, alcohol detoxification program. These patients all had a history of repeated hospital admissions for alcoholism, or were severe recidivists. They were divided into two groups, a treatment group receiving acupuncture at specific ear acupuncture points and a control group treated with sham acupuncture points on the ear. The patients were treated for 45 days from the date of their last acute alcoholism hospital admission.

Six months after the treatment program the control (sham) group had nearly twice as many drinking episodes and admissions to detox centers as the treatment groups (Bullock et al., 1989). These types of results have caught the attention of public agencies and criminal justice systems across the country who are concerned with the cost of managing the social impact of people with severe drug abuse behavior.

Promising early evidence suggests that acupuncture can be cost-effective in conventional medical practice settings as well. In France, for example, statistics from the insurance syndicate show that physicians whose practice is at least 50 percent acupuncture cost the system considerably less for laboratory examinations, hospitalizations, and medication prescriptions than their non-acupuncture-practicing colleagues (Helms, 1993). In the United States, a pilot study on followup of chronic pain patients receiving acupuncture in a managed-care setting demonstrated a reduction of clinic visits, physical therapy visits, telephone consultations, and prescription costs in the 6 months following a short course of acupuncture therapy (Erickson, 1992).

In Denmark a study was made involving the 58 patients on a county health system's waiting list for elective knee replacement surgery. Forty-eight of these patients were considered candidates for a controlled trial of acupuncture therapy, and two-thirds (32) participated in the study. The subgroup treated with acupuncture initially showed improvement in both objective and subjective measures of knee function and a 50-percent reduction in nonsteroidal anti-inflammatory drug (NSAID) use after six treatments when this group was compared with its own baseline findings and with the untreated subgroup. The untreated patients were then treated with acupuncture and also showed improvement. Five of these were called for their elective surgery, and the remaining 17 continued in long-term followup for 49 weeks with monthly acupuncture treatments for maintenance. At the 1-year followup point, NSAID use in the group as a whole was still 20 percent less than the baseline measurements, and 22 percent (seven) of the study group had responded so well that they no longer desired knee replacement surgery. These seven patients constituted 12 percent of the original elective surgery waiting list (Christensen et al., 1992). Taken as a whole, these results suggest that wider use of acupuncture in the United States might reduce health care costs significantly as well as improve outcomes of selected conditions.

Future research opportunities. Basic research is needed to examine the effects of acupuncture beyond the pain management field. This extended basic research in acupuncture should address the broad range of clinically observed effects of acupuncture treatments, including improved physical health, improved emotional stability and cognitive functioning, and overall improvement in quality of life. State-of-the-art techniques for monitoring and detecting changes in body physiology (e.g., electroencephalography, brain mapping, single-photon emission tomography scans, positron emission tomography scans, and electromyographic mapping) could be used. Such techniques are useful in evaluating medical conditions in which patients do not show gross changes in standard biochemical measures.

Basic research in the bioelectromagnetic effect of acupuncture on the physical and energetic phenomena of the human body might present another modern correlation to the traditional concept of qi. (See the "Bioelectromagnetics Applications in Medicine" and "Manual Healing Methods" chapters.) The alterations by acupuncture of the neuropeptide chemicals involved in the digestive and immune responses also could be studied. This biochemical research would parallel the existing studies on pain relief with acupuncture. Another promising area is research into disorders of the autonomic nervous system and their alteration or correction by acupuncture.

Acupuncture's traditionally reported effects on improving the well-being of the whole person should be investigated using established psychological and behavioral health measures as well as standardized measurements of health status and quality of life. Since acupuncture is a procedural therapy involving an intentional interaction between the practitioner and the patient, acupuncture research is an appropriate area in which to investigate the interpersonal and transpersonal aspects of mind-body healing. (See the "Mind-Body Interventions" chapter.)

Acupuncture research in clinical medicine is entering a challenging period. With a broad base of research and practice supporting the safety and promising results of acupuncture in many clinical conditions, studies now need to be done to firmly establish the efficacy of acupuncture in comparison with other medical interventions for relevant health problems. There are three appropriate questions for clinical studies of acupuncture: (1) Is acupuncture efficacious for the condition under study in comparison with conventional or other alternative treatments? (2) Is acupuncture more than a placebo intervention for the specific conditions being studied? (3) Is the mechanism of acupuncture more than that of a nonspecific irritant stimulation? That is, does it matter where you stick the needle? These levels of research, done as controlled clinical trials, are necessary to answer treatment efficacy questions that are equivalent to those being studied in Phase III drug treatment trials. These initial studies should assist in correcting the "experimental" designations imposed by the FDA and the AMA on the practice of acupuncture.

Key issues. Because of the entrenched skepticism in American medicine regarding acupuncture, an extremely high standard of biostatistical and clinical expertise will be required for these acupuncture clinical trials. Unfortunately, as an operator-dependent procedure—a type of procedure that has individualized treatment protocols—acupuncture can be studied in a full-scale, blinded, randomized, placebo-controlled fashion in only a limited number of clinical conditions. Suggested areas for such placebo-controlled acupuncture research studies include treatment of acute low back pain, chronic osteoarthritis of the knee, cancer chemotherapy-induced nausea and vomiting, and pain related to dental procedures. Issues for which existing studies have been criticized, such as sample bias, inadequate statistical power, lack of appropriate controls, practitioner incompetence, and inappropriate treatment design, must be addressed to ensure that the data generated in new clinical trials are of the highest possible quality (ter Riet et al., 1990).

Furthermore, the drug model of biomedical research is appropriate for only a limited range of acupuncture investigations. For most clinical applications, acupuncture research trials will have to compare clinical effectiveness, that is, compare the outcome of courses of acupuncture treatment with clinical outcomes in non-acupuncture-treated or conventionally treated patients. (See the "Research Methodologies" chapter.) The priority areas for these acupuncture research studies should be based on considerations of public health importance, the inadequacy of current treatment methods owing to excessive side effects or cost, and the existing promising data in the global acupuncture research base. Attention to specificity of the diagnostic, therapeutic, and outcome criteria is necessary to allow compelling conclusions to be drawn about the effectiveness of acupuncture in disorders such as chronic headaches, urinary system dysfunction, respiratory disorders, allergies, neurological and orthopedic problems, and substance abuse problems.

Since acupuncture treatments for many of these health problems are individually designed and directed at improving the function of the whole person, specific research methods must be involved that will not only document alterations in a specific disease process but also validate the improved quality-of-life outcomes reported by patients who have been treated by experienced acupuncture practitioners.

Ayurvedic Medicine

Overview. Ayurveda is the traditional, natural system of medicine of India, which has been practiced for more than 5,000 years. Ayurveda provides an integrated approach to the prevention and treatment of illness through lifestyle interventions and a wide range of natural therapies. The term *Ayurveda* has its origins in the Sanskrit roots *ayus,* which means "life," and *veda,* which means "knowledge."

Ayurvedic theory states that all imbalance and disease in the body begin with imbalance or stress in the awareness, or consciousness, of the individual. This mental stress leads to unhealthy lifestyles, which further promote ill health. Therefore, mental techniques such as meditation are considered essential to the promotion of healing and to prevention.

Ayurveda describes all physical manifestations of disease as due to the imbalance of three basic physiological principles in the body, called *doshas,* which are believed to govern all bodily functions. Evaluation of these three doshas—*vata, pitta,* and *kapha*—is accomplished primarily by feeling the patient's pulse at the radial artery, which is a detailed and systematic technique called *nadi vigyan.* This evaluation determines the types of herbs prescribed, and it guides the physician in the application of all other ayurvedic therapies.

Specific lifestyle interventions are a major preventive and therapeutic approach in Ayurveda as well. Each patient is prescribed an individualized dietary, eating, sleeping, and exercise program depending on his or her constitutional type and the nature of the underlying dosha imbalance at the source of the illness. The Ayurvedic practitioner uses a variety of precise body postures, all derived from the age-old discipline of yoga; breathing exercises; and meditative techniques. These postures are used to create an individualized self-care program to improve both physical health and personal consciousness. In addition, herbal preparations are added to the patient's diet for preventive and rejuvenative purposes as well as for the treatment of specific disorders.

In addition to mental factors, lifestyle, and dosha imbalance, Ayurveda identifies a fourth major factor in disease: the accumulation of metabolic byproducts and toxins in the body tissues. Ayurvedic physical therapy, called *panchakarma,* consists of physical applications, including herbalized oil massage, herbalized heat treatments, and elimination therapies (e.g., therapies to improve bowel movements), which promote internal cleansing and removal of such toxic metabolic wastes. Certain of the agents used in panchakarma therapy are proposed to have free-radical scavenging, or antioxidant, effects (Fields et al., 1990). Free radicals are naturally occurring atoms or molecules that are highly reactive with anything they come into contact with. A recently developed theory suggests that free radicals play important roles in causing a wide range of degenerative and chronic disorders, including cancer and aging. Thus, substances with antioxidant properties may be effective in preventing, or even treating, myriad conditions. (See the "Diet and Nutrition" chapter for more information on free radicals and antioxidants.)

Ayurveda emphasizes the interdependence of the health of the individual and the quality of societal life. Therefore, measures to ensure the collective health of society, such as pollution control, community hygiene, the collective practice of meditation programs, and appropriate living conditions, are supported.

There are currently approximately 10 Ayurveda clinics in North America, including one hospital-based clinic, which together have served an estimated 25,000 patients since 1985 (Lonsdorf, 1993). More than 200 physicians have received training as Ayurvedic practitioners through the American Association of Ayurvedic Medicine, have received continuing medical education credit for Ayurvedic training programs, and have incorporated Ayurveda into their clinical practices as an adjunct to modern medicine (Lonsdorf, 1993). A modern revitalization of Ayurveda now being practiced in the United States and internationally is known as Maharishi Ayurveda. This approach utilizes a full range of physical and mental therapies from the Ayurvedic tradition.

In India, Ayurvedic practitioners receive State-recognized and -institutionalized training along with their physician counterparts in the Indian state-supported systems for conventional Western biomedicine and homeopathic medicine. A number of these Indian-trained Ayurvedic physicians practice or teach Ayurveda in the United States.

Research base. There have been extensive studies of the physiological effects of meditative techniques and yoga postures in both the Indian medical literature and the Western psychological literature (Funderburk, 1977; Murphy, 1992a; Murphy and Donovan, 1988). For example, students in hatha yoga classes showed improvement in fitness measures, including flexibility, strength, equilibrium, and stamina (Jharote, 1973).

In addition, effects of yogic postures and breathing on finger blood flow showed consistent changes with various breathing practices, changes that were more pronounced in trained yogic practitioners (Gopal et al., 1973). Changes in endocrine hormone measurements also have been associated with certain Ayurvedic practices (Glaser et al., 1992; Udupa et al., 1971). Measurement of metabolic rate, oxygen exchange, lung capacity, and red and white blood cell counts have been found to be associated with general yogic training and in some cases with specific *asanas* (posture) (Gopal et al., 1974). Similar basic research on meditative practices has led to the development in Western medicine of biofeedback and relaxation training (see the "Mind-Body Interventions" chapter).

Yogic and meditative practices also have been studied as specific interventions for disease states such as asthma and hypertension (Bhole,

1967; Patel, 1973). A recent pilot study performed in Holland followed a group of patients who used a combination of Ayurvedic therapies. The study documented improvements with Ayurvedic therapies in 79 percent of patients who were studied for a 3-month treatment period with a number of chronic disease conditions, including rheumatoid arthritis, asthma, chronic bronchitis, eczema, psoriasis, hypertension, constipation, headaches, chronic sinusitis, and non-insulin-dependent diabetes mellitus (Janssen, 1989).

In addition, published studies have documented reductions in cardiovascular disease risk factors, including blood pressure, cholesterol, and reaction to stress, in individuals practicing Ayurvedic methods (Schneider et al., 1992) and have shown improvement in overall health care utilization measures among meditators (Orme-Johnson, 1988).

The "technology" of meditative practices has been subjected to studies showing physiological changes of heart rate, blood pressure, brain cortex activity, metabolism, respiration, muscle tension, lactate level, skin resistance, salivation, and pain and stress responses (improvement), and both negative and positive behavioral effects (Murphy, 1992a).

Further laboratory and clinical studies on Ayurvedic herbal preparations and other therapies have shown them to have a wide range of potentially beneficial effects for the prevention and treatment of certain cancers, including breast, lung, and colon cancers (Sharma et al., 1990). They have also been shown effective in the treatment of mental health (Alexander et al., 1989b) and infectious disease (Thyagarajan et al., 1988), in health promotion (Schneider et al., 1990), and in treatment of aging (Alexander et al., 1989a; Glaser et al., 1992). Mechanisms underlying these effects are believed to include free-radical scavenging effects (Fields et al., 1990), immune system modulation, brain neurotransmitter modulation, and hormonal effects (Glaser et al., 1992). The National Cancer Institute (NCI) has included Ayurvedic compounds on its list of potential chemopreventive agents and has recently funded a series of in vitro studies on the cancer-preventive properties of two Ayurvedic herbal compounds, *maharadis amrit kalash* 4 and 5 (MAK–4 and MAK–5). In preliminary studies, NCI researchers have demonstrated that MAK–4 and MAK–5 significantly inhibited cancer cell growth in both human tumor and rat tracheal epithelial cell systems (Arnold et al., 1991).

Future research opportunities and priorities. Because of the potential of ayurvedic therapies for treating conditions for which modern medicine has few, if any, effective treatments, this area is a fertile one for research opportunities. For example, when NCI researchers began testing MAK–4 and MAK–5 for effects against tumor cell growth, they also found that similar compounds such as ferulic acid, catechin, bioflavonoids, retinoic acid (vitamin A), ascorbyl palmitate, and glycyrrhetinic acid also showed chemopreventive activity (Arnold et al., 1991).

Known scientific data on the intrinsic rhythms and laterality (right side vs. left side) patterns in the autonomic nervous system can provide a model for understanding how stress disrupts healthy physical function. Certain meditative and yogic practices have been proposed as non-invasive "technologies" to self-regulate the neural matrices that couple mind and metabolism in the body (Shannahoff-Khalsa, 1991). Translation of the traditional concepts of yogic medicine into the language of modern medicine could stimulate creative research in the neurophysiology of stress and adaptation.

The following are the research opportunities as well as the priorities for investigations in this area of alternative medicine:

1. Performing a critical review of world literature to identify potentially useful Ayurvedic therapies for various conditions.
2. Conducting long-term health care utilization and cost effectiveness studies on individuals who use Ayurvedic therapies, lifestyle programs, and meditation regularly for prevention.
3. Studying the effectiveness of Ayurvedic therapies and lifestyle for the prevention and treatment of diseases such as cardiovascular disease, cancer, AIDS, osteoporosis, autoimmune disorders, Alzheimer's, and aging.
4. Assessing the cost and treatment effectiveness of Ayurvedic therapies in the treatment of specific functional or chronic disorders such as chronic fatigue syndrome, premenstrual syndrome, chronic pain, functional bowel and

digestive problems, insomnia, allergies, and neuromuscular disorders.

5. Identifying the mechanisms underlying therapeutic effects of herbal therapies, diet, Ayurvedic physical therapies such as panchakarma, meditation, yogic practices, and other treatment modalities.

6. Studying the effects of the collective practice of meditation on community health indices and health care costs in cities, the Nation, and other social groups.

Homeopathic Medicine

Overview. The term *homeopathy* is derived from the Greek words *homeo* (similar) and *pathos* (suffering from disease). The first basic principles of homeopathy were formulated by the German physician Samuel Hahnemann in the late 1700s. Curious about why quinine could cure malaria, Hahnemann ingested quinine bark and experienced alternating bouts of chills, fever, and weakness, the classic symptoms of malaria. From this experience he derived the principle of similars, or "like cures like": that is, a substance that can cause certain symptoms when given to a healthy person can cure those same symptoms in someone who is sick.

Hahnemann spent the rest of his life extensively testing, or "proving," many common herbal and medicinal substances to find out what symptoms they could cause. He also began treating sick people, prescribing the medicine that most closely matched the symptoms of their illness. The information from this experimentation has been carefully recorded and makes up the homeopathic materia medica, a listing of medicines and their indications for use. According to the *Homeopathic Pharmacopoeia of the United States*, homeopathic medicines, or remedies, are made from naturally occurring plant, animal, and mineral substances.

By the end of the 19th century, homeopathy was widely practiced in the United States, when there were 22 homeopathic medical schools, more than 100 homeopathic hospitals, and an estimated 15 percent of physicians practicing homeopathy. The practice of homeopathy (along with other types of alternative medicine) declined dramatically in the United States following the publication of the Flexner Report in 1910, which established guidelines for the funding of medical schools. These guidelines favored AMA-approved institutions and virtually crippled competing schools of medicine. In the past 15 years, however, there has been a resurgence of interest in homeopathy in this country. It is estimated that approximately 3,000 physicians and other health care practitioners currently use homeopathy, and a recent survey showed that 1 percent of the general population, or approximately 2.5 million people, had sought help from a homeopathic doctor in 1990 (Eisenberg et al., 1993).

Those who are licensed to practice homeopathy in the United States vary according to state-by-state "scope of practice" guidelines, but they include M.D.s, D.O.s, dentists, naturopaths (N.D.s), chiropractors, veterinarians, acupuncturists, nurse practitioners, and physician assistants. Three states now have specific licensing boards for homeopathic physicians: Arizona, Connecticut, and Nevada. Specialty certification diplomas for those prescribing homeopathic drugs are established through national boards of examination for M.D.s/D.O.s and N.D.s. Self-help as well as professional training courses in homeopathy are offered through the National Center for Homeopathy (NCH) in Alexandria, Virginia. NCH serves as an umbrella organization for consumer support of homeopathy as well as a focus for coordination among an increasing number of organizations and specialty societies offering lay and professional training programs in homeopathy.

Homeopathic medicine also is currently widely practiced worldwide, especially in Europe, Latin America, and Asia. In France, 32 percent of family physicians use homeopathy, while 42 percent of British physicians refer patients to homeopaths (Bouchayer, 1990; Wharton and Lewith, 1986). In India, homeopathy is practiced in the national health service, and there are more than 100 homeopathic medical colleges and more than 100,000 homeopathic physicians (Kishore, 1983).

In the United States today, the homeopathic drug market has grown to become a multimillion-dollar industry; a significant increase has occurred in the importation and domestic marketing of homeopathic drugs. Homeopathic remedies are recognized and regulated by the FDA and are manufactured by established pharmaceutical companies under strict guidelines established by the *Homeopathic Pharmacopoeia of the*

United States. Products that are offered for the treatment of serious conditions must be dispensed under the care of a licensed practitioner. Other products offered for the use of self-limiting conditions such as colds and allergies may be marketed as over-the-counter drugs.

Homeopathy is used to treat both acute and chronic health problems as well as for health prevention and promotion in healthy people. Homeopathic medicines are prescribed on the basis of a wide constellation of physical, emotional, and mental symptoms. The one remedy that most closely fits all of the symptoms of a given individual is called the *similimum* for that person. Thus, homeopathic treatment is individualized, and two or more people with the same diagnosis may be given different medicines, depending on the specific symptoms of illness in each person. A person with a sore throat, for instance, may need one of six or seven common remedies for sore throats, depending on whether the pain is worse on the right or left side, what time of day it is worse, what the person's mood is, and his or her body temperature, thirst, and appetite (Jouanny, 1980).

Hahnemann also discovered that if the homeopathic remedies were "potentized" by diluting them in a water-alcohol solution and then shaking, side effects could be diminished. He found that after the medicines were potentized to high dilutions, there was still a medicinal effect, and side effects were minimal. Some homeopathic medicines are diluted to concentrations as low as 10^{-30} to $10^{-20,000}$. This particular aspect of homeopathic theory and practice has caused many modern scientists to reject homeopathic medicine outright. Critics of homeopathy contend that such extreme dilutions of the medicines are beyond the point at which any molecules of the medicine can theoretically still be found in the solution (When to believe..., 1988).

On the other hand, scientists who accept the validity of homeopathic theory suggest several theories to explain how highly diluted homeopathic medicines may act. Using recent developments in quantum physics, they have proposed that electromagnetic energy may exist in the medicines and interact with the body on some level (Delinick, 1991). Researchers in physical chemistry have proposed the "memory of water" theory, whereby the structure of the water-alcohol solution is altered by the medicine during the process of dilution and retains this structure even after none of the actual substance remains (Davenas et al., 1988).

Recent research accomplishments. Basic science research in homeopathy has primarily involved investigations into the chemical and biological activity of highly diluted substances. The most thought-provoking research has involved observation of the physiological responses of living systems to homeopathically potentized solutions. For example, in the 1920s a German researcher conducted a series of studies spanning 12 years in which he showed periodic variations in the growth patterns of plants that had been exposed to a series of homeopathic dilutions of metallic salts (Kolisko, 1932). With the focus of modern biological laboratory research on cellular and organ function, homeopathic studies have more recently been conducted in this area. Such laboratory studies have shown positive effects of homeopathically prepared microdoses on mouse white blood cells (Davenas et al., 1987), arsenic excretion in the rat (Cazin et al., 1987), bleeding time with aspirin (Doutremepuich et al., 1987), and degranulation of human basophils—blood cells that mediate allergic reactions—(Davenas et al., 1988; Poitevin et al., 1988).

Furthermore, recent clinical trials in Europe have suggested a positive effect of homeopathic medicines on such conditions as allergic rhinitis (Reilly et al., 1986), fibrositis (Fisher et al., 1989), and influenza (Ferley et al., 1989), while an earlier study showed no apparent effect in the treatment of osteoarthritis by a homeopathic medicine (Shipley et al., 1983). The *British Medical Journal* published a meta-analysis in 1992 of homeopathic clinical trials, which found that 15 of 22 well-designed studies showed positive results. This study concluded that more methodologically rigorous trials should be done to address the question of efficacy of homeopathic treatment (Kleijnen et al., 1991). A recent double-blind study comparing homeopathic treatment with placebo in the treatment of acute childhood diarrhea found a statistically significant improvement in the group receiving the homeopathic treatment (Jacobs et al., 1993).

Homeopathic research study design has used different methodologies depending on the question being asked. One of the earliest studies of homeopathy in a peer-reviewed conventional medical journal asked the question, "Is the homeopathic medical system taken *as a whole* more effective or less detrimental than another treatment or placebo in the condition studied?" In this study, which focused on rheumatoid arthritis, 195 patients who had previously been treated with nonsteroidal anti-inflammatory drugs were allocated to placebo treatment or active treatment. The active-treatment population then was divided between aspirin and a homeopathic medication. The homeopathic doctors were allowed to prescribe any medication at whatever interval, frequency, or potency they considered appropriate.

The trial was conducted for a year, and by the end of the year almost 43 percent of the homeopathic treatment group had stopped other treatments and were judged to have improved since the beginning of the study. Another 24 percent of the homeopathic group improved, but they continued on their conventional medications. In contrast, only 15 percent of the aspirin group were maintained and improved on the treatment. The entire placebo group had dropped out within 6 weeks.

This study, however, was criticized on some methodological grounds—principally that the homeopathic prescribers were more committed to the treatment and the patients were easily able to determine who was in the placebo group (Gibson et al., 1978). Subsequently, the same researchers conducted another trial of this type, in which a specific disease was subjected to homeopathic treatment by any one of a number of clinically indicated homeopathic medications. This time, a placebo-controlled, double-blind study showed that the improvements among the homeopathically treated patients were statistically more significant than those of the placebo group (Gibson et al., 1980).

A second type of homeopathic study has been used to ask a more specific question, namely, Is a particular homeopathic medication more effective than another treatment or placebo for a particular disease? Fisher and colleagues (1989) asked this question in a study of primary fibromyalgia, a type of inflammation; patients who met recognized diagnostic criteria for fibromyalgia were further stratified as patients for whom a particular homeopathic medicine, rhus toxicodendron 6C, was homeopathically indicated. Patients with the active treatment were better on all variables, and a number of their tender points were reduced by 25 percent at the end of 4 weeks of active treatment in comparison with controls.

In a similar study, Reilly and colleagues (1986) used homeopathic medications with hay fever patients to address the issue of whether homeopathic medications are in fact placebos. The researchers directly treated matched groups of approximately 70 patients with a homeopathic medication made from mixed grass pollens at the dilution of one part in 10^{60}. This was done to address the assertion that a potency lacking in any of the original substances could act as more than a placebo. Patients took one tablet twice daily of either placebo or the test drug and were free to use a standard antihistamine at any time during the 5-week study. Only the homeopathically treated group showed a clear reduction in symptoms, and in comparison with the placebo-treated group, twice as many of the homeopathically treated patients had discontinued their antihistamines. This study also demonstrated that even a simple study design requires careful analysis of potential confounding variables, including the clinical observations that some homeopathically treated patients experience temporary aggravation of their symptoms before achieving a sustained improvement.

A third type of study simply looks at comparative utilization figures for homeopathic practitioners in a health care system with or without attention to the comparative clinical outcomes. For example, in France, research on cost-effectiveness has shown that the annual cost to the social security system for a homeopathic physician is 54 percent lower than the cost for a conventional physician. Moreover, the same study found that the price of the average homeopathic medicine is one-third that of standard drugs (CNAM, 1991).

Research opportunities. Research into the basic science areas of quantum physics, physical chemistry, and biochemistry may determine whether a homeopathic medicine's mechanism of action can be elucidated. Existing studies of the effects of the succussion process on the physical-energetic nature of medicinal dilutions should be repeated and extended (Smith and Boericke, 1967). Moreover, modern-day herbal, biological, or pharmaceutically synthesized agents should be subjected to homeopathic "provings." This scientific documentation of effects and side effects in healthy people would enable new homeopathic drug development.

Evaluating the clinical efficacy of homeopathy using randomized, double-blind clinical trials for the treatment of acute problems such as diarrhea, otitis media, and postoperative pain as well as for chronic illnesses is a fertile area for research. Existing studies should be repeated with different investigators, giving attention to rigorous methodology. Special emphasis should be given to research in areas where modern medicine does not have an established, satisfactory solution, such as arthritis, AIDS, asthma, headaches, and inflammatory bowel disease.

More clinical research also needs to be directed toward analyzing and improving the accuracy of the clinical data in the homeopathic literature, much of which is currently at least a century old. Indeed, homeopaths in Great Britain are currently establishing a system using a modern, computerized medical database and standardized subjective and objective outcome measures to analyze the outcomes of patients treated with various homeopathic medications (van Haseln and Fisher, 1990). This sort of study will help homeopathic clinicians to investigate the differential efficacy of various homeopathic medications and allow for an updating of the prescribing criteria for various medications in the homeopathic materia medica.

In addition to clinical trials on conditions with specific diagnoses, studies also need to be done to evaluate the possible benefits of long-term treatment with the system of homeopathic medicine. Since proponents of this discipline claim that homeopathy improves overall physical and mental health, health status indicators should be used to evaluate changes in health in patients treated this way for several months or years.

Recent surveys in the United States found that most homeopathic patients seek care for chronic illnesses (Jacobs and Crothers, 1991) and that homeopathic physicians spend twice as much time with their patients, order half as many laboratory tests and procedures, and prescribe fewer drugs (Jacobs, 1992). Since treatment of chronic illness accounts for a large proportion of health care expenditures in the United States, the cost-effectiveness of homeopathic medicine should be investigated by comparing homeopathy with conventional treatments for specific chronic illnesses such as recurrent childhood ear infections, allergies, arthritis, headaches, depression, and asthma. Clinical outcomes should be measured as well as such factors as utilization of health services, number of missed days of work or school, patient satisfaction, and overall cost of health care. This research will help determine whether incorporating homeopathy into the national health care scheme would significantly reduce health care costs.

Anthroposophically Extended Medicine

Overview. The foundations of anthroposophically extended medicine were laid down by the Austrian philosopher and spiritual scientist Rudolf Steiner, Ph.D. (1861–1925). Steiner's "anthroposophy" (*anthropos* [human]; *sophia* [wisdom]) proposed a philosophical or spiritual-scientific model of human individuality. He took rigorous precision and methodologies of scientific empiricism and extended them into the spiritual domain, into what he called the "supersensible world," the domain underlying all human life, thought, and physical well-being. Steiner's theories were applied to agriculture (biodynamics), education (Waldorf Schools), and social theories (threefold social order) as well as art, painting, sculpture, dance (eurythmy), architecture, music, and speech (e.g., for performance, education, and therapeutics).

In the 1920s Ita Wegman, M.D. (a Dutch physician, 1876–1943), and Steiner coauthored a foundational work for physicians seeking to broaden their medical practice according to these anthroposophical principles (Steiner and Wegman, 1925). Steiner's intention was to outline a "rationally exact medical mode of thinking" as part of his larger, lifelong program of approaching issues of spiritual knowledge as a scientist. He gave an extended series of lectures and training courses for physicians, nurses, social workers, and pastoral counselors. This effort to extend therapeutics through the anthroposophical paradigm was based on Steiner's 34 years of work with the scientific method and encompassed therapeutic efforts based on botany, anatomy, natural sciences, and the dynamics of healing. Steiner and his physician followers attempted to reorient medical therapeutics so that they would encompass the spiritual depths of human existence. "Medicine will be broadened by a spiritual conception of man to an *art of healing* or else it will remain a souless technology that removes only symptoms. Through the concrete inclusion of the spirit and soul of man, a humanization of medicine is possible" (Wolff, undated).

As an extension of Western medicine, anthroposophical medicine builds on three preexisting movements and therapeutics. The first is natural medicine or naturopathy, which involves the use of material substances in nondegraded, nonchemically separated forms. Naturopathy, established in Europe in the early 19th century, is now practiced in an increasing number of States in the United States (see below). The second foundation is homeopathy, introduced by the German physician Samuel Hahnemann in the 18th century (see the "Homeopathic Medicine" section). The third foundation for anthroposophical medicine is modern scientific medicine itself. Steiner insisted that anthroposophically extended medicine be practiced only on the foundation of a Western medical training and credentials, and thus only M.D.s could become anthroposophical physicians.

Estimates of the number of M.D.s who mainly or exclusively practice anthroposophical medicine range from 1,000 to 6,000 worldwide with between 30 and 100 such physicians in the United States (Ministry of Science and Technology, Federal Republic of Germany, 1992; Scharff, 1993). Most practitioners are concentrated in Switzerland, Germany, Sweden, and Holland, and there are more than a dozen hospitals and clinics in Europe specializing in anthroposophically extended medicine. The Witten-Herdecke Medical School, established in 1983 near Dortmund, Germany, teaches anthroposophical medicine and grants M.D. degrees. Efforts are under way to formally certify physicians with anthroposophical training, and the Board of the American College of Anthroposophically Extended Medicine has been established in the United States (Scharff, 1993).

Hundreds of uniquely formulated medications are used in anthroposophical practice. Some are prepared by a multiple dilution and succussion (potentization) process, which is similar to that used in standard homeopathic pharmaceuticals. About 85 percent of the remedies are such potentized preparations, and the remaining 15 percent are similar to other botanical or traditional herbal medicines. All the basic substances go through a standardized pharmaceutical process and are made into remedies according to the official pharmacopoeia of the country of manufacture. The preparation of medications seeks to match the "archetypal forces" in plants, animals, and minerals with disease processes in humans and, through this correspondence, to stimulate healing.

Two major pharmaceutical firms prepare anthroposophical medications for physicians around the world: Waleda and Wala, which are both located in Europe with subsidiaries in many countries, including the United States. Use of these products is not limited exclusively to anthroposophical medicine specialists. In the United States approximately 300 physicians regularly order anthroposophical pharmaceuticals, while in Germany up to 15,000 physicians prescribe these products, mainly preparations of the mistletoe plant for treatment of cancers (Ministry of Science and Technology, Federal Republic of Germany, 1992).

Today, anthroposophical physicians augment conventional science by including new scientific approaches to the living processes of nature, the soul, and the human spirit. One model for approaching this task is to identify three different interdependent aspects of a human's body-mind processes. First, the "sense-nerve" system, which includes the nervous system and the brain organization that support the mind and the thinking process. Second, there is the "rhythmic" system, which includes physical processes of a rhythmic or periodic nature (e.g., the pulse, breathing, intestinal rhythms) and supports the emotional or feeling processes. Third is the "metabolic-limb" system, which includes digestion, elimination, energetic metabolism, and the voluntary movement processes. This third system supports the aspects of human behavior that express the will.

This threefold model gives the physician a diagnostic scheme for understanding an illness as a deviation from the harmonious internal balance of the functions of the bodily self and the spiritual self. In this approach, a person's physical, human makeup is seen as continually interacting with the soul or spiritual nature of that person. This anthroposophical model is used by practitioners as a creative entry for therapeutic insight into what are now recognized as the processes of mind-body interactions in health and disease.

Research base. Much of the research in the field of anthroposophically extended medicine has been connected with attempts to understand the nature of disease, assess it qualitatively, and understand how the essential properties of the objects under investigation could be applied in therapy. For instance, Steiner suggested that mistletoe might have a role in cancer therapy. It was observed that mistletoe had unusual biological properties as a relatively undifferentiated plant as well as a tendency to show regular rhythmic changes in both a seasonal and a lunar cycle. From this observation came an extensive series of studies in Europe on iscador, iscucin, abnoba, vysorel, and helixor, cancer remedies made from mistletoe. This work suggests that these mistletoe remedies can stimulate the body's immunological defense systems and act as chemostatic agents to prevent further growth of tumors. Mistletoe extracts have been analyzed for their chemical fractions, which include lectins, polysaccharides, and proteins. A review of 36 controlled clinical trials using mistletoe in cancer therapy showed six as statistically significant, having results pointing to a life-extending effect (Keine, 1989). (See the "Pharmacological and Biological Treatments" chapter and the "Research Methodologies" chapter for further information on mistletoe research.)

In recent years, collaboration between anthroposophical scientists and established university-based researchers has led to improvement in the quality and mutual acceptability of "unconventional" anthroposophical research in Germany. Of particular note is the work done by Professor G. Hildebrandt and his colleagues at the University of Marburg. In the past 30 years they have contributed more than 500 papers to the world's scientific literature, placing particular emphasis on the chronobiology (biorhythms) of body physiology in stress, disease, and therapy (Hildebrandt and Hensel, 1982; Hildebrandt, 1986). An example of the application of this line of research is shown by the work of von Laue and Henn, who reported studies of the time rhythms of cancer patients and tumor growths and how these abnormal rhythmic functions in cancer could be altered with mistletoe therapy (von Laue and Henn, 1991).

The qualitative and analytical aspects of anthroposophical research are further illustrated in the psychosomatic field by the work of Fischer and Grosshans with colitis patients at Herdecke Hospital. They conducted a structured interview with 60 patients admitted with ulcerative colitis or Crohn's disease (inflammations of the bowel) for a 2-year period and found that in addition to the well-known physical characteristics of these two diseases, the patients displayed other characteristic behaviors, including distinct underlying mood tendencies, communication styles, self-perceptions, and typical attitudinal relationships to past and future events. These psychological responses differentiated the Crohn's disease and ulcerative colitis patients along a pattern that could be interpreted as a parallel to the clinical symptoms (Fischer and Grosshans, 1992).

Cost and effectiveness issues in health care delivery are important in European countries as well as the United States. In Germany, von Hauff and Praetorius, an economist and a political scientist, conducted a pilot study (1990) on the performance structure of alternative medical practices. They used a nonrandom poll of established practitioners of conventional, homeopathic, or anthroposophical practices and were able to qualitatively analyze the practices under consideration as well as show quantitative differences in health care utilization. They found that the patients being treated by homeopathic and anthroposophical practitioners claimed 30 percent to 50 percent fewer illness days, respectively, than patients being treated by conventional practitioners. Furthermore, the homeopathic and anthroposophical practices had fewer referrals for hospitalization, fewer referrals to specialists, and fewer laboratory tests.

Research opportunities. Anthroposophical physicians approach issues of medical research by stressing basic methodological issues. For instance, the current dominant model of medical practice based on classical physics is seen as inadequate for understanding the laws of living organisms. This criticism extends to clinical research, where anthroposophical principles emphasize the overall therapeutic strategies being studied and not the isolated effect of specific chemical medicines. A truly scientific research agenda, according to the anthroposophical approach, must match the study methods and questions posed with the subject under investigation. In other words, inorganic systems require one type of science, living organic systems require another, psychological processes another, and intellectual-spiritual activities yet another. Although a single rational scientific method may be valid throughout these various domains of human endeavor, the specific nature of the scientific approach must be different and appropriate to the context of each domain. A recent poll in Germany of anthroposophical physicians identified this methodological issue as the major problem for future medical research (Ministry of Science and Technology, Federal Republic of Germany, 1992).

Particular areas of recommended research for anthroposophical medicine include the following:

- Establishing comprehensive valid criteria for assessing quality-of-life outcomes in therapy trials.
- Conducting comparison trials of isolated active ingredients versus extracts from the whole plant.
- Comparing a single-therapy approach to a combination-therapy approach (e.g., medical treatment, diet, and curative eurythmy artistic therapies for groups of patients with given clinical conditions).
- Documenting the effect of the use of anthroposophical remedies from a chronobiological perspective.
- Prospectively evaluating the effect of using anthroposophical methods for early detection and correction of tendencies toward illness before they manifest as serious pathology requiring expensive medical interventions.

Naturopathic Medicine

Overview. As a distinct American health care profession, naturopathic medicine is almost 100 years old. It was founded as a formal health care system at the turn of the century by a variety of medical practitioners from various natural therapeutic disciplines. By the early 1900s there were more than 20 naturopathic medical schools, and naturopathic physicians, called "eclectic" physicians at the time, were licensed in most of the States. After the Flexner Report in 1910 and the rise in belief that pharmaceutical drugs could eliminate all disease, the practice of naturopathic medicine experienced a dramatic decline. It has experienced a resurgence in the past two decades, however, as a health-conscious public began to seek natural therapies delivered by professionals skilled in these modalities.

Today, there are more than 1,000 licensed naturopathic doctors (N.D.s) in the United States. Currently, there are two accredited U.S. naturopathic medical schools: the National College of Naturopathic Medicine (NCNM) in Portland, OR, and Bastyr College of Natural Sciences in Seattle, WA, which graduate approximately 50 physicians each per year. A third naturopathic medical school, Southwest College of Naturopathic Medicine in Scottsdale, AZ, began classes in September 1993. Seven U.S. States and four Canadian provinces grant licenses to practice naturopathic medicine. In addition, a number of other States have legal statutes that allow the practice of naturopathic medicine within a specific context. The American Association of Naturopathic Physicians publishes the *Journal of Naturopathic Medicine,* which includes articles on original research, research reviews, and news and review articles relating to naturopathic medicine.

As it is practiced today, naturopathic medicine integrates traditional natural therapeutics—including botanical medicine, clinical nutrition, homeopathy, acupuncture, traditional oriental medicine, hydrotherapy, and naturopathic manipulative therapy—with modern scientific medical diagnostic science and standards of care. Naturopathic physicians are trained in anatomy, cell biology, nutrition, physiology, pathology, neurosciences, histology, pharmacology, biostatistics, epidemiology, public health, and other conventional medical disciplines, and they receive specialized training in the alternative medicine disciplines. They integrate this knowledge into a cohesive medical practice and tailor their approaches to the needs of an individual patient according to these eight primary principles:

1. Recognition of the inherent healing ability of the body.
2. Identification and treatment of the cause of diseases rather than mere elimination or suppression of symptoms.

3. Use of therapies that do no harm.
4. The doctor's primary role as teacher.
5. Establishment and maintenance of optimal health and balance.
6. Treatment of the whole person.
7. Prevention of disease through a healthy lifestyle and control of risk factors.
8. Therapeutic use of nutrition to promote health and to combat chronic and degenerative diseases.

Research base. Medical research on naturopathic practice is based on the empirical documentation of treatments with case history observations, medical records, and summaries of practitioners' clinical experiences. Naturopathic physicians have conducted scientific research in natural medicines in China, Germany, India, France, and England as well as U.S. research in clinical nutrition.

The two current accredited naturopathic medical schools have active research departments. For example, NCNM participated in a 10-year nationwide study of the cervical cap as a method of birth control. Study conclusions were submitted to the FDA (National College of Naturopathic Medicine Clinical Faculty, 1991). Naturopathic researchers also have investigated the pharmacology and physiological effects of nutritional and natural therapeutic agents (Barrie et al., 1987a, 1987b; Mittman, 1990). Digestive tract stresses and their treatment with natural methods also have been a focus of study (Blair et al., 1991; Collins and Mittman, 1990; Thom, 1992), and naturopathic physicians have been active in the investigation of new homeopathic remedies (Brown and Lange, 1992).

Naturopathic medical researchers have shown a particular interest in the natural treatment of women's health problems. One series of clinical research studies evaluated a naturopathic treatment protocol for women with cervical dysplasia (abnormal Pap smears). All subjects received oral nutritional and botanical supplementation, local topical cleansings, and suppositories made from herbal and nutritional agents (Hudson, 1991). Eight distinct naturopathic protocols were used depending on the severity of the abnormal Pap smears. Treatment included topical applications of *Bromelia, Calendula,* zinc chloride, and *Sanguinaria.* Additional home treatments included vaginal suppositories with myrrh, *Echinacea, Usnea, Hydrastis, Althaea,* geranium, and yarrow. The patients also used vitamin A suppositories, vitamin C, beta-carotene, folic acid, selenium, and *Lomatium* systemically as well as a botanical formula including (a) *Trifolium,* (b) *Taraxacum,* (c) *Glycyrrhiza* and *Hydrastis,* or (d) *Thuja* plus *Echinacea* and *Ligustrum* (Hudson, 1993b).

Of the 43 women in the study, 38 returned to normal Pap smears and normal tissue biopsy. Three had partial improvement, two showed no change, and none progressed toward more advanced disease states during treatment (Hudson, 1993a). It was suggested that partial use of these protocols might also benefit the long-term outcome in patients undergoing conventional treatment of cervical dysplasia including cryosurgery, conization, or loop electrosurgical excision procedures.

The most recently completed naturopathic study in women's health tested the clinical and endocrine effects of a botanical formula as an alternative to estrogen replacement therapy. Results of this study suggest a clinically significant benefit (measured as reduction in the total number of menopausal symptoms) in 100 percent of the women versus 17 percent in the placebo group (Hudson and Standish, 1993).

Future research opportunities. The following areas in the field of naturopathy offer the best opportunities for yielding significant research results:

- Clinical trials on naturopathic botanical formulas as an alternative to hormone replacement therapy.
- Effects of individual herbs on specific disease, for example, *Glycyrrhiza* for peptic ulcer disease, *Crataegus* for hypertension, *Echinacea* as an antiviral, *Ulmus fulva* for irritable bowel, and *Taraxacum* as a diuretic.
- Evaluations of the postsurgical outcomes of patients who have used naturopathic medicine to accelerate healing and improve their recovery.
- Evaluations of naturopathic protocols for treatment of hyperlipidemia, cervical dysplasia, otitis media, diabetes, and hypertension.

- Clinical trials on the outcome of breast cancer patients who use naturopathic medicine with their conventional therapy versus patients who use only conventional treatment.
- Facilitation of research into ethnomedicines by documenting oral traditions and studying them in the context of their cultures—for example, hydrotherapy and European traditions, native plants of developing countries and their local use by native healers, and traditional diets of native peoples.
- Clinical trials to evaluate the effectiveness of combination naturopathic medical protocols and rigorous evaluation of single-agent botanical medicines and naturopathic modalities in the treatment of HIV and AIDS.

Environmental Medicine

Overview. Environmental medicine is an alternative system of medical practice based on the science of assessing the impact of environmental factors on health. It is the result of continuing study of the interfaces among chemicals, foods, and inhalants in the environment and the biological function of the individual.

Environmental medicine traces its roots to the practice of allergy treatment. In the 1940s Theron Randolph, the founding father of environmental medicine, identified a wide range of medical problems he believed were caused by food allergies. Working with the techniques developed by Herbert Rinkel, Randolph identified multiple symptoms due to a variety of common foods such as corn, wheat, milk, and eggs—symptoms previously unrecognized as caused by food exposure. Using Rinkel's method of unmasking food allergies by avoiding the suspect food for at least 4 days before challenging, Randolph was able to identify food-related triggers for symptoms such as arthritis, asthma, depression and anxiety, enuresis, colitis, fatigue, hyperactivity, and others (Randolph, 1962).

In the 1950s Randolph noted that in small amounts, chemicals such as natural gas, industrial solvents, pesticides, car exhaust, and formaldehyde were also responsible for significant and previously unrecognized health problems (Randolph, 1962). It was noted that certain individuals were more sensitive to these minute exposures and that illness could be triggered in such hypersensitive individuals by amounts of chemicals that most people could tolerate without apparent symptoms.

Many of the findings of Randolph and others were originally identified through the use of environmental control units (strictly controlled environments in hospitals). In these settings, patients' allergies and sensitivities were unmasked through fasting and complete avoidance of incitant chemicals. When foods or chemicals were introduced in a systematic fashion, cause and effect could be identified. Today there are several environmental control units in the United States and a Canadian Government-sponsored unit in Nova Scotia, Canada.

Through careful and detailed environmentally focused clinical observations of thousands of patients, Randolph and others developed a new model and associated clinical principles that helped explain and treat many of the complex problems seen in medical practice today. By assessing the interaction between the individual's internal state and exposure to external factors, the physician may understand the cause of an illness. This type of medical practice goes beyond traditional medical concepts because it emphasizes the effects of food and chemicals in health.

The problems treated by environmental medicine include both diagnosis of problems that are traditionally considered allergic problems—asthma, hay fever, allergic rhinoconjunctivitis, eczema, and anaphylactic food allergies mediated by immunoglobulin E (IgE) antibody as well as other factors—and other diagnoses for which the underlying immunological aspects are not yet understood: arthritis, colitis, depression, fatigue, attention deficit disorder, cardiovascular disease, migraine and other headaches, urinary tract disorders, and other functional illnesses.

Of particular importance is the recognition of the effects of chemicals in the home and workplace, such as in the "sick building syndrome." With the changing environment found in workplaces and homes as well as outdoors, the incidence of environmentally triggered illness has increased. Chemically induced environmental illness is already affecting 4 million to 5 million Americans, and it is estimated that no more than 5 percent have been identified and treated. If patients with problems stemming from environmental exposure are not seen by a physician knowledgeable in environmental illness, they are often misdiagnosed or told they have psychiatric problems or hypochondriases (Randolph and Moss, 1980; Rea and Mitchell, 1982).

In 1965, Randolph and his colleagues founded the Society for Clinical Ecology to further explore the connection between the environment and illness. Today, courses organized by the American Academy of Environmental Medicine are available for training in the techniques and principles of this field. This organization, the successor to the Society for Clinical Ecology, has annual scientific meetings to further research and education. It publishes the peer-reviewed journal *Environmental Medicine* (formerly *Clinical Ecology*).

Today, environmental medicine is a medical specialty practiced by more than 3,000 physicians worldwide, most of them in the United States, Canada, and Great Britain. Many of these clinicians and researchers are members of one of the following professional medical organizations: the American Academy of Environmental Medicine, the Pan American Allergy Society, or the American Academy of Otolaryngologic Allergy. More than 50 percent of the members in the American Academy of Environmental Medicine are board certified in one or more of 19 medical specialties. The binding factor in these diverse physicians' backgrounds is an expanded view of health and illness, including an emphasis on the role the environment plays in a wide variety of medical disorders. This view of health and illness allows environmental medicine to be considered as an "alternative system" of medical practices developed from within the Western heritage of biomedical science.

Principles of environmental medicine. Many complex problems in medicine are called *idiopathic:* there is no readily apparent cause for the illness. The conventional medical model holds that similar illnesses have the same cause in all patients and should be treated similarly. This is not the case in the paradigm of environmental medicine.

Environmental medicine recognizes that illness in the individual can be caused by a broad range of inciting substances, including foods; chemicals found in the home and workplace; chemicals in air, water, and food; and inhalant materials, including pollens, molds, dust, dust mites, and danders. Individual susceptibility to these exposures can vary widely. The response to these exposures over time is specific to each person's own level of susceptibility and can manifest differently from person to person. Therefore, the specific symptoms and illnesses developed depend on all these factors, and environmental medicine attempts to answer the question why a particular patient has a particular symptom at a particular time.

One key to understanding the diagnosis in environmental medicine is a detailed chronological history. The emphasis of this history is on environmentally focused events and stressors over time. A thorough medical history and a physical examination are also needed. The detail of the home and work environment is explored to identify possible incitants.

The factors contributing to the sensitivity of the patient are related to genetics, nutritional status, effectiveness of detoxification pathways, and total allergic and chemical load at the time. Biochemical individuality determines the adequacy of nutritional stores and influences the ability to operate the detoxification pathways effectively and thus contributes to the individual's degree of sensitivity. Other factors that can induce immune system dysfunction, such as emotional stress, may have a major impact on the outcome of an exposure to a chemical toxin, a food exposure, or an inhalant contact.

The onset of illness coincides with the person's inability to continue coping with the total *allergic load.* This onset can occur either with a large acute exposure or with low-level, gradual exposures. The total allergic load is defined as the total level of exposure to substances that the person can be sensitive to, and it varies significantly over time. The total allergic load is often the determining factor in maintaining health (homeostasis) versus falling ill.

Environmental medicine practitioners believe that large amounts of toxic substances affect all those exposed, but minute amounts affect only those who are susceptible to the material. This fact explains the varied response to a material such as formaldehyde; 10 percent of the population is highly sensitive to small amounts of this poison and 90 percent is not. Thus, a susceptible person may get sick from a small workplace exposure, while others who are not susceptible suffer no ill effects. This situation often leads to missing a diagnosis while ignoring the patient's individual susceptibility. Indeed, many patients and physicians are unaware of the effects of chemical exposures as a contributing factor in illnesses. As a result, patients are often labeled "hypochondriacs" or told their illness is psychosomatic ("all in their mind") (Choffres, 1987; Davis, 1985; Saifer and Saifer, 1987).

Another concept that can help to explain the course of events in environmental illnesses is *adaptation*. Adaptation is the process by which the body attempts to maintain homeostasis. There are four distinct phases of adaptation: *preadapted-nonadapted* (alarm), *adapted* (masked), *maladapted*, and *exhausted-nonadapted*. The first three stages occur sequentially and if left uninterrupted can lead to the *exhausted* stage, or the onset of disease.

An example of adaptation phenomena is a sensitivity to wheat. At first exposure, wheat might cause symptoms such as fatigue (preadapted phase). After further exposure, the homeostatic mechanism creates an adapted state with no reactions. On further and frequent exposure, however, overt symptoms can occur (maladapted phase); for example, headaches to wheat may be labeled migraine and treated with medication. Eventually, with continued exposure, more serious symptoms can occur (exhausted phase). If the person stops being exposed to the food for at least 4 days and challenging (deadaptation) then causes the symptoms to reappear, cause and effect have been observed clearly. This sequence can also be seen with low-level chemical exposures.

Another observed phenomenon in environmental medicine is the *spreading phenomenon*. There are two aspects: (1) new onset of acute or chronic susceptibility to previously tolerated substances, and (2) spreading of susceptibility to new target organs. These events can occur with a single large exposure to a chemical that damages particular biological mechanisms and causes sensitivity to occur to other chemicals in addition to the primary incitant substance. This phenomenon is frequently seen with solvent or pesticide exposure causing a person to become a "universal reactor" to many other chemicals.

The type of symptoms experienced in the reaction to an offending substance (food, chemical, or inhalant) is not specific to the substance but is determined by a combination of factors specific to the person. In contrast, all individuals exposed to a highly toxic chemical have similar symptoms (e.g., respiratory symptoms from exposure to formaldehyde). Symptoms of sensitivity to small levels of exposure can affect many target organs; widespread central nervous system effects such as fatigue, depression, anxiety, or poor memory and concentration may occur and can differ from person to person. This observation often makes the cause of these problems extremely difficult to identify and underlines the need for the multifactorial approach, which is the basis of environmental medicine.

The final pattern described in environmental medicine is labeled the *switch phenomenon*. In this situation, symptoms change and can affect different organ systems; symptoms may range from psychological (e.g., anxiety) to asthma, fatigue, and hyperactivity. This movement of symptoms was described by Randolph as bipolar and biphasic responses of the biological mechanism ranging from stimulatory phases (+1 to +4) to withdrawal phases (–1 to – 4). It is possible to range from stimulation to withdrawal in the course of the illness (Randolph, 1976).

Diagnostic and treatment techniques. Several aspects of the assessment and treatment approaches employed in environmental medicine are unique to this specialty. The key to proper treatment is an accurate environmental history. With a broader view of the connection between environment and illness, many illnesses that are attributed to other causes by traditional medicine are assessed in terms of environmental aspects.

The environmental history details the chronology of the symptoms as well as the current form of the illness. Using the chronological history and the assessment of the detailed circumstances of the symptoms can lead to a greater understanding of the etiology. There is a search for a history of adverse reactions to specific environmental substances, including biological inhalants, foods, and chemicals. A detailed description of the home, the workplace, and the effects of season, activity, and other environmental factors is necessary. A thorough understanding of the pathophysiology of the dysfunctioning systems is also required. The effects of total allergic load, the spreading phenomenon, the switch phenomenon, and biochemical individuality need to be recognized so that the etiology of the illness can be assessed.

The physical examination and laboratory assessment look for evidence of nutritional deficiencies, organ system dysfunction, and disorders of detoxification systems. Blood tests might include standard assessments such as chemistry panels, blood counts, and hormonal function tests. In addition, tests that further assess immune function are required, such as lymphocyte subset panels, immunoglobulin levels, autoantibody screens, viral and chemical antibody panels, and in vitro assessment of allergy to foods, inhalants, and chemicals. Furthermore, assessment of nutritional status is often included, involving in vitro analysis of minerals and vitamins through enzyme system activation, as well as serum, plasma, leukocyte, or erythrocyte levels. Levels of toxic chemicals and minerals may be measured in serum or other biological markers.

In-office testing for allergies and hypersensitivity is often the most important aspect of assessing a patient with environmental illness. The techniques employed include serial end-point titration, provocative neutralization, and bronchoprovocation. These techniques test a wide range of antigens including bacteria, foods, chemicals, and inhalants such as dust, mites, pollens, and molds. The antigen sources are the same ones used in traditional allergy testing, but these techniques can more effectively assess the non-IgE sensitivity reaction (King, 1989; McGovern, 1981; Miller, 1972; Morris, 1981; Rinkel, 1963). Although the validity of these techniques is controversial, a significant number of studies support these approaches (Brostoff, 1988; Gerdes, 1993; King, 1981).

Provocative testing is in essence a quantitative bioassay. Individual skin tests with progressively weaker blinded dilutions of extract can reproduce many of the patient's symptoms. Subjective and objective monitoring can show changes in heart rate, blood pressure, nasal patency, respiratory function, cognitive function, and handwriting during and after single allergy tests.

When complex patients cannot be evaluated as outpatients, inpatient environmental control units are available in several locations in the United States and Canada. In these settings, the patients are in hospital rooms that are environmentally controlled and are free of all common chemical exposures. They are fasted on water until all symptoms disappear. At this point, they are challenged with foods by mouth and with chemicals in inhalant booths. The symptomatic response to these substances can help clarify the cause of the illness.

Treatment approaches to these complex problems require a full understanding of the nature of environmentally induced illness. Immunotherapy based on the results of the in vivo allergy testing techniques can be used to reduce the sensitivity to these antigens through a variety of mechanisms, including modulation by T-suppressor cells and altering the ratio of antibody to antigen, which affects the formation of immune complexes and histamine release (Rapp, 1986).

Educating the patient is critical in environmental medicine. A thorough understanding of the factors contributing to illness must be emphasized for long-term improvement to occur. Emphasis is placed on environmental controls in the home and workplace to reduce exposure to inhalants as well as chemicals. Where possible, the patient is informed about alternatives to using chemicals such as pesticides in the home and the workplace.

Dietary management is based on avoidance of food antigens and on the 4-day rotary diversified diet. With the rotary diet and avoidance of repetitive food exposures, it is possible to reduce sensitivity to foods and hasten recovery from food allergies. Nutritional supplements are prescribed as indicated by both objective nutritional testing and symptomatology. Improving the xenobiotic detoxification pathways through therapeutic nutrition is often required. In this respect the practice of environmental medicine overlaps "orthomolecular" nutrition practices. (See the "Diet and Nutrition" chapter.)

Research accomplishments. Research in the field has been directed at both clinical treatment of ill patients and evaluation of the diagnostic and treatment techniques used by practitioners. Studies have been done that support the approach of environmental medicine in arthritis (Panush, 1986), asthma (Gerrard, 1989), chemical sensitivity (Rea, 1991), colitis (Lake, 1982), depression (Randolph, 1959), eczema (Atherton, 1988), eye allergy (Shirakawa and Rea, 1990), fatigue (Rowe, 1950), food allergy (Rapp, 1947), hyperactivity (Rapp, 1979), migraine (Munro et al., 1980), psychological complaints (Campbell, 1973), urticaria (August, 1989), and vascular disease (Rea, 1991). Published bibliographies on environmental medicine discuss other studies and background in this area (Oberg, 1990; Randolph, 1987; Rapp, 1981).

Rea et al. (1984) studied 20 patients with known food sensitivity. Using neutralization therapy in a double-blind study they found significant improvement ($p < 0.001$) in signs and symptoms of allergy reactions to those foods. Mabry (1982), treating women with premenstrual tension syndrome, used progesterone neutralization and found that 65 percent of them preferred the active treatment to placebo.

Gerdes (1993) performed critical reviews of 31 studies of the provocation-neutralization technique done between 1969 and 1988. Twenty-one studies showed evidence for the effectiveness of the technique, and 10 had negative results. Only 10 of the 31 studies reviewed were methodologically sound, however. Among these potentially replicable studies, 8 were supportive of the technique, 1 was not, and 1 could be cited by either side in the controversy. (See the "Diet and Nutrition" chapter for data on food allergy studies.)

Future directions for research. Despite its designation as an "alternative" professional specialty within the biomedical community, environmental medicine remains a controversial field. Practitioners of environmental medicine have been criticized for "nonstandard" diagnostic techniques and "unorthodox" treatment methods, as have other practitioners of alternative forms of medicine. The principal detractors have been the American Academy of Allergy and Immunology and the American College of Allergy and Immunology (Gerdes, 1993). Proponents claim, however, that the basic principles of environmental medicine are critical to designing the types of studies that could further validate the field. Research has also been hampered by application of the "unconventional" label to practices that attract patients who have failed to be helped by conventional internal medicine, allergy, and psychological approaches. The problem of chemical hypersensitivity and chemically induced illness and worker's disability led to a report by the New Jersey State Department of Health in 1989, which summarizes much of the controversy in this area (Ashford and Miller, 1989). Another major review of the complex medico-legal and social problems encountered with workers with multiple chemical sensitivities was published by Rosenstock and Cullen in 1994.

Although the belief that humans may get sick from accumulated low-level environmental stress is not well accepted in the conventional community, sick building syndrome and other diseases of the 20th century are being seen with greater frequency. Indeed, according to The National Research Council of the National Academy of Sciences, the U.S. population is exposed to at least 50,000 chemicals, most of which have not been studied sufficiently in relation to their effects on human health (National Research Council, 1975). Those that have been studied are assessed only in terms of their carcinogenicity in animal models and not in terms of a myriad of other aspects affecting human health. In addition, no work has been done on the additive effects of repeated low-level exposures to pesticides, solvents, formaldehyde, and the other common substances found in the immediate environment (Elkington, 1986).

Future occupational toxicology studies should include clinicians trained in environmental medicine. Peer review committees in allergy and toxicology grant review processes should not be dominated by persons whose belief system is threatened by the environmental medicine philosophy.

The testing techniques of environmental medicine need further validating studies, as do the various immunological and nutritional treatment methods. The research protocols must, however, actually test the paradigm. For example, food or chemical challenges in the exhausted stage of illness might yield different results if the study subjects were first deadapted (allowed to recover) before being challenged. Careful qualitative research might be needed to validate variable biological responses such as those described in the switch phenomenon.

Since quality-of-life issues surround many of the complex illnesses treated by environmental medicine, qualitative outcomes research comparing patients treated by these principles versus "orthodox medicine" could give insight into the best use of this approach in the U.S. health care system.

Summary. Environmental medicine offers an alternative view of the causation, prevention, and treatment of many common illnesses. It emphasizes self-care and the use of nonpharmaceutical approaches. Environmental medicine presents a dynamic and potentially cost-effective paradigm to deal with the many common illnesses seen in today's increasingly complex environment. It has been estimated by the U.S. Public Health Service (1990) that diet and environment play a role in 90 percent of cancers and cardiovascular disease. Environmental medicine is in a position to be a leading force in the investigation of ways to reduce the incidence of these and other disorders.

Community-Based Health Care Practices

Overview

All of the systems discussed in this section are community based in several ways. Most important, an individual's sickness is viewed as a sickness of the entire community. That is, when one person becomes sick, the whole community is believed to be in danger. Therefore, the treatment must address the whole community rather than just the patient.

Because the concepts of "medicine" and "religion" in these systems often are fused, no sickness can affect only one part of the body. Rather, it affects the whole network of existence, the natural world, and the spiritual world. Accordingly, in addition to their expertise in naturalistic healing (i.e., the use of herbs), community-based health care practitioners are expected to have expertise in dealing with relationships (between partners, between parents and children, etc.), mediating disputes and communicating with the spirit world. Also, health care is delivered in public, with members of the family and community present.

Community-based health care practices are varied and found throughout the United States, although many people would not consider that they were participating in such a system when they attend a healing service at a local church or go to a meeting of Weight Watchers. Like other health care specialists, community-based healers may emphasize naturalistic, personalistic, or energetic explanatory models or a combination. Traditional midwives and herbalists—and nowadays, pragmatic weight loss specialists—are probably the best known of community-based practitioners who follow the naturalistic model.[3]

Though most traditional healers will accept gifts, many refuse pay for their healing work. They believe they are the agents of God or the spirit world and that their power and skill should be used to help the needy. Most community-based healers do not advertise their skills, which are therefore mainly known locally. There are two types of personalistic healers: the shaman, and others who do not quite fit this model and whose practice can be called "shamanistic."

A *shaman* is a type of spiritual healer distinguished by the practice of *journeying* to nonordinary reality to make contact with the world of spirits, to ask their direction in bringing healing back to people and the community (Atkinson, 1987, 1992; Brown, 1988; Eliade, 1964; Halifax, 1979; Harner, 1990; Ingerman, 1991; Laderman, 1988; McClenon, 1993; Myerhoff, 1976). The *journey* is a controlled trance state that practitioners induce by using repetitive sound (drums, rattles) or movement (dancing) and occasionally by consuming plant substances (e.g., peyote or certain mushrooms). Characteristically experiential and cooperative, shamanic healing is found worldwide. It is fundamental to much traditional European, African, Asian, and Native American Indian folk practice and is rapidly gaining popularity among nonnative urban Americans, in which setting it is sometimes called neo-shamanism (Hufford, 1990).

Shamanic practices define healing broadly: not only are people to be healed of their spiritual and psychic wounds, but shamans also attempt to heal communities, modify the weather, and find lost objects. Many traditional shamans are also skilled in manipulative or herbal practices (Atkinson, 1987; Brown, 1988).

Clinical evidence of results is anecdotal, consisting of the stories successful shamans tell of their curing and healing activities (Black Elk and

[3]The Native American "medicine man" or "medicine woman" is a traditional healer with primarily naturalistic skills, that is, the skills of an herbalist in particular (Hultkrantz, 1985). Some medicine people are also shamans, in which case they are often distinguished as "holy" men and women. This distinction is usually not made in popular writing, though it is understandably important to the Native American Indian users.

Lyon, 1990; Harner, 1990; Ingerman, 1991; Yellowtail and Fitzgerald, 1991; Young, 1989). Some interpretations of shamanism have tended to categorize its effectiveness in the same range as psychotherapy, but wider interpretations may be more accurate (Atkinson, 1992; Brown, 1988; Laderman, 1988; McClenon, 1993).

Shamans are concerned with helping patients discover "meaning," but such meaning is not limited to the interior dialog. It expands to include the entire natural and spiritual community. For example, shamanic journeying and the precision with which shamans can "tell" a patient's life and concerns to a patient convince many that the spirit world is real and supportive. Also, shamans commonly help individual patients see their illness not as a personal failure but as a concern of the larger sociopolitical unit, thus drawing community support toward the sick. Shamanic care can also result in physical "curing." In summary, the shamanic approach is complex and paradigmatically quite different from mainstream Western explanatory models.

Personalistic specialists who do not practice journeying are not shamans. Nor can practices that depend on fixed rituals or charms, and thus are not experiential, be considered shamanic practices. However, to the extent that mediums, channelers, prayer healers, and others call on the unseen or on the spirit world to intervene for the benefit of people in the material world, they are "shamanistic."

In contrast to professionalized practitioners, community-based healers often do not have set locations—such as offices or clinics—for delivering care but do so in homes, at ceremonial sites, or even right where they stand. Community-based healing of the personalistic variety can also be "distant," that is, it does not require that practitioner and patient be in each other's presence. Prayers or shamanic journeys, for example, can be requested and "administered" at any time, and charm cures are sometimes delivered by telephone.

An example of rural community-based practitioners is the "powwowers." These are "wise women" or elders who by reason of birth or calling have been recognized as having the requisite "power" to say the verbal charms or prayers to cure trauma and disease in powwowing (Hostetler, 1976; Yoder, 1976). The term is borrowed from the Algonquin Indians, although the practices did not originate with the Native American Indian. Instead they date back many centuries in Europe. The original German dialect words, *brauche* or *braucherei,* are still sometimes used.

Powwowing closely resembles traditional European practices found elsewhere in the United States (Hufford, 1988, 1992; Kirkland, 1992; Reimansnyder, 1989; Wigginton, 1972; Wilkinson, 1987). "Granny women" deliver care in the Appalachians, *traiteurs* in Louisiana, and "power doctors" in the Ozarks, and similar ideas may be found in almost any State. A similar niche in African-American communities is filled by "rootwork." This community-based system is found throughout the Southern United States and in African-American communities elsewhere, sometimes under alternate names such as "conjure" and "hoo-doo" (Lichstein, 1992; Mathews, 1987, 1992; Snow, 1993; Terrell, 1990; Weidmann, 1978). Although not familiar to most urban peoples, these systems serve considerable numbers of rural Americans.

Meanwhile, community-based systems also thrive in urban areas. These systems include the popular weight loss programs and other 12-step programs. Often the practitioners rent office space and emphasize contact between client and practitioner, and they may charge considerable fees. Since these practitioners depend on their healing practice for their livelihood, they advertise and so may be easier to identify and contact for study purposes.

The following discusses the community-based health care practices of certain Native American Indian tribes, rural Latin American communities, and urban self-help systems.

Native American Indian Health Care Practices

Although each Native American Indian community-based medical system has its distinct characteristics, all share the following rituals and practices.

- *Sweating and purging.* Both techniques are intended to purify the body as well as the spirit. Herbal preparations, such as the famous "black drink" of the southeastern tribes, were formerly used to induce vomiting (Hudson, 1979). The goal was to strengthen the body and prepare it for challenges—a form of preventive medicine. Sweating continues to be widely practiced, often in special "sweat lodges" (McGaa, 1990). Typically, these are small conical structures where hot rocks are doused with water to create steam. Participants pray, sing, and drum to purify their spirits while sweating to cleanse their bodies. This practice is also considered a means of preventing imbalance and illness; in some cases it is also used to heal. In the Lakota community, a complete lodge ceremony lasts several hours and is recommended both for general purification (e.g., monthly for men, a kind of parallel to women's monthly menses) and for help in reaching major life decisions or dealing with major life challenges. In addition, praying in the sweat lodge commonly precedes and follows vision questing and sun dancing.

- *Herbal remedies.* All indigenous Americans depended on a variety of herbal remedies gathered from the surrounding environment and sometimes traded over long distances. The "Herbal Medicine" chapter gives more details on the types and applications of herbal remedies used by certain tribes.

- *Shamanic healing.* Shamanic healing is also an important part of virtually all Native American Indian health care. Most tribal people have one or more types of health care specialists in naturalistic or personalistic healing. Frequently, the two overlap—thus a midwife or a medicine man or woman might focus primarily on naturalistic explanations and healing but sometimes also uses prayer, suggestion, or other techniques characteristic of a personalistic framework. "Holy people" or shamans (each tribe has its own name for this specialist type) emphasize personalistic healing but often are also knowledgeable about herbs, massage, and other naturalistic techniques.

Shamanic practice is relatively well maintained in a number of tribes today and in several cases is expanding into the larger society. On the other hand, herbal and other practices have largely disappeared in many localities. There are some current efforts to save vanishing knowledge, and the next few years may see more young people apprentice themselves to elders and become naturalistic or personalistic healing specialists.

Below, major practices in two Native American Indian tribal communities are briefly outlined: the Lakota Sioux and the Dineh (Navajo). These two were selected because traditional healing practices have been relatively well maintained and well studied in these communities, and because they help to show the wide variety of practices used by Native American Indian peoples. There is a large literature on different groups, however, and the reader is also referred to sources such as Johnston, 1982; Morse et al., 1991; Naranjo and Swentzell, 1989; and Young, 1989.

Lakota practices. The Lakota—one of several branches of a tribe often called Sioux, who live primarily in North and South Dakota, Minnesota, and Manitoba—are perhaps unique in their recent efforts to inform the wider society of their psychosocial healing techniques (Black Elk and Lyon, 1990; McGaa, 1990; Neihardt, 1932; Powers, 1977, 1982). Though the Lakota have their own distinctive ways of practice, in broad outline their techniques are shared with other Plains tribes as well as with other groups from Wisconsin to Washington (Farrer, 1991; Harrod, 1992; Storm, 1972; Yellowtail and Fitzgerald, 1991).

Lakota techniques are based on the assumption of the absolute continuity of body and spirit; for the Lakota, "medicine" and "religion" are not separate. The two most famous Lakota religiomedical practices are the sweat lodge and the medicine wheel (sacred hoop.) Other techniques, such as the vision quest and sun dance, are familiar to many non-Native American Indians. Other practices, such as the *yuwipi* ceremony (Powers, 1982), are little known to outsiders.

All these healing ceremonials are led by specialists, usually called medicine women or men or holy men or women, who are essentially shamanic in their approach to healing (Hultkrantz, 1985). Some also have knowledge of herbal remedies or manipulative techniques. One usually discovers that one's path is to become a medicine person through a dream or vision, sometimes sought (as in the vision quest), sometimes unsought (appearing during the course of serious illness or in lucid dreaming). Shamanic skills also tend to run in families. Once called, one seeks training, usually by apprenticing oneself to a successful medicine man or woman, often for several years. Training is complete when the teacher says it is complete and when the candidate has practiced his or her skills publicly and with success.

The medicine wheel or sacred hoop is both a conceptual scheme and a major ceremonial. The wheel or hoop represents all of cosmology and life in a circle of four quarters, plus the directions of up, down, and center. Each of the four quarters has a character or power, which can be expressed in many ways; as an aspect of some form of wisdom, as an animal, as a color, as an energy, or as a season. The four quarters are separated by two "roads," one red for happiness, one black for sorrow. Everyone is born with the gift of one of the powers, and the thoughtful person will "journey" his or her life to develop the other forms of wisdom, know that happiness and sorrow come to everyone, and recognize the relatedness of the whole. This deeply ecological cosmology is expressed in virtually all Lakota prayer, and with the phrase "*Mitakuye oyasin*" ("Thanks to all our relatives"). The wheel or hoop is represented on much Lakota artwork; periodically it is represented as a stone circle on the ground, around which a ceremonial is held. Participation in the ceremonial is considered generally healing, and in addition, individuals can seek specific healing through prayer.

Dineh or Navajo practices. The Dineh are a herding people who have lived in the southwestern United States for some centuries; they are the largest tribe in North America today. Like the Lakota, in their traditional practice the Dineh make essentially no distinction between religious and medical practices. Here, discussion is limited to the famous Navajo healing "sings" or "chants" and the specialists who make them possible (Luckert and Cooke, 1979; Morgan, 1931/1977; Reichard, 1939, 1950; Sandner, 1979, 1991; Topper, 1987; Wyman and Haile, 1970).

A sing is a healing ceremonial that lasts from 2 to 9 days and nights. It is guided by a highly skilled specialist called a "singer." Although focused on helping an individual, sings are commonly attended by as many in the community as can come, for just being present is considered healing. Navajo cosmology teaches that health is present when all things are in harmony. The full concept is impossible to translate into English, so it is often rendered as the Navajo word *hozro*, which summarizes many things such as happiness, connection, and balance. Its opposite is something like "evil"; indeed, where there is disharmony, there is sickness and disease, and vice versa. A long-time student of Navajo singers notes:

> This "evil" must be controlled or banished and goodness restored. To implement this desired state of affairs, the Navajos have created a great body of symbolic rituals [that] attempt to placate or expel the destructive powers and attract the good, helpful ones. By doing this they reestablish the basic harmony, cure individual illness, and bring general blessing to the tribe (Sandner, 1979, p. 118).

There are three basic categories of chants: "holyway," "ghostway," and "lifeway." Holyway chants—including the most famous, called "blessingway"—are used to attract good, to cure, and to repair. Ghostway chants are used to remove evil and are often performed to heal Dineh who have had too much contact with strangers (non-Navajo), as in the armed forces or at college, or who have had contact with dead bodies. Lifeway chants are used to treat what westerners would call "physical" injuries and accidents; such treatment includes both restoring cosmological harmony and repairing trauma—by setting broken bones, for example.

The two kinds of healing specialists among the Dineh are the "diagnosticians" and the aforementioned singers. Diagnosticians are usually "called" to their profession by nonordinary experiences and receive little formal training in their skill. They diagnose deep cause by going into trance. While in trance, "hand tremblers" pass their shaking hands over the body of the patient; when the hands stop trembling, the locale of the illness is shown and the cause is usually nameable. "Star gazers" also enter trance to read cause in the stars. "Listeners" do not go into trance but listen to the patient's story and on that basis diagnose deep cause. Once cause is known—and it is always phrased in terms of harmony and disharmony—patients seek a singer who can provide the indicated treatment.

Singers are specialists of symbology who have a good deal in common both with priests and with psychotherapists; in addition, their moral probity and high intellectual powers mean that they usually perform as community leaders as well. They are not shamans and are not "called" by supernatural powers to their profession. Instead, interest and patience are the prerequisites, as well as demonstrated dependability and economic success. To learn a single chant can take up to several years, for the performance of each chant involves memorizing what amounts to a long epic poem (one that takes 2 to 9 nights to repeat) along with the recipes for the accompanying herbal preparations and sand paintings. The singer must also know where to find the herbs, how to prepare them, and how to use them. He must know where to find the colored sands necessary for the sand paintings, and he must learn to make—without error—the intricate sand paintings specific to the chant he is learning. Because the training is so arduous, most singers learn only a few chants in a lifetime.

The Dineh have depended on singers and chants for many centuries; today they are used in combination with conventional medicine. It remains common for Dineh both on and off the reservation to seek sings to treat conditions that conventional medicine does not recognize and to use sings for healing along with conventional medicine used curatively.

Numerous observers have asked why the sings "work." Topper (1987, p. 248) remarks that sings are restorative: "They restore an individual's ego functions and integrate the patient back into the social setting from which he or she has become estranged." Sandner (1979, 1991) analyzes the process further: First, the herbal remedies often have requisite physiological effects. Second, the patient's expectation is encouraged time and again during the chant by its intricate psychological structure. Third, the patient is socially supported by the entire community, who are centrally concerned since, by Navajo cosmology, the well-being of all is threatened by disharmony in one. Fourth, the chant wordings guide the sick person to finding culturally appropriate answers to difficult cosmological problems, such as the management of evil and the inevitability of death.

Formal research into the healing ceremonies and herbal medicines conducted and used by bona fide Native American Indian healers or holy people is almost nonexistent, even though Native American Indians believe they positively cure both the mind and body. Ailments and diseases such as heart disease, diabetes, thyroid conditions, cancer, skin rashes, and asthma reportedly have been cured by Native American Indian doctors who are knowledgeable about the complex ceremonies. Among Native American Indians living today there are many stories about seemingly impossible cures that have been wrought by holy people. However, the information on what was done is closely guarded and not readily rendered to non-Native American Indian investigators. It has been suggested that if Congress restored religious freedom to Native American Indians, then collaborative research into Native American Indian healing and healing practices could be possible (Locke, 1993).

Latin American Rural Practices

Curanderismo is a folk system used in Latin America and among many Hispanic-Americans in the United States. Hispanic-American refers to Americans of Spanish or Spanish-American descent; in the United States most trace their roots to Mexico (63 percent), Puerto Rico (12 percent), and Cuba, but increasing numbers of immigrants are arriving from Central America (Wright, 1990). The population of Hispanics is rapidly growing in the United States, and today about 22 million people call themselves Hispanic. More than half of this population lives in Texas and California, and large populations are also in Colorado, Arizona, Florida, Illinois, New Jersey, New Mexico, and New York.

Curanderismo typically includes two distinct components, a humoral model for classifying activity, food, drugs, and illness; and a series of folk illnesses such as "evil eye," "fright," "blockage," and "fallen fontanelle." Curanderismo as described herein is most characteristic of Mexican-Americans, especially those who are little assimilated; variants on the humoral component typify most of Latin America, while the folk diseases and the treatment modalities reflect national background. Thus the Cuban-American folk system is not curanderismo, but *santeria*, and it is African influenced.

Although no formal effectiveness studies seem to have been done on this system, its wide popularity and the research suggesting the relevance of the folk diagnoses for biomedical practice indicate the need for further demographic and effectiveness studies.

In the humoral component of curanderismo things could be classified as having qualitative (not literal) characteristics of hot or cold, dry or moist. (Harwood, 1971; Messer, 1981; Weller, 1983). According to this theory, good health is maintained by maintaining a balance of hot and cold. Thus, a good meal will contain both hot and cold foods, and a person with a hot disease must be given cold remedies and vice versa. Again, a person who is exposed to cold when excessively hot may "take cold" and become ill.

While this model is simple in theory, how people perceive in practice the hotness or coldness of substances varies greatly by region. Thus, while most can be expected to classify chili peppers as "hot" and milk as "cold," the classification of pork or penicillin is not so predictable.

The second component, the folk illnesses, is actively in use in much of Mexico and among less educated Hispanic U.S. citizens (Rubel, 1960, 1964; Rubel et al., 1984; Young, 1981). Trotter (1985) did more than 2,000 clinic interviews in Texas, Arizona, and New Mexico and found that 32 percent to 96 percent of Mexican-American households (more frequent in the less Americanized communities) treated members for Hispanic folk illnesses. Baer and colleagues found similarly high use patterns among Mexican migrant workers in Florida and Mexico (Baer and Penzell, 1993; Baer and Bustillo, 1993).

Four important Mexican-American folk illnesses are *mal de ojo, susto, empacho,* and *caida de mollera.* Mal de ojo, or evil eye, is a worldwide disease concept in which a person can make another sick by looking at him or her. The one who gets sick, typically an infant, is usually "weak." The one who causes the illness is usually thought not to do it on purpose—the person just has the misfortune to have a "piercing" glance. Typical symptoms of mal de ojo include fussiness, refusal to eat, and refusal to sleep. Infants are protected from evil eye with amulets or by having their faces covered in the presence of strangers. Treatment is primarily symbolic.

Caida de mollera, or fallen fontanelle, is an illness of infants before the anterior fontanelle (crown of the head) closes. Common symptoms include diarrhea, excessive crying, fever, loss of appetite, and irritability. Usual folk treatments focus on raising the fontanelle by, for example, pushing up on the palate.

Empacho is thought to be caused by something getting stuck in the intestines, causing blockage. Common symptoms are diarrhea, constipation, indigestion, vomiting, and bloating. The commonest treatment is massage along with herbal teas; the former is for dislodging the blockage, and the latter is for washing it out.

Susto, or fright (sometimes called magical fright), develops when a person has had a sudden shock—a mother may develop fright if she sees her child nearly drown, or someone may experience fright after participating in an unusually intense argument. The sick person experiences such symptoms as daytime sleepiness combined with nighttime insomnia, irritability and easy startling, palpitations, inability to stop thinking about the shocking event, anxiety that it will be repeated, and sometimes a sense of loss or a sadness that will not leave. The mild form is treated with herb tea; more severe cases are treated with ritual cleansings (barridas) to restore the harmony of body and soul.

When mild, these folk illnesses are commonly treated at home, but if they persist, the help of specialists—curanderos (men) or curanderas (women)—is sought. The training of curanderos and curanderas varies widely. Most practice a combination of shamanic healing and herbal or practical first aid healing. Most are also astute at manipulating symbols and "reading" the prevailing psychological and social indicators. Some curanderas specialize in midwifery and infant care. In some areas, becoming a healer is a matter of inheritance; the skills are passed from mother to daughter or perhaps aunt to niece. In some areas it is a matter of being called. Typically, curanderos and curanderas spend several years in apprenticeship; their subsequent reputation depends on the number of their patients and how successful their patients judge them.

Treatment techniques, usually a combination of the shamanic and the naturalistic, vary widely; interested readers should consult specialist texts. An issue of concern is that some curanderismo treatments, particularly for empacho, involve feeding lead- or mercury-based remedies. Investigators' efforts to test whether the amounts ingested were causing medical complications were inconclusive. Although curanderas were found to be largely aware of the danger of the remedies and used them sparingly, intervention programs to limit use of these remedies were begun (Baer et al., 1989; Trotter, 1985).

Trotter (1985) collected symptomatology lists from more than 2,000 interviews and submitted symptom clusters to medical doctors for "blind" diagnoses. He found, for example, that caida de mollera appears to be symptomatic of serious dehydration secondary to gastroenteritis or respiratory infection. Trotter also found that people who are sicker than average are more likely to be diagnosed with susto. Baer and Penzell (1993) similarly report that migrant workers most affected in a pesticide poisoning incident were also those most likely to report suffering from susto. Susto fits the pattern of "soul loss" (Ingerman, 1991), a shamanically recognized disorder known worldwide that resembles several serious psychotherapeutically recognized conditions, including depression and posttraumatic stress syndrome. Therefore, people being treated for folk diseases could be considered to have conventional illnesses that are being treated outside the conventional biomedical health care system.

Urban Community-Based Systems

Alcoholics Anonymous (AA) is a community-based healing system for helping people whose lives are damaged by the consumption of alcohol to stop drinking (Encyclopaedia Britannica, 1990; Scott, 1993; Trice and Staudenmeier, 1989). Founded in 1935 by Bob Smith, M.D., and Bill Wilson, two alcoholics, it is a patient-centered self-help fellowship of men and women. AA has burgeoned and today is widely considered the most successful existing method for supporting sobriety.

Habitual excessive drinking or craving for alcohol was first proposed as constituting a disease by Magnus Huss in 1849. Currently many definitions of the condition exist, but most emphasize that the drinker has "lost control" (is addicted or dependent) and that alcohol use is causing physical, social, mental, or economic harm to the drinker. The concept of loss of control is especially important to AA, which requires its members, as the first step toward sobriety, to comprehend the extent to which they have lost control of their lives. Only then—when they have understood that "playing God" has led them to their sickness, that in fact they are limited human beings in need of salvation—can they begin the breakthroughs that support sobriety (Scott, 1993).

In contrast to most community-based systems, a very large literature exists analyzing AA. Several models attempt to explain its success. One popular psychometric model interprets AA as a "cult" and the achievement of sobriety as a "conversion experience" (Galanter, 1990; Greil and Rudy, 1983; Rudy, 1987). Another model accepts AA's interpretation of itself (Hufford, 1988; Kurtz, 1982; Scott, 1993): members recover by integrating their own experiences with alcohol with those of others in the group and by learning and practicing some new ways to behave. Through these new ways, AA members feel as if they are living apart from the urban materialist norm; that the cause of alcoholism is not at issue; that people should share, not compete; and that the individual need not rise above the rest (spiritual anonymity). In contrast to the "conversion" theory of AA membership, learning to live in the "new way" is not achieved through catharsis but is an intellectual and educational process requiring considerable work and perseverance. As Kurtz comments, "AA addresses itself not to alcoholism, but to the alcoholic" (Kurtz, 1982).

AA, by most accounts, is more successful than any other system aimed at helping individuals to achieve sobriety. Estimates put membership at about a half-million members worldwide, and although it was originally an American urban phenomenon, AA has found its way into isolated and rural communities of completely different cultural backgrounds (Slagle and Weibel-Orlando, 1986; Sutro, 1989). Recently, AA has seen a rise in membership proportions of women, people younger than 30, and people dually addicted to alcohol and drugs (Emrick, 1987). Studies have concluded that active AA membership allows 60 percent to 68 percent of alcoholics to drink less or not at all for up to a year, and 40 percent to 50 percent to achieve sobriety for many years (Emrick, 1987). More active or dedicated members (those who attend meetings more often) remain sober longer. However, because AA defines alcoholism as a disease controllable only by the cessation of drinking, it is a less appropriate choice for those who simply want to cut down on their drinking (Ogborne, 1989).

Despite these interesting effectiveness data, some authors argue that no appropriate controlled studies of AA effectiveness have been done (Peele, 1990); others hold that difficult research design issues have not been sufficiently addressed, such as how to measure psychosocial functioning before and after AA, or the effects of AA plus some other intervention (Glaser and Ogborne, 1982). Given the popularity and the apparent success rates of AA, further careful research on AA seems highly appropriate. The research design issues applicable to studying AA's effectiveness would be relevant to other alternative practices that include an individual's commitment to a shared belief system and a social behavior pattern.

Research Opportunities

Community-based health practices are specific to many subcultural groups in the United States, including immigrant, rural, and Native American communities. The first step in research would be to categorize and characterize these forms of ethnomedicine practices using qualitative research methods developed in the field of anthropology. Clinical research could begin promptly on those systems that have already been well described and are used widely and in which practitioners of the systems are open to dialog.

A study of various symbolic or nonmaterial concepts of healing such as shamanic healing might identify effective principles of body-mind intervention that would be useful to integrate in the training of future primary care practitioners in the general community. Herbal agents and ethnic herbal practitioners deserve study to identify fruitful clinical areas for research in phytopharmaceutics (pharmacology of plants). Practices and techniques that are rapidly spreading beyond their original cultural confines, such as AA and the sweat lodge, would be candidates for outcomes research. Careful investigation of tribal and folk practices may illuminate larger issues of health care and provide guidelines for low-cost alternatives to existing conventional biomedical interventions. Utilization studies of tribal and folk health care practices could develop a realistic sense of the self-care patterns used by the Nation's ethnic and cultural minorities and inform national public health policies about these minority communities.

Research Barriers

To effectively research and study the alternative health practices people are using, it is necessary to recognize that the operating assumptions of the conventional biomedical way of thinking have led to these alternative systems being ignored or suppressed. Historically the practices of these systems have been scorned as cultic, superstitious, or sectarian, and these systems have been suppressed economically, politically, and scientifically.

From an economic standpoint it is not surprising that the institutions and agents charged with maintaining the exclusive professional mandates of the biomedical system have sought to eliminate competition from alternative professionalized systems as well as folk and tribal practitioners. This anticompetitive tendency is also extended to popular health practices. Popular self-help health books now routinely have a "consult your professional" disclaimer to protect the authors from law suits for practicing "unscientific" medicine in the media without a license.

In the political arena, current concerns about FDA regulation of the health food industry have resulted from an attempt to extend a level of governmental control mandated for a professionalized drug-dispensing health care system into a whole system of self-help and demand-driven popular health care. In addition, the suppression of the tribal health care practices of Native American Indian groups has been primarily due to the dominant political and cultural view that it is in the best interest of these peoples to be forcibly assimilated into the mainstream.

Community-based practitioners themselves may present barriers to research: some may not want to share their knowledge. In some cases the explanatory model of the folk system states that to share the knowledge, except under particular circumstances, is to lose one's power, even to call down punishment on one's head. In other cases, especially among Native American Indians, it is felt that the sharing of traditional secular and sacred knowledge has resulted in the misuse of that knowledge, especially when it has been applied without sufficient awareness of the social and environmental context.

Key Research Issues

In the current climate of concern about the adequacy of the U.S. health care delivery system, a culturally sensitive and scientifically grounded dialog about alternative systems of health care is required. Therefore, cross-cultural researchers must heed the insights of professionals who do health care outreach.

The concept of cultural sensitivity means that issues of conflicts between basic paradigms, worldviews, or belief systems are recognized and openly dealt with when a dominant culture tries to study, influence, or assist a different culture or subculture. The goal of cultural sensitivity—to find common ground among different cultures—has been widely understood among outreach specialists for perhaps 20 years. Cultural sensitivity is a worthy and necessary goal, but it is not easy to achieve. Hufford (1992) notes that understanding the other's position does not imply acceptance or agreement. Nor does it imply that bridging models to accomplish good research is easy. These studies require patience and often extensive negotiation. In addition, the tendency to see differences can sometimes overwhelm the ability to see similarities, thereby unnecessarily focusing people on conflict and negotiation.

Most published studies in these areas have been done by social scientists, folklorists, and historians. Literature on the topic is extensive, including books (e.g., Harwood, 1981; Pedersen et al., 1989) and many articles. From this database one can begin exploring the role of nonprofessionalized health care in the human community.

The first job is, of course, to establish that significant differences exist, and then to detail them. For example, Aitken (1990), speaking as an insider, claims that Native American Indians have distinctive values, and researchers such as Dubray (1985) and Fox (1992) find ways to measure the differences. Often, researchers do their best to identify the differences, and outreach proceeds with certain assumed values, for example, that clients should be asked to help in designing programs intended to benefit them (e.g., Broken Nose, 1992).

Subsequently, evaluations can show which research or outreach models were most successful in given locales. For example, May (1986) and May and Smith (1988) report that alcoholism is better controlled on reservations when indigenous concepts are included in treatment plans; Guilmet and Whited (1987), Marburg (1983), and Manson and colleagues (1987) compare mental health outreach programs among Native American Indians and conclude that the most effective ones reflect indigenous value systems, such as team-based approaches in using group and family therapy rather than individual one-on-one counseling. Beauvais and LaBoueff (1985) state that the control of drug and alcohol abuse will come about through "bolstering the spirit of the community."

Thus, doing clinical research in community-based health care requires questioning certain common assumptions of researchers who are schooled in the biomedical model. These assumptions include (1) that community-based systems are disappearing and are not delivering health care to many people; (2) that the care they deliver is psychosomatic or not really significant, an idea made more sensible by the segregation of body and mind that is characteristic of mainstream medicine; and (3) that existing clinical research methods are sufficient to analyze community-based practices.

A careful, culturally sensitive analysis of the function and intent of various community-based practices will help sort out the psychic from the somatic aspects of health care. While similarities between systems may allow researchers to pose interesting questions, the research must take into account the particularities of the folk or tribal system being studied. For example, Navajo singers share some characteristics with psychotherapists, *but they are not psychotherapists.* Likewise, members of AA share their experiences and thus "counsel" other members, *but they are not alcohol counselors.* Researchers must resist trying to fit these systems into their existing categories.

Research Priorities

The following are general recommendations and priorities for research in the area of alternative professionalized medical systems and community-based practices:

1. Establish a database with descriptive information about traditional medical practice from medical and nonmedical sources. Included should be a review of existing scientific data, including a meta-analysis of studies in selected disciplines.

2. Promote and publish consumer-based surveys describing which alternative systems and traditional ethnic medical practices are being used and for what illnesses.

3. Explore alternative and ethnic medical systems, including historical traditions that may not be replicable in the biomedical model, and recognizing the role of body, mind, spirit, and environmental factors in health and disease.

4. Conduct basic science research to investigate the existence, nature, and role of "energy" (chi, vital force) as a phenomenon active in health and disease.

5. Develop cross-agency guidelines to facilitate research on alternative systems and traditional practices by reducing legal barriers for research that may already exist in other Federal agencies; encourage best case series research, as has been done by NCI in other Federal research agencies; and create an ongoing database of activities in alternative systems and traditional medical practices.

6. Initiate an evaluation program for traditional remedies and herbal medicines, including a global ethnobotany inventory, investigation into issues of toxicity and safety, and creation of an appropriate regulatory category for herbal therapeutic agents.

7. Establish collaboration standards for alternative medical practice research to ensure that the research team respects the paradigm under study; that there is joint involvement of representatives of alternative and traditional practitioners along with existing biomedical research institutions; and that joint involvement occurs at all stages of the research project: conception, method design, funding, data collection, evaluation, and publication.

8. Support the legislative intent of Congress in creating the Office of Alternative Medicine by focusing on socially and economically critical health conditions through cost-effectiveness research.

9. Encourage the addition of alternative systems or ethnomedicine research components to current clinical studies sponsored by the National Institutes of Health; for example, adding traditional Asian therapy, naturopathic, or homeopathic interventions to current studies in the Women's Health Initiative.

10. Expand studies such as the International Cooperative Biodiversity Group so that whole plant material is used rather than isolating an active ingredient for pharmaceutical usage.

References

Aitken, L. 1990. The cultural basis of Indian medicine. In L. Aitken and E. Haller, eds. Two Cultures Meet: Pathways for American Indians to Medicine. Garrett Park Press, Garrett Park, Md.

Alexander, C.N., E.J. Langer, J.L. Davies, H.M. Chandler, and R.I. Newman. 1989a. Transcendental meditation, mindfulness and longevity: an experimental study with the elderly. J. Pers. Soc. Psychol. 57:950–964.

Alexander, C.N., M.V. Rainworth, and P. Gelderloos. 1989b. Transcendental meditation, self-actualization, and psychological health: a conceptual overview and statistical meta-analysis. J. Soc. Behav. Pers. 6(5):189–247.

American Foundation of Medical Acupuncture. 1993. Clinical research in medical acupuncture: a literature review. In Biomedical Research on Acupuncture: An Agenda for the 1990s. Conference Summary. Los Angeles, Calif.

Arnold, J.T., E.A. Korytynski, B.P. Wilkinson, and V.E. Steele. 1991. Chemopreventive activity of Maharishi Amrit Kalash and related agents in rat tracheal epithelial and human tumor cells. Journal of Proceedings of the American Association for Cancer Research, 32:128–151.

Ashford, A.A., and C.S. Miller. 1989. Chemical sensitivity: a report to the New Jersey State Department of Health.

Atherton, D. 1988. Role of diet in treating atopic eczema: diet can be beneficial. Br. Med. J. 297:145–146.

Atkinson, J.M. 1987. The effectiveness of shamans in an Indonesian ritual. American Anthropologist 89:342–355.

Atkinson, J.M. 1992. Shamanisms today. Annual Review of Anthropology 21:307–330.

August, P. 1989. Urticaria successfully treated by desensitization with grass pollen extract. Br. J. Dermatol. 120:409–410.

Baer, R., et al. 1989. Lead-based remedies for empacho: patterns and consequences. Soc. Sci. Med. 29:1373–1379.

Baer, R., and M. Bustillo. 1993. Susto and mal de ojo among Florida farmworkers: emic and etic perspectives. Medical Anthropology Quarterly 7:90–100.

Baer, R., and D. Penzell. 1993. Research report: susto and pesticide poisoning among Florida farmworkers. Cult. Med. Psychiatry 17:321–327.

Barrie, S.A., J.V. Wright, and J.E. Pizzorno. 1987a. Effects of garlic oil on platelet aggregation, serum lipids, and blood pressure in humans. Journal of Orthomolecular Medicine 2:15–21.

Barrie, S.A., J.V. Wright, J.E. Pizzorno, E. Kitter, and P.C. Barron. 1987b. Comparative absorption of zinc picolinate, zinc citrate, and zinc gulconate in humans. Agents and Actions 21:223–228.

Beauvais, F., and S. LaBoueff. 1985. Drug and alcohol abuse intervention in American Indian communities. Int. J. Addict. 20:139–171.

Bensky, D., and A. Gamble. 1986. Chinese Herbal Medicine: Materia Medica. Eastland Press, Seattle, Wash.

Bhole, M.V. 1967. Treatment of bronchial asthma by yogic methods. Yoga-Mimamfa 9(3):33–41.

Birch, S. 1993. Some thoughts on the nature and timing of currently proposed changes in the acupuncture field. Unpublished paper.

Black Elk, W., and W.S. Lyon. 1990. Black Elk, The Sacred Ways of a Lakota. Harper & Row, San Francisco.

Blair, D.M., C.S. Hangee-Bauer, and C. Calabrese. 1991. Intestinal candidiasis, L. acidophilus supplementation, and Crook's questionnaires. Journal of Naturopathic Medicine 2:33–36.

Bouchayer, F. 1990. Alternative medicines: a general approach to the French situation. Complementary Medical Research 4:4–8.

Broken Nose, M. 1992. Working with the Aoglala Lakota: an outsider's perspective. Fam. Soc. 73:380–384.

Brostoff, J. 1988. Double-blind sublingual treatment and immunological studies. Department of Immunology, Middlesex Hospital. (Abstract presented at 6th Annual International Symposium on Man and His Environment, Dallas.)

Brown, D., and A. Lange. 1992. A homeopathic proving of Candida parapsilosis. Homeopathic Links 5:21–22.

Brown, M.F. 1988. Shamanism and its discontents. Medical Anthropology Quarterly 2:102–120.

Bullock, M., P. Culliton, and R. Olander. 1989. Controlled trial of acupuncture for severe recidivist alcoholism. Lancet 1:1435–1439.

Campbell, M.B. 1973. Neurological manifestations of allergic disease. Ann. Allergy 31:485–498.

Cassidy, C. 1994. Survey of acupuncture clinic patients at the Traditional Acupuncture Institute, Columbia, Md. Unpublished.

Cassileth, B., E. Lusk, R. Strouse, and B. Bodenheimer. 1984. Contemporary unorthodox treatments in cancer medicine: a study of patients, treatments, and practitioners. Ann. Intern. Med. 101:105–112.

Cazin, J., M. Cazin, and J.L. Gaborit, et al. 1987. A study of the effect of decimal and centesimal dilutions of arsenic on the retention and mobilization of arsenic in the rat. Hum. Toxicol. 6:315–320.

Chapman, C.R., and C.C. Gunn. 1990. Acupuncture. In J.J. Bonniker, ed. The Management of Pain. Lea and Febiger, Philadelphia.

Chen, J.Y.T. 1973. Acupuncture anesthesia in the People's Republic of China. DHEW Pub. (NIH)75–759. National Institutes of Health, Bethesda, Md.

Choffres, E.R. 1987. Neurotoxic effects of pesticides critical to health. Nation's Health APHA (April).

Christensen, B.V., I.U. Iuhl, H.H. Vilvek, H.H. Bulow, N.C. Dreijer, and H.F. Rasmussen. 1992. Acupuncture treatment of severe knee osteoarthrosis: a long-term study. Acta Anaesthesiol. Scand. 36:519–525.

CNAM. 1991. Healthcare Professionals in Private Practice in 1990. CNAM Pub No. 61. Social Security Statistics, Paris, France.

Collins, J.C., and P.J. Mittman. 1990. The physiological effects of colon hydrotherapy. Journal of Naturopathic Medicine 1:4–9.

Davenas, E., F. Beauvais, and J. Amara. 1988. Human basophil degranulation triggered by very dilute antiserum against IgE. Nature 333:816–818.

Davenas, E., B. Poitevan, and J. Benveniste. 1987. Effect on mouse peritoneal macrophages of orally administered very high dilutions of silica. Eur. J. Pharmacol. 135:313–319.

Davis, E.S. 1985. The new victims. Ecological Illness Law Report (July–October).

Dean, K. 1981. Self-care responses to illness: a selected review. Soc. Sci. Med. 15A:673–687.

Delinick, A.N. 1991. A hypothesis on how homeopathic remedies work on the organism. Berlin Journal on Research in Homeopathy 1:249–253.

Dickens, E., and G. Lewith. 1989. A single-blind controlled and randomized clinical trial to evaluate the effect of acupuncture in the treatment of trapezio-metacarpal osteoarthritis. Complementary Medical Research 3:5–8.

Doutremepuich, C., et al. 1987. Template bleeding time after ingestion of ultralow dosages of acetylsalicylic acid in healthy subjects. Thromb. Res. 48:501–504.

Dubray, W.H. 1985. American Indian values: critical factor in casework. Soc. Casework 66:30–37.

Dundee, J.W., et al. 1989. Acupuncture prophylaxis and cancer chemotherapy-induced sickness. R. Soc. Med. 82:268–271.

Dundee, R.G., K.N. Ghaly, W.N. Bill, K.T.J. Chestnutt, Fitzpatrick and A.G.A. Lynas. 1989. Effect of stimulation of the P6 antiemetic point on postoperative nausea and vomiting. Br. J. Anaesth. 63:612–618.

Eisenberg, D.M., R.C. Kessler, C. Foster, F.E. Norlock, D.R. Calkins, and T.L. Delbanco. 1993. Unconventional medicine in the United States. N. Engl. J. Med. 328:246–252.

Eliade, M. 1964. Shamanism: Archaic Techniques of Ecstasy. Princeton University Press, Princeton, N.J.

Elkington, J. 1986. The Poisoned Womb. Penguin Books, Middlesex, England.

Emrick, C.D. 1987. Alcoholics Anonymous: affiliative processes and effectiveness as treatment. Alcohol. Clin. Exp. Res. 11:416–423.

Encyclopaedia Britannica. 1990. Alcohol and alcoholism. Macropaedia, Vol. 13:216–229.

Erickson, R.J. 1992. Acupuncture for chronic pain treatment: its effects on office visits and the use of analgesics in a pre-paid health plan—a feasibility study. American Academy of Medical Acupuncture Review 4(2):2–6.

Farrer, C.R. 1991. Living Life's Circle: Mescalero Apache Cosmovision. University of New Mexico Press, Albuquerque, N.M.

Ferley, J.P., D. Smirou, D. D'Adhemar, and F. Balducci. 1989. A controlled evaluation of a homeopathic preparation in the treatment of influenza-like syndromes. Br. J. Clin. Pharmacol. 27:329–335.

Fields, J.Z., P.A. Rawal, J.F. Hagen, et al. 1990. Oxygen free radical scavenging effects of an anti-carcinogenic natural product, Maharishi Amrit Kalash (MAK). The Pharmacologist 32:155.

Fischer, K., and S. Grosshans (trans. A.R. Meuss). 1992. Psychology and biography of patients with ulcerative colitis and Crohn's disease: a study (parts 1 and 2). J. Anthroposophical Medicine 9, autumn and winter.

Fisher, P., A. Greenwood, E.C. Huskisson, P. Turner, and P. Belon. 1989. Effect of homeopathic treatment on fibrositis (primary fibromyalgia). Br. Med. J. 299:365–366.

Flaws, B. 1993. On the historical relationship of acupuncture and herbal medicine in China and what this means politically in the United States. American Journal of Acupuncture 21(3):267–278.

Fox, E. 1992. Crossing the bridge: adaptive strategies among Navajo health care workers. Free Inquiry in Creative Sociology 20: 25–34.

Funderburk, J. 1977. Science Studies Yoga—A Review of Physiologic Data. Himalayan Institute of Yoga Science and Philosophy of U.S.A.

Fung, K.P., and O.K.W. Chow. 1986. Attenuation of exercise-induced asthma by acupuncture. Lancet 14–1422.

Galanter, M. 1990. Culture and zealous self-help: a psychiatric perspective. Am. J. Psychiatry 147:28–40.

Gerdes, K.A. 1993. Provocation/neutralization testing: state of the art 1993. Environmental Medicine 9(1).

Gerrard, J. 1989. A double-blind study on the value of low-dose immunotherapy in the treatment of asthma and allergic rhinitis. Clinical Ecology 6:43–46.

Gibson, R.D., et al. 1980. The place for non-pharmaceutical therapy in chronic R.A.: a critical study of homeopathy. British Homeopathy Journal 69:121–123.

Gibson, R.G., S.L.M. Gibson, A.D. MacNeill, G.H. Gray, W.C. Dick, and W. Buchanan. 1978. Salicylates and homeopathy in rheumatoid arthritis: preliminary observations. Br. J. Clin. Pharmacol. 6:391–395.

Glaser, F.B., and A.C. Ogborne. 1982. Does AA really work? Br. J. Addict. 77:123–129.

Glaser J.L., J.L. Brind, J.H. Vogelman, et al. 1992. Elevated serum DHEAS levels in practitioners of the transcendental meditation (TM) and TM-Sidhi programs. J. Behav. Med. 15(4):327–341.

Gopal, K.S., V. Anatharaman, S. Balachander, and S.D. Nishith. 1973. The cardiorespiratory adjustments in "pranayama," with and without "bandhas" in "Vajrasana." Indian J. Med. Sci. 27(9):686–692.

Gopal, K.S., A. Natarajan, and S. Ramakrishnan. 1974. Biochemical studies in foreign volunteers practicing hatha yoga. Journal of Research in Indian Medicine 9(3):1–8.

Greil, A., and D. Rudy. 1983. Conversion to the world view of Alcoholics Anonymous: a refinement of conversion theory. Qualitative Sociology 6:5–28.

Guilmet, G., and D. Whited. 1987. Cultural lessons for clinical mental health practice: the Puyallup tribal community. Am. Indian and Alsk. Native Ment. Health Res. 1:32–49.

Gunn and Milbrandt. 1980. Dry needling of muscle motor points for chronic low back pain. Spine 15:279–291.

Halifax, J. 1979. Shamanic Voices: A Survey of Visionary Narratives. E.P. Dutton, New York.

Han, J.S. 1987. The Neurochemical Basis of Pain Relief by Acupuncture. Beijing Medical University, Beijing, People's Republic of China.

Harner, M. 1990. The Way of the Shaman: A Guide to Power and Healing. Harper and Row, San Francisco.

Harrod, H.L. 1992. Renewing the World. University of Arizona Press, Tucson, Ariz.

Harwood, A. 1971. The hot-cold theory of disease: implications for treatment of Puerto Rican patients. JAMA 216:1153–1158.

Harwood, A., ed. 1981. Ethnicity and Medical Care. Harvard University Press, Cambridge, Mass.

Helms, J. 1987. Acupuncture for the management of primary dysmenorrhea. Obstet. Gynecol. 69:51–56.

Helms, J. 1993. Physicians and Acupuncture in the 1990s. Report for the Subcommittee on Labor, Health and Human Services, and Education of the Appropriations Committee, U.S. Senate, 24 June, 1993. American Academy of Medical Acupuncture Review 5:1–6.

Hildebrandt, G. 1986. Die Bedeutung der Medizinischen Cronobiologie für Diagnostik und Therapie. Heilkunst 99:506–518.

Hildebrandt, G., and H. Hensel, eds. 1982. Biological Adaptation. Thieme-Verlag, Stuttgart, Germany.

Hiller, S.M., and J.A. Jewel. 1983. Health Care and Traditional Medicine in China: 1800 to 1982. Routledge and Kegan Paul, London, England.

Hirayama, C., et al. 1989. A multicenter randomized controlled clinical trial of shosaikoto in chronic active hepatitis. Gastroenterol. Jpn. 24:715–719.

Hostetler, J. 1976. Folk medicine and sympathy healing among the Amish. In W. Hand, ed. American Folk Medicine, a Symposium (pp. 249–258). University of California Press, Berkeley, Calif.

Hsu, H.Y., et. al. 1982. Chemical Constituents of Oriental Herbs, Vol. 1. Oriental Healing Arts Press, Long Beach, Calif.

Hsu, H.Y., et al. 1985. Chemical Constituents of Oriental Herbs, Vol. 2. Oriental Healing Arts Press, Long Beach, Calif.

Hudson, C. 1979. Black Drink, a Native American Tea. University of Georgia Press, Athens, Ga.

Hudson, T. 1991. Consecutive case study research of carcinoma in situ of cervix employing local escharotic treatment combined with nutritional therapy. Journal of Naturopathic Medicine 2:6–10.

Hudson, T. 1993a. Escharotic treatment for cervical dysplasia and carcinoma. Journal of Naturopathic Medicine 4(1):23.

Hudson, T. 1993b. Gynecology and Naturopathic Medicine: A Treatment Manual (2nd ed.). C.K.E. Publications, Olympia, Wash.

Hudson, T., and L. Standish. 1993. Clinical and endocrinologic effects of a menopausal formula. Presented at American Association of Naturopathic Physicians Convention, Portland, Ore.

Hufford, D.J. 1988. Contemporary folk medicine. In N. Gevitz, ed. Other Healers, Unorthodox Medicine in America. Johns Hopkins University Press, Baltimore, Md.

Hufford, D.J. 1990. Psychosocial Background and Prevalence of Unconventional Cancer Treatments; Selected Practitioners. Report to the U.S. Office of Technology Assessment. U.S. Government Printing Office, Washington, D.C.

Hufford, D.J. 1992. Folk medicine in contemporary America. In J. Kirkland, H. Mathews, C. Sullivan III, and K. Baldwin, eds. Herbal and Magical Medicine, Traditional Healing Today. Duke University Press, Durham, N.C.

Hultkrantz, A. 1985. The shaman and the medicine man. Soc. Sci. Med. 20:511–515.

Hwang, Y.C., and E.M. Jenkins. 1988. Effect of acupuncture on young pigs with induced enteropathogenic Escherichia coli diarrhea. Am. J. Vet. Res. 49:1641–1643.

Ingerman, S. 1991. Soul Retrieval: Mending the Fragmented Self. Harper, San Francisco.

Jacobs, J. 1992. Unpublished survey data. American Institute of Homeopathy.

Jacobs, J., and C. Crothers. 1991. Who sees homeopaths? British Homeopathic Journal 80:57–58.

Jacobs, J., M. Jiménez, S. Gloyd, F. Carares, G. Paniagua, and D. Crothers. 1993. Homeopathic treatment of acute childhood diarrhea. British Homeopathic Journal 82:83–86.

Janssen, G.W.H.M. 1989. The application of Maharishi Ayur-Veda in the treatment of ten chronic diseases: a pilot study. Nederlands Tijdschrift Voor Integrale Geneeskunde 5:586–594.

Jharote, M.L. 1973. Effect of yoga training on physical fitness. Yoga-Mimamsa 15(40):31–35.

Johnston, B. 1982. Ojibway Ceremonies. University of Nebraska Press, Lincoln, Neb.

Jouanny, J. 1980. The Essentials of Homeopathic Therapeutics. Laboratoires Boiron, Ste-Foy-les-Lyon, France.

Keine, H. 1989. Klinische Studien zur Misteltherapie karzinomatöser Erkrankungen, Eine Übersicht. Therapeutikon 3:347–353.

King, D.S. 1981. Can allergic exposure provoke psychological symptoms? A double-blind test. Biol. Psychiatry 16:3–19.

King, W.P. 1989. Diagnostic and therapeutic techniques for chemical-environmental allergy and hypersensitivity. In H.F. Krause, ed. Otolaryngologic Allergy and Immunology. W.B. Saunders, Philadelphia.

Kirby, M. 1992. Moving toward a holistic lifestyle. Lightworks (August):11.

Kirkland, J. 1992. Talking fire out of burns: a magicoreligious healing tradition. In J. Kirkland, H. Mathews, C. Sullivan III, and K. Baldwin, eds. Herbal and Magical Medicine, Traditional Healing Today. Duke University Press, Durham, N.C.

Kishore, J. 1983. Homeopathy: the Indian experience. World Health Forum 4:105–107.

Kleijnen, J., P. Knipschild, and G. ter Riet. 1991. Clinical trials of homeopathy. BMJ 302:316–323.

Kleinman, A. 1980. Patients and Healers in the Context of Culture. University of California Press, Berkeley, Calif.

Kolisko, L. 1932. Physiologic Proof of the Activity of Smallest Entities. Mitteilungen des Biologischen Instituts am Goetheanum, Nr 1. Medizinische Sektion am Goetheanum, Orient Occident Verlag, Stuttgart, Germany. (Translated by H. Jurgens, Mercury Press, Spring Valley, N.Y., 1990.)

Kurtz, E. 1982. Why AA works: the intellectual significance of Alcoholics Anonymous. J. Stud. Alcohol 43:38–80.

Laderman, C. 1988. Wayward winds: Malay archetypes, and theory of personality in the context of shamanism. Soc. Sci. Med. 27:799–810.

Lake, A. 1982. Dietary protein-induced colitis in breastfed infants. J. Pediatr. 101:906–910.

Lee, M.H.M., and S.J. Liao. 1990. Acupuncture in physiatry. In Cottke and Leahmann, eds. Kruse's Handbook of Physical Medicine and Rehabilitation. W.B. Saunders, Philadelphia.

Lichstein, P.R. 1992. Rootwork from the clinician's perspective. In J. Kirland, H. Mathews, C. Sullivan III, and K. Baldwin, eds. Herbal and Magical Medicine, Traditional Healing Today. Duke University Press, Durham, N.C.

Locke, P. 1993. Declaration of War 1993, Lakota, Dakota, Nakota traditionalists. Personal communication.

Lonsdorf, N. 1993. Personal communication.

Luckert, K.W., and J.C. Cooke. 1979. Coyoteway, a Navajo Holyway Healing Ceremonial. University of Arizona Press, Tuscon, Ariz.

Lytle, C.D. 1993. An Overview of Acupuncture. Center for Devices and Radiological Health, U.S. Department of

Health and Human Services, Public Health Service, Food and Drug Administration.

Mabry, C.R. 1982. Treatment of common gynecologic symptoms by allergy management procedures. Obstet. Gynecol. 59:560–564.

Manson, S., R. Walker, and D. Kivlahan. 1987. Psychiatric assessment and treatment of American Indians and Alaska Natives. Hosp. Community Psychiatry 38:165–173.

Marburg, G.S. 1983. Mental health and Native Americans: responding to the challenge of the biopsychosocial model. White Cloud Journal of American Indian Mental Health 3:43–52.

Mathews, H.F. 1987. Rootwork: description of an ethnomedical system in the American South. South. Med. J. 80(7):885–891.

Mathews, H. 1992. Doctors and root doctors: patients who use both. In J. Kirkland, H. Mathews, C. Sullivan III, and K. Baldwin, eds. Herbal and Magical Medicine, Traditional Healing Today. Duke University Press, Durham, N.C.

May, P. 1986. Alcohol and drug misuse prevention programs for American Indians: needs and opportunities. J. Stud. Alcohol 47:187–195.

May, P., and M.B. Smith. 1988. Some Navajo opinions about alcohol abuse and prohibition: a survey and recommendations for policy. J. Stud. Alcohol 49:324–334.

McCaleb, E.R. 1993. Into the mainstream: rational use and regulation of herb products in the United States. Journal of the Acupuncture Society of New York 1(1):16–19.

McClenon, J. 1993. The experiential foundations of shamanic healing. J. Med. Philos. 18:107–128.

McGaa, E. (Eagle Man). 1990. Mother Earth Spirituality: Native American Paths to Healing Ourselves and Our World. Harper & Row, San Francisco.

McGovern, J.J. 1981. The provocative sublingual method (letter). Ann. of Allergy 46:44–47.

Messer, E. 1981. Hot-cold classification: theoretical and practical implications of a Mexican study. Soc. Sci. Med. 15B:133–145.

Miller, J.B. 1972. Food Allergy, Provocation Testing and Injection Therapy. Charles C. Thomas, Springfield, Ill.

Ministry of Science and Technology, Federal Republic of Germany, Bonn. 1992. Anthroposophical medicine. In Unkonventionelle Medizinische Richtungun, Bestandsaufnahme zur Forschungssituation [Unconventional Medical Orientations, Assessment of Scientific Status; H. Jurgens, trans.]. Fellowship Community Associates, Spring Valley, N.Y.

Mittman P. 1990. Double blind randomized study of Urtica dioica in the treatment of allergic rhinitis. Planta Med. 56:44–47.

Monro, J., J. Brostoff, C. Carini, and K. Zilkha. 1980. Food allergy in migraine. Study of dietary exclusion and RAST. Lancet 2(8184):1–4.

Morgan, W. 1931/1977. Navaho treatment of sickness: diagnosticians. In D. Landy, ed. Culture, Disease, and Healing: Studies in Medical Anthropology. Macmillan, New York.

Morris, D.L. 1981. Formaldehyde sensitivity and toxicity (letter). JAMA 246:329.

Morse, J., D. Young, and L. Swartz. 1991. Cree Indian healing practices and Western health care: a comparative analysis. Soc. Sci. Med. 32:1361–1366.

Murphy, M. 1992a. Scientific studies of contemplative experience. In The Future of the Body, Jeremy Tarcher, Los Angeles, Calif., pp. 527–529.

Murphy, M. 1992b. Appendix C, scientific meditation studies. In The Future of the Body. Jeremy Tarcher, Los Angeles, Calif., pp. 603–611.

Murphy, M., and S. Donovan. 1988. The Physical and Psychological Effects of Meditation—A Review of Contemporary Meditation Research with a Comprehensive Bibliography 1931–1988. Esalen Institute Study of Exceptional Functioning, San Rafael, Calif.

Myerhoff, B. 1976. Shamanic equilibrium: balance and mediation in known and unknown worlds. In W. Hand, ed. American Folk Medicine: A Symposium (pp. 99–108). University of California Press, Berkeley.

Naranjo, T., and R. Swentzell. 1989. Healing spaces in the Tewa Pueblo world. American Indian Culture and Research Journal 13:257–265.

National College of Naturopathic Medicine Clinical Faculty. 1991. Safety and Efficacy of Cervical Caps.

National Council Against Health Fraud. 1991. Acupuncture: the position paper of the National Council Against Health Fraud. Clin. J. Pain 7(2):162–166.

National Research Council. 1975. Working Conference on Principles of Protocols for Evaluating Chemicals in the Environment. Committee on Toxicology/Environmental Studies Board. National Academy of Sciences, Washington, D.C.

Neihardt, J.G. 1932. Black Elk Speaks: Being the Life Story of a Holy Man of the Oglala Sioux. Pocket Books, New York.

New Mexico Association of Acupuncture and Oriental Medicine. 1993. Scope of Practice in New Mexico—Background Information on the Scope of Practice of Doctors of Oriental Medicine in the State of New Mexico. (P.O. Box 5882, Santa Fe, NM 87502.)

Ng, T.H., et al. 1991. Encephalopathy and neuropathy following ingestion of Chinese herbal broth containing podophyllin. J. Neurol. Sci. 101:107–113.

Oberg, G.R. 1990. An overview of the philosophy of the American Academy of Environmental Medicine. (Available from AAEM, P.O. Box 16106, Denver, CO 80216.)

Ogborne, A.C. 1989. Some limitations of Alcoholics Anonymous. In M. Galanter, ed. Recent Developments in Alcoholism, Vol. 7: Treatment Research. Plenum Press, New York.

Orme-Johnson, D.W. 1988. Medical care utilization and the Transcendental Meditation program. Psychosom. Med. 49(5):493–507.

Panush, R. 1986. Food-induced allergic arthritis. Arthritis Rheum. 29:220–226.

Patel, C.H. 1973. Yoga and biofeedback in the management of hypertension. Lancet 2(837):1053–1055.

Patel, M., F. Gutzwiller, F. Paccaud, and A. Marazzi. 1989. A meta-analysis of acupuncture for chronic pain. Int. J. Epidemiol. 18:900–906.

Pedersen, P., J. Draguns, W. Lonner, and J. Trimble. 1989. Counseling Across Cultures (3rd ed.). University of Hawaii Press, Honolulu.

Peele, S. 1990. Research issues in assessing addiction treatment efficacy: how cost-effective are Alcoholics Anonymous and private treatment centers? Drug Alcohol Depend. 25:179–182.

Phillip, T., J.R. Shah, and H.L. Worth. 1988. Acupuncture in the treatment of bladder instability. Br. J. Urol. 61:490–493.

Poitevin, B., E. Davenas, and J. Benveniste. 1988. In vitro immunological degranulation of human basophils is modulated by lung histamine and apis mellifica. Br. J. Clin. Pharmacol. 25:439–444.

Pomeranz, B. 1986. Scientific basis of acupuncture. In Stux and Pomeranz, eds. Acupuncture: Textbook and Atlas. Springer-Verlag, Berlin.

Powers, W. 1977. Oglala Religion. University of Nebraska Press, Lincoln, Neb.

Powers, W. 1982. Yuwipi: Vision and Experience in Oglala Ritual. University of Nebraska Press, Lincoln, Neb.

Quinn, J.R., ed. 1972. Medicine and Public Health in the Peoples Republic of China. DHEW pub. no. (NIH)72-67. National Institutes of Health, Bethesda, Md.

Randolph, T. 1959. Ecologic mental illness. J. Lab. Clin. Med. 54:936.

Randolph, T. 1962. Human Ecology and Susceptibility to the Chemical Environment. Charles C. Thomas, Springfield, Ill.

Randolph, T. 1976. Stimulatory and withdrawal levels of manifestation. In L. Dickey, ed. Clinical Ecology. Charles C. Thomas, Springfield, Ill.

Randolph, T. 1987. Environmental Medicine Beginnings and Bibliographies of Clinical Ecology. Clinical Ecology Publications, Fort Collins, Colo.

Randolph, T., and R.W. Moss. 1980. An Alternative Approach to Allergies. Lippincott and Crowell, New York.

Rapp, D. 1947. Bibliography of Environmental Medicine. (Available from Practical Allergy Research Foundation, P.O. Box 60, Buffalo, NY 14223–0060.)

Rapp, D. 1979. Food allergy treatment for hyperkinesis. Journal of Learning Disabilities 12:42–50.

Rapp, D. 1981. A prototype for food sensitivity studies in children. Ann. Allergy 47:123–124.

Rapp, D. 1986. Environmental medicine: an expanded approach. Buffalo Physician February issue.

Rea, W.J. 1991. Chemical Sensitivity. Lewis Publishers, Boca Raton, Fla.

Rea, W.J., and M.J. Mitchell. 1982. Chemical sensitivity in the environment. Journal of Immunology and Allergy Practice (September/October):21–31.

Rea, W.J., R.N. Podell, M.L. Williams, E. Fenyves, D.E. Sprague, and A.R. Johnson. 1984. Elimination of oral food challenge reaction by injection of food extracts: a double-blind evaluation. Arch. Otolaryngol. 110(4):248–252.

Reichard, G.A. 1939. Navaho Medicine Man. J.J. Augustin, New York.

Reichard, G.A. 1950. Navaho Religion: A Study of Symbolism. Princeton University Press, Princeton, N.J.

Reilly, D.T., M.A. Taylor, C. McSharry, and T. Aitchison. 1986. Is homeopathy a placebo response? Controlled trial of homeopathic potency, with pollen in hayfever as model. Lancet 2(8512):881–886.

Reimansnyder, B.L. 1989. Powwowing in Union Country: A Study of Pennsylvania German Folk Medicine in Context. AMS Press Inc., New York.

Rinkel, H.J. 1963. Archives of Otolaryngol. 77:302–326.

Romanuicci-Ross, L. 1969. The hierarchy of resort in curative practices: the Admiralty Islands, Melanesia. J. Health Soc. Behav. 10(3):201–209.

Rosenstock, L., and M. Cullen. 1994. Textbook of Clinical, Occupational, and Environmental Medicine. Saunders, Philadelphia.

Rowe, A. 1950. Allergic toxemia and fatigue. Ann. Allergy 8:72–79.

Rubel, A. 1960. Concepts of disease in Mexican-American culture. American Anthropologist 62:795–814.

Rubel, A. 1964. The epidemiology of a folk illness: susto in Hispanic America. Ethnology 3:268–283.

Rubel, A., C.W. O'Neill, and R.C. Ardon. 1984. Susto: a folk illness. University of California Press, Berkeley, Calif.

Rudy, D. 1987. Taking the pledge: the commitment process in Alcoholics Anonymous. J. Stud. Alcohol 41:727–732.

Saifer, P., and M. Saifer. 1987. Clinical detection of sensitivity to preservatives and chemicals. In Food Allergy and Intolerance. W.B. Saunders, Philadelphia. pp. 416–424.

Sancier, K.M. 1991 (fall). Reports from the Qi Gong Institute. San Francisco, Calif.

Sancier. K.M. 1993 (spring). Reports from the Qi Gong Institute. San Francisco, Calif.

Sancier, K.M., and B. Hu. 1991. Medical applications of qi gong and emitted qi on humans, animals, cell cultures, and plants: review of selected scientific research. American Journal of Acupuncture 19:367–377.

Sandner, D.F. 1979. Navaho Indian medicine and medicine men. In D.S. Sobel, ed. Ways of Health. Harcourt Brace Jovanovich, New York.

Sandner, D.F. 1991. Navajo Symbols of Healing: A Jungian Exploration of Ritual, Image, and Medicine. Healing Arts Press, Rochester, Vt.

Scharff, P. 1993. Personal communication. Board of the American College of Anthroposophically Extended Medicine, Spring Valley, N.Y.

Schneider, R.H., C.N. Alexander, and R.K. Wallace. 1992. In search of an optimal behavioral treatment for hypertension: a review and focus on transcendental meditation. In E.H. Johnson, W.D. Gentry, and S. Julius, eds. Personality, Elevated Blood Pressure, and Hypertension. Hemisphere Publishing Corp., Washington, D.C.

Schneider, R.H., K.L. Cavanaugh, A.H.S. Kasture, et al. 1990. Health promotion with a traditional system of natural health care: Maharishi Ayur-Veda. Journal of Social Behavior and Personality 5(3):1–27.

Scott, A.W. 1993. Masters of the Ordinary: Integrating Personal Experience and Vernacular Knowledge in Alcoholics Anonymous. Ph.D. dissertation. Michigan Microfilms, Ann Arbor, Mich.

Shannahoff-Khalsa, X. 1991. Stress technology medicine: a new paradigm for stress and considerations for self-regulation. In M. Brown, G.F. Koob, and C. Rivier, eds. Stress—Neurobiology and Neuroendocrinology. Marcel Dekker, New York.

Sharma, H.M., C. Dwivedi, B.C. Satter, H.A. Gudehitihlu, W. Malarkey, and G.A. Tejwani. 1990. Antineoplastic properties of Maharishi 4, against DMBA-induced mammary tumors in rats. Journal of Pharmacology, Biochemistry, and Behavior 35:767–773.

Sheehan, M.P., and J. Atherton. 1992. A controlled clinical trial of traditional Chinese medicinal plants in widespread, non-exudative atopic eczema. Br. J. Dermatol. 126(2):179–184.

Shipley, M., H. Berry, and G. Broster, et al. 1983. Controlled trial of homeopathic treatment of osteoarthritis. Lancet 1(8316):97–98.

Shirakawa, S., and W. Rea. 1990. Evaluation of the autonomic nervous system response by puppilo-graphical study in the chemically sensitive patient. Clinical Ecology 7(2).

Slagle, A., and J. Weibel-Orlando. 1986. The Indian Shaker church and Alcoholics Anonymous: revitalistic curing cults. Hum. Organ. 45:310–319.

Smith, M.O. 1987. Chinese Medical Treatment for AIDS. Results of Five Years of Experience. World Congress of Acupuncture and Natural Medicine, Beijing, People's Republic of China.

Smith, M. 1988. An acupuncture programme for the treatment of drug-addicted persons. Bull. Narc. 11:35–41.

Smith, R.B., and G.W. Boericke. 1967. Continued research with modern instrumentation for the evaluation of homeopathic drug structure. Journal of the American Institute of Homeopathy (Sep/Oct.):259–272.

Snow, L. 1993. Walkin' over Medicine. Westview Press, Boulder, Colo.

Sonoda, K. 1988. Health and Illness in Changing Japanese Society. Tokyo University Press, Tokyo, Japan.

Steiner, R., and I. Wegman. 1925. Fundamentals of Therapy: An Extension of the Art of Healing Through Spiritual Knowledge. Anthroposophic Press, Spring Valley, N.Y.

Storm, H. 1972. Seven Arrows. Harper & Row, San Francisco.

Sun, Y. 1988. The realm of traditional Chinese medicine in supportive care of cancer patients. Recent Results Cancer Res. 108:327–334.

Sutro, L. 1989. Alcoholics Anonymous in a Mexican peasant-Indian village. Hum. Organ. 48:180–186.

Tao, X.L., et al. 1989. A prospective controlled double blind crossover study of terptertygium wilfodil hook F in treatment of rheumatoid arthritis. Chin. Med. J. 102(5):327–332.

ter Riet, G., et al. 1990. Acupuncture in chronic pain: a criteria-based meta analysis. J. Clin. Epidemiol. 43:1191–1199.

Terrell, S.J. 1990. This Other Kind of Doctors: Traditional Medical Systems in Black Neighborhoods in Austin, Texas. AMD Press, Inc., New York.

Thom, D. 1992. Clinical Assessment of Food Sensitivities. Presented at American Association of Naturopathic Physicians Convention, Whistler, British Columbia, Canada.

Thyagarajan, S.P., S. Subramanian, T. Thirunalasundari, P.S. Venkateswaran, and B.S. Blumberg. 1988. Effect of phyllanthus amarus on chronic carriers of hepatitis B virus. Lancet 2(8614):764–766.

Topper, M.D. 1987. The traditional Navajo medicine man: therapist, counselor, and community leader. Journal of Psychoanalytic Anthropology 10:217–250.

Trice, H.M., and W.J. Staudenmeier. 1989. A sociocultural history of Alcoholics Anonymous. In M. Galanter, ed. Recent Developments in Alcoholism, Vol. 7: Treatment Research. Plenum Press, New York.

Trotter, R.T. 1985. Folk medicine in the Southwest: myths and medical facts. Postgrad. Med. 78:167–179.

Tsutani, K. 1993. Evaluation of herbal medicine: an East Asian perspective. In G.T. Lewith and D. Aldridge, eds. Clinical Research Methodology for Complementary Therapy. Hodder and Stoughton, London.

Udupa, K.N., R.H. Singh, and R.M. Settiwar. 1971. Studies in physiologic, endocrine, and metabolic response to the practice of yoga in young, normal volunteers. Journal of Research in Indian Medicine 6:345–355.

Unschuld, P.U. 1985. Medicine in China: History of Ideas. University of California Press, Berkeley, Calif.

Unschuld, P.U. 1986. Medicine in China: History of Pharmaceutics. University of California Press, Berkeley, Calif.

Unschuld, P.U. 1992. Epistemological issues in changing legitimization: traditional Chinese medicine in the 20th Century. In C. Leslie, and A. Young. eds. Paths to Asian Medical Knowledge. University of California Press, Berkeley, Calif.

U.S. Public Health Service. 1990. Healthy People 2000: National Health Promotion and Disease Prevention Objectives. U.S. Department of Health and Human Services, Washington, D.C.

van Haseln, R., and P. Fisher. 1990. Analyzing homeopathic prescribing using the Read Classification and Information technology. British Homeopathic Journal 79:74–81.

Vincent, C. 1990. A controlled trial in the treatment of migraine by acupuncture. Clin. J. Pain 5:305–312.

von Hauff, M., and R. Praetorius. 1990. The Performance Structure of Alternative Medical Practices—A Public Health Structure Analysis—A Pilot Study. University of Stuttgart. (Published by Soziale Hygiene, Verein Für ein Erweiteres Heilwesen, Bad Liebenzell, 1991; Translation by H. Jurgens, Anthroposophical Therapy and Hygiene Association, 1993.)

von Laue, H.B., and W. Henn. 1991. Chronological phenomena in cancerous diseases. Der Merkurstab 44(Jan–Feb):1,5. (Translation by H. Jurgens in Journal of Anthroposophical Medicine 8(1):1–18, 1991.)

Weidman, H. 1978. Southern black health profile. Miami Health Ecology Project, University of Miami (offprint).

Weller, S. 1983. New data on intracultural variability: the hot-cold concept of medicine and illness. Hum. Organ. 42:249–257.

Wharton, R., and G. Lewith. 1986. Complementary medicine and the general practitioner. Br. Med. J. 292:1490–1500.

When to believe the unbelievable. 1988. Nature 333:787.

Wigginton, E. 1972. The Foxfire Book. Anchor Books, New York.

Wilkinson, D. 1987. Traditional medicine in American families: reliance on the wisdom of elders. Marriage and Family Review 11:65–76.

Williams, B. Personal Communication. American Academy of American Acupuncture, Los Angeles, Calif.

Wiseman, N., et al., trans. 1985. Fundamentals of Chinese Medicine. Paradigm Publications, Brookline, Mass.

Wolff, O. n.d. The Anthroposophical Approach to Medicine, Vol. 1. Anthroposophic Press, Spring Valley, New York.

Wong, N.D., et al. 1991. A comparison of Chinese traditional and Western medical approaches for the treatment of mild hypertension. Yale J. Biol. Med. 64(1):79–87.

Wright, J.W., ed. 1990. The Universal Almanac. Andrews and McMeel, Kansas City, Mo.

Wyman, L., and B. Haile. 1970. Blessingway. University of Arizona Press, Tuscon. Ariz.

Xu, G.Z., et al. 1989. Chinese herb "destagnation" series, 1: combination of radiation with destagnation in treatment of nasopharyngeal carcinoma (NPC), a prospective randomized trial in 188 cases. Int. J. Radiat. Oncol. Biol. Phys. 16(2):297–300.

Yellowtail, T., and M. Fitzgerald. 1991. Yellowtail, Crow Medicine Man and Sun Dance Chief: An Autobiography. University of Oklahoma Press, Norman, Okla.

Yoder, D. 1976. Hohman and Romanus: origins and diffusion of the Pennsylvania German powwow manual. In W. Hand, ed. American Folk Medicine, A Symposium (pp. 235–248). University of California Press, Berkeley, Calif.

Young, J.C. 1981. Medical Choice in a Mexican Village. Rutgers University Press, New Brunswick, N.J.

Young, M. 1989. Cry of the Eagle: Encounters with a Cree Healer. University of Toronto Press, Buffalo, N.Y.

Zhao, H.Y., et al. 1993. Effects of Kampo (Japanese herbal) medicine FHO-Saiko-To on DNA-synthesizing enzyme activity in 1,2-dimethylhydrazine-induced colonic carcinomas in rats. Planta Med. 59(2):152–154.

Zmiewski, P. 1994. Introduction. In G. Soulie de Morant. L'Acuponcture Chinoise (English ed.). Redwing Books, Brookline, Mass.

Manual Healing Methods

PANEL MEMBERS

Barbara Brennan, M.S.—Cochair
Anthony Rosner, Ph.D.—Cochair
Alan Demmerle, M.S.E.E.
Michael Patterson, Ph.D.
Nelda Samarel, R.N., Ed.D.

CONTRIBUTING AUTHORS

Beverly Rubik, Ph.D.—Lead Author
Richard Pavek—Lead Author

Osteopathy
Robert Ward, D.O.
Massage
Elliott Greene, M.A.
Cranial-Sacral
John Upledger, D.O.
Chiropractic
Dana Lawrence,D.C.
Biofield Therapeutics
Richard Pavek
Physical Therapy
Elsa Ramsden, Ed.D.

Introduction

Touch and manipulation with the hands have been in use in health and medical practice since the beginning of medical care. Whether in comforting a child by stroking or rubbing a body stiffened by the cold, touch was the first and foremost of all diagnostic and therapeutic devices. Hippocrates discussed the benefits of therapeutic massage and instructed his students in its use and in spinal manipulation. The Chinese also included massage in its ancient healing practices and touch in its diagnostic methods (see "Alternative Systems of Medicine" chapter); the practitioner's taking of the pulse with the fingertips was considered to be the most important diagnostic tool of the ancient Chinese physician (Veith, 1949). Entire healing systems of touch based on the meridian system (see the glossary) were developed centuries ago and remain in use today in the United States as well as in Asia.

The hands once were the physician's greatest and most important diagnostic and therapeutic tool. Today the medical and health practitioner retreats further and further from physical contact with the patient, ever more distanced by banks of diagnostic equipment, legal constraints, and time factors. Psychotherapists are admonished not to touch their clients, and the price of medical doctors' time is now so high that they cannot even massage the stiffness from a patient's back; instead, the doctor or psychotherapist must write a prescription for a massage therapist, a person with therapeutic skills no longer taught in medical schools. It is skills of this type—ancient traditional healing skills that are now called "alternative"—that this chapter addresses.

All the manual healing methods addressed in this chapter rely on the practitioner's hands as a primary modality both to access information from (that is, to diagnose) and to treat the patient. Nevertheless, many manual healing methods are highly individualized; there is much art in this field, much individualization. Many practitioners have developed unique systems, in some cases teaching them to others. Consequently, there are many more systems than can be discussed here; no slight is intended by the omissions.

This chapter is divided into four sections. The first discusses methods that use physical touch, pressure, and movement. The second discusses those that are described as using a biofield, or "energy." Therapies that appear to rely on both physical and biofield elements are described in the third section. The fourth section illustrates how manual healing methods are becoming included in mainstream health care. Recommendations and references follow at the end.

Physical Healing Methods

All the biomechanical therapies—grouped here as "physical healing methods"—are based on the understanding that dysfunction of any discrete body part often affects secondarily the function of other discrete, not necessarily directly connected, body parts, both in close proximity and at a distance. The various manual medicines have developed theories and processes that treat these secondary dysfunctions through a variety of methods that manipulate the soft tissues or realign the body parts. Overcoming these misalignments and manipulating soft tissues bring the individual parts back to optimal function and return the body to health.

Osteopathic Medicine

One of the earliest systems of health care in the United States to use manual healing methods was osteopathic medicine. To its practitioners and to much of the public, the manual healing methods of osteopathic medicine are mainstream processes, but some people consider them alternative.

The principles and philosophy of osteopathy integrate health and illness, emphasizing four major areas:

- Structure and function are interdependent. Furthermore, behavior is an intermingled complex in which psychosocial influences can affect both anatomy (structure) and physiology (function). All these relationships are fundamentally designed to work in harmony.
- The body has the ability to heal itself, and the role of the osteopathic physician is to enhance the healing process as much as possible.
- Diseases, impairments, and disabilities arise from disruptions of the normal interactions of anatomy, physiology, and behavior.
- Appropriate treatment is based on the ability to understand, diagnose, and treat—by whatever methods are available—including manually applied procedures. When hands-on procedures are used to identify somatic dysfunction (see the glossary), the practitioner then determines whether the pattern of somatic dysfunction that is observed can be related to any visceral (that is, related to the internal body organs), neuromusculoskeletal, or—occasionally—behavioral dysfunction.

History and context. American osteopathic medicine was begun by Andrew Taylor Still (1828–1917). Still was a physician of his period, trained mainly through apprenticeships. It is said that he attended a medical school in Kansas City, MO, for one semester but found it boring and irrelevant (Gevitz, 1980). As a result of many adverse experiences with then contemporary medical practices, including the death of several family members from untreatable meningitis and pneumonia, Still began a personal search for improved methods to treat diseases and restore health (Gevitz, 1980; Schiotz, 1958). This empirical approach continues to be used by many osteopathic physicians.

Development and use of osteopathically oriented manipulative skills began around the time of Still's search (Carlson, 1975; Gevitz, 1980), but how he developed his system that combined "lightning bone setting" with the magnetic healing concepts of Mesmer is not clear (Hood, 1871).

> It seems likely that his knowledge (of manipulation) was derived from simply observing the work of another practitioner in the field. However he learned these methods, Still soon afterwards made an important discovery, namely, that the sudden flexion and extension procedures peculiar to the spinal area were not limited to orthopedic problems; furthermore, they constituted a more reliable means of healing than simply rubbing the spine (Gevitz, 1980).

Whatever the circumstances, Still began his new health profession in 1874, before beginning his use of manipulation, which he was reported to use somewhat later in that decade (Gevitz, 1980). After advertising and working as both a magnetic healer and a lightning bone setter, he began writing about his ideas (Still, 1899). Ultimately, he founded his first school, the American School of Osteopathy, in 1892 at Kirksville, MO, to improve on existing surgical and obstetrical practices. The original emphasis was on observing the relationship between structure and function. He incorporated assumptions that manual restoration of normal anatomic relationships leads to physiological improvements. This reasoning included by definition a spectrum not only of health issues but of specific recommendations for disease and obstetrical interventions. Some examples from osteopathic literature include discussions dealing with labor and delivery, postoperative ileus (bowel) paralysis, asthma, otitis media (middle ear infection), hypertension, coronary artery disease, back pain, neck pain, diabetes, trauma of all kinds, migraine headache, and stress-related illnesses (Downing, 1935; Kuchera and Kuchera, 1990; Sleszynski and Kelso, 1993).

Osteopathy spread to England in the 1920s when John Littlejohn emigrated from Chicago to London, establishing the British School of Osteopathy, the first of several such schools. The expansion continued as continental European practitioners studied at the British schools in the 1930s and 1940s.

Historically, many currently popular manual medical techniques—with the exceptions of "energy" techniques, massage, and high-velocity maneuvers (Hood, 1871)—originated within American osteopathy and spread elsewhere. Among those techniques are manual methods applied in other medically oriented systems and also activities of alternative health care providers. Examples include muscle energy and postisometric relaxation concepts, which were originally developed and codified by Fred Mitchell, Sr. and Paul Kimberly; fascial-myofascial release and visceral techniques, developed by A.T. Still and others, including Charles Neidner; cranial-craniosacral techniques, William G. Sutherland (Sutherland, 1990); strain and counterstrain, Lawrence Jones; and thoracic pump and lymphatic techniques, A.T. Still, Gordon Zink, and several contemporaries. (Most of these techniques are described briefly in the "Osteopathic Education" section.)

In many instances, contemporary practices of these methods throughout the world are extensions and refinements of original osteopathic concepts. Other systems, such as chiropractic, Swedish massage, Cyriax (Great Britain), Mennell (Great Britain), Lewit (Czech Republic), Dvorak (Switzerland), and several German systems also have influenced current practices, both in the United States and elsewhere. Two current osteopathically based examples are advances in myofascial release and fascial unwinding maneuvers and in "energy"-based practices arising from basic cranial concepts, codified by both Sutherland and Harold Magoun, Sr. (Magoun, 1976; Sutherland, 1990).

Demographics. As of 1993, this country had more than 32,000 American-educated and licensed doctors of osteopathy (D.O.s), some in every State. They perform all aspects of medical care, including all specialties and family practice. Sixteen colleges and schools graduate approximately 1,500 D.O.s annually. While graduates make up about 5 percent of the country's physician population, the profession is responsible for approximately 10 percent of total health care delivery in the United States. More than 60 percent of osteopathic physicians are involved in primary care areas—family medicine, pediatrics, internal medicine, and obstetrics-gynecology (Annual Directory, 1993).

Many osteopathic physicians from a variety of disciplines regularly incorporate structural diagnosis of abnormalities of musculoskeletal function and manual medical treatments in their day-to-day activities.[1] Ironically, because of current attitudes among third-party payers toward physician use of manual medicine, many are not paid for these services. Much of the reluctance to pay is based on a lack of adequately funded research, particularly relating to outcome measures. From an osteopathic perspective, what is considered "alternative" by most of the medical and research establishment is mainstream for the average D.O. (Gevitz, 1980; Grad, 1979; Schiotz, 1958).

Osteopathic education. Basic American osteopathic education (Gershenow, 1985) includes substantial emphasis on osteopathic philosophy and principles including extensive manually oriented training designed to develop *manual medicine* diagnosis and treatment skills. The profession generally refers to the latter as *structural diagnosis* and *manipulative treatment*. These skills have been used by osteopathic physicians for more than 100 years in a context of total patient care.

---

[1]Robert Ward, an experienced osteopathic physician-researcher, estimated that 10 percent of osteopathic physicians use manual diagnosis and treatment a great deal and that some 60 percent use them in selected cases. Ward believes most patients receiving primary care from osteopaths probably receive a diagnostic workup involving manual diagnosis at some time, particularly if neuromusculoskeletal problems have been reported (Ward, 1994).

The Education Council on Osteopathic Principles, representing the 16 osteopathic colleges, is currently contributing to osteopathic education through three principal projects: the 1982 publication of an updated glossary of osteopathic terminology; development of a core curriculum for osteopathic principles; and development of state-of-the-art textbook chapters highlighting the uses of palpatory diagnosis (use of touch) and manipulative treatment in multiple clinical disciplines.

Basic palpation and structural diagnosis and treatment skills are emphasized in preclinical American osteopathic education, and eight major manual medical methods are taught in osteopathic colleges. These eight methods are as follows:

1. *Soft-tissue techniques* that enhance muscle relaxation and circulation of body fluids.
2. *Isometric and isotonic techniques* (often referred to as muscle energy or postisometric relaxation) that focus primarily on restoring physiological movements to altered joint mechanics.
3. *Articulatory techniques* (also called joint play and manipulation without impulse) that emphasize restoration of intrinsic joint mobility.
4. *High-velocity, low-amplitude techniques* (also called manipulation with impulse), designed to restore the symmetry of the movements associated with the vertebral joints.
5. *Myofascial release techniques* (also called fascial release techniques) that use combinations of so-called direct and indirect methods (see the glossary) to modify problems of individual and interactively related muscle groups and surrounding or covering (myofascial) tissues.
6. *Functional techniques* that emphasize treatment of restrictive patterns in joint, myofascial, and neural systems, using "ease," "bind," "sensing," and "motor" hands (see the glossary) as proprioceptive (see the glossary) diagnostic concepts.
7. *Strain and counterstrain techniques,* designed to locate sore places at specific sites on the body, tender points that relate to specific patterns of abnormal joint movement. The points are "turned off" by moving the body or limb to a treatment position that quiets painful feedback. The position is held for 90 seconds. Reevaluation typically reveals improvement in movement and a decrease in local pain.
8. *Cranial techniques* (also called craniosacral techniques) that highlight the manual ability to assess and release tensions associated with subtle, reciprocating cranial (head) and sacral (tailbone) oscillations. These movements are thought to arise from a complex combination of dural (covering) and ligamentous (fibrous connecting tissue) relationships in the spinal network. Adams and Heisey have documented movement of cranial bones in studies using cats. They found cerebrospinal fluid waves having various frequencies and amplitudes (Adams et al., 1992; Heisey and Adams, 1993). Opportunities for research in this area abound.

A number of continuously evolving diagnostic and treatment systems that are osteopathically oriented and manually based incorporate various of these eight manual techniques. Some systems are meant to stand on their own, while others are integrated to a greater or lesser extent with medically (i.e., allopathically) oriented decisionmaking.

Postdoctoral training, certification, and fellowship status in manual medicine are available to American osteopathic graduates, approximately 35 postdoctoral positions are available each year. Programs last 1 to 4 years. One-year fellowships are available for D.O.s and M.D.s who have finished a previously approved residency. Standalone 2-year programs leading to manual medicine certification are available in several colleges. Interdisciplinary 3- and 4-year programs that combine some of the many specialties and subspecialties are also available. The most popular are combinations of manual medicine with either family practice or physical medicine and rehabilitation.

Total patient care. Osteopathic physicians are involved in all aspects of total patient care (Northup, 1966), including structural diagnosis and manipulative treatment. Manipulative treatment is commonly used, especially by osteopathic family physicians, as adjunctive care for systemic illness and for various neuromusculoskeletal problems, such as low back, head, and neck pain. In this context, a wide variety of hands-on and—in some situations—"energy" applications are used in a range of disciplines, including family practice, pediatrics, geriatrics, physical medicine, surgery of all kinds, physical medicine and rehabilitation, neurology, rheumatology, pulmonology, and sometimes behavioral medicine and psychiatry. A few disciplines have conducted research using manual methods (Reynolds et al., 1993; Sleszynski and Kelso, 1993), but many questions remain.

Research base. Since its inception, the osteopathic profession has maintained and pursued active research in many areas. This work has usually been published in the *Journal of the American Osteopathic Association*, which until recently was not listed in *Index Medicus*. Present activities designing research tend to be directed toward evaluating (1) long-term effects of somatic dysfunctions and facilitated segments in disease states and (2) the outcome resulting from the use of manipulative treatment.

An extensive body of work supports a physiological basis for using osteopathic techniques in both musculoskeletal and nonmusculoskeletal problems. Of particular interest are studies dealing with

- interactions between internal body organs and neuromuscular structures,
- alterations in reflex thresholds,
- reliability of physician palpatory skills (interrater reliability studies), and
- effects of manipulative treatments on disease processes and a variety of physiological functions.

Early work performed by Louisa Burns demonstrated that spinal strain has adverse effects on both functional and motor neuron levels (Burns, 1917). Later work by Denslow and Korr demonstrated long-lasting, highly individual patterns of spinal hyperexcitability associated with neuromuscular and various visceral dysfunctions. This research led to the concept of the "facilitated segment" (fig. 1; also see "facilitation" in the glossary), which has been associated with a variety of clinical problems (Denslow et al., 1947; Korr, 1947, 1955). The concept of the facilitated segment is that repeated stimulation produces hyperactive responses, resulting in improper functioning of some body part.

By considering function along with structure, osteopathic theory has included conjecture on the role of the body's communication systems—nervous, circulatory, and endocrine—in initiating somatic dysfunction and causing additional responses in the body. Some early research (Northup, 1970) supports this supposition with regard to reflexes having a role in mediating both the origin of somatic dysfunctions and the effects of manipulative treatment. Osteopathic medicine needs continuing basic research on the role of the nervous system in establishing and maintaining somatic dysfunctions and effecting interactions with the rest of the body.

Figure 1 demonstrates potential effects of repeated facilitation; that is, inducing a hyperactive response, leading to somatic dysfunction. The term *facilitation* is usually used to describe enhancement or reinforcement of otherwise subthreshold neuronal activities that stimulate effector units to inappropriately carry out whatever action they are programmed to do. Examples of effector sites are muscle bundles, muscle groups, viscera, and other neural units and networks. Osteopathic treatment is designed to raise these stimulus thresholds so that the stimulatory event is less likely to occur.

More recent examples of osteopathic research include a preliminary assessment of the effectiveness of manipulative treatment for paresthesias (abnormal sensations) with peripheral nerve involvement (Larson et al., 1980) and thermographic studies of skin temperature in patients receiving manipulative treatment for peripheral nerve problems (Kappler and Kelso, 1984; Larson, 1984). Thermography was selected as a promising method to study segmental facilitation of sympathetic nerves without invading the body (as would be required if needle electrodes were used). Initial studies have been complicated, however, by the number of variables affecting skin-level circulation, including circulatory patterns, local influences, and local shunting. If methods can be developed to identify the effects of these variables, then thermography may prove useful for detecting changes in the sympathetic nervous system that affect skin-level circulation.

Other current clinical research projects that examine the effects of manual treatments have researched their effects on postoperative pulmonary flow rates (Sleszinski and Kelso, 1993), pain management (Zhu et al., 1993), and electromyographic changes associated with manual treatments. If vibration is applied to muscles near the spine or these paraspinal muscles contract volun-

Figure 1. Role of Facilitation in Somatic Dysfunction

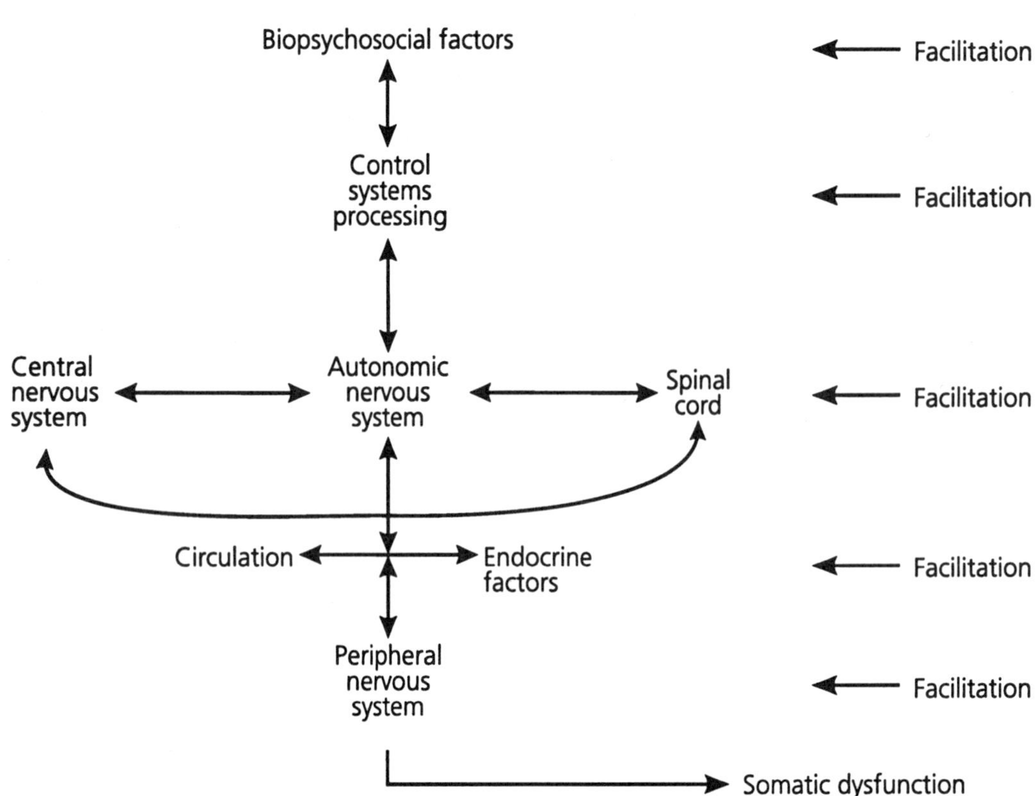

tarily, weakened electrical potentials are observed in the cerebrum, the main part of the human brain. This finding suggests that muscle spindle receptors are responsible for providing signals that cause the early components of magnetically evoked brain potentials. The brain's evoked potentials return to normal amplitude (1) when the muscle spasm subsides after a period of time and (2) after spinal manipulative therapy is applied (Zhu et al., 1993).

Additional research on the interaction of visceral and somatic structures (Eble, 1960) has supported clinical findings that palpation of neuromuscular structures can help identify visceral disturbances (Johnston, 1992; Kelso et al., 1980) and that manual procedures can help restore both visceral and neuromuscular (somatic) functions (Buerger and Greenman, 1985; Korr, 1978; Northup, 1970). The latter include situations involving low back pain (Hoehler et al., 1981), neurological development in children (Frymann et al., 1992), carpal tunnel syndrome (Sucher, 1993), postoperative collapsed lung (Sleszynski and Kelso, 1993), and burning pain in an extremity (Levine, 1991). Moreover, in some preliminary observations with cadavers, Reynolds and Ward (Ward, 1994) found that palpatory diagnoses tended to correlate with radiographic and autopsy data.

One example of the diagnostic potential of osteopathic palpation is the studies of Johnston and colleagues (Johnston et al., 1980, 1982b), comparing subjects with normal and high blood pressure. A significant number of the hypertensive patients were shown to have a stable pattern of musculoskeletal findings in the cervicothoracic spinal region. This finding suggests that osteopathic diagnoses could contribute to identifying internal difficulties.

Another issue that osteopathic researchers have addressed is the accuracy of their examinations of patients before and after manipulative treatment, including whether such observations are consistent among a group of osteopathic physicians. Several studies (Beal et al., 1980, 1982; Johnston, 1982a; Johnston et al., 1982a, 1982c, 1983; McConnell et al., 1980) have been conducted in which osteopathic physicians working independently have used a mutually agreed-upon test procedure. These studies of *inter-rater reliability* look for correlations in the observations of two or more independent raters. Results suggest that when there is prior training or agreement on which tests to use and what is clinically significant with respect to findings, inter-rater agreement can be achieved consistently. This ability to reach agreement becomes particularly important as the basis for establishing a method of setting up controlled clinical trials to determine the success of manipulative treatments.

Virtually all osteopathically oriented research has been funded from the private sector, mainly through the bureau of research of the American Osteopathic Association. The largest grant to date, $400,000, is for evaluating outcomes associated with the use of manipulation for back pain in a Chicago health maintenance organization population. This is a 3-year prospective study conducted by two osteopathic physicians specializing in musculoskeletal medicine. Patients having acute back pain with and without sciatica (pain radiating downward into the leg) are randomized into the project so that some receive manipulative care while others receive "standard" medical care. Clinical outcomes are evaluated by uninvolved clinicians. Preliminary data are expected in late 1994.

Barriers and key issues. Historically, Federal research initiatives relevant to osteopathic medicine (for example, from the National Institute of Neurological Disorders and Stroke at the National Institutes of Health (NIH) or from the Centers for Disease Control and Prevention) have been controlled by traditionally defined disciplines and their expert panels. Manual-methods research panels are not among them, and the result is a lack of genuine peer review capability. This sociological fact of life has inhibited development and understanding of the manual medicine field, even though public acceptance has been and continues to be high throughout the world.

Some major issues to be considered in trying to improve osteopathic research opportunities are the following:

- Selecting appropriate patient populations in which to study the effects of manual manipulation.
- Arranging for knowledgeable peer review and research guidance, including (1) ensuring that persons with osteopathic experience serve on peer review panels (see also the "Peer Review" chapter) and (2) determining appropriate procedures for measuring success of osteopathic treatments.
- Establishing whether previous inter-rater agreement studies support the use of the inter-rater agreement method in osteopathic and other kinds of research.
- Making previous osteopathic research more accessible (for example, the recent inclusion of the *Journal of the American Osteopathic Association* in *Index Medicus*), which could educate other investigators about osteopathic issues and possibly lead to collaborative research. (See also the "Research Databases" chapter.)
- Ensuring that osteopathic clinician-researchers are part of any research team so that persons inexperienced with osteopathic diagnosis and treatment do not conduct the work improperly. Additional training in planning, conducting, evaluating, and reporting clinical research should be made available to the osteopathic clinicians.
- Setting up a review process to integrate available information from outside the osteopathic profession with osteopathically based research on the structure-function relationship. Included would be research, for example, on homeostasis; short-, intermediate-, and long-term responses to different stressors; and adaptation to changes in internal and external environment. Useful new research questions are likely to result.
- Documenting anecdotal observations of patients and osteopathic clinicians who treat the somatic component of medical and health-related problems to tabulate patient benefits that include relief from stress and improvement in function and well-being. Attention should be paid to *all* patient health outcomes, not just short-term benefits from manipulation; for example, reducing health risks, improving health maintenance, and modifying adaptive responses would be included.

- Designing and conducting research to support or refute the use of palpatory examination and manipulative treatment for the somatic component of dysfunction and illness. Also researching the role of the somatic system; identifying the nature and effects of somatic dysfunctions and their incidence, prevalence, and effects on acute illness and long-term health; and any changes in those effects resulting from treatment.
- Developing alternative research designs for safety and efficacy studies that do not require blind controls for manual procedures. (See also the "Research Methodologies" chapter.) There are both practical and ethical reasons not to use blind controls for a hands-on procedure. One alternative is to use naive patients who lack any expectation that the treatment will be beneficial.
- Developing and integrating cost-benefit research that compares the use of palpatory examination and manipulative treatment with mainstream health care and disease management procedures. Common examples include headaches of all kinds, back pain, allergy, asthma, many orthopedic problems, postoperative and posttraumatic effects of all kinds, and various rheumatologic diseases.

Chiropractic

Chiropractic science is concerned with investigating the relationship between structure (primarily of the spine) and function (primarily of the nervous system) of the human body in order to restore and preserve health. Chiropractic medicine addresses how to apply this knowledge to diagnose and treat structural dysfunctions that affect the nervous system.

Chiropractic philosophy and practice emphasize four major points:

- The human body has an innate self-healing ability and seeks to maintain homeostasis (see the glossary), or balance.
- The nervous system is highly developed in humans and influences all other systems in the body, thereby playing a significant role in health and disease.
- The presence of joint dysfunction and subluxation (see the glossary) may interfere with the ability of the neuromusculoskeletal system to act efficiently and may lead to or be a concomitant of disease.
- Treatment is based on the chiropractic physician's ability to diagnose and treat existing pathologies and dysfunctions by appropriate manual and physiological procedures.

The chiropractic physician relies heavily on hands-on procedures using touch (palpation) to determine both structural and functional joint "dysrelationships." These hands-on procedures are carried out alongside more traditional forms of diagnostic assessment. By training and by law, chiropractic physicians use manual procedures and interventions, not surgical or chemotherapeutic ones.

History and context. While manipulative medicine has been practiced for millennia, the chiropractic profession is only now preparing for its centennial. The profession was founded in the 1890s when Daniel David (D.D.) Palmer, a grocer and magnetic healer, applied his knowledge of the nervous system and manual therapies, thrusting on a thoracic vertebra to restore the hearing of Harvey Lillard, a local janitor. While Palmer was not the first to practice manual thrusting, he was the first to use the bony projections, or processes, of the vertebrae (specifically, the spinous and transverse processes) as levers for the manual contact.

Within 2 years of this initial discovery, Palmer had founded his Chiropractic School and Cure, while at the same time developing the concept of subluxation, a type of partial joint dislocation, as a causal factor in disease. For these reasons, D.D. Palmer is known as the Founder.

By 1902, Palmer's son Bartlett Joshua (B.J.) had enrolled in his father's school; he gained operational control by late 1904, and by 1906, D.D. Palmer was no longer associated with the college he had founded. The year 1906 also saw the development of the schism that still exists in the profession today; several faculty members, including John Howard, left Palmer College because of deep differences with B.J. Palmer (who came to be known as the Developer) over the role of subluxation in disease. By that time, B.J. was espousing subluxation as the cause of all disease; John Howard, however, saw a need for what he considered to be a more rational alternative to such thinking and focused his new National

School of Chiropractic around a broad-based educational program incorporating basic and clinical sciences, laboratory work, dissection, and clinical care (Beideman, 1983).

From 1910 to 1920, many other chiropractic colleges came into existence; some followed the lead of B.J. Palmer in a "straight" form of chiropractic, while others followed the lead of Howard in developing "mixer" programs. The development of the profession could not have occurred without the missionary zeal of B.J. Palmer, who led his namesake college for 54 years. But others helped to advance the profession as well, including Carl Cleveland, Earl Homewood, Fred Illi, Joseph Janse, Herbert Lee, and Claude Watkins.

What these innovators did—in addition to all their educational and scientific advancements—was to place disease in a different context involving the concept of subluxation (Bergmann et al., 1993). Some factors are common to chiropractic and allopathic medicine. Both recognize the existence of bacteria and other "germs" and their role in creating disease; both mandate that a susceptible host be present along with the germ. Both also accept that the host's susceptibility depends on many factors. But only in the chiropractic model is the presence of subluxation stressed as an important factor; the contention of chiropractic is that since the subluxation can serve as a noxious irritant to the body, its removal becomes critical for restoring optimal health.

Chiropractors are responsible for the development and refinement of manual therapies, particularly those known as high velocity, short amplitude. Within the purview of these therapies, many systems have been developed concerning how to apply the various procedures. Examples include:

- *sacrooccipital technique,* originally developed by Major B. De Jarnette;
- *activator technique,* developed and advanced by Arlan Fuhr;
- *diversified technique,* which comes from many sources—including manual medicine (physician John Mennell), and various chiropractors, including Arnold Hauser and Joseph Janse—and which was developed largely in the National College of Chiropractic;
- *Thompson terminal point technique,* developed by J. Clay Thompson;
- *flexion-distraction technique,* developed from original osteopathic concepts by James Cox (this is not a traditional thrusting procedure);
- *Gonstead technique,* developed by Clarence Gonstead; and
- *applied kinesiology,* developed by George Goodheart.

This list is by no means exhaustive; other innovators include L. John Fay, Henri Gillet, and John Grostic.

Today's common chiropractic procedures are refinements of systems developed during the past half-century, both in diagnosis (the motion palpation of Fay and Gillet, for example [Gillet and Liekens, 1984; Schaefer and Fay, 1989]) and in therapy.

Today chiropractic procedures are being examined by researchers from most of the chiropractic colleges, who also are receiving input from field-based chiropractors. Standards of care are being determined by coalitions of chiropractors, including practitioners, academics, researchers, and administrators. One group has already produced a set of guidelines called the Mercy Conference guidelines (Haldeman et al., 1992).

In reaching their decisions concerning practice parameters and standards of care, the various groups of chiropractors have been participating in consensus-development procedures (Hansen et al., 1992).

Demographics. In 1993 more than 45,000 licensed chiropractors were practicing in the United States alone. Licensing occurs in every State in the Union as well as in many foreign countries. Chiropractors provide various aspects of health care but cannot use surgery or drugs; they have several specialty areas, such as radiology, orthopedics, neurology, and sports medicine. Seventeen American chiropractic colleges graduate more than 2,000 chiropractors annually; colleges also exist in Canada, Australia, England, France, and Japan. Some other foreign countries are considering them (e.g., South Africa, Italy, and Germany). Chiropractors currently see 12 percent to 15 percent of the U.S. population, and most professionals practice in private office settings, usually solo.

Most chiropractic physicians incorporate structural diagnosis into their practice and use manual adjusting therapies as their main treatment mode. Today, most third-party payers accept chiropractic services, though they did not always. Increased chiropractic research has helped to allay the reluctance of insurance companies toward chiropractic, and the recent development of professional standards of care has opened new avenues for chiropractic coverage.

Chiropractic education. Today's chiropractic educational program is a 5-year curriculum that emphasizes chiropractic philosophy, basic and clinical science, and clinical care in outpatient settings. Standard forms of medical diagnosis are heavily detailed, with additional workloads in structural and functional diagnosis and chiropractic technique. All chiropractic colleges require at least 2 years of college education prior to matriculation, as well as a series of courses (e.g., chemistry, physics) meeting criteria set by the Council of Chiropractic Education (CCE).

Manual therapies include any procedure during which the hands are used to palpate, diagnose, mobilize, adjust, or manipulate the somatic or visceral structures of the body. There are two broad groups—joint manipulation procedures and soft-tissue manipulation procedures. Adjustments are the most commonly applied chiropractic therapy within either group. The most common forms of adjustment taught in chiropractic colleges are the diversified, Gonstead, activator, and sacrooccipital techniques.

Today CCE accredits chiropractic colleges on the professional level, while regional accreditation also occurs. All CCE-accredited colleges teach a comprehensive program that incorporates elements of basic science (physiology, anatomy, and biochemistry); clinical science (such as laboratory diagnosis, radiology, orthopedics, and nutrition); and clinical experience (e.g., patient management in the clinical setting). In addition, the profession offers postdoctoral training in a wide range of disciplines, with orthopedics and radiology the most popular. In this country, some hospital training has recently become available to chiropractic students and residents; such training has been available in Canada since 1975.

Research base. The chiropractic profession has performed rigorous research since its early days. However, at least in one sense, the research within the profession is still very much in its infancy, because the profession "lost" much of its early work for lack of an appropriate forum in which to publish it. Today the *Journal of Manipulative and Physiological Therapeutics* is the sole chiropractic research publication indexed in *Index Medicus, Current Contents, BIOSIS,* and *Excerpta Medica.* However, other journals such as *Spine,* which is indexed in the major medical data bases, do public chiropractic-related research.

Current chiropractic research interests include back and other pain, somatovisceral disorders, and reliability studies.

Back and other pain. Recent emphasis in research trials has been on manipulation and back pain, manipulation and various organic disturbances, and reliability and validity. In 1984, Brunarski identified 50 trials of spinal manipulation (Brunarski, 1985); the number has increased since then. Studies by Bergquist-Ullman and Larsson (1977), Godfrey et al. (1984), Hadler et al. (1987), Mathews et al. (1987), and Waagen et al. (1986) were all important in establishing a definitive role for manipulation in the management of low back pain. The argument for including chiropractic in British National Health Service coverage was based on recent work by Meade et al. (1990), comparing chiropractic care to hospital outpatient care. The research of Koes (1992) served a similar role in the Netherlands. Further, the RAND report (cited in Haldeman et al., 1992), a recent and large undertaking examining all published literature on the use of manipulation for low back pain, made definitive comments regarding its use in specific situations.

The RAND report found that manipulation was effective in the following five situations: (1) acute low back pain without evidence of neurological involvement or sciatic nerve irritation; (2) acute low back pain with sciatic nerve irritation; (3) acute low back pain with minor neurological findings and sciatic nerve root irritation (although there was some conflicting evidence); (4) subacute low back pain with no evidence of neurological involvement or sciatic irritation; and (5) subacute low back pain with minor neurological findings and major neurological findings. In other situations, the literature was found to present too many conflicts to determine effectiveness of manipulation.

Besides these trials, research has examined patient perceptual issues in the use of chiropractic care. Notable here is the research of Cherkin and MacCornack (1989), who reported that patients seeing chiropractors for low back pain were happier with the treatment they received than were similar patients seeing medical doctors for similar problems.

Studies examining manipulation for pain other than low back pain include work of Barker (1983) on thoracic pain; Molea et al. (1987) on postexercise muscle soreness; Terrett and Vernon (1984) on paraspinal cutaneous pain tolerance; Vernon (1982) on headache; Jirout (1985) on C2–C3 vertebral dysfunction; and Parker et al. (1978) on migraine.

Somatovisceral disorders. One area that is gaining in research interest is the type O disorder (*O* for organic, as opposed to *M* for musculoskeletal). Much of the early impetus for studies of type O disorders came from osteopathic research examining somatic dysfunction. Examples of this work include studies by Johnston et al. (1985) and Vorro and Johnston (1987) using kinematic and electromyographic instrumentation to investigate clinical signs of somatic dysfunction. Johnston developed a way to detect "mirror image asymmetries," a presumed indicator of the presence of somatic dysfunction (the osteopathic spinal lesion). He laid out palpatory procedures to look for these asymmetries and later refined his concepts in a series of three papers (Johnston, 1988a, 1988b, 1988c) discussing palpatory diagnosis.

Studies that have examined manipulation in treating hypertension include work of Fichera and Celander (1969), Morgan et al. (1985), and Plaugher and Bachman (1994). All of these studies demonstrated changes in blood pressure following spinal manipulation, but the changes were relatively transient. Kokjohn et al. (1992) examined manipulation to treat dysmenorrhea.

Reliability studies. Clinical trials are simply not possible unless their assessment procedures have themselves been tested and found reliable. A procedure is said to be reliable if it gives similar results when applied more than once to the same object it is measuring or when it gives similar results when applied to a series of objects with similar qualities. (See also the "Research Methodologies" chapter.) Reliability tests within chiropractic are commonly used to evaluate specific diagnostic procedures, such as motion palpation.

Motion palpation (examination for presence or absence of joint play) was first advanced by Gillet and Fay as a diagnostic procedure; it has since become a well-studied, common diagnostic procedure. Gonnella et al. (1982) used a seven-point scale to evaluate interexaminer and intraexaminer reliability, while Boline et al. (1988), Love and Brodeur (1987), Mior et al. (1985), Mootz et al. (1989), Nansel et al. (1989), and Wiles (1980) examined simple reproducibility. Beattie et al. (1987) studied the attraction method of measuring motion, and Lovell et al. (1989) used a flexible ruler to assess lumbar lordosis (spinal curvature, such as swayback).

Besides doing clinical studies of various chiropractic procedures, Haas (Haas, 1991; Haas et al., 1993) has made several important additions to reliability literature, even going so far as to study the reliability of reliability. Lawrence (1985) published a critique of reliability studies for measuring leg length, and Frymoyer et al. (1986) have looked at radiographic interpretation. (This list is by no means all-inclusive.)

The research described above has been accomplished largely without any Federal funding. The largest funding agency in the chiropractic profession is the Foundation for Chiropractic Education and Research, which generally has an annual research budget well below $1 million. Chiropractors have made an impressive addition to scientific knowledge despite the lack of encouragement and support by government agencies and medical personnel outside the chiropractic profession.

Barriers and key issues. Several barriers and key issues need to be addressed so that chiropractic research can progress:

- Lack of access to Federal funds has negatively affected the chiropractic research enterprise. Ways must be found to make funds available for chiropractic research through the various agencies. To date, no chiropractic research has been funded by NIH, although several approved studies later failed to meet funding cutoff guidelines. A Small Business Administration innovative research grant funded one study. One approach to alleviating this situation is through the workshops the Office of Alternative Medicine (OAM) is conducting on grant writing and research design. OAM's ability to fund small-scale projects is also a help. If research resources could be increased, much more could be accomplished.

- Lack of access to previous chiropractic research through indexing and databases also hampers research. As mentioned earlier, only a single solely chiropractic research publication is internationally indexed. (The *Journal of Manipulative and Physiological Therapeutics* is indexed in the former Soviet Union as well as in the Western publications previously cited.) Because other chiropractic research journals are unlikely to gain the status of indexing in a conventional database, it is necessary to consider including chiropractic research in an alternative medicine database. Meanwhile, the inclusion of CHIROLARS (Chiropractic Literature and Retrieval System) in BRS Colleague as a sub-database may help to make chiropractic literature more accessible. (For information about research databases see the "Research Databases" chapter.)

- Philosophical differences (the straight-vs.-mixer controversy) continue to split the profession without any obvious solution. Unification is a goal that may still be years away.

- Inclusion of chiropractic in any of the proposed reforms of the health care system, such as those proposed by the Clinton administration, is not assured. It may be that the decision whether to include chiropractic in a national health care plan will be driven by congressional action. Major efforts are already under way to make contact with politicians regarding this issue, and chiropractic input was provided to the President's Health Care Task Force.

New avenues for the chiropractic profession have become available as a result of the decision against "biomedicine's" restraint of trade in the 1991 judgment rendered in *Wilk et al.* v. *the American Medical Association* (AMA) (see the "Introduction"). While it is likely to take many years to overcome the AMA's history of opposition to chiropractic, continuing quality research and patient care will negate this opposition. The current processes by which chiropractors are reviewing standards of care and chiropractic procedures should help solidify the public standing of this field.

Massage Therapy

Massage therapy is one of the oldest methods in the gallery of health care practices. References to massage are found in Chinese medical texts 4,000 years old. Massage has been advocated in Western health care practices in an almost unbroken line since the time of Hippocrates, the "father of medicine." In the 4th century B.C., Hippocrates wrote, "The physician must be acquainted with many things and assuredly with rubbing" (the ancient Greek and Roman term for massage).

Some of the greatest physicians in history advocated massage, including Celsus (25 B.C.–50 A.D.), who wrote *De Medicinia*, an encyclopedia of Roman medical knowledge that dealt extensively with prevention and therapeutics using massage; Galen (131–200), the most influential physician in the ancient, medieval, and Renaissance worlds, who addressed techniques and indications for massage in his book *De Sanitate Tuenda* (which is translated as *The Hygiene*, meaning prevention); and Avicenna (980–1037), a Persian physician who wrote extensively about massage in his *Canon of Medicine*, which was considered the authoritative medical text in Europe for several centuries. A sampling of other noted advocates includes Ambrose Paré, who wrote the first modern textbook of surgery; William Harvey, who demonstrated the circulation of the blood; and Herman Boerhaave, who introduced the clinical method of teaching medicine.

Modern, scientific massage therapy was introduced in the United States in the 1850s by two New York physicians, brothers George and Charles Taylor, who had studied in Sweden. The first massage therapy clinics in this country were opened by two Swedes after the Civil War: Baron Nils Posse ran the Posse Institute in Boston, and Hartwig Nissen opened the Swedish Health Institute near the U.S. Capitol in Washington, DC. Several members of Congress and U.S. Presidents, including Benjamin Harrison and Ulysses S. Grant, were among the massage therapy clientele.

As the health care system in the United States became more influenced by biomedicine and technology in the early 1900s, physicians began assigning massage duties (which were also labor-intensive, requiring more time to be spent with patients) to assistants, nurses, and physical therapists. In turn, in the 1930s and 1940s, nurses and physical therapists lost interest in massage therapy, virtually abandoning it. However, a small number of massage therapists carried on until the 1970s, when a new surge of interest in massage therapy revitalized the field, albeit in the realm of alternative health care. That interest has continued to the present.

Basic approach. Massage therapy is the scientific manipulation of the soft tissues of the body to normalize those tissues. It consists of a group of manual techniques that include applying fixed or movable pressure, holding, and/or causing movement of or to the body, using primarily the hands but sometimes other areas such as forearms, elbows, or feet. These techniques affect the musculoskeletal, circulatory-lymphatic, nervous, and other systems of the body. The basic philosophy of massage therapy encompasses the concept of *vis medicatrix naturae*—that is, aiding the ability of the body to heal itself—and is aimed at achieving or increasing health and well-being.

Touch is the fundamental medium of massage therapy. While massage methods can be described in terms of a series of techniques to be performed, it is important to understand that touch is not used solely in a mechanistic way in massage therapy; there is also an artistic component. Because massage usually involves applying touch with some degree of pressure, the massage therapist must use touch with sensitivity to determine the optimal amount of pressure appropriate for each person. Touch used with sensitivity also allows the massage therapist to receive useful information about the body, such as locating areas of muscle tension and other soft-tissue problems. Because touch is also a form of communication, sensitive touch can convey a sense of caring—which is an essential element in the therapeutic relationship—to the person receiving massage. Using the wrong kind of touch—sometimes thought of as "toxic touch"—is counterproductive, tending to render a technique ineffective and to cause the body to defend or guard itself, which in turn introduces greater tension.

Demographics. The advancement of higher standards and the development of a system of professional credentials have paralleled the dynamic growth of the massage therapy profession. Massage therapists are currently licensed by 19 States and a number of localities; additional States are expected to adopt licensing acts in the near future. Most States require 500 or more hours of education from a recognized school program and a licensing examination. While some States require continuing education, most massage therapists voluntarily take additional courses and workshops on a regular basis during their careers.

The National Certification Exam, a professional certification program accredited by the National Commission for Certifying Agencies in December 1993 and currently administered by the Psychological Corporation, was inaugurated in June 1992. More than 9,000 people nationwide were certified as of July 1994. Six States have already adopted the exam as their licensing exam, and more States are expected to follow suit.

The Commission on Massage Training Accreditation/Approval, a national accreditation agency that was set up in accord with the guidelines of the U.S. Department of Education, currently recognizes 60 school programs. Curriculums must consist of 500 or more hours and include specified hours of anatomy, physiology, massage theory and practice, and ethics.

The primary sponsor of the national certification and accreditation programs is the American Massage Therapy Association (AMTA), the largest and oldest national professional membership association for massage professionals. AMTA currently has more than 20,000 members and publishes the *Massage Therapy Journal*. The association recently founded the public, charitable AMTA Foundation to fund projects for research, education, and outreach; the foundation awarded its first grants in June 1993.

Each of a number of other national nonprofit membership associations for massage professionals has between 200 and 1,500 members. These groups usually are formed for practitioners of specific methods. To alleviate the competition and infighting that are sometimes found among various professional groups, an innovative coalition known as the Federation of Therapeutic Massage and Bodywork Organizations was formed in 1991 by the AMTA, the American Oriental Bodywork Therapy Association, the American Polarity Therapy Association, the Rolf Institute, and the Trager Institute. The federation fosters greater communication and cooperation among its members.

The number of massage therapists in the United States can only be estimated, because no formal census has been taken. Furthermore, a census or estimate would be affected by the criteria for inclusion, which would involve such variables as extent of training, number of hours worked, and whether methods used by an individual are considered forms of massage. It is estimated that there are approximately 50,000 qualified massage therapists in the United States, providing some 45 million 1-hour massage sessions per year. The number of massage therapists appears to be increasing rapidly along with a corresponding increase in use by the American public. An estimated 20 million Americans have received massage therapy. Indeed, in the study by Eisenberg and colleagues (1993)—which found that 34 percent of the American public used alternative health care—relaxation techniques, chiropractic, and massage were the most frequently used forms of alternative health care.

Methods. Some 80 different methods may be classified as massage therapy, and approximately 60 of them are less than 20 years old. There are several reasons why this is the case.

The period of the 1940s to the mid-1970s was relatively dormant for the massage therapy profession. Little standardization was established in the field. Then in the 1970s, stimulated by changes in society such as greater interest in fitness, healthier lifestyles, personal improvement, and alternative methods of health care to complement conventional medicine, interest in massage therapy increased. An influx of new practitioners brought with them a wave of new ideas and creativity regarding ways to use hands-on techniques. Since there was little standardization, these techniques sometimes developed into freestanding methods rather than being incorporated into an existing system of classification.

Another source of new techniques was the various forms of massage native to most cultures around the world but not previously described outside each culture. For example, many of the forms of massage that come from Asia are based on concepts of anatomy, physiology, and diagnosis that differ from Western concepts.

The proliferation of methods has slowed. It is expected—as has happened in the development of other professions—that as the development of standards and credentials continues, there will be some consolidation and integration of methods.

The forms of massage therapy described in this section are either among the most widely used or representative of a group of similar practices. Several forms that include additional techniques besides massage are listed briefly here and discussed in more detail in the following sections. In actual practice, many massage therapists use more than one method in their work and sometimes combine several.

Swedish massage uses a system of long gliding strokes, kneading, and friction techniques on the more superficial layers of muscles, generally in the direction of blood flow toward the heart, sometimes combined with active and passive movements of the joints. This system is used to promote general relaxation, improve circulation and range of motion, and relieve muscle tension. Swedish massage is the most common form of massage.

Deep-tissue massage is used to release chronic patterns of muscular tension using slow strokes, direct pressure, or friction directed across the grain of the muscles with the fingers, thumbs, or elbows. It is applied with greater pressure and to deeper layers of muscle than Swedish massage.

Sports massage uses techniques that are similar to Swedish and deep-tissue massage but are specially adapted to deal with the needs of athletes and the effects of athletic performance on the body.

Neuromuscular massage is a form of deep massage that is applied specifically to individual muscles. It is used to increase blood flow, release trigger points (intense knots of muscle tension that refer pain to other parts of the body), and release pressure on nerves caused by soft tissues. It is often used to reduce pain. *Trigger point massage* and *myotherapy* are similar forms.

Manual lymph drainage improves the flow of lymph by using light, rhythmic strokes. It is primarily used for conditions related to poor lymph flow, such as edema, inflammation, and neuropathies.

The reflexology, zone therapy, tuina, acupressure, rolfing (structural integration), Trager, Feldenkrais, and Alexander methods are addressed in the following sections.

The various methods of massage therapy can be divided into two major groupings:[2]

1. *Traditional European methods* based on traditional Western concepts of anatomy and physiology, using five basic categories of soft-tissue manipulation: effleurage (gliding strokes), petrissage (kneading), friction (rubbing), tapotement (percussion), and vibration. Swedish massage is the main example.

2. *Contemporary Western methods* based on modern Western concepts of human functioning, using a wide variety of manipulative techniques. These may include broad applications for personal growth; emotional release; and balance of the mind, body, and spirit in addition to traditional applications. These methods go beyond the original framework of Swedish massage and include neuromuscular, sports, and deep-tissue massage; and myofascial release, myotherapy, Bindegewebsmassage, Esalen, and manual Lymph Drainage.

In addition, there are structural, functional, and movement integration methods that organize and integrate the body in relationship to gravity through manipulating the soft tissues or through correcting inappropriate patterns of movement; methods that bring about a more balanced use of the nervous system through creating new, integrated possibilities of movement. Examples are Rolfing, Hellerwork, Aston patterning, Trager, Feldenkrais, and Alexander.

Current research. From 1873, when the term *massage* first entered the Anglo-American medical lexicon, through 1939, more than 600 journal articles appeared in mainline English language journals of medicine, including the *Journal of the American Medical Association, Archives of Surgery,* and the *British Medical Journal.* During the past 50 years, reports on nearly 100 clinical trials have been published in the medical and allied health literature. Many well-designed studies have documented the benefits of several methods of massage therapy for the treatment of acute and chronic pain; acute and chronic inflammation; chronic lymphedema; nausea; muscle spasm; various soft-tissue dysfunctions; grand mal epileptic seizures; anxiety; and depression, insomnia, and psychoemotional stress, which may aggravate significant mental illness. A larger number of studies also have been carried out in Europe, particularly in the former Soviet Union and East Germany. Unfortunately, the published reports on most of these have not been translated into English.

Research base. The following studies reflect the versatility of massage therapy and its broad and diverse range of applications.

Premature infants treated with daily massage therapy gain more weight and have shorter hospital stays than infants who are not massaged. A study of 40 babies with low birth weight found that the 20 massaged babies had 47-percent greater weight gain per day and stayed in the hospital an average of 6 fewer days than 20 similar infants who did not receive massage; the cost saving was approximately $3,000 per infant (Field et al., 1986). Cocaine-exposed preterm infants given massages three times daily for a 10-day period showed significant improvement. Results indicated that massaged infants had fewer postnatal complications and exhibited fewer stress behaviors during the 10-day period, had 28-percent greater daily weight gain, and demonstrated more mature motor behaviors at the end of the 10-day course of massage therapy (Field, 1993).

A study comparing 52 hospitalized depressed and adjustment-disorder children and adolescents with a control group that viewed relaxation videotapes found that the massage therapy subjects were less depressed and anxious and had lower saliva cortisol levels (an indicator of less depression) (Field et al., 1992).

Another study showed that massage therapy produced relaxation in 18 elderly subjects. This

[2]*The* energetic *and* oriental *manual techniques are categorized by some as massage techniques. However, in this chapter the energetic techniques are addressed in the "Biofields Therapeutics" section and the "Combined Physical and Biofield Methods" section, and the oriental techniques are addressed in the remainder of the "Physical Healing Methods" section. The energetic methods are considered to affect the biofield—a field that is described as surrounding and infusing the human body—by pressure and/or manipulation of the physical body or by the passage or placement of the hands in, or through, that energetic field. These methods are based on traditional Ayurvedic, Eastern or Western esoteric, modern therapeutic, or other recognized and accepted systems of healing. Examples are polarity therapy and therapeutic touch. The oriental methods of treatment use pressure and manipulation based on traditional East Asian medical principles to assess and evaluate the energetic system (Jwing-Ming, 1992) or to provide actual treatment that affects and balances the energetic system. Examples are tuina (or tui-na), shiatsu, acupressure, an-mo, and jin shin do.*

study demonstrated physiological signs of relaxation in measures such as decreased blood pressure and heart rate and increased skin temperature (Fakouri and Jones, 1987).

A combination of Swedish massage, shiatsu, and trigger point suppression in 52 subjects with traumatically induced spinal pain led to significant alleviations of acute and chronic pain and increased muscle flexibility and tone. This study also found massage therapy to be extremely cost-effective in comparison with other therapies, with savings ranging from 15 percent to 50 percent (Weintraub, 1992a, 1992b). Massage has also been shown to stimulate the body's ability to control pain naturally; in one study, massage stimulated the brain to produce endorphins, the neurochemicals that control pain (Kaarda and Tosteinbo, 1989). Fibromyalgia, a painful type of inflammation, is an example of a condition that may be favorably affected by this mechanism.

A pilot study of five subjects with symptoms of tension and anxiety found a significant response to massage therapy based on one or more psychophysiological parameters, including heart rate, frontalis and forearm extensor electromyograms, and skin resistance; these changes denote relaxation of muscle tension and reduced anxiety (McKechnie et al., 1983).

Another study found that massage therapy can have a powerful effect on psychoemotional distress in persons suffering from chronic inflammatory bowel disease. Stress can worsen the symptoms of ulcerative colitis and Crohn's disease (ileitis), which can cause great pain and bleeding and even lead to hospitalization or death. Massage therapy was effective in reducing the frequency of episodes of pain and disability in these patients (Joachim, 1983).

Lymph drainage massage has been shown to be more effective than mechanized methods or diuretic drugs to control lymphedema (a form of swelling) secondary to radical mastectomy (removal of breast tissues). It is expected that using massage to control lymphedema will significantly lower treatment costs (Zanolla et al., 1984).

Research opportunities. The pace of research in the United States involving massage therapy appears to be increasing, and the activities of OAM may play a supportive role. A list of studies (directed by Tiffany Field) under way at the Touch Research Institute of the University of Miami Medical School illustrates the range of possibilities for research:

- Infant studies—infants exposed to human immunodeficiency virus (HIV), depressed infants, infant colic, sleep disorders, and pediatric oncology.
- Child studies—asthma, autism, posttraumatic stress disorder following natural disasters, neglected and abused children in shelters, preschool behavior, pediatric skin disorders, diabetes, and juvenile rheumatoid arthritis.
- Adolescent studies—depressed adolescent mothers, adolescent mothers after childbirth, and eating disorders.
- Adult studies—job performance and stress, eating disorders, pregnancy and neonatal outcome, hypertension, HIV-positive adults, spinal cord injuries, fibromyalgia syndrome, rape and spouse abuse victims, and couples therapy.
- Elderly studies—volunteer foster grandparents giving and receiving massage, and arthritis.

Research recommendations. The preceding section indicates the diversity and breadth of applications of massage therapy and suggests the range of possibilities for future research.

General studies of the efficacy and effectiveness of massage therapy are still needed. Outcome studies are recommended that would allow massage therapists to work in a manner and setting that approximate actual working conditions as much as is possible. Cost-effectiveness studies also are needed. Several of the studies cited in this report have indicated that massage therapy provides substantial cost savings; this is a critical issue related to health care reform. To verify the savings, some of the more recent studies should be replicated as part of this approach.

There are numerous possibilities for studying effects of massage on many health conditions:

- Since massage therapy is especially effective with soft-tissue problems, studies involving muscle strains, sprains, tendinitis, problems related to acute and chronic muscle tension, and other such conditions would be useful, as would studies of the effect of massage on the tissue healing process.

- Because research offers mounting evidence that a significant percentage of health problems can be attributed to stress and that stress reduction can be a powerful means of preventing or treating such problems, studies of the stress-reduction effects of massage therapy would be valuable.

- Another question that needs to be addressed is whether massage can cause cancerous tumors to metastasize.

- The various subject areas under investigation at the Touch Research Institute are also examples of areas that merit further study.

Barriers and key issues. Several barriers and key issues need to be addressed to make research on massage therapy more productive:

- *Study design.* A key issue related to research is the need for researchers to collaborate with massage therapists during the design stage of a study. Some previous studies used massage in an inappropriate or ineffective manner. For example, the duration of massage is an important factor; a common error is use of massage sessions that are too brief to be effective. Another error is the choice of techniques that are not effective.

- *Appropriate use of therapists.* Properly qualified and skilled massage therapists should be used in each study. Some studies have been carried out in which individuals who were untrained or undertrained applied massage; it then became impossible to discern whether any negative results meant that massage was ineffective or that it was not applied properly.

- *Collaborations.* Since few individuals are both doctorate-level researchers and massage therapists, it is recommended that NIH facilitate collaboration between researchers and massage therapists. Researchers would benefit by knowing more about interesting and promising possibilities for research, resources available from the massage therapy profession, and massage therapy itself. Massage therapists would benefit by being able to locate researchers with whom to collaborate (1) to pursue study ideas and (2) to have a better understanding of the needs of researchers and the research process itself.

- *Translations.* Because many studies are in foreign languages, translations of such studies are needed.

- *Regulatory barriers.* Another key issue is the existence of barriers to practice that hinder massage therapists; these must be removed. In some States, regulatory boards use powers granted through licensing laws to limit the practice of legitimate massage therapy by qualified massage therapists. These barriers also restrict the ability to conduct research on massage therapy in traditional settings, such as clinics and hospitals, thereby hampering research efforts.

If regulatory, insurance payment, and research barriers are not removed, they will inhibit progress regarding massage therapy, along with other forms of alternative health care.

Pressure Point Therapies

Pressure point therapies use finger pressure on specific points—usually related to the oriental meridian points (see the glossary), but also other neurological release points—to reduce pain and treat various disease states. There are antecedents in Europe, Asia, and the United States. Adamus and A'tatis described a pressure system in 1582, and the sculptor Cellini (1500–71) wrote of using pressure points to relieve pain. In 1770 the Jesuit Amiat contributed to European understanding with an article on Chinese pressure point "massage." This article influenced the Swedish therapeutic massage pioneer Ling. In turn, Swedish therapeutic massage influenced traditional Japanese folk massage in the early 20th century, and this cross-fertilization became known as shiatsu. About 1913, Fitzgerald, an American, developed what came to be known as zone therapy. Fitzgerald had been influenced by Bressler in Europe. The use of pressure points has evolved under several systems, some of which are discussed below.

Reflexology. Fitzgerald's work with hand reflex points was developed and promoted by Ingram in the United States and Marquardt in Europe. Because in this system specific "zones" on the feet are related to specific organs, the system is often called zone therapy. There is a related system of hand zone therapy as well. The results reported for the process include relief of pain;

release of kidney stones; and recovery from the effects of stroke, sinusitis, sciatica, and menstrual and other disorders (Marquardt, 1983).

Traditional Chinese massage. Traditional Chinese remedial massage methods were described in the texts of the Han period (202 B.C. to circa 220 A.D.). By the Tang Dynasty (618–907 A.D.), these systems were taught in special institutes. Both "tonification" (energizing) and "sedation" techniques are used to treat and relieve many medical conditions. Major techniques in use are

- *ma,* rubbing with palm or finger tips;
- *pai,* tapping with palm or finger tips;
- *tao,* strong pinching with thumb and fingertip;
- *an,* rapid and rhythmical pressing with thumb, palm, or back of the clenched hand;
- *nie,* twisting, with both thumbs and tips of the index fingers grasping and twisting the area being treated;
- *ning,* pinching and lifting in a stationary position;
- *na,* moving while performing ning; and
- *tui,* pushing, often with slight vibratory effect.

These techniques are usually used in combinations. Two prominent groupings of techniques are known as an-mo and tui-na.

Widely varying illnesses and conditions are treated with traditional Chinese massage, including the common cold, sleeplessness, leg cramps, painful menses, whooping cough, diarrhea, abdominal pains, headache, asthma, rheumatic pains, stiff neck, colic, bed-wetting, nasal bleeding, lumbago, and throat pains.

Acupressure systems. Currently, four systems in which the fingers manipulate the oriental meridian system are in widespread use in the United States. In all these systems, pressure is applied to meridian points (acupuncture points on the meridians; also called acupoints) to stimulate or sedate them. Amounts of pressure and length of application vary according to the system, the ailment, and the intent. All of these systems—shiatsu, tsubo, jin shin jyutsu, and jin shin do—rely on traditional oriental medical theory (see the "Alternative Systems of Medical Practice" chapter), although their treatment methods vary considerably.

Shiatsu and tsubo rely largely on sequenced applications of pressure applied from one end of each meridian to the other. The patient reclines, usually lying on the back and then the front for approximately equal periods as the practitioner uses thumb pressure to stimulate the point through a combination of direct pressure and transference of qi (see the glossary) to the point from the practitioner's thumb. "Barefoot shiatsu" is a form that uses foot pressure to stimulate the meridian points. Sessions typically treat the meridians of the entire body in an attempt to bring relaxation, harmony, and balance to the patient. Shiatsu, which is traditional in Japan, has been used in the United States quite extensively for about 20 years. Therapy sessions have a strong focus on long-term health improvement. Procedures include specific treatments for a variety of functional disorders as well as postural, stress-related, and emotional problems. Conditions that have been improved include headache, asthma, bronchitis, diarrhea, depression, and circulatory problems (Namikoshi, 1969).

Jin shin jyutsu and jin shin do have developed sequences of meridian point pressure applications that are specific to the ailment being addressed. These systems are used more often than shiatsu and tsubo as alternative treatment approaches. Jin shin jyutsu, the "art of circulation awakening," was developed in Japan by Jiro Murai in the early 1900s and brought to the United States in the 1960s by Mary Iino Burmeister. It is the antecedent of jin shin do, which was developed in the United States by Iona Teeguarden in the 1980s. Sessions are primarily for treatment of specific problems. The approach is similar to that of acupuncture, as the meridian connections to the organs are understood and applied, but from somewhat different application perspectives. Pressure is applied to the meridian points, which are then held in specific patterns, to tonify or detonify (energize or enervate) the meridian qi. Conditions addressed include a wide range of organic dysfunctions (Teeguarden, 1987).

Postural Reeducation Therapies

Three prominent therapies in the United States use as their approach the reeducation of the body through movement and physical touch. In all three systems—Alexander, Feldenkrais, and Trager—

patients are taught how to retrain their bodies to come into alignment to release and change postural faults, to improve coordination and balance, and to relieve structural and functional stress. A major principle underlying the three methods is that awareness has to be experienced rather than taught verbally. The awareness may then lead to more effective use of one's whole self.

Alexander technique. The Alexander method is a system of body dynamics, especially in respect to the head, neck, and shoulders. The technique was developed by the actor F.M. Alexander, who created the method after concluding that bad posture was responsible for his chronic periods of voice loss (Maisel, 1989). The technique includes simple movements that improve balance, posture, and coordination and relieve pain. During a session the client typically goes through a series of standing and seated exercises while the practitioner applies light pressure to points of contraction in the body. These pressures are intended to awaken kinesthetic response (sensitivity to motion by the muscles) and retrain the kinesthetic organs in the joints to their proper spatial relationship. The process is taught in many drama schools and is popular with performers. The techniques help clients learn how to use their bodies with less tension and more awareness and efficiency.

Alexander practitioners report success with neck and back pain, postural disorders, whiplash injury, breathing problems, myalgia, rheumatica, repetitive strain injury, hypertension, anxiety, stress, and other chronic conditions.

Feldenkrais method. The Feldenkrais method was developed by Moshe Feldenkrais, a Russian-born Israeli physicist, who turned his attention to the study of human functioning. His work integrated an understanding of the physics of the body's movement patterns with an awareness of the way people learn to move, behave, and interact (Feldenkrais, 1949, 1972, 1981, 1985). He began teaching his method in North America in the early 1970s. The Feldenkrais method consists of two branches—"awareness through movement" and "functional integration."

- *Awareness through movement.* This verbally directed form of the Feldenkrais method consists of gentle exploratory movement sequences organized around a specific human function (such as reaching, bending, or walking) with the intention of increasing awareness of multiple possibilities of action. A group of students may be standing, sitting, or lying on the floor. Thinking, sensory perception, and imagery are also involved in examining each function.

- *Functional integration.* This method involves the practitioner's use of words and gentle, noninvasive touch to guide an individual student to an awareness of existing and alternative movement patterns. The teacher communicates to the student—who may be lying, sitting, standing, kneeling, or in motion—how she or he organizes herself or himself and suggests additional choices for functional movement patterns. The use of touch is for communication, not correction, and there are no special techniques of pressing or stroking. Any changes in functioning result from the student's actions.

Practitioners report success with a variety of postural and functional disorders in such diverse applications as sports performance, equine training, physiotherapeutics, zoo animal rehabilitation, the performing arts, neurological and orthopedic physical therapy practice, pain management, and habilitation of developmentally impaired children.

Currently, the North American Feldenkrais Guild has approximately 1,000 members. As of January 1994, 31 training programs lasting 3 to 4 years were available around the world for Feldenkrais practitioners.

The method is a synthesis of modern ideas and basic research findings in perception, motor learning, neural plasticity, and sensory integration (Edelman, 1987; Georgopolus, 1986; Jacobson, 1964; Jenkins and Merzenic, 1987; Jenkins et al., 1990; Kaas, 1991; Kandel and Hawkins, 1992; Seitz and Wilson, 1987; and Sweigard, 1974). Only limited clinical research studies have been conducted to document the Feldenkrais method. Clinical successes have been cited in several review articles and clinical guidelines for physical therapy and pain management (DeRosa and Porterfield, 1992; Jackson, 1991; Lake, 1985; and Shenkman and Butler, 1989) and have included reports on exercise for the elderly and for persons recovering from spinal injury (Ginsberg, 1986; Gutman, 1977).

In one research study, Jackson-Wyatt and colleagues (1992) used video analysis to measure the kinetics of the change in motor ability in a vertical jump test in a subject who completed eight 5-day weeks of 6-hour training days in a Feldenkrais practitioner training program. Dramatic improvement in power, velocity, and movement efficiency were demonstrated.

Narula (1993) similarly examined the sit-to-stand movement, walking speed, and grip strength of four subjects with class 2 rheumatoid arthritis. After attending a twice-weekly 75-minute class for 6 weeks, all subjects showed decreased pain, improved walking performance, and improved kinetics of the sit-to-stand movement, but no improvement in grip strength. The results suggest that lessons in awareness through movement could be used by individuals to improve their functions despite long-term disabling medical conditions.

Ruth and Kegerries (1992) used a 25-minute, four-step process to test the flexion range of neck motion in college students before and after half the group received a 15-minute sequence from the awareness through movement methods. Compared with the control group, students experiencing this sequence showed measurably improved neck flexion motion and a decrease in the perceived effort to accomplish this motion.

Since Feldenkrais's functional integration method involves a highly individual interaction between practitioner and client, outcomes research should be long-term, using both subjective and objective measures. Such studies could establish whether various applications of the Feldenkrais method are useful both for medical care and in educational systems.

Trager psychophysical integration. The Trager method uses light, rhythmic rocking and shaking movements that loosen joints, ease movement, and release chronic patterns of tension. This method was developed by a Hawaiian physician, Milton Trager, on the basis of his experience as a trainer for the sport of boxing. The Trager practitioner uses his or her hands with the aim of influencing deep-seated psychophysiological patterns in the client's mind and interrupting the projection of those patterns into body tissues.

This method of movement reeducation is distinguished by compressions, elongations, and light bounces as well as rocking motions. These actions cause patients or clients to begin to experience freedom of movement of their body parts. Since practitioners believe they are affecting the inhibiting patterns at their source, it is expected that clients can experience long-lasting gains.

The goal of Trager work is general functional improvement, partly by creating a feeling of pleasure in being able to move body parts more freely. The process incorporates a meditative state called "hookup," which is intended to enhance sensory, kinesthetic, and other pleasurable experiences for the client.

Several case histories describe long-term improvement in movement function for persons with multiple sclerosis; in chest mobility with lung disease (Witt and MacKinnon, 1986); and in trunk mobility with childhood cerebral palsy (Witt and Parr, 1986). Other reports suggest success in treating chronic pain of various sorts, headaches, muscular dystrophy, muscle spasms, temporomandibular joint pain, recovery from stroke, spinal cord injuries, and polio.

The Trager method also includes Trager "mentastics," a system of mentally directed physical movements developed to maintain and enhance a sense of lightness, freedom, and flexibility. Mentastics is used by Trager practitioners and is taught to clients to enhance results.

There are now more than 800 certified Trager practitioners around the world. Training is available in the United States and several other countries.

Structural Integration (Rolfing)

Unlike most systems of body manipulation, which are concerned with the muscular system or the skeletal systems or both, structural integration focuses on the fascias, which are sheets of connective tissue. Ida Rolf, whose work was the foundation of the various systems of structural integration, noted that while bones support the body and muscles connect the bones. It is the enwrapping fascias that support and hold the muscle-bone combinations in place. Rolf's second precept was that the fascias would maintain not only the normal relationship of bone and muscle but also whatever postural misalignment the body might adopt. This misalignment could incorporate effects of trauma as well as poor posture.

Later theorists have used renowned architect and designer Buckminster Fuller's "tensegrity mast" as an explanatory model for the relationship of the bones and fascias. In this structure, none of the solid elements are connected directly together but are held by tensioned wires. The structure becomes a model for the body if the solid segments are called the bones and the flexible wires are called the fascias (Robie, 1977).

When the body attempts to distribute the stress of an injury, the result is likely to be shortened and thickened fascias, which may in turn lead to symptoms somewhere other than the site of the original trauma. Structural integration is a system to "unwind" and stretch the distorted fascias back to their normal condition, thereby allowing the bones and muscles to come back to normal alignment and the body to return to normal functioning. Structural integration, or "Rolfing," involves stretching the fascia sheaths by applying sliding pressure to the affected area with fingers, thumbs, and occasionally elbows. In its early days, the process was known to be quite painful, but later refinements in technique have made Rolfing considerably more comfortable.

Rolf postulated that the plasticity of the fascias in the body could offset the aging process (Rolf, 1973). Research in Rolfing has suggested beneficial results with cerebral palsy in children (Perry et al., 1981), state-trait anxiety (i.e., a person's current anxiety state or level is measured against his or her anxiety traits) (Weinberg and Hunt, 1979), the stress and symptoms of lower back pain and whiplash (Rolf, 1977), and changes in parasympathetic tone (degree of vigor and tension of muscles innervated by parasympathetic nerves) (Cottingham et al., 1988a, 1988b). Changes in psychological and physiological function have also been measured (Silverman et al., 1973).

The Rolf Institute, the first school to teach the principles of structural integration, offers a post-bachelor's degree training program requiring 28 weeks of classroom work. Today there are also three other schools based on Rolf's work and 1,500 practitioners who treat an estimated 150,000 individuals per year. Licensing requirements differ in various States.

Aston patterning, developed by Judith Aston, and Hellerwork, developed by Joseph Heller, are major offshoots of structural integration. Both incorporate movement reeducation training to bring the body into fuller activity and expression.

Bioenergetical Systems

Several therapeutic systems using manual healing are designed to release bodily held emotions through various combinations of activity on the part of the client and applied pressure or holding on the part of the practitioner. These systems derive from Wilhelm Reich's original observations about bodily held emotions and his work with patients and clients to release emotion (Reich, 1973). In this work, the client assumes and holds one of several different postures, either seated or reclining. Simultaneously, the practitioner applies pressure to areas of abnormal stress that are revealed by the posture. The client may then be invited to breathe deeply into the stressed area. The combination of external, inwardly directed pressure and outwardly directed breath exaggerates holding patterns that have become so deeply imbedded that the client is no longer aware of them. Release of the emotion can be quite pronounced, resulting in spontaneously revealed insight, increased freedom of movement, and new social postures. Individual releases during the process may be accompanied by pronounced but brief periods characterized by increased body heat, tingles, and reported rushes of "energy."

Bioenergetics, core energetics, Lowenwork, neo-Reichian therapy, radix, and some other methods derive from Reich's basic approach.

Although some psychotherapists incorporate various forms of this work into their practices, there are constraints in some States because of ethical questions about touching the client. Discussions with various psychotherapists indicate that some would like to include these therapies but fear to do so at this time, when the legal and ethical considerations have not been resolved. Those who do the work operate in a dual capacity—as psychotherapist and bioenergetic body worker. However, they do not apply touch during straight psychotherapy sessions, and the straightforward touch used during the body work is clinically applied pressure and not sensually evocative.

Biofield Therapeutics

Overview

Biofield (see the glossary) therapeutics, often called energy healing or laying on of hands, is one of the oldest forms of healing known to humankind. Discovery, partial characterization, and use of the biofield have risen independently among peoples and cultures in every sector of the world (see table 1).

The earliest Eastern references are in the *Huang Ti Nei Ching Su Wên* (*The Yellow Emperor's Classic of Internal Medicine*), variously dated between 2,500 and 5,000 years ago (Veith, 1949). The earliest Western references are in hieroglyphics and in depictions of biofield healings dating from Egypt's Third Dynasty.[3] Hippocrates, a major figure in Western medicine, referred to the biofield as "the force which flows from many people's hands" (Schiegl, 1983). Franz von Mesmer, an Austrian physician who investigated and popularized this process in the late 18th century, referred to the biofield as "animal magnetism" to differentiate it from "metal magnetism," which he understood to be a similar but different medium (Mesmer, 1980). In the United States, use increased after Mesmer's "magnetic healing" became popular in the 1830s. (Among others, both Andrew Still (founder of osteopathy) and Daniel Palmer (founder of chiropractic) practiced for a time as magnetic healers (Gevitz, 1993).

Historically, beliefs about causation in this type of healing have clustered around two views that remain active today. The first is that the "healing force" comes from a source other than the practitioner, such as God, the cosmos, or another supernatural entity. The second is that a human biofield, directed, modified, or amplified in some fashion by the practitioner, is the operative mechanism. Some of the terms presented in table 1 are devoid of religious or spiritual overtones, while others carry religious aspects common to the culture in which they were or are used.

Therapeutic application of the biofield is a process during which the practitioner places his or her hands either directly on or very near the physical body of the person being treated. In so doing, the practitioner engages the perceived biofield from his or her hands with the recipient's perceived biofield either to promote general health or to treat a specific dysfunction. The person being treated, who is usually clothed, reclines in some forms of the process but is seated in others.

The process is not instantaneous, as it is in "faith healing." (Faith is not a factor in the biofield process.) Treatment sessions may take

Table 1. Some Equivalent Terms for *Biofield*

Term	Source
Ankh	Ancient Egypt
Animal magnetism	Mesmer
Arunquiltha	Australian aborigine
Bioenergy	United States, United Kingdom
Biomagnetism	United States, United Kingdom
Gana	South America
Ki	Japan
Life force	General usage
Mana	Polynesia
Manitou	Algonquia
M'gbe	Hiru pygmy
Mulungu	Ghana
Mumia	Paracelsus
Ntoro	Ashanti
Ntu	Bantu
Oki	Huron
Orenda	Iroquois
Pneuma	Ancient Greece
Prana	India
Qi (chi)	China
Subtle energy	United States, United Kingdom
Sila	Inuit
Tane	Hawaii
Ton	Dakota
Wakan	Lakota

Source: Provided courtesy of the Biofield Research Institute.

[3] *These depictions can be seen in the Third Dynasty exhibit in the National Museum, Cairo, Egypt.*

from 20 minutes to an hour or more; a series of sessions is often needed to complete treatment of some disorders.

The ability to perform biofield healing appears to be universal, although most people seem unaware of possessing the talent. As with any innate talent, practice and learning appropriate techniques improve results.

There is consensus among practitioners that the biofield that permeates the physical body also extends outward from the body for several inches. Therefore, no real difference is seen between placing the hands directly on the body (either by direct skin contact or through clothing) or in close proximity to the body. In either case, the practitioner's biofield is understood to come into confluence with the recipient's biofield. There are advantages and disadvantages to each approach in clinical applications.[4]

Extension of the external portion of the biofield is considered variable and dependent on the person's emotional state and state of health. Practitioners describe the external portion, sometimes called the "aura," as tactilely detectable (see the "Biofield Diagnostics" section) and less dense than the portion permeating the physical body.

Biofield practitioners have a holistic focus, for most treatment sessions produce results that encompass more than one aspect of the person's health. Within that focus there is, however, a range of therapeutic intents:

- *General* (e.g., stress relief, improvement of general health and vitality).
- *Biologic* (e.g., reduction of inflammation, edema, chronic and acute pain; change in hematocrit and T-cell levels; and acceleration of wound healing and fracture repair).
- *Vegetative functions* (e.g., improvement of appetite, digestion, and sleep patterns).
- *Emotional states* (e.g., changes in anxiety, grief, depression, and feelings of self-worth).
- *Dysfunctions often classified psychosomatic* (e.g., treatment of eating disorders, irritable bowel syndrome, premenstrual syndrome, and post-traumatic stress disorder).

Some practitioners incorporate mental healing, or focused intent to heal, as part of their biofield treatments. This is also called psychic healing, distant healing, nonlocal healing, and absent healing. Mental healing can also be performed by itself at a considerable distance from the recipient. It is an active process on the practitioner's part, involving centered, focused concentration; it may include various imagery (visualization) techniques as well. (See the "Imagery" section and the "Prayer and Mental Healing" section in the "Mind-Body Interventions" chapter.)

A related mind effect sometimes used in biofield healing is described as the practitioner, by effort of will, extending the biofield (principally from the hands) into the recipient's body with increased force, sometimes from a distance of several feet. Chinese qigong masters are considered especially adept at this. The process appears to be draining; interviews with practitioners who do this procedure indicate they are limited in the number of treatments they can perform in a day.

Some practitioners meditate before giving a treatment in order to enter a so-called healing space; some others maintain a meditative state during treatment.

Biofield diagnostics. Detailed diagnostic methods have been developed to determine the condition of the patient's general health and present disorder by sensing, with touch, subtle perturbations in the biofield (clairsentience). Janet Quinn, researcher of the therapeutic touch method, writes that "assessment [of the external portion] focuses on perceiving the way this energy is flowing and is distributed in the patient" (Krieger, 1992). Patricia Heidt adds that areas of "accumulated tension" or "congested energy" are detected (Heidt, 1981b). Barbara Brennan,

[4]*The differences between direct and indirect contact are analogous to the two methods of illuminating a neon light. The first is to place the neon bulb in a strong electromagnetic field. This is the simpler way, as it requires no wiring or particular orientation; the bulb will glow wherever it is placed. However, a great deal of power is required for a given light output, and the light fluctuates sharply with small fluctuations in the field. The second method is to connect the neon bulb into an electric circuit. This method requires wires and knowledge of how to connect the bulb correctly; it produces much more light with far less power, but the light is less likely to fluctuate. Similarly, the biofield is described as having both external field and internal circuitry.*

developer of the healing science method, describes the use of "high sense perception," which includes other subtle perceptions of the external biofield (Brennan, 1987).

Biofield researcher Richard Pavek writes of similar subtle tactile cues detected when the hands are placed directly on the body during SHEN®[5] therapy as "changes in temperature . . ., tingles, prickles, 'electricity' (sensation of light static), pressure or 'magnetism' . . . sensations are usually different over an area of physical pain, inflammation, tension and/or when release of emotion occurs" (Pavek, 1987, p. 57).

Many practitioners develop their treatment plans entirely by interpreting these various tactile sensations. Others use biofield diagnostics to supplement conventional methods, such as nursing diagnostic forms or chronic pain evaluation forms.

Current status. Considerable interchange of technique occurs between Europe and the United States and some between the United States and Asia.

United States. The process of using biofields has been treated with a reflexive mixture of awe and disgust, reverence and fear, and belief and disbelief, but this situation appears to be changing as more and more people seriously investigate the process from a critically neutral perspective.

No formal census is available, but reasonable estimates suggest that some 50,000 practitioners in the United States provide about 120 million sessions annually (Pavek, 1994). Of these, about 30,000 have trained in therapeutic touch (Benor, 1994). For some, it is a major part of their vocational activity; others use the process occasionally to help family and friends. Many practitioners have had no formal training in the process, and many have independently discovered biofield effects. Others learned rudimentary techniques from friends or trained in one of several schools that teach various forms of the process. Reviews of school enrollment records indicate that most practitioners are women.

Some practitioners, often those who have independently discovered the process, and some teachers ascribe to it a religious or spiritual basis. A few link the process with specific religious activities.

No State has licensing requirements for biofield practitioners. Because legal constraints in many States prohibit the use of the terms *patient* and *treatment*, most practitioners use the terms *receiver* and *session* in describing their work.

Some, possibly because they fear being charged with practicing medicine without a license, have cloaked themselves by incorporating under the name of a healing church. They often deny attempting to treat biological disorders and describe their process as "healing the spirit," from which "healing of the physical" will follow.

In the past 20 years or so, formal training in the process has emerged in considerable strength in this country. At this time several teaching establishments with standardized training programs teach different forms of the process; most grant certificates. Schools differ considerably in curriculum, focus, length of training, extent of internship, and certification requirements. Some schools are semistructured associations of instructors trained in a particular method; others are more centrally organized.

The major biofield therapies used in the United States are summarized in table 2.

At least four forms of biofield therapy—healing science, healing touch, SHEN® therapy, and therapeutic touch—have been taught in a number of medical establishments. Currently, student nurses are trained in one or another system in more than 90 colleges and universities around the world. Acupuncturists, massage practitioners, and nurses who pass these courses receive continuing education credit from several State bureaus for training in these four forms.

Most of the practitioners of this process work independent of conventional medical and health practitioners. The conventional practitioner may occasionally be aware that his or her patient-client is seeing a biofield practitioner collaterally, but most are not.

However, while much of the current activity in this discipline can be considered separate and alternative, the process is beginning to seep upward

[5]SHEN® stands for Specific Human Energy Nexus. SHEN® therapy is described by Pavek as a biofield method of treating the so-called psychosomatic and related disorders by releasing repressed and suppressed debilitating emotions directly from the body.

Table 2. Brief Features of the Major Biofield Therapies in the United States

Therapy	Year originated	Developer	Theoretical basis	Diagnostic procedures	Certification	Placement of hands	Mental healing at a distance	Therapeutic intent
Healing science	1978	Barbara Brennan	Open system, incorporates chakras and psychic layers	High sense perception	Yes, after completion of advanced study	Both on and near the body	Yes	Treat the whole person and specific disorders
Healing touch	1981	American Holistic Nurses Association	Elements of therapeutic touch, healing science, and Brugh Joy's and other work	Tactile assessment	Yes	Both on and off the body	Yes	Whole person, specific disorders
Huna	Traditional Hawaiian		Involves mana (universal force) and aka (universal substance)	Various	No	Both on and near the body	Yes	Heal mind and body
Mari-el	1983	Ethel Lombardi	Vibrational energy is transmitted from a higher source through the practitioner to the patient, affecting cellular memory and the endocrine system	Tactile assessment	No	Usually off the body	Yes	Heal and harmonize the life of the individual
Natural healing	1974	Rosalyn Bruyere	Operates on a belief in a universal principle of energy	Tactile assessment	Graduates are ordained			Effect symptomatic relief, assists in proper use of energy
Qigong	Traditional Chinese		Qi flows through the body in meridians and other patterns; Qi is delivered with great force by many practitioners called qigong masters	Varies with practitioners	Not usually	At the meridian points or at a short distance from the body	Yes	Healing of biological disorders

Table 2. Brief Features of the Major Biofield Therapies in the United States (cont.)

Therapy	Year originated	Developer	Theoretical basis	Diagnostic procedures	Certification	Placement of hands	Mental healing at a distance	Therapeutic intent
Reiki	Japan, 1800s; USA, 1936	Mikao Usui (introduced by Hawayo Takata)	Spiritual energy with innate intelligence, channeled through the practitioner; the spiritual body is healed, it in turn is expected to heal the physical; Uses rituals, symbols, spirit guides	Varies	Spiritual initiation (i.e., the power to heal is given after training)	A few standard hand placements (usually side by side; on the physical body)	Yes	
SHEN® therapy	1977	Richard Pavek	Biofield conforming to natural laws of physics, with a discernable flux pattern through the body	Conventional medical and psychotherapy instruments with questions designed to discover repressed emotional states	Yes, after internship. Practitioners meet requirements of U.S. Department of Labor Occupational Code 076.264–640.	Sequence of paired-hand placements, directly on the body, arranged according to flux patterns, usually with one on top and one underneath	No	Primarily emotional disorders and somatopsychic dysfunctions
Therapeutic touch	1972	Dora Kunz and Dolores Kreiger	Practitioner restores correct vibrational component to the patient's universal, unitary field	Tactile assessment	None	Generally near the body	Yes	Nonprescriptive healing of the whole person

Note: Polarity therapy was omitted from this table but is discussed in the "Combined Physical and Biofield Methods" section of this chapter.

into mainstream medical and health practices. It is likely that several thousand practitioners of conventional therapies currently combine one or another of the biofield therapy processes with their primary approaches. Among these are nurses, counselors, psychotherapists, chiropractors, and massage practitioners who at least occasionally use a form of biofield therapy as an adjunct.

At least three forms are currently in use in hospitals: healing touch and therapeutic touch are used for a variety of reasons in several hospitals (Quinn, 1981, 1993), and SHEN® therapy is used in alcohol abuse, drug abuse, and codependent recovery programs in a few hospitals (Sunshine and Wright, 1986).

Europe. The United States falls far behind other countries in legal recognition of biofield therapy. Currently, more than 8,500 registered healers in the United Kingdom (British Medical Association, 1993) "are permitted to 'give healing' (a term for the process in common usage in the United Kingdom) at the request of patients" (p. 92). Approval has been obtained to use the process at the 1,500 government hospitals. In some situations, biofield healers are paid under the U.K. National Health Service (Benor, 1993). Physicians receive postgraduate education credits for attending courses in the biofield process, and healers are able to purchase liability insurance policies similar to those covering physicians (Benor, 1992).

In Poland and Russia, biofield healing is being incorporated into conventional medical practice; some medical schools include instruction in the process in the curriculum. In Russia, the process is under investigation by the Academy of Science. In Bulgaria, a government-appointed scientific body assesses abilities and recommends licensing for those who pass rigorous examinations (Benor, 1992).

Asia. China leads the rest of the world in research on therapeutic application and methods of increasing biofield effects. Biofield healing is called wei qi liao fa, or "medical qigong" (chi kung), in China, where proficient practitioners are called "qigong masters." Qigong masters are described as having developed their qi (biofield) to a high degree through qigong exercises.[6] (A few qigong masters are reported to be able to anesthetize patients for surgery solely with this method [Houshen, 1988]). Reduction of secondary cancers by medical qigong masters is commonly reported; there are clinics for that purpose alone.

Departments of medical qigong research exist in every college of traditional Chinese medicine in China. Both national and regional governments sponsor periodic international conferences on medical qigong. American researchers are frequently invited to present papers at these conferences.

Explanatory models. No generally accepted theory accounts for the phenomena of biofields. As one might expect of a discipline often perceived as bordering between superstition and random process on the one hand and science and technique on the other, there are profound differences—both inside the discipline among practitioners and researchers, and outside among theoreticians—as to the exact nature of the phenomena. In many cases, the view of the biofield is not a clearly defined one; it often mixes concepts of physics and metaphysics, or ancient and modern wisdoms (see the glossary).

The current major hypotheses are that the biofield is

- metaphysical (outside the four dimensions of space and time and untestable),
- an electromagnetic field effect, and
- a presently undefined but potentially quantifiable field effect in physics.

There are three metaphysical approaches:

- *Spiritual energy.* Practitioners of some methods believe that they are channeling a spiritual energy that has innate intelligence or logic and knows where and to what extent it is required (Baginski and Sharamon, 1988). Reiki and also "radiance," a form of reiki, are examples of this view (Ray, 1987). Reiki teaches that the practitioner is merely a conduit for spiritual energy. After training, the practitioner is initiated and given the power to heal; sacred symbols are often used to give added power to the process

[6] *Qigong exercises are repetitive physical motions coordinated with breath and mental efforts to move the qi through meridians and other "channels." They are gaining popularity in the United States. (See the "Combined Physical and Biofield Methods" section.)*

(Jarrell, 1992). Another system with a similar approach, mari-el, incorporates the use of angels or spiritual guides in the healing practice.

- *Interacting human and universal energy fields.* Heidt and others have postulated that both the healer and the healed are vibrating fields of energy (Heidt, 1981b) that interact with the environmental energy field around them for healing purposes. Brennan describes a similar process as one of "harmonic induction" (Brennan, 1987).
- *Repatterning of resonant vibratory fields.* Going further, Quinn and nurse-theorist Rogers state that

> current assumptions (about Therapeutic Touch), which remain "untested" and "untestable," [are that] people are energy fields. We are not saying that people have energy fields in addition to what they are. . . . [Instead they are] open systems engaged in continuous interaction with the environmental energy field. [Therefore] when a person is "sick" there is an imbalance in the person's energy field, [and] when a person uses his or her intent to help or heal a person, the energy field of the person may repattern towards greater wellness. . . . The Therapeutic Touch practitioner knowingly participates in . . . "a healing meditation," facilitates repatterning of the recipient's energy field through a process of resonance, rather than "energy exchange or transfer" (Quinn, 1993).

The healing intervention is seen as a "purposive patterning of energy fields, a mutual process in which the nurse uses his or her hands as a mediating focus in the continuing patterning of the mutual patient-environment energy field process" (Rogers, 1990).

In addition, certain models in physics may offer some explanation of biofield phenomena. Although quantum physics, the branch of physics that treats atomic and subatomic particles, has been proposed to explain the effects of a related phenomenon, mental healing at a distance (see the "Mind-Body Interventions" chapter), it has not proved to be a useful model to explain biofield healing. For example, Brennan states, "I am quite unable to explain these experiences without using the old [classical physics] frameworks" (Brennan, 1987, p. 26).

Classical physics is a model that is applied with high precision to large-scale phenomena involving relatively slow motion, such as the flow of fluids, electromagnetic currents and waves, hydraulics, aerodynamics, and atmospheric physics. It appears to be a reasonable model to apply in studying biofield phenomena.

Indeed, much of the terminology used by biofield practitioners to describe their work—while somewhat imprecise and variable—clearly describes quantitative and qualitative factors similar to those in fields of classical physics. For example, qi appears to be equivalent to flux in electromagnetic fields, for it describes direction and quantity of field. Polarity between the hands and between different bodily regions appears to be equivalent to polar difference in electromagnetic fields and to pressure differential in hydrodynamics. Pavek describes the biofield as having "circulating [flux] patterns . . . similar in formation and function to magnetic fields or electrostatic fields" (Pavek, 1987, p. 61). (See table 3 for other analogies.)

Around 1850, Karl von Reichenbach (discoverer of kerosene and paraffin) demonstrated apparent biofield polarities and determined apparent velocity through a copper rod to be about 4 meters per second (von Reichenbach, 1851).[7] In 1947, L.E. Eeman demonstrated a polarity through the arms and hands and another through the spine with his device known as an Eeman screen (Eeman, 1947). (See fig. 2.)

In about 1950 Randolph Stone, developer of polarity therapy, determined that flux density showed polarities within the physical body (Stone, 1986).

In 1978, Pavek compared paired-hand placements and reversed paired-hand placements on patients by hundreds of trained and untrained practitioners; he noted that one arrangement consistently resulted in relaxation and feelings of well-being but that the other set consistently produced agitation and anxiety. From this he deduced normal (healthy) qi polarities and movement patterns in the body (Pavek, 1987). (See fig. 3.)

In 1985 Pavek expanded on these findings by demonstrating coherent linkages between qi patterns, emotional holding patterns, and autocontractile pain response while developing biofield

[7]*Flow is much slower through human tissue and varies with the person's health and emotional state.*

Table 3. Rough Equivalencies in Applied Physics

Atmospheric Physics	Biofield Physics[a]	Electromagnetics	Hydrodynamics
Air	Qi	Flux	Liquid
Density	Denseness	Charge	Viscosity
Wind	Flow	Current	Stream
High pressure	Sending hand[b]	Negative terminal	Source
Low pressure	Receiving hand[b]	Positive terminal	Slump
Friction	Resistance	Reluctance	Friction
System	Biofield	Field	Flow-field
Pressure	Force	Electromagnetic field	Pressure
Pressure gradient	Polarity	Polar difference	Pressure differential

Source: Provided courtesy of the Biofield Research Institute.
[a]Proposed category
[b]In some systems

treatments for disorders often classified as psychosomatic (Pavek, 1988b; Pavek and Daily, 1990) and correlating emotional holding patterns with Chinese five-phase theory (Pavek, 1988a).

In 1992, Isaacs conducted a double-blind study using Eeman screens, which confirmed polarity at the spine and arms (Isaacs, 1991).

It is unclear at this time whether the biofield is electromagnetic or some other presently unmeasured but potentially quantifiable medium. It is popularly hypothesized that the biofield is a form of bioelectricity, biomagnetism, or bioelectromagnetism.[8] This may well be the case but has yet to be established. Some researchers discount the possibility.[9]

Some Chinese researchers have conducted experiments indicating that when *wei qi* (the external biofield) is used in fa qi (healing), electro-magnetic radiation in the infrared range is produced; others found indications of infrasonic waves. However, both phenomena appear to be minor secondary effects (Shen, 1988; Xin et al., 1988).

Figure 2. Arm and Spine Polarities

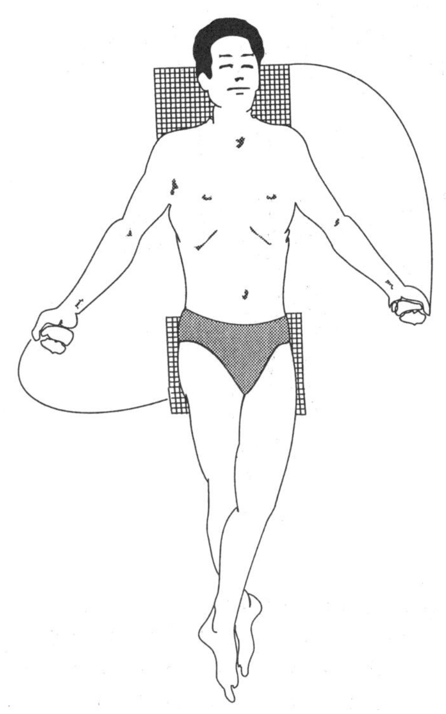

[8]*An erroneous report, "New Technologies Detect Effects of Healing Hands," in* Brain/Mind Bulletin, *vol. 10, no. 16, contributed to this supposition when it stated that one researcher, John Zimmerman, had measured electromagnetic effects of healers' hands during healing with a SQUID (superconducting quantum interference device); actually, he made his measurements at the healers' heads while measuring very low-amplitude electromagnetic brainwave activity.*

[9]*No one has yet been able to detect either current flow or electromagnetic flux emanating from the hands of a practitioner. Dry skin electrical impedance at the hands is quite high, ≥10 megohms (10 million ohms). Silver/silver chloride electrodes, as used in biofeedback, measure skin conduction, not flux emanations.*

Figure 3. Normal Qi Patterns in the Body

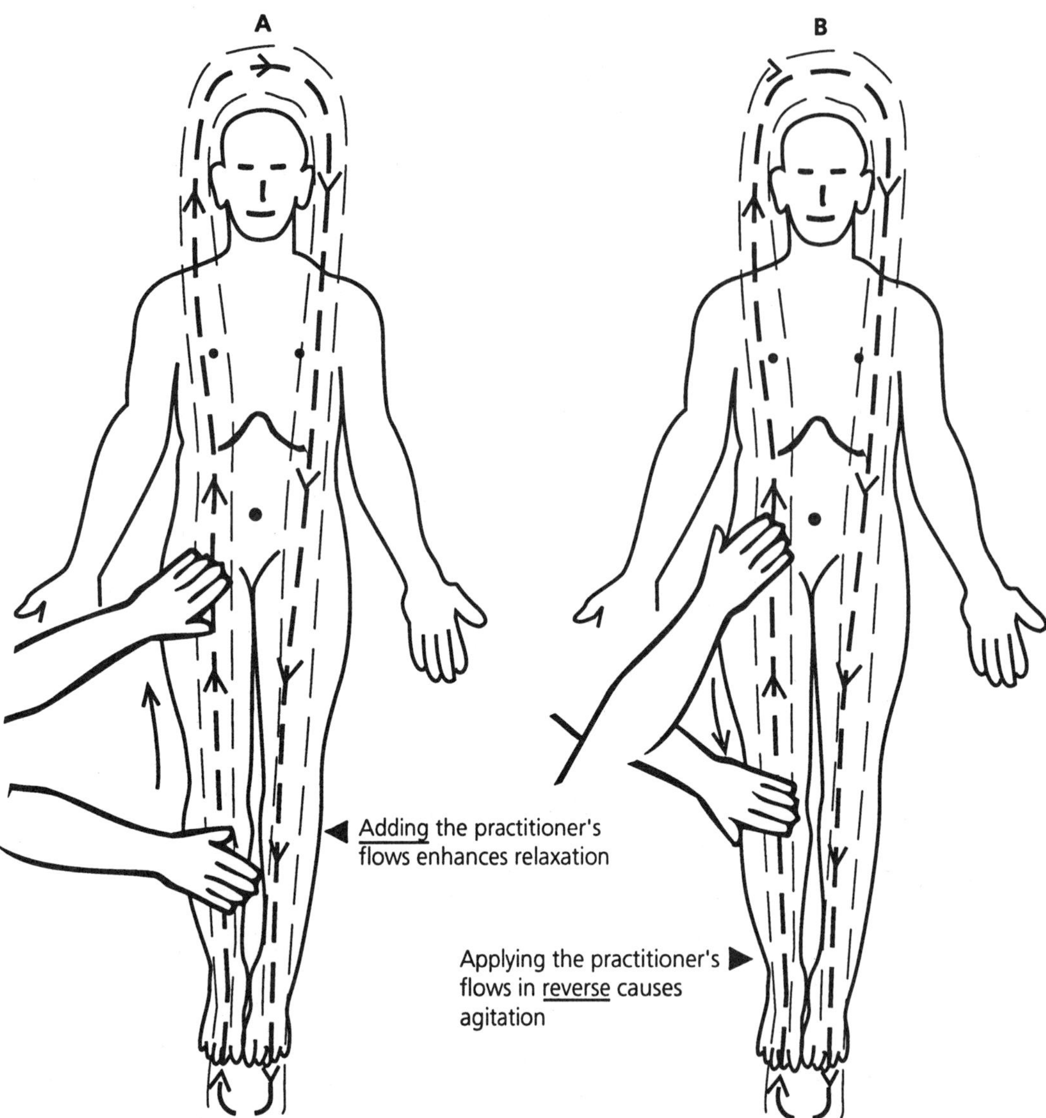
A
B
Adding the practitioner's flows enhances relaxation
Applying the practitioner's flows in reverse causes agitation

Research base. Rigorous research on biofield healing has been hindered by the belief, held by many, that nothing more than a placebo effect is the operative factor. This belief has affected funding, publishing, and status of researchers. Because funding organizations and scientific communities believed that any effects obtained were largely placebo effects, not real effects of biofields, research has been considered pointless. Moreover, many researchers have been unwilling to study biofield effects that they would otherwise be interested in, because they fear being ostracized by other researchers. Publication of research by the journals has been limited for similar reasons.

Notwithstanding these limitations, a number of studies have been implemented. In the United States, there are more than 17 published studies on biofield therapeutics.

Published U.S. studies. Because no comprehensive database of studies on biofield therapeutics exists, the following are considered to be only a sampling.

In two controlled studies on therapeutic touch, Krieger found significant change in hemoglobin levels in hospitalized patients (Krieger, 1975, 1973). In a similar study, Wetzel found significant change in hematocrit and hemoglobin levels of 48 subjects receiving reiki, and no significant change with 10 controls (Wetzel, 1989).

Wirth found significant change in the healing rate of full-thickness skin wounds in a carefully controlled, double-blind study of therapeutic touch (Wirth, 1990), while Keller and Bzdek found highly significant decreases in pain scores recorded on the McGill-Melzak Pain Questionnaire by patients with tension headache in a controlled study of therapeutic touch (Keller, 1993; Keller and Bzdek, 1986).

Although Meehan found no significant difference on the Visual Analog Scale and Pain Intensity Descriptor Form between postoperative patients receiving therapeutic touch and controls, secondary analysis showed patients receiving therapeutic touch waited longer before requesting analgesia (Meehan, 1985, 1988). Similarly, Heidt found significant changes in anxiety levels of hospitalized cardiovascular patients receiving therapeutic touch versus controls as measured on the A-State Self-evaluation Questionnaire (Heidt, 1979, 1981a; Spielberger et al., 1983). Quinn (1983) found similar results in a study of therapeutic touch versus mimic therapeutic touch without centering and intention to assist.

In a replication study on patients before and after open heart surgery, using therapeutic touch versus mimic therapeutic touch and no-treatment groups, Quinn found no significant differences between the groups. Yet changes occurred in the expected direction, and there was a significant reduction in diastolic blood pressure among the therapeutic touch group that was not seen in the no-treatment group (Quinn, 1989). In another study of therapeutic touch versus mimic therapeutic touch, Parkes showed no significant differences among elderly hospitalized patients (Parkes, 1985).

Collins (1983), Fedoruk (1984), and Ferguson (1986) found significant relaxation effects of therapeutic touch with various subjects in different studies, and Quinn (1992), in a pilot study of four bereaved people, found significant reduction of suppressor T cells in all four after therapeutic touch. Moreover, Kramer found significant differences in stress reduction between treatment and control groups in a study of therapeutic touch with hospitalized children (Kramer, 1990).

Other U.S. studies. A number of pilot and case studies in fruitful areas have shown interesting results that are worthy of further investigation. These studies were conducted without controls, usually because of the severe limitations on funding.

In four uncontrolled cases, Pavek found that white cell decrease during chemotherapy reversed and rose significantly after single SHEN® therapy treatments at the thymus gland (Pavek, unpublished, 1984–85). In a pilot study on SHEN® therapy and premenstrual syndrome, Pavek noted significant long-term symptom relief and behavioral change with 11 of 13 subjects (Pavek, unpublished, 1986).

Beal, in an unpublished study of 12 hospitalized major depressives, found no statistical difference in time of release from the hospital between 6 subjects randomized to receive SHEN® therapy and 6 controls receiving sham SHEN® therapy. However, in analyzing both subject and counselor reports, Pavek found significant change in dreaming, emotional expressiveness, and interpersonal contact with subjects receiving SHEN® therapy and much less change among controls (Beal and Pavek, 1985).

Other therapeutic touch research with promising indications includes research on rehabilitation (Payne, 1989), helping patients to rest (Heidt, 1991), mental patients (Hill and Oliver, 1993), symptom control in acquired immunodeficiency syndrome (AIDS) (Newshan, 1989), and severe burn patients (Pavek, unpublished observations).

Promising research with SHEN® therapy includes research with occupational therapy clients, third-trimester abdominal pain, reduction of pain during birthing without pain medication, irritable bowel syndrome, posttraumatic stress disorder, anorexia, bulimia, phobias, and chronic migraine.

International research. There has been considerable research on biofield therapeutics in other countries. In China, more than 30 controlled studies on effects of fa qi on both humans and animals were reported in the proceedings of just one meeting, the First World Conference for the Academic Exchange of Medical Qigong. At the same meeting, 32 studies were presented on effects on health of qigong exercises that raise qi (Proceedings, 1988).

In an overview report, Daniel Benor has compiled data on 151 healing studies from around the world (Benor, 1992). In many of these studies, mental healing efforts were combined with the biofield processes. However, 61 were controlled, published studies of biofield healing effects without the confounding factors of mental intent. These studies are shown in tables 4 and 5.

Table 4. Controlled Studies of Biofield Therapeutics With Humans

Subject	No. of studies	Significant results[a]
Anxiety	9	4 (+2)
Hemoglobin	4	4
Skin wounds	1	1
Asthma and bronchitis	1	0
Tension headache	1	1
Postoperative pain	1	0
Neck and back pain	1	(?+1)[b]
Total	18	10 (2)
Percent of total		56% (11%)

Source: Benor, 1993.

[a]Significance $p<.01$; for values in parentheses, $p<.02-.05$.

[b]Possibly significant results, but faulty reporting or design prevented proper evaluation of the studies.

Research Recommendations

Promising clinical results. While technique, focus, and range of treatments attempted vary considerably, a number of results are common to all forms of the biofield process:

- Acceleration of wound healing.
- Reduction of the pain of thermal burns and acceleration of healing time.
- Reduction of sunburn pain and coloration.
- Reduction of acute and chronic pain.
- Reduction of anxiety.
- Release of pent-up grief.

In addition, practitioners of some forms of the process report consistently good results with

- recurrent panic attacks;
- premenstrual syndrome;
- posttraumatic stress disorder;
- irritable bowel syndrome;
- nonbiological sexual dysfunction;
- drug, alcohol, and codependence recovery;
- migraine;
- anorexia and bulimia; and
- third-trimester pregnancy and birthing.

Characterization of the biofield. That the biofield has definable form, flux pattern, and polarities seems clear to practitioners from the wealth of empirical evidence available. However, characterization of the biofield is far from complete, and determining its nature is paramount to its further development among the healing arts.

Two hypotheses should be tested: first, that the biofield is a field in physics other than an already known field, and, second, that the biofield is bioelectromagnetism. One approach that would support the first hypothesis would be development of a device (transducer) that would react with the biofield so as to exclude the possibility of bioelectromagnetism. Research projects in China have shown that application of the biofield affects lithium fluoride thermoluminesence detectors, polarized light beams, Van de Graff generators, and silicone crystal plates (Proceedings, 1988). These preliminary experiments suggest possible approaches toward further characterization.

Research design considerations. The following should be considered in planning well-designed studies to evaluate potential effects of biofields on health:

- *Mental healing techniques.* Since mental healing techniques are often mixed with biofield techniques, care must be taken in all research designs to separate out the two factors. Unless

Table 5. Other Controlled Biofield Studies

Subject	No. of studies	Significant results[a]		
Enzymes	8	3	(+2)	(?+3)[b]
Fungus/yeast	6	4	(+1)	(?+1)[b]
Bacteria	2	?		
Red blood cells	1	1		
Cancer cells	3	1		(?+2)[b]
Snail pacemaker cells	4	4		
Plants	10	7		(?+2)[b]
Motility				
Flagellates	2	0		(?+1)[b]
Algae	2	1		
Moth larvae	1	1		
Mice				
Skin wounds	2	2		
Retardation of goiter growth	2	2		
Total	43	26	(3)	
Percent of total		61%	(7%)	

Source: Benor, 1993.

[a]Significance $p<.01$; for values in parentheses, $p<.02$–$.05$.

[b]Possibly significant results, but faulty reporting or design prevented proper evaluation of the studies.

this is done, unclear results will prevent reasonable analysis.

- *Sham treatments.* Unlike placebo pills, biofield healing cannot be faked. According to the observations of practitioners, it is not possible to touch subjects in a clinical study in a purely physical way for any period of time without resulting in some effect from the practitioner's biofield. Nor is there a way to shield the biofield emitted by one person from another person's; this renders the notion of a "sham control" meaningless. This particular confounding factor has adversely affected results in several studies of biofield therapeutics (Beal and Pavek, 1985; Meehan, 1988; Parkes, 1985; Quinn, 1989). In these studies, controls were established by effecting a mimic, or sham, of the primary method. The practitioners' hands were brought into close proximity with the subject in a "sham treatment." In all such cases, some positive effect was obtained with the mimic or sham treatments that was greater than could be reasonably expected from no-treatment controls.

- *Double-blind studies.* Although it is not possible for a biofield healing practitioner to perform in a strict double-blind situation, it is possible to design studies in which the evaluators are blinded to the treatment method and subjects are blinded to the method and to the specific intended outcome.

- *Science and metaphysics.* Because the metaphysical model lies, by both definition and practice, outside the usual confines of science, research on metaphysical explanatory models will be difficult. However, outcome studies of clinical effect could be designed and executed.

- *Collaborations.* The process could be speeded up if experienced researchers sympathetic to energy healing work together with researchers experienced in developing appropriate criteria. These criteria must (1) provide the established medical and health communities with valid, reproducible data and (2) be constructed so as not to negate the operative treatment mechanism.

Barriers and Key Issues

Hindrances. For various reasons, biofield healing has been hindered from reaching its fullest potential. Principal among these reasons are the following:

- Until recently, few testable hypotheses.
- Few theoreticians who are also practitioners.
- The disdain of currently established scientists.
- Lack of a solid research base.
- Lack of an adequate outcomes database.
- Unsystematic accumulation of empirical evidence.
- Obscuring of the extent of efficacy by a plethora of conceptual confusions and conflicting claims as to causal factors, best methods, and procedures.

Placebo and efficacy. Some people have attributed any successful applications of biofield therapeutic to a high probability of placebo effect. This assumption has inhibited reviewers and editors from accepting as valid the usual, smaller pilot studies that would be acceptable for other types of therapy.

No studies that have been done, however, indicate that placebo factors are any higher with biofield therapies than with other healing methods. In fact, a number of situations in which placebo effects would have been highly unlikely cast doubt on the concern. Some such studies have had marked, positive results (Benor, 1992) with animals and with small children below the age of reason. There are also numerous anecdotal reports of children receiving treatments while asleep and awakening with marked change. Fevers have broken during such treatments, panic attacks have ceased, and comas have ended (Pavek, 1988).

Such evidence suggests that the reason why biofield treatments are effective is other than the placebo effect.

Peer review. At this time, there are no peer review groups that actually include "peers." True peers, who have a hands-on understanding of biofield therapeutics, should be included on review committees. (See the "Peer Review" chapter.)

Recommendations

Because the stigma associated with "faith healing" has been attached to biofield therapy, it has not been seriously considered as a viable treatment method. Consequently, the discipline languishes in a research doldrum. The following steps are recommended:

1. The biofield should be characterized. Reasonable approaches exist, some of which have been described in this report.
2. Simple and appropriate instruments should be developed to begin the process systematically collecting clinical data. With properly designed forms, individual case studies could be statistically sorted and grouped by disorder, treatment process, and results. This sorting would begin to establish relative efficacy in the various categories, suggesting productive avenues for future research. To implement this process, OAM should establish a small study group, including members familiar with intake and outcome forms and data collection and representative members of the discipline.
3. Studies should be undertaken to determine how much of biofield therapeutics is attributable to mental healing and how much is attributable to quantity and proper directional application of the biofield flows.
4. Appropriate review panels with actual peers should be established.
5. A number of open technical questions in the discipline should be resolved. OAM should invite the leaders of the various systems to a general meeting to discuss and compare techniques and methods and to begin resolving these questions. Resolving these differences will enhance the techniques of all biofield healing methods.
6. A number of clinical studies that have been done in Europe and in Asia could be replicated here. Replication is necessary to assure the American research community that the studies are valid and to point the way for further research here.
7. A wealth of serious study proposals are available. These should be reviewed, and the most promising should be implemented.

Conclusion

Biofield therapeutics and diagnostics have been struggling to cross the border from metaphysics to physics and gain mainstream acceptance for a long time. In spite of considerable difficulties, biofield methods are gaining acceptance from health professionals and the general public in two areas—(1) the medical clinic and (2) hospital and psychotherapeutic settings. In both, biofield treatments are reported to be of benefit for many people.

Biofield therapeutics are a low-cost, noninvasive, nondrug approach, and applications have been reported in many medical and health situations as alternatives or as complements to mainstream medicine. The potential reward-to-risk ratio is great, and relatively small amounts of money are needed to start a validation process, which should be done with dispatch.

Combined Physical and Biofield Methods

The following methods are described by their practitioners as combining physical and biofield aspects. The list, which is not all-inclusive, tends to be descriptive; little research is available as a basis for judging the usefulness of these methods. Most of them would benefit from research on their efficacy and their scientific bases.

Applied Kinesiology

Applied kinesiology, or "touch for health," consists of both a diagnostic method of determining dysfunctional states of the body and related therapeutics. Based on principles of physiology and the meridian system mentioned earlier, it was developed in the 1960s by George Goodheart. It uses both the meridian qi and the biofield qi in its diagnostics and therapeutics.

Neurolymphatic holding points, neurovascular holding points, meridian holding points, and the biofield external qi are all said to be incorporated in the process. A session starts with various "muscle testings" that are used to determine the state of qi flow through the meridians. Muscle testings give an indication of the area to be worked on and are a necessary part of the treatment.

A number of applied kinesiology practitioners use the process in conjunction with more established practices, such as chiropractic.

Network Chiropractic Spinal Analysis

Network chiropractic spinal analysis (NCSA) merges conventional chiropractic mechanical or structural approaches with biofield approaches to evaluate and correct anomalies of the spine and nervous system. At the clinical core of NCSA is the classification of spinal subluxations into two categories: (1) structural subluxation that involves mechanical dislocation of spinal sections and (2) soft-tissue subluxation that involves tension in the muscles and other soft tissue connected to the spinal sections. NCSA does not address structural subluxations until after a reduction of soft-tissue subluxations has occurred. (It has been noted that structural subluxations often self-correct shortly after soft-tissue subluxations have been adjusted.) Application of the biofield is included for the soft-tissue adjustments and is applied first. Conventional chiropractic adjustments follow, as required, for structural adjustments.

The clinician uses a phased system to introduce order to the subluxated segments. Since the body often creates movement from a tense, restricted state, a spontaneous discharge of tension often occurs as the spinal distortions are resolved; this is a common occurrence. A wide range of responses is then observed with certain common elements. Among the unique individual responses typically seen is a period of deep and full respirations; other responses include periods of muscular movements and naturally occurring postures as the body and mind seek to purge mechanical tension or stored memories of traumatic experiences.

Polarity Therapy

Polarity therapy is a natural health system based on the idea of a "human energy field." Drawing from oriental and Indian sources, it asserts that well-being and health are conditions determined by the nature of the flow of this human energy field and that the flow can be affected by various natural methods. Polarity therapy incorporates a variety of strategies to enhance the flow of the energy field, including touch, diet, movement, and self-awareness. (Polarity practitioners generally believe that the energy field that they are enhancing is electromagnetic, but this point has not been established.)

The central concepts of polarity therapy are as follows:

- All phenomena have a fundamental structure involving charged particles in a relationship of expansion-contraction or attraction-repulsion. In East Asia this relationship is called the tao, or relationship of opposites (yin and yang).
- An "energy anatomy" precedes and creates physical anatomy, and this energy anatomy exists in several layers that are affected, and possibly distorted, by life experience.
- These distortions may be corrected by several methods, including touch, holding pressure points, and using the practitioner's hands to link various "polarities" in the client's body.

Commonly reported benefits of "polarity energy balancing" include relaxation, pain reduction, reduction of nervous conditions, heightened self-awareness, and improvement in range of motion.

Polarity therapy was developed in the 1950s by Randolph Stone, a chiropractor, osteopath, and naturopath. Today the American Polarity Therapy Association, which was founded in 1983, organizes and supports training and certification of practitioners; the association also is developing a research arm. At present there are more than 500 practitioners of polarity therapy, trained at several levels of proficiency.

Qigong Longevity Exercises

The qigong longevity or health exercises are a fairly recent addition to alternative health practices in the United States. Qigong exercises are similar in appearance to tijijuan (tai chi chuan), a rhythmical nonaerobic form of exercise; however, this appearance is only superficial. Qigong movement exercises do not flow from one position to another as in tai chi; they are done in shorter movement groups that are repeated many times. This, however, is not the essence of the practice, but only the visible form.

Qigong exercises combine repetitions of coordinated physical motions with mental concentration and directive efforts to move the qi in the body. During these exercises, which are based on slow, repetitive movements of the arms, legs, and torso, the exerciser's mind is focused on moving the qi (biofield flux) through the meridian pathways and nonmeridian pathways that were developed by the ancient Taoist (Daoist) sages.

This mental effort is coordinated with specific movements; for example, qi may be directed up the back as the arms are raised and down the front as the arms are lowered. Large amounts of internal qi are said to be developed in the process. It is estimated that there are more than 100 different forms of qigong health exercises. There are considerable differences in the styles, but all consider the mental effort to be crucial. Qigong exercises are used daily for health improvement by several million Chinese, both in the People's Republic and in Chinese communities throughout Southeast Asia.

Qigong exercises are also used by qigong masters (see the "Biofield Therapeutics" section) to increase the quantity of qi available for healing; some use it in various forms of martial arts such as gongfu (kung fu).

In China, qigong exercises have been under study for their long-term effects on a number of medical conditions, such as cancer and arthritis, and for their effects on general health. More than 32 studies were recently presented at just one major conference on the effects on general and specific states of health of exercises enhancing qigong qi (Proceedings, 1988).

Several schools and organizations in this country focus entirely on these practices. The principal ones are China Advocates, the Chinese National Chi Kung Institute, the Qigong Academy, and the Qigong Institute. The practice of qigong is gaining in popularity in the United States, both with Asians and non-Asians.

Craniosacral Therapy

Craniosacral therapy is a gentle, hands-on treatment method that focuses on alleviating restrictions to physiological motion of all the bones of the skull, including the face and mouth, as well as the vertebral column, sacrum, coccyx, and pelvis. Concurrently, the craniosacral therapist focuses as well on normalizing abnormal tensions and stresses in the meningeal membrane, with special attention to the outermost membrane, the dura mater, and its fascial connections. Attention is also paid to alleviating any obstacles to free movement by the cerebrospinal fluid within its membrane compartment and to normalizing and balancing perceived related energy fields. This approach is derived from experiments of John Upledger, an osteopathic physician and researcher (for example, see Upledger, 1977a and 1977b, which are discussed below).

As usually practiced, this therapy is a noninvasive treatment process that requires an uninterrupted treatment session of at least 30 minutes; often the session is extended beyond an hour. Practitioners indicate that successful treatment relies largely on the therapist's ability to facilitate the patient's own self-corrective processes within the craniosacral system. Postgraduate training in craniosacral therapy has been undertaken by a wide variety of physicians, dentists, and therapists. In the United States during 1993, 2,738 health care professionals completed the Upledger Institute's introductory-level workshop and seminar; 1,827 received training at the intermediate level, and 80 completed the advanced level. Training outside this country is available through the Upledger Institute Europe in the Netherlands and on a smaller scale in Japan, New Zealand, France, and Norway by American Upledger Institute teachers.

The most powerful effects of craniosacral therapy are considered to be on the function of the central nervous system, the immune system, the endocrine system, and the visceral organs via the autonomic nervous system. This therapy has been used with reported success in many cases of brain and spinal cord dysfunction. Although these successes have not been documented in formal studies, they have been observed subjectively or anecdotally by both patients and therapists. Most prominent among these success reports are cases of brain injury resulting in symptoms of spastic paralysis and seizure. Other areas of claimed success include cerebral palsy, learning disabilities, seizure disorders, depressive reactions, menstrual dysfunction, motor dysfunction, strabismus (a vision disorder), temporomandibular joint problems, various headaches, chronic pain problems, and chronic fatigue syndrome.

Research on tissues has documented the potential for movement between skull bones in adult humans, and pilot work with live primates has shown rhythmical movement of their skull bones. Interrater reliability studies, which look for correlations in the observations of two or more independent raters (see the "Osteopathic Medicine" section), have shown agreement between "blinded" therapists evaluating preschool-aged children ("blinding" means that the therapists making the observations did not know which children had received craniosacral therapy, nor did they know the history or problems of the children) (Upledger, 1977a). Controlled studies have shown high correlation between schoolchildren with various brain dysfunctions and specific dysfunctions of the craniosacral system; that is, the craniosacral exam scores correlated with recorded school teacher and psychologist opinions of "not normal," behavioral problems, motor coordination problems, learning disabilities, and obstetrical complications (Upledger, 1977b). Moreover, Upledger reports that a few pilot studies by dentists have demonstrated significant changes in the transverse dimension of the hard palate as well as in occlusion in response to craniosacral therapy.

At present, work is under way that appears to demonstrate fluctuations in what are called energy measurements in circuits between craniosacral therapists and patients. The circuits are established by attaching electrodes to the patient and the therapist with an ohmmeter and a voltmeter interposed in the circuits. In observations with 22 patients, measurements have ranged from more than 30 million ohms at the start of a treatment session to 448 ohms with a brain-injured child; voltages have fluctuated between 10 and 254 millivolts. Upledger's interpretation is that the elevation in resistances read with the ohmmeter correlate with the palpable resistances that craniosacral therapists feel with their hands and that the energy put into overcoming these resistances is reflected by elevations in the millivolt readings. On the basis of these preliminary studies, plans are under way to explore further whether the energetic changes measured in the circuits accompany specific landmarks in treatment processes.

Physical Therapy: An Example of Transition to Mainstream Health Care

Physical therapists are health care professionals who diagnose and treat problems related to physical function. While physical therapy is considered to be a part of mainstream medicine in this country, its practitioners frequently use manual healing methods that are categorized as alternative. Many of the methods identified in other sections of this chapter are part of the standard repertoire of physical therapy. The development of the profession and its transition into mainstream health care are discussed in this section. Some of the alternative procedures and the difficulties encountered in training for them are noted.

Background

Physical therapy is a relatively young profession in comparison with medicine and nursing, although its roots lie in ancient Rome and Greece. Its modern embodiment appeared at about the time of World War I, through the creation of the Women's Auxiliary Medical Aides, renamed Medical Aides and then again Reconstruction Aides, in the Office of the Surgeon General of the Army. Physical therapy training programs existed in France and England at this time under the name *physiotherapy*, a term that is still used in most Western nations outside the United States.

It quickly became apparent that the United States also needed to train its own people in new ways to assist the war wounded. Few, if any, professionals who were trained in medicine or nursing at that time could deal with physical, vocational, and psychological problems associated with injuries sustained in war (Ramsden, 1978).

Educational preparation in 1917 consisted of 4-month sessions after graduation from high school but quickly moved to 12-month sessions that followed preparation in nursing or physical education. Since the 1920s, preparation for practice has shifted from an apprentice model to an academic model and from clinic-based education to universities. Currently, 50 percent of entry-level degrees are awarded at the master's degree level. Not included are master's degrees in physical therapy awarded to people already trained in the field. The professional doctorate—the D.P.T.—is available at three universities.

Adversity stimulated the growth of the profession, with major spurts during both world wars and during the polio epidemics in 1914, 1916, and the 1940s. Then a new creativity in prosthetics and orthotics in conjunction with physical therapy treatment evolved in response to the problems of thalidomide-affected babies after the belated recognition in 1961 that thalidomide was a teratogen (a substance affecting embryonic development). Thalidomide was given to pregnant women, primarily in Great Britain, to treat nausea, or "morning sickness."

The startling growth of physical therapy as a profession in the 1980s and 1990s may be explained by many factors, including documented effectiveness of treatment of patients of all ages. The targets of treatment include virtually all problems affecting normal function resulting from trauma and illness as well as those resulting from genetically transmitted disease, trauma sustained in childbirth, developmental delay, and normal and abnormal consequences of aging.

The number of schools in the United States preparing men and women for the profession of physical therapy is now 140, with approximately 5,000 graduates each year (American Physical Therapy Association, 1993). There are additional schools at various stages in the accreditation process. Previously made up entirely of women from physical education and nursing, the professional ranks today include approximately 30 percent men. The curriculums draw applicants from a wide variety of academic backgrounds, including fine arts, basic science, humanities, behavioral sciences, engineering, and business. Membership in the American Physical Therapy Association is approximately 60,000, which is half the total number of practicing physical therapists in the United States.

The number of graduates from academic programs does not begin to meet society's need for physical therapy services. Because professional practice is relatively autonomous, physical therapists frequently work in private practice. Growing sophistication and autonomy have led to a nationwide effort by members of the profession to seek legislative changes in State practice acts to permit practice without referral. Twenty-eight States have enacted such legislation. Real shortages of physical therapists exist in many health care institutions; it is one of the professions having the greatest number of vacant positions in the Nation.

Current Practice

Physical therapists are licensed health care professionals. The therapist's normal scope of work for any given client involves evaluating the patient, identifying potential problems, and determining the diagnoses that are related to physical function; then the therapist establishes objectives or goals, provides treatment services, evaluates the effectiveness of treatment, and makes any modifications necessary to achieve the desired outcome.

Therapeutic interventions focus on posture, movement, strength, endurance, cardiopulmonary function, balance, coordination, joint mobility, flexibility, pain, healing and repair, and functional ability in daily living skills, including work.

Among the therapeutic activities included are therapeutic exercise; application of assistive devices; physical agents, such as heat and cold; ultrasound; electricity, such as electromyography and electrical muscle stimulation; manual procedures, such as joint and soft-tissue mobilization; neuromuscular reeducation; bronchopulmonary hygiene; and ambulation training with and without assistive devices.

This professional activity may take place in a wide variety of settings, including neonatal nurseries, intensive care units, bedside acute care, rehabilitation units, outpatient clinics, private offices, private homes, physical fitness or sports facilities, and schools. In addition to providing direct service, physical therapists are also involved in health maintenance programs and illness prevention programs, health policy development, administration, education, research, consultation, and other advisory services.

Physical therapists also apply many of the therapeutic interventions identified and discussed elsewhere in this chapter. Therapists using these procedures consider them fundamental tools in their repertoire. Among these procedures are acupressure, myofascial release, craniosacral therapy, massage techniques, Alexander technique, Feldenkrais method, and therapeutic touch.

Such procedures are rarely included in the academic preparation of physical therapy students. Rather, they may be learned through special programs with a select group of practitioners who conduct continuing education experiences throughout the country. Perhaps the inclusion of these procedures in the clinical practice of physical therapy is evidence of the belief by a growing segment in the profession that mind and body are connected, but we do not know or understand all the connections.

Several of these systems seem to share common threads. The therapy is aimed at restoring the homeostasis of a person's body-mind-spirit, using a comprehensive and holistic approach. The emphasis is on promotion of health, prevention of illness, and education approaches.

Philosophy

The philosophy of physical therapy is based on an educational model; the objective is to help individual patients help themselves to attain the maximum level of function they are capable of. The decisions about treatment—what to do, when to do it, and how much—are not made only on the basis of experience with what "works." A general understanding of the effects of an approach for a given condition is not adequate justification for applying that method.

The professional literature of physical therapy that appears in several refereed journals documents evidence of the efficacy, or lack thereof, of particular treatment interventions. Both quantitative and qualitative research methods are used with increasing sophistication. A major effort by physical therapists in academic and clinical leadership positions and by the professional association has contributed to the prominence of this kind of documentation for a wide variety of physical therapy interventions.

Current Research

Responding to a research mandate may be difficult for some physical therapists who are using procedures that are less well-known and not generally included in the traditional academic preparation (Hariharan, 1993). Research may be even more difficult for therapists whose work is entirely clinical and whose academic preparation did not include training in research methodology appropriate for clinical practice (Soderberg, 1991). Nevertheless, the research mandate for the profession today is clear: do it if it works, document carefully what has been done, develop careful research studies to determine the mechanisms involved, publish the results, and continue the research until everyone understands what is being done and why. As a corollary, a corresponding need has arisen for physical therapists to obtain training in research methodology.

Physical therapist researchers currently publish in major medical journals as well as the journal *Physical Therapy*. The research covers a wide range of subjects related to clinical practice and the underlying mechanisms of function (Bohannon, 1986). Recently published work on the following subjects illustrates the range: physical therapy treatment of peripheral vestibular dysfunction based on clinical case reports; impact of three posting methods on controlling abnormal subtalar pronation; a comparison of three different respiratory exercises in prevention of postoperative pulmonary complications after upper abdominal surgery; motor unit behavior in Parkinson's disease; a study of age and training on skeletal muscle physiology and on performance; a study of the factors associated with burnout of physical therapists working in a specific work environment; and a study of the discrete behaviors that differentiate the expert from the novice physical therapist.

Summary

Physical therapy began with a few women who trained briefly and learned on the job how to help care for seriously injured soldiers. The group grew dramatically, and the length of training increased as the scope of work became apparent and the amount of knowledge to impart expanded. With the knowledge and technology explosions, physical therapy became more sophisticated and moved into the mainstream of health care, contributing in significant ways to patient care and to the literature of research and practice.

Overall Recommendations

Research on manual healing methods is needed in four parallel and interactive directions:

- To determine the range of clinical benefits for the many common physical complaints and problems treated by therapists using these methods (e.g., back pain, headache, whiplash, and chronic fatigue syndrome).
- To determine the degree to which a general sense of well-being is enhanced by the various manual healing methods.
- To evaluate the effect of structural manipulation on body awareness (both visceral and external); regulation of motion; range of movement; ability to cope with stress; muscle tone and flexibility; growth, development, and aging; autonomic function (neural control systems); electrical patterns in muscles; immune system response; and cardiovascular and respiratory function.
- To determine the physiological and neurological mechanisms associated with specific manual healing methods.

References

Adams T., R. Heisey, M.C. Smith, and B. Briner. 1992. Parietal bone mobility in the anesthetized cat. J. Am. Osteopath. Assoc. 92:599–622.

American Physical Therapy Association. 1993. Post-Entry Level Programs for Physical Therapists. Department for Education, American Physical Therapy Association, Alexandria, Va.

Annual Directory, J. Am. Osteopath. Assoc. 1993. Pp. 537–548.

Baginski, B.J., and S. Sharamon. 1988. Reiki Universal Life Energy. LifeRhythm, Mendicino, Calif.

Barker, M.E. 1983. Manipulation in general medical practice for thoracic pain syndromes. British Osteopathic Journal 15:95.

Beal, M., and R. Pavek. 1985. An uncompleted controlled study of SHEN and major depression. Milwaukee County Mental Health Center.

Beal, M.C., J.P. Goodridge, W.L. Johnston, et al. 1980. Interexaminer agreement on long-term patient improvement: an exercise in research design. J. Am. Osteopath. Assoc. 79:432–440.

Beal, M.C., J.P. Goodridge, W.L. Johnston, et al. 1982. Interexaminer agreement on patient improvement after negotiated selection of tests. J. Am. Osteopath. Assoc. 81:322–328.

Beattie, P., J.M. Rothstein, and R.L. Lamb. 1987. Reliability of the attraction method for measuring lumbar spine backward bending. Phys. Ther. 77:364.

Beideman, R.P. 1983. Seeking the rational alternative: the National College of Chiropractic 1906 to 1982. Chiropractic History 3:17.

Benor, D.J. 1992. Healing research. Helix Verlag 1.

Benor, D.J. 1993. Healers and a changing medical paradigm. Frontier Perspectives 3:33–40.

Benor, D.J. 1994. Personal communication to the editorial review board via Richard Pavek.

Bergmann, T.F., D.H. Peterson, and D.J. Lawrence. 1993. Chiropractic Technique, vol. 5. Churchill Livingstone, New York.

Bergquist-Ullman, M., and U. Larsson. 1977. Acute low back pain in industry. Acta Orthop. Scand. Suppl. 170:1–117.

Bohannon, R.W., and D.F. Gibson. 1986. Citation analysis of physical therapy. Phys. Ther. 66:540–541.

Boline, P.D., J.C. Keating, J. Brist, et al. 1988. Interexaminer reliability of palpatory evaluation of the lumbar spine. Am. J. Chiro. Med. 1:5.

Brennan, B. 1987. Hands of Light. Bantam Books, New York.

British Medical Association. 1993. Complementary Medicine: New Approaches to Good Practice. Oxford University Press, Oxford, England.

Brunarski, D.J. 1985. Clinical trials of spinal manipulation: a critical appraisal and review of the literature. J. Manipulative Physiol. Ther. 7:243.

Buerger, A.A., and P.E. Greenman. 1985. Empirical Approaches to the Validation of Spinal Manipulation. Charles C. Thomas, Springfield, Ill.

Burns, L. 1917. Further contributions to the study of the effects of lumbar lesions. Bulletin 5, A.T. Still Research Institute, Chicago.

Carlson, R.J. 1975. The End of Medicine: Why Modern Medicine Fails to Produce Better Health for Americans. John Wiley and Sons, New York.

Cherkin, D.C., and F.A. MacCornack. 1989. Patient evaluations of low back pain care from family physicians and chiropractors. West J. Med. 150:351–355.

Collins, J.W. 1983. The Effect of Non-Contact Therapeutic Touch on the Relaxation Response. Unpublished master's thesis, Vanderbilt University.

Cottingham, J.T., S.W. Porges, and T. Lynn. 1988a. Effects of soft tissue manipulation (Rolfing pelvic lift) on parasympathetic tone in two age groups. Journal of the American Physical Therapy Association 68:352–356.

Cottingham, J.T., S.W. Porges, and K. Richmond. 1988b. Shifts in pelvic inclination angle and parasympathetic tone produced by Rolfing soft tissue manipulation. Journal of the American Physical Therapy Association 68:1364–1370.

Denslow, J.S., I.M. Korr, and A.D. Krems. 1947. Quantitative studies of chronic facilitation in human motoneuron pools. Am. J. Physiol. 150:229–238.

DeRosa, C., and J. Porterfield. 1992. A physical therapy model for the treatment of low back pain. Phys. Ther. 72:261–272.

Downing, C.H. 1935. Osteopathic Principles in Disease, R.J. Orozco, San Francisco, Calif.

Eble, J.N. 1960. Patterns of response of musculature to visceral stimuli. Am. J. Physiol. 198:429–433.

Edelman, G.M. 1987. Neural Darwinism: The Theory of Neuronal Group Selection. Basic Books, Inc., New York.

Eeman, L.E. 1947. Cooperative Healing. Fredric Muller, London.

Eisenberg, D., R. Kessler, C. Foster, F.E. Norlock, D.R. Calkins, and T.L. Delbanco. 1993. Unconventional medicine in the U.S.: prevalence, costs, and patterns of use. N. Engl. J. Med. 328:246–252.

Fakouri, C., and P. Jones. 1987. Relaxation Rx: slow stroke back rub. J. Gerontological Nursing 13:32–35.

Fedoruk, R.B. 1984. Transfer of the Relaxation Response: Therapeutic Touch as a Method for the Reduction of Stress in Premature Neonates. Unpublished Ph.D. dissertation, University of Maryland.

Feldenkrais, M. 1949. Body and Mature Behavior: A Study of Anxiety, Sex, Gravitation, and Learning. International Universities Press, Inc., New York.

Feldenkrais, M. 1972. Awareness Through Movement: Health Exercises for Personal Growth. Harper and Row, New York.

Feldenkrais, M. 1981. The Elusive Obvious. Meta Publications, Cupertino, Calif.

Feldenkrais, M. 1985. The Potent Self: A Guide to Spontaneity or Learning to Learn. Harper and Row, New York.

Ferguson, C.K. 1986. Subjective Experience of Therapeutic Touch (SETT): Psychometric Examination of an Instrument. Unpublished Ph.D. dissertation, University of Texas at Austin.

Fichera, A.P., and D.R. Celander. 1969. Effect of osteopathic manipulative therapy on autonomic tone as evidenced by blood pressure changes and activity of the fibrinolytic system. J. Am. Osteopath. Assoc. 67:1036–1038.

Field, T. 1993. Personal communication to Elliott Greene, president, American Massage Therapy Association.

Field, T., C. Morrow, C. Valdeon, et al. 1992. Massage reduces anxiety in child and adolescent psychiatric patients. J. Am. Acad. Child Adolesc. Psychiatry 31:125–131.

Field, T., S. Schanberg, F. Scafidi, et al. 1986. Tactile/kinesthetic stimulation effects on preterm neonates. Pediatrics 77:654–658.

Frymann, V.M., R.E. Carney, and P. Springall. 1992. Effect of osteopathic medical management on neurological development in children. J. Am. Osteopath. Assoc. 92:729–744.

Frymoyer, J.W., R.B. Phillips, A.H. Newberg, et al. 1986. A comparative analysis of the interpretations of lumbar spinal radiographs by chiropractors and medical doctors. Spine 11:1020–1023.

Georgopolus, A.P., et al. 1986. Neuronal population coding of movement direction. Science 243:1416–1419.

Gershenow, R.P. 1985. The Education of the Osteopathic Physician. American Association of Colleges of Osteopathic Medicine, Rockville, Md.

Gevitz, N. 1980. The DOs: A social history of osteopathic medicine. Unpublished Ph.D. dissertation, University of Chicago.

Gevitz, N. 1993. Orthodox medicine has been enriched by the challenge posed by its competition. Advances 9.

Gillet, H., and M. Liekens. 1984. Belgian chiropractic research notes. Motion Palpation Institute, Huntington Beach, Calif.

Ginsberg, C. 1986. The shake-a-leg body awareness training program: dealing with spinal injury and recovery in a new setting. Somatics, Spring/Summer:31–42.

Godfrey, C.M., P.P. Morgan, and J. Schatzker. 1984. A randomized trial of manipulation for low-back pain in a medical setting. Spine 9:301–304.

Gonnella, C., S.V. Paris, and M. Kutner. 1982. Reliability in evaluating passive intervertebral motion. Phys. Ther. 62:436–444.

Grad, B. 1979. Healing by the laying on of hands: a review of experiments. In D.S. Sobel, ed. Ways of Health. Harcourt Brace Jovanovich, New York, pp. 267–287.

Gutman, G., C. Herbert, and S. Brown. 1977. Feldenkrais vs. conventional exercise for the elderly. J. Gerontol. 32:562–572.

Haas, M. 1991. The reliability of reliability. J. Manipulative Physiol. Ther. 14:199–208.

Haas, M., D.H. Peterson, D. Panzer, et al. 1993. Reactivity of leg alignment to articular pressure testing: evaluation of a diagnostic test using a randomized crossover clinical trial approach. J. Manipulative Physiol. Ther. 16:220–227.

Hadler, N.M., P. Curtis, D.B. Gillings, et al. 1987. A benefit of spinal manipulation as adjunctive therapy for acute low-back pain: a stratified controlled trial. Spine 12:702–706.

Haldeman, S., D. Chapman-Smith, and D.M. Peterson. 1992. Guidelines for chiropractic quality assurance and practice parameters. Aspen Publishers, Gaithersburg, Md.

Hansen, D.T., A.H. Adams, W.C. Meeker, et al. 1992. Proposal for establishing structure and process in the development of implicit chiropractic standards of care and practice guidelines. J. Manipulative Physiol. Ther. 15:430–438.

Hariharan, V. 1993. Non-orthodox health care. Australian Physiotherapy 39:1.

Heidt, P. 1979. An Investigation of the Effect of Therapeutic Touch on the Anxiety of Hospitalized Patients. Unpublished Ph.D. dissertation, New York University.

Heidt, P. 1981a. Effects of therapeutic touch on anxiety level of hospitalized patients. Nurs. Res. 1:32–37.

Heidt, P. 1981b. Scientific research and therapeutic touch. In M.D. Borelli and P. Heidt, eds. Therapeutic Touch. Springer, New York, pp. 3–12.

Heidt, P. 1991. Helping patients to rest: clinical studies in therapeutic touch. Holistic Nursing Practice 5:57–66.

Heisey, R.S., and T. Adams. 1993. Role of cranial bone mobility in cranial compliance. Neurosurgery 33:1–9.

Hill, L., and N. Oliver. 1993. Technique integration: therapeutic touch and theory based mental health nursing. J. Psychosoc. Nurs. Ment. Health Serv. 31(2):19–22.

Hoehler, F.K., J.S. Tobis, and A.A. Buerger. 1981. Spinal manipulation for low back pain. JAMA 245:1835–1839.

Hood, W. 1871. On Bonesetting, So-Called, and Its Relation to the Treatment of Joints Crippled by Injury. MacMillan and Co., London.

Houshen, L. 1988. A Clinical and Laboratory Study of the Effect of Qigong Anaesthesia on Thyroidectomy. Proceedings of the First World Conference for Academic Exchange of Medical Qigong, Beijing, pp. 84–85.

Isaacs, J. 1991. A double blind study of the "Biocircuit," a putative subtle-energy-based relaxation device. Subtle Energies 2.

Jackson, O. 1991. The Feldenkrais Method: a personalized learning model. In M. Lister, ed. Contemporary Management of Motor Control Problems. Proceedings of the II-Step Conference. Foundation for Physical Therapy, pp. 131–135.

Jackson-Wyatt, O., D. Gula, A. Kireta, et al. 1992. Effects of Feldenkrais practitioner training program on motor ability: a videoanalysis. Phys. Ther. 72(suppl):S86.

Jacobson, E. 1964. Anxiety and Tension Control. Lippincott, New York.

Jarrell, D.G. 1992. Reiki Plus Professional Practitioner's Manual. Hibernia West, Celina, Tenn.

Jenkins, W.M., and M.M. Merzenich. 1987. Reorganization of neocortical representations after brain injury: a neurophysiological model of the basis of recovery from stroke. Prog. Brain Res. 71:249–266.

Jenkins, W.M., M.M. Merzenich, M.T. Ochs, et al. 1990. Functional reorganization of primary somatosensory cortex in adult owl monkeys after behaviorally controlled tactile stimulation. J. Neurophysiol. 63:82–104.

Jirout, J. 1985. Comments regarding the diagnosis and treatment of dysfunctions in the C2–C3 segment. Manual Med. 2:62.

Joachim, G. 1983. The effects of two stress management techniques on feelings of well-being in patients with inflammatory bowel disease. Nursing Papers 15:5–18.

Johnston, W.L. 1982a. Interexaminer reliability studies: spanning a gap in medical research. Louisa Burns Memorial Lecture. J. Am. Osteopath. Assoc. 81:819–829.

Johnston, W.L. 1982b. Passive gross motion testing. Part I. Its role in physical examination. J. Am. Osteopath. Assoc. 81:298–303.

Johnston, W.L. 1988a. Segmental definition. Part 1. A focal point for diagnosis of somatic dysfunction. J. Am. Osteopath. Assoc. 88:99–105.

Johnston, W.L. 1988b. Segmental definition. Part 2. Application of an indirect method in osteopathic manipulative treatment. J. Am. Osteopath. Assoc. 88:211–217.

Johnston, W.L. 1988c. Segmental definition. Part 3. Definitive basis for distinguishing somatic findings of visceral reflex origin. J. Am. Osteopath. Assoc. 88:347–353.

Johnston, W.L. 1992. Osteopathic clinical aspects of somatovisceral/viscerosomatic interaction. In M.M. Patterson and J.N. Howel, eds. The central connection: somatovisceral interaction. 1989 International Symposium. Sponsored by American Academy of Osteopathy, Indianapolis, Ind. University Classics Ltd., Athens, Ohio, pp. 30–52.

Johnston, W.L., B.R. Allan, J.L. Hendra, et al. 1983. Interexaminer study of palpation in detecting location of spinal segmental dysfunction. J. Am. Osteopath. Assoc. 82:839–845.

Johnston, W.L., M.C. Beal, G.A. Blum, et al. 1982a. Passive gross motion testing. Part III. Examiner agreement on selected subjects. J. Am. Osteopath. Assoc. 81:309–313.

Johnston, W.L., J.L. Hill, M.L. Elkiss, et al. 1982b. Identification of stable somatic findings in hypertensive subjects by trained examiners using palpatory examination. J. Am. Osteopath. Assoc. 8:830–836.

Johnston, W.L., M.L. Elkiss, R.V. Marino, et al. 1982c. Passive gross motion testing. Part II. A study of interexaminer agreement. J. Am. Osteopath. Assoc. 81(5):304–308.

Johnston, W.L., J.L. Hill, J.W. Sealey, et al. 1980. Palpatory findings in the cervicothoracic region: variations in normotensive and hypertensive subjects. A preliminary report. J. Am. Osteopath. Assoc. 79:300–308.

Johnston, W.L., J. Vorro, and R.P. Hubbard. 1985. Clinical/biomechanic correlates for cervical function. Part 1. A kinematic study. J. Am. Osteopath. Assoc. 85:429.

Jwing-Ming, Y. 1992. Chinese Qigong Massage. YMMA Publication Center, Jamaica Plain, N.Y.

Kaarda, B., and O. Tosteinbo. 1989. Increase of plasma beta-endorphins in connective tissue massage. Gen. pharmacol. 20:487–489.

Kaas, J. 1991. Plasticity of sensory and motor maps in adult mammals. Ann. Rev. Neurosci. 14:137–167.

Kandel, E.R., and R.D. Hawkins. 1992. The biological basis of learning and individuality. Sci. Am. 267:78–88.

Kappler, R.E., and A.F. Kelso. 1984. Thermographic studies of skin temperature in patients receiving osteopathic manipulative treatment for peripheral nerve problems. J. Am. Osteopath. Assoc. 84:126.

Keller, E. 1993. The Effects of Therapeutic Touch on Tension Headache Pain. Master's thesis, University of Missouri—Columbia.

Keller, E., and V.M. Bzdek. 1986. Effects of therapeutic touch on tension headache pain. Nurs. Res. 35:101–105.

Kelso, A.F., N.J. Larson, and R.E. Kappler. 1980. A clinical investigation of the osteopathic structural examination. J. Am. Osteopath. Assoc. 79:460–467.

Koes, B.W. 1992. Efficacy of Manual Therapy and Physiotherapy for Back and Neck Complaints. Cip-Gegevans Koninklije Bibliotheek, the Hague.

Kokjohn, K., D.M. Schmid, J.J. Triano, et al. 1992. The effects of spinal manipulation on pain and prostaglandin levels in women with primary dysmenorrhea. J. Manipulative Physiol. Ther. 15:278–279.

Korr, I.M. 1947. The neural basis of the osteopathic lesion. J. Am. Osteopath. Assoc. 47:191–198.

Korr, I.M. 1955. The concept of facilitation and its origins. J. Am. Osteopath. Assoc. 54(5):265–268.

Korr, I.M. 1978. The Neurologic Mechanisms in Manipulative Therapy. Plenum, New York.

Kramer, N.A. 1990. Comparison of therapeutic touch and casual touch in stress reduction of hospitalized children. Pediatric Nursing 16:483–485.

Krieger, D. 1973. Relationship of touch with the intent to help or heal subject's in-vivo hemoglobin values. Paper presented to the American Nursing Association, Kansas City, Mo., March 21.

Krieger, D. 1975. Therapeutic touch: the imprimatur of nursing. American Journal of Nursing 7:767–784.

Krieger, D. 1992. The potentials of therapeutic touch. In D.S. Rogo, ed. New Techniques of Inner Healing. Paragon House, New York.

Kuchera, M., and W. Kuchera. 1990. Osteopathic Considerations in Systemic Dysfunction, second edition. K.C.O.M. Press, Kirksville, Mo.

Lake, B. 1985. Acute back pain: treatment by the application of Feldenkrais principles. Aust. Fam. Physician 14(11):1175–1178.

Larson, N.J. 1984. Functional vasomotor hemiparesthesia syndrome. Academy of Applied Osteopathy Year Book of Selected Osteopathic Papers 70:39–44.

Larson, N.J., M.W. Walton, and A.F. Kelso. 1980. Effectiveness of manipulative treatment for paresthesias with peripheral nerve involvement. J. Am. Osteopath. Assoc. 80(3):114.

Lawrence, D.J. 1985. Chiropractic concepts of the short leg: a critical review. J. Manipulative Physiol. Ther. 8:157–161.

Levine, D.Z. 1991. Burning pain in an extremity. Postgrad. Med. 90:175–185.

Love, R.M., and B.R. Brodeur. 1987. Inter- and intraexaminer reliability for motion palpation of the thoracic spine. J. Manipulative Physiol. Ther. 10:1–4.

Lovell, F.W., J.M. Rothstein, and W.J. Peronius. 1989. Reliability of clinical measurements of lumbar lordosis taken with a flexible ruler. Phys. Ther. 69:96–105.

Magoun, H.I. 1976. Osteopathy in the Cranial Field, third edition. The Journal Printing Co., Kirksville, Mo.

Maisel, E. 1989. The Alexander Technique. New York University Books, New York.

Marquardt, H. 1983. Reflex Zone Therapy of the Feet: A Textbook for Therapists. Thorsons, London.

Mathews, J.A., S.B. Mills, V.M. Jenkins, et al. 1987. Back pain and sciatica: controlled trials of manipulation, traction, sclerosant, and epidural injections. Br. J. Rheumatol. 26:416–423.

McConnell, D.G., M.C. Beal, U. Dinnar, et al. 1980. Low agreement of findings in neuromusculoskeletal examinations by a group of osteopathic physicians using their own procedures. J. Am. Osteopath. Assoc. 79:441–50.

McKechnie, A., F. Wilson, N. Watson, et al. 1983. Anxiety states: a preliminary report on the value of connective tissue massage. Journal of Psychosomatic Research 27(2):125–129.

Meade, T.R., S. Dyer, W. Browne, et al. 1990. Low back pain of mechanical origin: randomised comparison of chiropractic and hospital outpatient treatment. Br. Med. J. 300:1431–1437.

Meehan, T.C. 1985. An Abstract of the Effect of Therapeutic Touch on the Experience of Acute Pain in Post-operative Patients. Unpublished Ph.D. dissertation, New York University.

Meehan, T.C. 1988. The effect of therapeutic touch on experience of acute pain in postoperative patients. Ph.D. dissertation, New York University.

Mesmer, F.A. 1980. Mesmerism. G.J. Bloch, translator. William Kaufmann, Los Altos, Calif.

Mior, S.A., R.S. King, M. McGregor, et al. 1985. Intra- and interexaminer reliability of motion palpation in the cervical spine. Journal of Canadian Chiropractic Association 29:195–198.

Molea, D., B. Murcek, C. Blanken, et al. 1987. Evaluation of two manipulative techniques in the treatment of postexercise muscle soreness. J. Am. Osteopath. Assoc. 87:477–483.

Mootz, R.D., J.C. Keating, H.P. Kontz, et al. 1989. Intra- and interobserver reliability of passive motion palpation of the lumbar spine. J. Manipulative Physiol. Ther. 12:440–445.

Morgan, J.P., J.L. Dickey, H.H. Hunt, et al. 1985. A controlled trial of spinal manipulation in the management of hypertension. J. Am. Osteopath. Assoc. 85:308–313.

Namikoshi, T. 1969. Shiatsu. Japan Publications, San Francisco.

Nansel, D.D., A.L. Peneff, R.D. Jansen, et al. 1989. Interexaminer concordance in detecting joint-play asymmetries in the cervical spine of otherwise asymptomatic patients. J. Manipulative Physiol. Ther. 12:428–433.

Narula, M. 1993. Effect of the Six-Week Awareness Through Movement Lessons—The Feldenkrais Method on Selected Functional Movement Parameters in Individuals With Rheumatoid Arthritis. Unpublished Master's thesis, Oakland University, Rochester, Mich.

Newshan, G. 1989. Therapeutic touch for symptom control in persons with AIDS. Holistic Nursing Practice 3(4):45–51.

Northup, G.W. 1966. Osteopathic Medicine: An American Reformation. American Osteopathic Association, Chicago.

Northup, G.W., moderator. 1970. Symposium on the Physiologic Basis of Osteopathic Medicine. The Postgraduate Institute of Osteopathic Medicine and Surgery, New York (based on a 1967 seminar). [Available through the American Academy of Osteopathy, Indianapolis.]

Parker, G.B., H. Tupling, and D.S. Pryor. 1978. A controlled trial of cervical manipulation for migraine. Aust. N.Z. J. Med. 8:589.

Parkes, B.S. 1985. Therapeutic Touch as an Intervention to Reduce Anxiety in Elderly Hospitalized Patients. Unpublished Ph.D. dissertation, University of Texas at Austin.

Pavek, R. 1984, 1985, 1986. Unpublished pilot studies. The SHEN Therapy Institute, Sausalito, Calif.

Pavek, R.R. 1987. Handbook of SHEN. The SHEN Therapy Institute, Sausalito, Calif.

Pavek, R.R. 1988a. Proceedings of the First World Conference for Academic Exchange of Medical Qigong, Beijing, pp. 150–152.

Pavek, R.R. 1988b. Effects of SHEN Qigong on Psychosomatic and Other Physio-Emotional Disorders. Proceedings of the First World Conference for Academic Exchange of Medical Qigong, Beijing.

Pavek, R.R., and T. Daily. 1990. SHEN physioemotional release therapy: disruption of the autocontractile pain response. Occupational Therapy Practice 1(3):53–61.

Pavek, R.R. 1994. Personal communication to the editorial review board. A compilation of school estimates obtained from several sources.

Payne, M.B. 1989. The use of therapeutic touch with rehabilitation clients. Rehabilitation Nursing 14(2):69–72.

Perry, J., M.H. Jones, and L. Thomas. 1981. Functional evaluation of Rolfing in cerebral palsy. Dev. Med. Child Neurol. 23:717–729.

Plaugher, G. and T.R. Bachman. 1994. Chiropractic management of a hypertensic patient. J. Manipulative Physiol. Ther. 16:544–549.

Proceedings of the First World Conference for Academic Exchange of Medical Qigong, Beijing. 1988.

Quinn, J. 1981. An Investigation of the Effect of Therapeutic Touch Without Physical Contact on State Anxiety of Hospitalized Cardiovascular Patients. Unpublished Ph.D. dissertation, New York University.

Quinn, J. 1983. Therapeutic touch as energy exchange: testing the theory. ANS 6:42–49.

Quinn, J. 1989. Therapeutic touch as energy exchange: replication and extension. Nursing Science Quarterly, 12:78–87.

Quinn, J. 1992. Psychoimmunologic effects of therapeutic touch on practitioners and recently bereaved recipients: a pilot study. ANS 15(4):13–26.

Quinn, J. 1993. Therapeutic touch. ISSSEEM Newsletter 4(1).

Ramsden, E.L. 1978. Physical therapy in the United States of America—Physiotherapy Practice. Longman Group, U.K. Limited, United Kingdom, p. 3.

Ray, B. 1987. The Expanded Reference Manual of Radiance Technique. Radiance Associates, St. Petersburg, Fla.

Reich, W. 1973. Selected Writings. Farrar, Straus & Giroux, New York.

Reynolds, H.M., M.C. Beal, and R.C. Hallgren. 1993. Quantifying passive resistance to motion in the straight leg raising test on asymptomatic subjects. J. Am. Osteopath. Assoc. 93:913–920.

Reynolds, H., and R. Ward. 1994. Unpublished observations, early 1980s. Personal communication by Ward to editorial review board.

Robie, D.L. 1977. Tensional forces in the human body. Orthop. Rev. 6(11):45–48.

Rogers, M.E. 1990. Nursing: science of unitary, irreducible, human beings: update 1990. In E.A.M. Barret, ed. Visions of Rogers Science-based Nursing. National League of Nursing, New York, pp. 5–11.

Rolf, I. 1973. Structural integration: a contribution to the understanding of stress. Confina Psychiatrica 16:69–79.

Rolf, I.P. 1977. Rolfing: The Integration of Human Structures. Dennis-Landman, Santa Monica, Calif.

Ruth, S., and S. Kegerries. 1992. Facilitating cervical flexion using a Feldenkrais method: awareness through movement. Journal Sports and Physical Therapy 16:25–29.

Schaefer, R.C., and L.J. Fay. 1989. Motion Palpation and Chiropractic Technic. Motion Palpation Institute, Huntington Beach, Calif.

Schiegl, H. 1983. Healing Magnetism. Herman Verlag KG, Freiburg, Germany.

Schiotz, E.H. 1958. Manipulation treatment of the spinal column from the medical-historical viewpoint. Tidsskr Nor Laegeforen 78:429–438. [NIH Library Translation NIH-75-23C.]

Seitz, R.H. and C.L. Wilson. 1987. Effect on gait of motor task learning in a sitting position. Phys. Ther. 67:1089–1094.

Shen, H.C. 1988. Photographic presentation at the Founding Conference of the Chinese Society of Behavioral Medicine, Tainjin, People's Republic of China.

Shenkman, M., and R. Butler. 1989. A model for multisystem evaluation, interpretation, and treatment of individuals with neurologic dysfunction. Phys. Ther. 69:538–547.

Silverman, J., M. Rappaport, H.K. Hopkins, et al. 1973. Stress, stimulus intensity control, and the structural integration technique. Confina Psychiatrica 16:201–219.

Sleszynski, S.L., and A.F. Kelso. 1993. Comparison of thoracic manipulation with incentive spirometry in preventing postoperative atelectasis. J. Am. Osteopath. Assoc. 93:834–845.

Soderberg, G.I., and J.M. Walter. 1991. Modeling physical therapy clinical research centers. Phys. Ther. 71:734–745.

Spielberger, C.D., R.L. Gorsuch, et al. 1983. Manual for the State-Trait Anxiety Inventory. Consulting Psychologists Press, Palo Alto, Calif.

Still, A.T. 1899. Philosophy of Osteopathy. A.T. Still, Kirksville, Mo. [Available through the American Academy of Osteopathy, Indianapolis, Ind.]

Stone, R. 1986. Polarity Therapy, Vol. 1. CRCS Publications, Sebastopol, Calif.

Sucher, B.M. 1993. Myofascial release of carpal tunnel syndrome. J. Am. Osteopath. Assoc. 93:92–101.

Sunshine, L., and J.W. Wright. 1986. The 100 Best Treatment Centers for Alcoholism and Drug Abuse. Avon, New York.

Sutherland, W.G. 1990. Teachings in the Science of Osteopathy. A. Wales, ed. Rudra Press, Cambridge, Mass.

Sweigard, L. 1974. Human Movement Potential: Its Ideokinetic Facilitation. Harper and Row, New York.

Teeguarden, I.M. 1987. The Joy of Feeling Body-Mind: Acupressure—Jin Shin Do. Japan Publications USA, Briarcliff Manor, N.Y.

Terrett, A.C.J., and H. Vernon. 1984. A controlled study of the effect of spinal manipulation on paraspinal cutaneous pain tolerance levels. Am. J. Phys. Med. Rehabil. 63:217–225.

Upledger, J.E. 1977a. The reproducibility of craniosacral examination findings: a statistical analysis. J. Am. Osteopath. Assoc. 76:890–899.

Upledger, J.E. 1977b. The relationship of craniosacral examination findings in grade school children with developmental problems. J. Am. Osteopath. Assoc. 77:760–774.

Veith, I., trans. 1949. Huang Ti Nei Nei Ching Su Wên. The Yellow Emperor's Classic of Internal Medicine. University of California Press, Berkeley, Calif.

Vernon, H. 1982. Manipulative therapy in the chiropractic treatment of headaches: a retrospective and prospective study. J. Manipulative Physiol. Ther. 5:109–112.

von Reichenbach, C. 1851. Physico-Physiological Researches on the Dynamics of Magnetism, Electricity, Heat, Light, Crystallization and Chemism in Their Relation to the Vital Force. Clinton-Hall, New York.

Vorro, J., and W.L. Johnston. 1987. Clinical/biomechanic correlates of cervical function. Part 2. A myoelectric study. J. Am. Osteopath. Assoc. 87:353–367.

Waagen, G.N., S. Haldeman, G. Cook, et al. 1986. Short-term trial of chiropractic adjustments for the relief of chronic low back pain. Manual Medicine 2:63–67.

Ward, R.C. 1994. Personal communication to the editorial review board.

Weinberg, R.S., and V.V. Hunt. 1979. Effects of structural integration on state-trait anxiety. J. Clin. Psychol. 35:319–322.

Weintraub, M. 1992a. Alternative medical care: Shiatsu, Swedish muscle massage, and trigger point suppression in spinal pain syndrome. Am. J. Pain Mgmt. 2(2):74–78.

Weintraub, M. 1992b. Shiatsu, Swedish muscle massage, and trigger point suppression in spinal pain syndrome. Am. Massage Therapy J. 31(3):99–109.

Wetzel, W. 1989. Reiki healing: a physiologic perspective. Journal of Holistic Nursing 7:47–54.

Wiles, M.R. 1980. Reproducibility and interexaminer correlation of motion palpation findings of the sacroiliac joint. J. Can. Chiro. Assoc. 24:59–66.

Wirth, D. 1990. The effect of non-contact therapeutic touch on the healing rate of full-thickness surgical wounds. Subtle Energies 1:1–20.

Witt, P., and J. MacKinnon. 1986. Trager psychosocial integration: A method to improve chest mobility of patients with chronic lung disease. Phys. Ther. 66:214–217.

Witt, P., and C. Parr. 1986. Effectiveness of Trager psychosocial integration in promoting trunk mobility in a child with cerebral palsy: a case report. Physical and Occupational Therapy in Pediatrics 8:75–93.

Xin, N., L. Guolong, and Y. Shiming. 1988. In Proceedings of the First World Conference for Academic Exchange of Medical Qigong, Beijing, pp. 181–183.

Zanolla, R., C. Mizeglio, and A. Balzarini. 1984. Evaluation of the results of three different methods of postmastectomy lymphedema treatment. J. Surg. Oncol. 26:210–213.

Zhu, V., S. Haldeman, A. Stan, et al. 1993. Paraspinal muscle cerebral-evoked potentials in patients with unilateral low back pain. Spine 18:1096–1101.

Pharmacological and Biological Treatments

PANEL MEMBERS

Ralph W. Moss, Ph.D.—Cochair
Frank D. Wiewel—Cochair

Berkley Bedell	*John M. Ellis, M.D.*
Richard A. Bloch	*Helga Fallis*
Seymour Brenner, M.D.	*Natalie Golos*
Stanislaw R. Burzynski, M.D., Ph.D.	*Gary Johnson*
James A. Caplan	*Joseph Latino, Ph.D.*
Barrie Cassileth, Ph.D.	*Floyd Leaders, Jr., Ph.D.*
Peter B. Chowka	*Edward Sopcak*
Serafina Corsello, M.D.	*John Stegmeier*
Harris Coulter, Ph.D.	*Morton Walker, D.P.M.*
Michael Culbert, D.Sc.	*Michael F. Ziff, D.D.S.*

CONTRIBUTING AUTHORS

Ralph W. Moss, Ph.D.
Linda Silversmith, Ph.D.
Leanna Standish, N.D., Ph.D.
Frank Wiewel

Overview

The alternative pharmacological and biological treatments discussed in this chapter are an assortment of drugs and vaccines that have not yet been accepted by mainstream medicine. If and when they are accepted, many of these drugs and vaccines will fit into conventional medicine as it is practiced today. Thus, these treatments differ from other alternative health measures in this report because, by and large, they do not represent an entirely new theory or unified approach to health and disease.

Despite their diversity, the alternative pharmacological approaches share some or all of the following themes:

- Unlike many mainstream drugs, most unconventional substances are believed to be nontoxic.
- Many are directed not toward eradicating a specific disease entity but toward stimulating the patient's immune system to fight the onslaught of a pathological condition or organism. Frequently, these methods may have to be tailored to individual patients to be effective.
- For other approaches, practitioners may postulate an entirely new defense system altogether.
- Other alternative substances are derived from old Native American herbal remedies or are turn-of-the-century remedies that were cast aside during the rapid advance of biomedicine.

Hundreds of alternative drugs and vaccines could have been included in this report. The ones that are included were chosen because they met one or more of the following criteria:

- *Therapeutic promise.* Available evidence suggests that they may be effective.
- *Wide use.* Because they are now used by many people, public health considerations indicate that they should be investigated. If any of these products prove harmful, that news needs to be spread quickly; if any prove effective, this should be officially recognized and they should be put to further use. An up-to-date example is the use of cartilage products

for acquired immune deficiency syndrome (AIDS), cancer, and arthritis. Since a "60 Minutes" television program about them in late February 1993, some 50,000 Americans are currently reported to be taking shark cartilage even though properly designed trials have not yet been conducted. (Another consideration besides safety and effectiveness for the users is that demand for these products entails destroying many sharks.) Ozone is another example of a substance now being used widely—particularly as a self-medication in the AIDS community—without solid evidence of its usefulness.

- *Subject of controversy.* Some other pharmacological or biological products have been the subject of long-standing controversies that need to be resolved. This point is particularly true for certain medicines derived from Native American remedies, such as the Hoxsey method and Essiac.

- *Former use or use elsewhere.* Some products have been tested and well documented in the scientific literature but for various reasons have fallen by the wayside. An example is Coley's toxins, an immunotherapy for cancer that was developed at the turn of the century by a New York bone surgeon and which is currently being used in China and Germany. Similarly MTH-68, a nontoxic, biological vaccine, is reported to buttress the immune system against cancer. Another example is the use of a local anesthetic (often, novocaine) for neural therapy to combat chronic pain, allergies, and other problems; this approach is in wide use in Europe.

A major impediment to full investigation of alternative pharmacological treatments is the high expense of conducting the trials necessary to meet Food and Drug Administration (FDA) approval. Nearly every one of the few drugs that FDA approves each year is marketed by one of the major pharmaceutical companies. Nevertheless, even well-capitalized biotechnology firms have sometimes been driven out of the marketplace by the difficulty in meeting FDA requirements.

Another problem for many alternative materials—such as herbs, nutrients, and common chemicals—is their lack of sponsorship. Because they are in the public domain and therefore inexpensive and not patentable, drug companies understandably lack interest in investing the enormous sums required for full trials. Therefore, most such alternatives lack both sponsors and funding for clinical trials of their safety and effectiveness.

Marketing most of the substances discussed in this chapter is not allowed by FDA on the basis of its interpretation of Title 21, article 355, of the U.S. Code, which states that unless a developer has presented "substantial evidence" of a drug's safety and efficacy, the FDA can deny approval for marketing that substance. "Substantial evidence" is defined as "adequate and well-controlled investigations, including clinical investigations, by experts qualified by scientific training and experience to evaluate the effectiveness of the drug involved."

Many alternative medical practitioners have attempted to market new drugs or vaccines under this statute, but few have succeeded. The failure often occurs because "qualified experts" are defined as those who adhere to mainstream medical practices. To be an alternative practitioner has, until now, been reason enough to disqualify a person to evaluate the usefulness of the drug in question.

Moreover, "clinical investigations" are generally interpreted to mean randomized, double-blind, placebo-controlled studies (see the "Research Methodologies" chapter) of the kind that only pharmaceutical companies and major medical centers can afford to conduct. This is true despite a declaration by Jay Moskowitz, former deputy director of the National Institutes of Health in September 1992, that "not all alternative medical practices are amenable to traditional scientific evaluation, and some may require development of new methods to evaluate their efficacy and safety." Thus, the reluctance of conventional medicine to accept for examination and possible use the materials assessed here appears to be tied to measuring them with the wrong yardstick.

The remaining sections of this chapter deal with the existing research base for 14 specific treatments, future research opportunities for these 14 treatments, and key issues and recommendations that are relevant to all such biological and pharmacological treatments. Each treatment fits one or more of the criteria cited earlier—such as wide use, controversy, and therapeutic promise—and may require selection or development of appropriate methodologies for proper evaluation.

Research Base for Specific Treatments

Hundreds of potentially useful alternative drugs or vaccines are supported by data indicating that they may be useful in the treatment of such diseases as cancer, AIDS, heart disease, hepatitis, and other major health problems. What follows is only a sampling of the many products available for study.

Antineoplastons

Antineoplastons are peptide fractions originally derived from normal human blood and urine, although a method for synthesizing them was subsequently developed by Dr. Stanislaw Burzynski. Burzynski has named some of these peptides A2, A5, A10, and AS2–1. He first discovered antineoplastons as a graduate student in Poland in 1967 (Moss, 1989) when he compared normal urine and urine from people with cancer and noted an anomalous streak on electrophoresis of the normal urine that was not present in the urine of cancer patients. He then chemically defined these antineoplastons at Baylor College of Medicine in Houston (Burzynski, 1973, 1976, 1986; Burzkynski and Kubove, 1986a, 1986b; Moss, 1992). He depicts these substances as a newly discovered, natural form of anticancer protection, apart from the lymphocyte system.

Burzynski reported that the antineoplaston peptides are essentially nontoxic (Burzynski, 1986) and that preliminary clinical results indicated tumor responses (shrinkages) in a number of difficult cases, most of which involved subjects who had exhausted conventional treatments (Burzynski, 1986; Moss, 1992). He also reported at the 1992 International Conference on AIDS that some patients infected with human immunodeficiency virus (HIV) responded to antineoplastons by a marked increase in certain white blood cells (CD4+ lymphocytes); other observations included increases of energy and weight and a decrease of opportunistic infections.

Although antineoplastons have been employed against a wide variety of tumors, the greatest interest has been generated by using them with otherwise incurable brain cancers. Burzynski reports that he has been most successful treating prostate cancer and brain cancer (specifically, several forms of childhood glioma) and has had good results with (in descending order) non-Hodgkins lymphomas and pancreatic cancers, breast cancer, lung cancer, and colon cancer. Burzynski has published scores of medical articles in peer-reviewed journals, mostly in Europe (Bertelli, 1990; Bertelli and Mathe, 1985, 1987; Kuemmerle, 1988). At the 18th International Congress of Chemotherapy in Stockholm on July 1, 1993, more than a dozen papers were presented by researchers from Brazil, Holland, Japan, Poland, and the United States in a special session on antineoplastons.

In the late 1970s, controversy began swirling around Burzynski when he left a position at Baylor College of Medicine during a disagreement about an interdepartmental transfer, research freedom, research funding, and maintenance of a private medical practice. Since then, Burzynski has worked independently, paying for his research from patients' fees. Some research physicians are fascinated by his work, but many others have attacked it. On one hand, after conducting a review of a "best case series" (see app. F), including a site visit in October 1991, the National Cancer Institute (NCI) concluded that antitumor activity by antineoplastons may have been demonstrated by Burzynski in seven cases of incurable brain cancer (confirmation by NCI communication, 1994). Consequently, NCI agreed that conducting confirmatory trials would be a worthwhile effort. On the other hand, Saul Green, formerly a researcher at Memorial Sloan-Kettering Cancer Research Center, attacked treatments with antineoplastons in the *Journal of the American Medical Association* (Green, 1992).

The trials that NCI proposed are Phase II studies (that is, small-scale clinical trials), in which researchers examine the effectiveness of a potential treatment in some 25 to 40 subjects. The Office of Alternative Medicine (OAM) has contributed to the funding of these trials; Burzynski has participated in the planning steps and provided a supply of synthetic antineoplastons A10 and AS2–1. (He informed NCI that he no longer uses urine-derived products.) In late 1993 and early 1994, three sites opened enrollment for these trials: Memorial Sloan-Kettering in New York, the Mayo Clinic in Minnesota, and the Clinical Pharmacology Branch of NCI in Maryland. The subjects to receive antineoplastons are patients with two types of brain tumors, gliomas and astrocytomas. They are required to have a particularly small tumor, at Burzynski's request.

Because of the possible promise of some of Burzynski's products and the controversy surrounding them, further research should be conducted.

Cartilage Products

Investigations of cartilage to improve health began with a graduate student wondering whether cartilage could assist wound healing. Physician-researcher John Prudden decided to find out, using a powdered and washed cartilage product. There is now a long list of reported effects of cartilage preparations, including accelerating wound healing, possessing topical anti-inflammatory capability, alleviating autoimmune diseases, relieving osteoarthritic pain, alleviating scleroderma (a disease in which the skin hardens), easing skin symptoms of herpesvirus infections, alleviating psoriasis (a chronic, scaly skin disease), and inhibiting a wide spectrum of cancers (Prudden, 1985). A recent report adds relieving swollen and tender joints of patients with rheumatoid arthritis (Trentham et al., 1993). This study bolsters previous anecdotal reports that cartilage products can palliate the painful effects of rheumatoid arthritis.

The various cartilage products under study or reported on anecdotally derive from cattle, sheep, sharks, and chicken cartilage; some products, such as Prudden's "Catrix," are a form of repeatedly powdered and cleaned cartilage; others are relatively pure substances, such as the type II collagen used by Trentham et al. (1993) in a randomized double-blind trial. (See app. F for types of trials.)

The popularity of cartilage products increased dramatically after the television program "60 Minutes" produced a segment on the possible benefits of shark cartilage in late February 1993, citing a 16-week clinical trial in Cuba with some allegedly positive results. Medical centers have since been inundated with calls about the effectiveness of shark cartilage in treating AIDS, cancer, and arthritis. Since the show, this product has been aggressively marketed in the United States, and some 50,000 Americans are said to be currently taking shark cartilage at an individual cost of approximately $7,000 or more per year. The numbers of persons and amount of money they are spending are together sufficient reason to undertake an evaluation of the safety and effectiveness of shark cartilage treatments.

As for one or more scientific bases, a scientific hypothesis for the effectiveness of cartilage products as anticancer agents relates to their effects on blood vessel formation. A substance present in very small amounts in cartilage is believed to act by inhibiting angiogenesis, or interfering with the ability of a tumor to create a network of new blood vessels. It has been shown that if a tumor cannot establish a new blood network, it cannot grow any larger than the point of a pencil (Brem and Folkman, 1975; Folkman, 1976; Langer et al., 1976). Thus it has been proposed that cartilage, and appropriate substances purified from cartilage, may act against cancer through angiogenesis-inhibiting effects.

A researcher at NCI has proposed another anticancer mechanism involving a class of proteins that are produced in normal tissues such as cartilage and bone (Liotta, 1992). These proteins are called tissue inhibitors of metalloproteinases (TIMPs); TIMPs appear to block the action of certain metal-containing enzymes (the metalloproteinases) that help tumor cells to invade surrounding tissue.

A detailed explanation for the successful treatment of rheumatoid arthritis with type II collagen (Trentham et al., 1993) is still being sought. A working hypothesis is that the large amount of collagen taken by mouth (in daily doses in orange juice) suppresses autoimmune reactions; this observation was made in previous studies with animal models of autoimmune diseases and in small pilot human studies of patients with multiple sclerosis and with rheumatoid arthritis. Possibly the collagen stimulates certain immune system cells to produce anti-inflammatory cytokines.

In reviewing the scientific literature on cartilage, Prudden (1985) described other health-promoting activities studied by other researchers. Wound-healing activity is attributed to a polymer of N-acetyl glucosamine. Inhibition of cell division and inflammation appear to be attributable to a different "fraction" of cartilage. Although practitioners of alternative medicine tend to prefer dealing with natural substances, such as cartilage, the more conventional academic view is that such mixtures must be separated into identifiable, pure products.

The most recent work with cartilage itself, rather than purified products, is probably the anticancer shark cartilage studies. NCI informally reviewed the results of the 16-week Cuban study that "60 Minutes" cited when the chief Cuban investigator presented a seminar in the United States. Staffers from NCI's Cancer Treatment Effectiveness Program noted the uncertainty of accurate drug delivery by enemas (apparently enemas had to be used because the preparation's taste was so bad that subjects would not eat it) and what they called the lack of any clear benefits in the cases described. Nevertheless, the NCI staff indicated that it would be willing to reconsider this product if additional data should prove positive.

Charles Simone—an oncologist from Lawrenceville, NJ, who has NCI research experience—examined the results of the Cuban study for "60 Minutes" and was guardedly optimistic. In his own practice, he has treated some patients who initiated self-medication with cartilage. He has said that some of his patients experienced dramatic improvement, including the clearing of liver metastases and rapid reduction in certain prostate antigens in prostate cancer (Simone, 1993). Simone provided OAM with a copy of a protocol (study plan) and has begun a prospective study (see the glossary and app. F) on shark cartilage. In early 1994, he received IND (investigational new drug) approval from FDA for shark cartilage.

Most previous studies with cartilage have used bovine cartilage. Catrix, a trade-named product derived from the tracheal rings of cattle, was developed by John Prudden, who holds a patent on the use of all cartilage products (including shark) and an FDA IND permit to conduct research studies. Prudden was formerly a surgeon at Columbia-Presbyterian Hospital in New York and associate professor of clinical surgery at Columbia University. He has published more than 60 papers on the use of cartilage, mostly to accelerate wound healing but also to treat psoriasis, cancer, and rheumatoid arthritis. In 1985, Prudden reported on results of a study in which 31 cancer patients were treated continually with Catrix. The overall response rate, measured as a greater than 50-percent reduction in tumor size, was reported as an unusually high 90 percent; 61 percent had complete disappearance of tumors.[1] Both oral and injectable forms of Catrix were used, and Prudden concluded that the oral route was superior.

Clinical trials using Catrix in kidney (renal cell) cancer patients are currently under way at Westchester Medical Center in Valhalla, NY, and Royal Victoria Hospital in Montreal. Renal cell cancer is an intractable tumor, resistant to cure, relief, and control; response rates with Catrix are said to be about 25 percent (Prudden, 1993).

The proposed usefulness of cartilage for AIDS patients would be for treatment of AIDS-related cancers such as Kaposi's sarcoma and AIDS-related lymphoma and for opportunistic infections caused by viruses other than HIV. Although cartilage is reported to have activity against herpes infections, it does not directly affect herpesviruses (Prudden, 1993). Prudden proposes that the antiviral effects result from stimulation of patients' immune systems; this point should be explored in more detail.

EDTA Chelation Therapy

Chelation is the major form of alternative therapy for cardiovascular disease and one of the most popular alternative pharmacological treatments. Chelation employs ethylene diamine tetraacetic acid (EDTA), a material that readily binds to metallic ions. EDTA is used in standard medicine as the preferred treatment for lead poisoning as well as for removing more than a dozen other toxic metals ranging from cadmium to zinc (Berkow, 1992).

Since shortly after EDTA was synthesized in the 1950s, its use has been suggested to treat heart disease and circulatory problems, including atherosclerosis (Clarke et al., 1955), high blood pressure (Schroeder and Perry, 1955), angina pectoris (Clarke et al., 1956), occlusive vascular disease (Clarke, 1960), and porphyria (Peters, 1960). Chelation has also been suggested as a potential treatment for rheumatoid arthritis

[1]*Prudden noted in his report that he was providing data only on the 31 patients who "took Catrix consistently and followed instructions completely." If the number of patients who stopped treatment are included (approximately another 60 patients), the recalculated response rates (approximately 30 percent responding and 20 percent complete) are still satisfactory. However, cancer therapy studies usually deal with one type of cancer at a time, and Prudden's patients had at least nine different types.*

(Boyle et al., 1963) and even as a preventive for cancer (Blumer and Cranton, 1989).

Several mechanisms have been proposed for the therapeutic action of EDTA. Since the molecule is known to be able to incorporate a metal ion into its own ring structure, it may maintain cellular health by removing those ions that cause harmful peroxidation of lipids (fatty materials). EDTA is also believed to remove calcium particles deposited in the arterial wall—various kinds of plaques—by analogy to its standard use in heavy-metal poisoning. But it may also lower the ionized calcium levels by blocking the slow calcium currents in the arterial wall, thus functioning as a kind of "calcium-blocking agent," a category of drugs known to have potent coronary vasodilating effects (Casdorph, 1981). EDTA has also been identified as acting to increase the concentration of a vasodilator (Cranton and Frackelton, 1989).

Most recently, the various mechanisms proposed for EDTA's therapeutic action have been brought together under a unified but controversial theory that they all involve protective effects against detrimental actions of free radicals (Cranton and Frackelton, 1989). This protection may lead indirectly to such activities as removing deposits from the walls of arteries or dilating blocked arteries.

Various peer-reviewed articles support the use of EDTA chelation in heart disease because of the observed effects on the health of patients, but clear demonstration of physiological change has been possible only in the past few years. In the early 1980s, the problem was how to directly measure arterial effects of EDTA, because measurements of the size (diameter) of arteries were accurate within only 25 percent (Cranton and Frackelton, 1982); yet dilations of 10 to 15 percent may have significant (doubling) effects on blood flow (Cranton, 1985; Olszewer and Carter, 1989). One 1982 study did report decreased blockage of arteries in 88 percent of 57 patients by means of a noninvasive analysis (McDonagh et al., 1982) that relies on a technique developed by Langham and To'mey (1978). Later research involving some of the same investigators (Rudolph et al., 1991) using ultrasound showed a decrease in blockage of carotid arteries using chelation therapy that was statistically significant in both males and females and was an average of 21 percent lower than initial values. The investigators calculated large improvements in blood flow as a result of the decreased blockage.

Furthermore, a large retrospective study of 2,870 patients in Brazil showed that 89 percent of the patients treated with EDTA had marked or good improvement (Olszewer and Carter, 1989). Olszewer et al. (1990) followed the retrospective study with a small, randomized, double-blind clinical trial of EDTA treatments for 10 men with peripheral vascular disease. After 10 of 20 intended EDTA treatments, it was clear that some patients were showing dramatic improvements. When the code that identified which patients were receiving medication was broken, the group that had improved were all identified as persons who received EDTA. All patients were then placed on EDTA treatment, and the ones previously receiving placebo showed improvement comparable to that of the first EDTA group. The group continuing on EDTA showed additional improvements as well, although later progress was not as dramatic as the initial changes.

Chelation is currently available in nearly every State of the United States as well as many foreign countries. In the United States, the four major organizations promoting acceptance of chelation therapy are the American Board of Chelation Therapy, the American College for Advancement in Medicine, the Great Lakes Association of Clinical Medicine, and the International Bioxidative Medicine Association. Chelation therapy is administered as an outpatient treatment, costing $75 to $120 per visit; the average cost for a course of 20 to 30 treatments is approximately $3,000. Since 1960, 500,000 patients have received chelation in more than 5 million treatments.

The toxicity of EDTA is a matter of some dispute. Advocates claim that it is essentially nontoxic, with approximately the same "danger" as that of normal doses of aspirin. They explain that early adverse effects, especially on the kidney, resulted from preexisting kidney disease or from using greater doses and rates of administration than those now recommended (the protocol available from the American College of Advancement in Medicine for use of intravenous EDTA also includes dietary supplements with multivitamins and trace elements). Although some reports claimed EDTA-related deaths, proponents state that these claims were erroneous, explaining, for example, that some deaths resulted from heavy-metal toxicity. See Cranton and Frackelton (1989) for references reviewing the field.

Hundreds of physicians are convinced that EDTA chelation therapy is of greater benefit to their patients than conventional treatments that are more dangerous and costly, such as bypass operations or toxic cardiotonic drugs such as digoxin. For example, Cranton (1985) compared 4,000 deaths from bypass surgery over a 30-year period with fewer than 20 associated with EDTA treatment (both procedures had approximately 300,000 patients during that time). Proponents also note that in issuing an IND permit to the American College of Advancement in Medicine to study EDTA to treat peripheral vascular disease, FDA officials indicated that "safety is not an issue" (Olszewer and Carter, 1989).

A double-blind, placebo-controlled study that might have settled the question of the usefulness of EDTA treatment was begun at three military hospitals in the 1980s under the FDA-approved IND application cited in the preceding paragraph. This study was dropped in November 1991, reportedly because of the exigencies of Operation Desert Storm in the Persian Gulf. At that time, 31 patients had completed their dosages, but the double-blind code was not broken.

At present, it is estimated that the study could be resumed by an interested sponsor at a cost of $3.75 million for the remaining 150 patients, or $25,000 per patient. Since EDTA is an unpatented drug in the public domain, no drug company is likely to sponsor this research or develop it for sale. Proponents of alternative medicine believe that EDTA could and should be evaluated in less costly ways. (See the "Future Research Opportunities" section.)

Ozone

Anecdotal claims abound for ozone therapy among persons infected with HIV (the virus causing AIDS). Yet there have been only a few test tube (in vitro) and clinical evaluations of ozone as an antiviral therapy.

One such study (Wells et al., 1991) showed that ozone caused test tube inactivation of HIV by inhibiting an enzyme called reverse transcriptase and by disrupting viral particles and viral attachment to target cells. Ozone in nontoxic concentrations (4.0 μg/mL) was also shown to inactivate this virus in both serum (Freeburg and Carpendale, 1988) and whole blood (Wagner et al., 1988). These test tube results appeared promising, but that was true for a number of other proposed AIDS treatments that were not subsequently successful for treating human beings.

More recently, two small sets of clinical trials using ozone-treated blood have been described in published reports (Garber et al., 1991; Hooker and Gazzard, 1992) and one clinical study using rectal administration of ozone (Carpendale et al., 1993). Garber and colleagues reported on withdrawing blood from patients infected with HIV, treating the blood with ozone, and returning the blood to the patient. Their hypothesis was that this technique would return killed HIV to patients that could then stimulate their immune systems.[2] In a Phase I study, which examines safety of the treatment in a small number of subjects, ozone therapy was reported to be safe and also *possibly* effective; the latter was suggested because 3 of 10 patients showed some improvement in various measurements associated with HIV infection. (Study participants were HIV-infected persons who either refused or could not tolerate zidovudine [AZT] treatments.) Next, a Phase II randomized, double-blind study was initiated to look for signs of effective treatment in 14 subjects. On the basis of this 12-week study and blood, biochemical, and clinical laboratory tests, the authors reported that ozone had no significant effect.

Although a suggestion has been made that different dosing or other procedural variations might have produced positive results, the work of Hooker and Gazzard corroborates the negative results discussed above. Hooker and Gazzard conducted an open study of nine patients, using a procedure like that of Garber and colleagues and following the participants for 12 weeks. These researchers concluded, "We agree with Garber et al. that there is no evidence to support a belief that ozone, used by this method, is beneficial during HIV infection."

Nevertheless, persons applying or receiving ozone therapy tend to rely on the test tube results

[2]*Some other researchers are interested in ozone's ability to stimulate production of interferon (Bocci and Paulesu, 1991).*

concerning ozone killing HIV and stimulating interferon, and on anecdotal information such as the following: To obtain additional information on ozone therapy in actual practice, the Research Department of Bastyr College of Natural Health Sciences in Seattle collected anecdotal data in 1993 from three physicians who used ozone in the treatment of their HIV and AIDS patients. In examining the case records of nine cases of HIV-positive patients treated with ozone by a physician in Washington State, Bastyr scientists concluded that some patients with CD4 counts above 500 showed increased counts of these cells after several weeks of treatment.[3] Patients with CD4 counts of 200 and below (more critical levels) did not seem to respond, although the doctor reported anecdotally that these patients were doing well clinically. Bastyr's researchers expressed interest in conducting a clinical trial.

A physician with a 5-year history of interest in ozone therapy, John Pittman, recently announced plans to open the North Carolina Bio-Oxidative Health Center in August 1994 and provide there a holistic treatment approach that includes ozone therapy. Previously, Pittman had closed his office to comply with an order from the State board of medical examiners, which considered ozone use nonconventional. North Carolina subsequently passed a "freedom of medicine law" that allows physicans choice among therapies so long as they have not been proved ineffective or dangerous. Pittman has indicated that the center will collect data on the effectiveness of its treatments.

A different approach to ozone use by AIDS patients appears to deserve further exploration. This application is not for attacking HIV, but for treating a debilitating and deleterious symptom—diarrhea. Carpendale et al. (1993) treated five patients with AIDS-related, intractable diarrhea using rectal administration of ozone gas daily for 3 to 4 weeks. This choice of treatment was based on reports from the 1930s that ozone was effective for three kinds of diarrhea. Diarrhea in three of the five patients was resolved, and one other patient improved as well. The ozone had no toxic effects. The authors suggest that further investigation is warranted, that longer treatment periods and different doses be studied, and that attention be paid to whether good results depend on the initial immunological state of the patients.

The fact that many people are receiving some kind of ozone treatment and that some practitioners continue to regularly apply such treatments is sufficient reason to recommend that definitive studies be undertaken to determine whether these treatments have any utility. Possibly, Pittman's new center will be able to provide this information.

Immunoaugmentative Therapy

Immunoaugmentative therapy, which was developed by Lawrence Burton, is "one of the most widely used unconventional cancer treatments," according to the Office of Technology Assessment (OTA)(Office of Technology Assessment, 1990). It has also been one of the most bitterly contested. The process is patented, and some details of it appear to have been kept secret, although this situation may change since Burton's death in early 1993. The attempt to achieve a fair evaluation of immunoaugmentative therapy led some of its proponents, such as Frank Wiewel of People Against Cancer, to work for the establishment of OAM (Mason, 1992).

Essentially, immunoaugmentative therapy is an experimental form of cancer immunotherapy consisting of daily injections of processed blood products. Several blood fractions recovered by means of centrifugation are used in an attempt to restore normal immune function to the person with cancer. These fractions are said to include the following substances: (1) deblocking protein—an alpha-2 macroglobulin derived from the pooled blood serum of health donors; (2) tumor antibody 1 (TA1)—a combination of alpha-2 macroglobulin with other immune proteins (IgG and IgA) derived from the pooled blood serum of healthy donors; and (3) tumor antibody 2 (TA2)—also derived from healthy blood serum but differing in potency (and possibly in composition) from TA1.

Proponents of immunoaugmentative therapy hypothesize that the tumor antibodies attack the tumors and that the deblocking proteins remove

[3] *The quantity of CD4 cells, a type of white blood cell, usually decreases sharply as the condition of a patient with AIDS worsens.*

a "blocking factor" that prevents the patient's immune system from detecting the cancer.

Originally a New Yorker with a clinic in Great Neck, Long Island, Burton established a new base in Freeport, the Bahamas, in the late 1970s after he failed to obtain FDA approval for his blood fraction medications. This move followed nearly 20 years of work with tumor-inducing and tumor-inhibiting factors at various institutions. During the 1960s and 1970s, Burton and a colleague, Frank Friedman, reported discovering cancer-inhibiting factors in mice (Friedman et al., 1962). In one experiment, daily administration of these factors was said to eliminate palpable disease in 26 of 50 mice with leukemia. The treated animals appeared to survive significantly longer than the controls. In another experiment, Burton reported that 37 of 68 experimental animals survived for an average of 131 days without any evidence of leukemia, versus a 12-day average survival of untreated mice (Office of Technology Assessment, 1990). Burton concluded that the study of the biological action and interaction of these components in mice suggests the existence of an inhibitory system involved in the genesis of tumors and capable of causing specific tumor cell breakdown.

In July 1985, Burton's Freeport clinic was suddenly closed by the Bahamian health authorities and the Pan American Health Organization on charges of contamination with HIV (then called HTLV–III) and hepatitis virus. Despite alarming stories in the media, no patient has yet been found who became HIV positive or succumbed to AIDS because of Burton's treatment. Investigations by the Immunoaugmentative Therapy Patients Association (now People Against Cancer) suggest that there may never have been any HIV contamination (Moss, 1989). Some 500 patients were receiving 8 to 10 injections per day; during the year after the clinic was closed, several hundred all tested negative for HIV (Wiewel, 1994). Additional standard HIV tests of serum and blood supply used to prepare the treatment were all negative as well.

The Freeport clinic, which reopened in January 1986 through the actions of Burton's patients and some members of the U.S. Congress, remains open at present despite Burton's death. More than 5,000 patients have received immunoaugmentative therapy in Freeport.

In spite of the many patients treated and the stories of remissions, extensions of life, and improvements in the quality of life, very little documentation exists of either the methods or the results of Burton's therapy. After the hostile reaction by the cancer establishment in the 1970s, Burton retaliated by withdrawing from his former colleagues and ignoring the basic requirements of scientific documentation. A standoff resulted, which OTA was unable to resolve. It is possible that the Freeport clinic, now led by R.J. Clement, and the other existing clinic in Germany will be more willing to cooperate in concrete studies and that serious investigations of immunoaugmentative therapy can now be launched.

714–X

The ideas of French-born Gaston Naessens are a controversial area on the fringe of modern medicine. Naessens, a microbiologist whose formal education was interrupted by World War II before he could earn an advanced degree, has proposed a theory that cancer cells are deficient in nitrogen and can become normal cells if they receive it. Naessen's treatment to provide the nitrogen is a mixture of camphor and nitrogen called 714–X. The camphor is present reputedly to help deliver the nitrogen when 714–X is injected into the lymph system in the region of the abdomen. Naessens also uses the treatment for AIDS. To find out whether the 714–X treatment is working, Naessens uses a special microscope that he invented, called a somatoscope. The somatoscope has been described as an altered dark-field microscope. Naessens claims it can visualize living things at magnifications unattainable through the ordinary light microscope. He monitors improvement in his patients by the status of their "somatids," variable particles that he has described in his viewings with the somatosocope.

In the 1980s in Quebec, Naessens was prosecuted for health fraud and threatened with life imprisonment. He was acquitted, however, after many people testified not only to his character, but also to beneficial results from using 714–X. Some of the individuals claiming cures for cancer and AIDS are quoted in *Galileo of the Microscope* (Bird, 1989).

Many Americans, including former congressman Berkley Bedell (Bedell, 1993), have used 714–X as an unconventional treatment for cancer.[4] It has penetrated a number of alternative clinics that concentrate on other treatments. Stories are circulating of dramatic improvements or, with AIDS, of conversion from HIV positive to HIV negative. However, Naessens has not published in peer-reviewed literature. Without impartial scientific evaluation, it is difficult to reach conclusions on his work.

Hoxsey Method

The Hoxsey treatments are among the oldest U.S. alternative therapies for cancer and have been some of the most controversial. Like Essiac (see next section), they use a mixture of powerful herbs. These mixtures were probably derived from early Native American Indian medicines, although that connection is not as well established as with Essiac. Some of the same herbs are included in the formulas for both methods.

In the early part of the century Harry Hoxsey, an uncredentialed layman, marketed several cancer treatments in his clinics across the South. He claimed his remedies had been passed down to him by his father and grandfather, and he kept the ingredients secret until 1950. Eventually U.S. authorities shut down Hoxsey's clinics, but the treatment is still available at the Bio-Medical Center in Tijuana, Mexico, which is headed by Mildred Nelson, Hoxsey's former nurse assistant. Hoxsey indicated that some of his herbal components were present to necrotize tumors and others, as purgatives, to carry away the waste.

Hoxsey's remedies basically consist of an external salve and an herbal potion. The external medicine is an escharotic—a kind of burning paste—composed of zinc chloride, antimony, trisulfide, and bloodroot; its purpose is to corrode cancers. The paste is used principally for skin cancer (usually basal cell carcinomas), and many ambitious claims have been made for it. However, few reports on its efficacy (or lack thereof) exist in peer-reviewed literature. Moh's micrographic surgery, an orthodox procedure that bears some relationship to the Hoxsey treatment, is cited (Swanson, 1983): Moh's method consists of the use of zinc chloride paste to "fix" the tumor in place; the tumor is then removed in a series of steps.

The internal medication, which is the primary concern here, is made up of various herbs added to a base of potassium iodide and cascara, which is a bark preparation. The principal herbs are pokeweed root, burdock root, barberry (*Berberis*), buckthorn bark, stillingia root, and prickly ash. As Patricia Spain Ward noted in a contract report to OTA for its Unorthodox Cancer Treatments project, many of these roots and barks are now known to have anticancer and immunostimulatory effects.[5] The following items discuss several:

- *Pokeweed.* Pokeweed root *(Phytolacca americana)* has several effects on the immune system including stimulation of the production of two cytokines (see the glossary), interleukin 1 (IL–1) and tumor necrosis factor (TNF) (Bodger et al., 1979a, 1979b). Boosting the immune system is generally thought to help the body fight cancer.[6] Although pokeweed root is poisonous, it apparently has been used without serious toxicity problems since the mid-18th century.
- *Burdock root.* Burdock root *(Arctium lappa)* contains what Japanese scientists have called the "burdock factor" (Morita et al., 1984), which is reputed to act as a desmutagen, that is, a substance that reduces mutations. Burdock also has been shown to inhibit HIV, according to the World Health Organization (1989). In Japanese and macrobiotic diets young burdock roots are eaten as a vegetable called "gobo."
- *Buckthorn.* Buckthorn contains emodin, which has shown antileukemia activity in the laboratory (Kupchan and Karim, 1976).

It is noteworthy that, despite intense opposition, the Hoxsey formula has persisted as a cancer treatment for almost 100 years (Chowka, 1985). Among numerous anecdotal accounts of its effectiveness, some are hard to dismiss out of

---

[4] *Congressman Bedell previously had surgery and radiation treatment for prostate cancer. At public meetings and hearings, he attributes to 714–X the stopping of a recurrence of this cancer 2 years after surgery. (No medical confirmation of the recurrence has been provided publicly.)*

[5] *Ward, P.S. 1988. History of Hoxsey Treatment (contract report for the Office of Technology Assessment).*

[6] *For example, the Merck Manual (Berkow, 1992) indicates that "the presence of immunogenic surface structures on human neoplastic cells permits their recognition by immunocompetent host cells as well as their interaction with humoral antibodies."*

hand; it therefore warrants investigation. Despite decades of controversy, no clinical trials have ever been performed by either supporters or detractors of the Hoxsey therapies.[7] But since the Hoxsey formula contains the poisonous substance pokeweed, testing the formula is also a public health concern.

Essiac

Like Hoxsey therapy, Essiac is an herbal treatment. Reported to be of Native American (Ojibwa) origin, it was first brought to public attention in 1922 by an Ontario nurse named Renée Caisse (*Essiac* is *Caisse* spelled backward). Caisse was impressed by the case of a local woman who claimed to have been cured of breast cancer by a local Native American healer. Caisse set up a clinic in Bainbridge and treated thousands of patients before being shut down by the Canadian medical authorities in 1942. One problem was that Caisse never made the formula public during her lifetime (1888–1978).

In 1982 a Canadian government report concluded, "No clinical evidence exists to support the claims that Essiac is an effective treatment for cancer." Nevertheless, the relevant government agency, Health and Welfare Canada (equivalent to FDA in the United States), agreed to make this medication legally available to advanced cancer patients under Canada's Emergency Drug Regulations. It is currently produced as a trademarked product in Canada. This and other versions of Essiac are also widely available through the "cancer underground" in the United States.

There are several different Essiac products, each of which claims to be the one and only authentic Caisse formula. According to author Gary L. Glum, a Los Angeles chiropractor, authentic Essiac contains four ingredients: (1) sheep sorrel (*Rumex acetosella*); (2) burdock (*Arctium lappa*); (3) slippery elm inner bark (*Ulmus fulva*); and (4) Turkey rhubarb (*Rheum palmatum*) (Glum, 1988).

- *Sheep sorrel.* The main ingredient, sheep sorrel—not to be confused with the more readily available vegetable garden sorrel, also known as "sour grass"—contains vitamins, minerals, carotenoids, and chlorophyll, all of which supposedly have anticancer effects either directly or through immunological or antimutagenic activity (Moss, 1992). Sorrel was the basis of a celebrated cancer "cure" in Virginia in the 1740s, and as *jiwisi* it was a noted remedy of the Algonquin Ojibwa (Snow, 1993). In folk tradition it is reputed to have many other medicinal qualities as well.

  Sorrel also contains generous amounts of oxalic acid as well as emodin, which has been shown to have "significant antileukemia activity" (see discussion of buckthorn in the "Hoxsey Method" section).

- *Burdock.* (See also the "Hoxsey Method" section.) That the two long standing remedies of Hoxsey and Caisse have burdock in common is suggestive, although both formulas were long held in secret, and it is unlikely that Hoxsey and Caisse communicated or even knew of each other's existence. Burdock has been shown to be bioactive in a number of experiments (Dombradi and Foldeak, 1966; Foldeak and Dombradi, 1964; Morita et al., 1984; World Health Organization, 1989).

- *Slippery elm inner bark.* Slippery elm inner bark was tested by NCI without producing any sign of anticancer activity. Slippery elm lozenges, powdered bark, and slippery elm extracts are often available in health food stores and catalogs, with a wide range of curative and restorative claims listed for them.

- *Rhubarb.* Rhubarb has been used in Chinese medicine since at least 220 B.C. It is believed to exert a beneficial effect on the liver and gastrointestinal tract. Rhubarb extract showed anticancer activity in the sarcoma 37 test system (Belkin and Fitzgerald, 1952). It contains rhein, an anthraquinone, which has been shown to have antitumor effects (Office of Technology Assessment, 1990).

Essiac is widely used throughout North America, although, unlike ushe of Hoxsey's formula, use of Essiac is not associated with any particular clinic (Snow, 1993).

---

[7] *Indeed, Patricia Ward notes in her research paper that the American Cancer Society listed Hoxsey's remedy in 1971 on its unproven methods list without citing any research basis for this listing.*

Coley's Toxins

Like many of the other pharmacological and biological treatments, Coley's toxins have attracted considerable medical and political controversy. More than 100 years ago, a New York bone surgeon at Memorial Hospital, William B. Coley, was investigating new approaches to curing cancer after his surgery failed to save a 19-year-old cancer patient. Coley chose to buttress a patient's immune system by giving him a bacterial infection that would cause a high fever and potently mobilize the patient's immune system to fight the cancer cells. Today, Coley is widely recognized as the first pioneer of immunotherapy—an approach that was virtually unknown in the 1890s.

The preparations that Coley developed were a mixture of killed cultures of bacteria from *Streptococcus pyogenes* and *Serratia marcescens.* Although not all patients responded to Coley's toxins, his treatment is reported to have shown dramatic curative effects on various cancers for many patients (Coley, 1894). These results were documented by Coley's daughter, Helen Coley Nauts, in a series of articles and monographs (Nauts, 1976, 1982, 1989.) Helen Nauts also founded the Cancer Research Institute in New York in 1953; this institute devotes itself to "the immunological approaches to the diagnosis, treatment, and prevention of cancer."

Nauts's monographs outline remarkable cures from the use of Coley's methods. Lloyd Old, an immunologist at Memorial Sloan-Kettering Cancer Research Center and a colleague, wrote, "Those who have scrutinized Dr. Coley's records have little doubt that the bacterial products that came to be known as Coley's toxins were in some instances highly effective" (Old and Boyse, 1973).

Over the years, Coley's work led to other discoveries. For instance, in the course of work on Coley's toxins in the 1940s, M.J. Shear of NCI discovered lipopolysaccharide (LPS), a component of bacterial cell walls. By injecting LPS into mice previously treated with bacillus Calmette-Guérin, Old discovered TNF (Old, 1987, 1988; Oettgen, 1980).

The original Coley formulas are no longer being used, even experimentally, in the United States. Until the 1980s, they were being tested at Temple University, Pennsylvania (Havas et al., 1958; Havas et al., 1990). In his 1990 paper, Havas pointed out that using purified LPS to evoke immune reactions is problematic because of its toxicity and proposed returning to a cruder mixture, a mixed bacterial vaccine similar to Coley's toxins. The research reported in that paper showed the mixed bacterial vaccine to have anticancer and immunostimulatory properties at nontoxic levels in animals with tumors. The authors concluded that the vaccine "compares favorably with other biological response modifiers."

Outside the United States, Coley's toxins are being used in Beijing Children's Hospital, the People's Republic of China, and Germany (Kölmel et al., 1991).

MTH–68

The MTH–68 vaccine is a form of immunotherapy that employs a little-known biological product against viral diseases and various kinds of cancer. Developed by Lászlo K. Csatáry, a Hungarian-American physician who currently resides in Ft. Lauderdale, FL, MTH–68 therapy is based on the idea that certain nonpathogenic viruses can be used to interfere with the growth of cancer in humans and the activity of harmful viruses.

MTH–68 is a modified attenuated strain of the Newcastle disease virus of chickens (paramyxovirus). In poultry, it causes an acute, fever-causing, generally fatal disease. In humans, however, the worst it does is trigger an acute but transient conjunctivitis (pinkeye), but this side effect is rare (Moss, 1992).

While Csatáry was searching for a virus that would be harmless to humans but would attack cancer viruses, it came to his attention that a chicken farmer in Hungary with advanced metastatic gastric carcinoma had undergone a complete regression of his cancer after his flock experienced an epidemic of Newcastle disease. Csatáry published his early observation in the British medical journal *Lancet* (Csatáry, 1971). In 1982, 1984, and 1985 he published study results and a general article on interference between pathogenic and nonpathogenic viruses (Csatáry et al., 1982, 1984, 1985).

Researchers in Hungary—under the direction of Sandor Eckhardt, the 1990–94 president of the International Union Against Cancer and the director of the Institute of Oncology—completed a multicenter, Phase II, double-blind, placebo-controlled clinical trial with terminal cancer patients (Csatáry et al., 1990; Moss, 1992). According to the statistical analysis in internal reports on the Phase II study, "the number of cases with stabilization or regression was significantly higher in the MTH–68/N group; favorable response in subjective parameters, such as pain relief, occurred in a significantly higher percentage in the MTH–68/N group; and performance status improved in the MTH–68/N group and significantly deteriorated in the placebo group."

Patients in Phase II received MTH–68/N by nasal drops or by inhalation (MTH–68/N is a live virus vaccine derived from the attenuated strain). The researchers say that the treatment has proved to be nontoxic and devoid of side effects. Currently, the Hungarian research team is still waiting for financial arrangements for Phase III trials.

A recently published report provides more details concerning the Phase II study (Csatáry et al., 1993). The study subjects had advanced cancers with multiple and widely distributed metastases. The duration of the protocol was 6 months, but those patients who had reacted favorably to treatment were continued on therapy. Further evaluation about survival was done after 1 and 2 years.

There were 59 patients in the study—33 in the MTH–68/N group and 26 in the placebo group. Their tumor types included lung, pancreas, kidney, sigmoid colon, and stomach cancer. In the MTH–68/N group, 2 patients experienced complete remissions, 5 experienced partial remission, 1 had moderate remission, and 10 had stabilization, for a total of 18 positive responses. Median survival time was significantly extended beyond that of the placebo group, which had only 2 stabilizations.

In addition, 26 subjects in the MTH–68/N group versus only 7 in the placebo group had either unchanged or increased weight. In the MTH–68/N group, 15 subjects had a sense of better well-being, 13 reported increased appetite, and 11 reported decreased pain; no one in the placebo group reported these effects (Csatáry et al., 1993).

Csatáry is currently negotiating with an American biotechnology company to speed development in the United States, and he has expressed willingness to have OAM conduct clinical trials of his product. He does not treat patients in the United States. Csatáry's explanation of how MTH–68 works is based on his belief that many human cancers are of viral origin.

Three possible mechanisms of antitumor action by the nonpathogenic avian viruses include direct cytolysis (cell killing), tumor-specific immune enhancement, and cytokine (see the glossary) stimulation. Thus, the avian viruses may modify tumor cells and enhance tumor-specific immunity (Schirrmacher et al., 1986). Or they may selectively kill cancer cells. Or they may stimulate a wide variety of cytokines (Csatáry, 1986, 1989), such as TNF (Lorence et al., 1988), interferons (Wheelock, 1966), and interleukins (Van Damme et al., 1989).

Neural Therapy

Neural therapy is a healing technique for attempting to deal with chronic pain and other longstanding illnesses and conditions. It involves injecting local anesthetics into autonomic ganglia (nerve cell bodies), peripheral nerves, scars, glands, acupuncture points, trigger points (points that produce a sharp pain when pressed), and other tissues and anatomical sites. Though unfamiliar to most American practitioners—and therefore part of alternative medicine—neural therapy is apparently quite widely used in Europe, especially for the treatment of chronic pain. According to its advocates, such as the American Academy of Neural Therapy, this "gentle healing technique" can instantly and lastingly resolve chronic problems when correctly applied (Klinghardt, 1991).

The history of neural therapy began with the discovery of local anesthetics in the late 19th century. In 1883, the Russian physiologist Ivan Petrov (1849–1936) laid the basis for the entire field when he hypothesized that the nervous system exercises a coordinating influence over all organic functions. Before he developed psychoanalysis, Sigmund Freud (1856–1939) discovered the anesthetic effect of cocaine on mucous membranes. In 1890, abdominal surgery was first performed using a 0.2-percent solution of cocaine. In 1903, a French surgeon first employed cocaine as an epidural anesthetic.

One obvious problem with cocaine, however, was its potential to be addictive. In 1904, Alfred Einhorn discovered procaine (novocaine), still widely used in medicine. In 1906, G. Spiess observed that wounds and inflammations subsided with fewer complications if they were first injected with novocaine. In 1925, a French surgeon, René Leriche, used this compound for treating chronic intractable arm pain. He called novocaine "the surgeon's bloodless knife." In the same year, two German physicians described another local effect, claiming that an intravenous injection of novocaine could abolish migraine headaches (Dorman and Raven, 1991; Dosch, 1984).

A key development came in 1940, when Ferdinand Huneke discovered an instant healing reaction—what is now called the "lightning reaction" or the "Huneke phenomenon." First, Huneke injected novocaine into the shoulder joint of a woman with a severely painful, frozen right shoulder, but without any beneficial local effect. Instead, unexpectedly, the woman developed severe itching in a seemingly unrelated and relatively distant scar on her lower left leg. On a hunch, Huneke then injected novocaine into the itching scar, and within seconds the woman obtained full and painless range of motion in her right shoulder. The woman's scar dated from an operation on an infected tibia (shin bone). Although the leg operation was a "success," the woman soon afterward developed the frozen shoulder on the opposite side of her body. The initial scar had become, in neural therapy terminology, an interference field (Huneke, F., 1950; Huneke, W., 1952).

By combining the use of local anesthetics with the treatment of such (inferred) interference fields, Huneke and colleagues created an entirely new healing system they called neural therapy (Dosch, 1985). Neural therapy is said to be widely used for pain control in Europe, Russia, and Latin America and by 35 percent of all Western German physicians.

At first sight, it seems improbable that a scar on the left leg could cause a pain in the right shoulder or be resolved by an injection of local anesthetic into a scar at a site so distant from the shoulder. Dietrich Klinghardt offers several possible explanations for this phenomenon (Klinghardt, 1991), including one that he calls the "nervous system theory." Klinghardt's teacher, A. Fleckenstein, demonstrated that normal body cells and cells in scar tissue have a different electric potential across the cell membrane. In cells that have lost normal potential, the ion flux across the membrane stops (Fleckenstein, 1950). This means that toxic substances and abnormal minerals build up inside the cell. In turn, the cell becomes unable to heal itself and resume normal functioning. Treatment with local anesthetic may help restore ion flux for 1 to 2 hours, which could be enough time for the cell to partially repair itself and resume normal activity.

Another theory is that scar tissue can become, in effect, a "battery" of about 1.5 volts in the body. This scar "battery" sends forth abnormal electrical signals that disturb the autonomic nerve fibers (which lack the protective myelin coating possessed by most other nerve cells in the body). This electrical abnormality can disturb the overall autonomic nervous system, leading to systemic, and often severe, bodily dysfunction.

Also proposed is what Klinghardt calls the "fascial continuity theory." According to this theory, the fascia, or sheaths of connective tissues, are all interconnected. If scar tissue is present anywhere in this system, fascial movement can become impaired. Klinghardt claims that back pain, for instance, can sometimes be completely resolved by injecting a local anesthetic (novocaine or lidocaine without epinephrine) into a scar, such as that from an appendectomy or gallbladder operation.

In addition to its antipain functions, neural therapy has been used to treat allergies, chronic bowel problems, kidney disease, prostate and female urogenital problems, infertility, and tinnitus (Brand, 1983), as well as other problems (Pischinger, 1991). Klinghardt contends that although many diseases and conditions can be successfully treated by a variety of healing techniques, some conditions can be treated successfully *only* with neural therapy.

If it is an effective method, why is neural therapy not more widely accepted in the United States? One explanation may be that it does not lend itself to a double-blind study. According to Klinghardt, "each patient with low back pain needs to be treated in a different way." In addition, neural therapy also requires a meticulous injection technique and detailed history taking, both of which are time-consuming.

Apitherapy

Apitherapy is the medicinal use of various products of *Apis mellifera*—the common honeybee—including raw honey, pollen, royal jelly, wax, propolis (bee glue), and venom. Various studies attribute antifungal, antibacterial, anti-inflammatory, antiproliferative, and cancer-drug-potentiating properties to honey (*Science News,* 1993). In China, for example, raw honey is applied to burns as an antiseptic and a painkiller. Recently, propolis (the bee product that cements a hive together) has been identified as containing substances called caffeic esters that inhibit the development of precancerous changes in the colon of rats given a known carcinogen (Rao et al., 1993). Preparations from pieces of honeycomb containing pollen are reported to be successful for treating allergies, and bee pollen is touted as an excellent food. This section focuses on bee venom to treat chronic inflammatory illness because of the popularity of this treatment and the availability of related research material.

That forms of apitherapy have been used since ancient times is not remarkable, because bees formed an important part of many early economies. Ancient writers as diverse as Hesiod (ca. 800 B.C.), Aristophanes (ca. 450–ca. 388 B.C.), Varro (166–27 B.C.), and Columella (1st century A.D.) all wrote on the cultivation of the hive, and Charlemagne (742–814 A.D.) is said to have had himself treated with beestings. The Koran (XVI: 71) refers to bee products in the following terms: "There proceeded from their bellies a liquor wherein is a medicine for men" (Kim, 1986). For apiculture and the scientific understanding of bees, real progress began about 100 years ago when physician Phillip Terc of Austria advocated the deliberate use of beestings in his 1888 work, *Report about a Peculiar Connection Between the Beestings and Rheumatism.*

Today's proponents of apitherapy cite the benefits of bee venom for alleviating chronic pain and for treating many ailments including various rheumatic diseases involving inflammation and degeneration of connective tissue (e.g., several types of arthritis), neurological disease (e.g., multiple sclerosis, low back pain, migraine), and dermatological conditions (e.g., eczema, psoriasis, herpesvirus infections).

In one sample description of the use of bee venom therapy, a physician reported anecdotally that among 128 patients with a wide spectrum of illnesses, all but 11 appeared to improve (Klinghardt, 1990). (Of the 11 who did not improve, 1 was worse and 10 were unchanged.) This report is typical of anecdotal apitherapy reports that begin with stories of beekeepers recounting various health improvements after receiving accidental multiple stings from their bees. Klinghardt's patients had diagnoses of gout, rheumatoid arthritis, fibromyalgia, spinal strain or sprain, spinal disc injuries, postlaminectomy pain, bunion, postherpetic neuralgia, incomplete healing of a fractured bone, intractable pain from large burn wounds, osteoarthritis, ankylosing spondylitis, vertigo, and multiple sclerosis. Earlier, Steigerwaldt and colleagues (1966) reported improvement among 84 percent of 50 cases of arthritis in a controlled study.

In contrast, interest in bees has been sporadic in conventional medicine, focusing mainly on three areas unrelated to the therapeutic uses proposed above. These areas are (1) the danger of hypersensitivity reactions, including anaphylactic shock, from the sting of insects of the genus *Apis;* (2) the use of bee venom itself as immunotherapy for allergic reaction to such stings, especially to prevent life-threatening anaphylactic reactions in adults; and (3) the danger of infants contracting botulism from ingesting raw honey—possibly one death every 2 to 5 years (Wyngaarden and Smith, 1988).

The modern movement promoting apitherapy is spearheaded by veteran beekeeper Charles Mraz of Vermont and physician Bradford Weeks of Washington State, assisted by other members of the American Apitherapy Society. They cite studies identifying various biological properties for semipurified fractions of bee venom and for more purified products to help explain the curative properties attributed to this venom. Table 1, adapted from Klinghardt (1990), summarizes these properties, which include pronounced anti-inflammatory, analgesic, and immunostimulatory properties.

The American Apitherapy Society contends that hypersensitivity reactions to bee venom therapy are very rare, occuring mostly from stings by related species but not by the honeybee. The procedures the society recommends include always testing a new patient first with a small amount of venom to look for possible allergic reactions and never using bee venom without an emergency beesting kit (containing epinephrine) available.

In practice, proponents say that the best results are obtained when there is a "good reaction"—considerable swelling and inflammation—at the

Table 1. Analysis of Bee Venom

Component	Action	Effect on pain/painful joint
Hyaluronidase and isoenzymes	Depolymerizes hyaluronic acid (the "glue" of the body).	Allows other components of bee venom to penetrate deep into tissues, inside cells, and inside joints.
Compound X	Lowers surface tension of all fluids (surfactant).	"Wets" cell walls with bee venom, allows better penetration.
Phospholipase A (20% of venom)	Converts lecithin (from cell walls) into lyso-lecithin, which acts as emulsifier, causes hemolysis in high doses. Most toxic component of venom.	Emulsifies debris within joints and other tissues, increases local pain briefly; counterirritant.
Melittin—a major component of venom; a peptide containing 26 amino acids	Stimulates ACTH secretion in the pituitary (cortisol). Protects lysosomal membranes. Powerful antibacterial agent. Causes lysis of mast cells. Also may be membrane-active, superoxide-production-inhibiting enzyme.	Strong anti-inflammatory effect and long-acting. Short-acting histamine effects—increased capillary permeability, edema, temperature elevation, itching pain, increased vitality and sense of well-being.
Apamin—a peptide containing 18 amino acids	Stimulates central secretion of serotonin and dopamine. Blocks nerve signal crossings in periphery.	Increases central and peripheral nervous system pain threshold; decreased pain, increased sense of well-being.
Mast cell degenerating protein (also called peptide 401)	Strong anti-inflammatory action (approximately 100 times more than hydrocortisone).	Reduces inflammation and pain through local action on tissue inflammation.
Other components:		
Acid phosphatase, α-glucosidase, phospholipase B, several peptides	Inhibition of complement, kinines, proteases, substance P, and other effects.	Anti-inflammatory, pain reducing.

Source: Adapted from Klinghardt (1990).

site of sting. Mraz believes that the optimal means of delivering venom is through a hypodermic needle administered by a licensed physician. However, since most medical practitioners do not recognize the benefits of bee venom, practicing apitherapists almost always use "the original hypodermic needle developed by Mother Nature and the honeybee some 30 million years ago: the bee stinger." Procedures for obtaining and purifying venom have been developed, but of course this product in liquid or dried form costs more than using live bees.

The usual treatment involves stinging the patient at a specific site relative to the illness and repeating the stings over a period of time. For example, it is suggested that the venom be injected into arthritic patients at trigger points in a daily course of treatment that lasts 4 to 8 weeks. Proponents indicate that there are typical patterns of responsiveness, depending on the ailment. A 50-year-old patient with arthritis might note pain relief in 2 weeks, mobility in 3 weeks, and freedom from symptoms in 4 weeks (Weeks, 1994).

Research on bee venom has included studies of whole venom and venom products. For example, in the 1960s and 1970s, studies on bee venom to treat rheumatic diseases were conducted by William H. Shipman of the U.S. Navy Radiological Defense Laboratory, James Vick of the Walter Reed Army Hospital Medical Research Center, and Gerald Weissman of New York University Hospital and their colleagues, with funding by private and public sources. One finding was that whole bee venom could suppress the development of an induced arthritis in rats, although it could not alleviate the illness after it had started (Zurier et al., 1973). Treatment with separate fractions of bee venom had no positive effect.

In later studies in which the components of bee venom were purified further, the various properties, such as anti-inflammatory and antibacterial activity (see table 1), began to be associated with specific materials.

In a more recent study (Kim, 1992), a randomized, controlled trial was conducted comparing true honeybee venom therapy with a "sham" product for 180 patients suffering from chronic pain and inflammation; solutions were injected twice weekly for 6 weeks. Significant posttreatment reductions in pain and inflammation were recorded in the true bee venom therapy group and were maintained at 6-month followups.

The American Apitherapy Society endeavors to coordinate information on bee venom research. Starting with 100 citations 12 years ago, when patients in his medical practice first interested him in the subject, Bradford Weeks, the society's president, has now acquired more than 12,000 case reports on persons treated with bee venom (Weeks, 1994). Together, these 12,000 reports are the basis for the ongoing National Multicenter Apitherapy Study. Approximately 200 physicians and 200 beekeepers voluntarily contribute reports.

At this time, the database for the multicenter study contains mostly anecdotal information, such as "I had an illness; I was stung by bees; my health improved." As Weeks notes, there is no proof in such reports that a person really had the specified illness and really improved because of the bee venom treatment.

The American Apitherapy Society would like to obtain research funds to improve the collection of both retrospective (past) information and prospective (future) data. Funding could provide research staff to search out medical records for proof of illness, training for research staff and bee venom therapists on how to gather data, and support for statistical analyses.

Meanwhile, the multicenter study has in its database some 1,300 reports on patients with multiple sclerosis (subjectively reporting increased sensation and bowel and bladder control), 2,800 with rheumatoid arthritis, and other groupings of data on such problems as gout, viral illnesses, and premenstrual syndrome—nearly 100 percent of 40 women being treated for premenstrual syndrome by apitherapy became symptom free, according to Weeks (1993).

In some ways, apitherapy is a classic alternative therapy. It has ancient roots and, although discarded by mainstream medicine, has survived in folk practice.

Iscador/Mistletoe

Iscador is a liquid extract from the mistletoe plant (*Viscum album*) that has been used to treat tumors for more than 60 years (Hajto et al., 1990a). A complex mixture, iscador has two properties that are thought to make it effective against tumors.

Iscador is cytostatic and sometimes cytotoxic—that is, it can stop cell growth, sometimes even killing cells. In addition, iscador has immunostimulatory properties, affecting the immune system. Two protein components of the mistletoe extracts appear to be the major active ingredients, viscotoxins and lectins (Jung et al., 1990).

The mistletoe lectins have been studied in more detail than the viscotoxins. In general, lectins are a group of sugar-containing proteins that are able to bind specifically to the branching sugar molecules of complex proteins and lipids on the surface of cells. Certain lectins have both cell-killing and immunostimulatory activity. Their toxic effect occurs because they can stop protein synthesis in cells.

Viscotoxins can kill cells but do not act on the immune system. They act by injuring cell membranes. Considering the toxic properties of both major active ingredients of mistletoe extracts, it is not surprising that mistletoe itself can be poisonous and that proponents of iscador provide cautions about how much to take.

One study examined a lectin from a proprietary mistletoe extract that has been reported to show ability to affect the immune system in rabbits (Hajto et al., 1989). When a tissue culture of certain white blood cells was exposed to this lectin, increased secretion of certain immune system products resulted, including TNF alpha and interleukins 1 and 6, which are cytokines (see the glossary). In turn, there was an increase in the number and activity of certain types of white blood cells. A corroborating increase was seen in cytokine levels in serum of patients after injection of lectin doses (Hajto et al., 1990b).

Both the cell-killing and the immunostimulatory activities of iscador could potentially affect tumor cells. Whether iscador is an appropriate treatment for cancer has been the subject of at least 46 published clinical studies (6 collective reports, 5 small historical studies, 9 large historical studies, 14 retrospective studies, 10 prospective studies, and 2 randomized studies), which were reviewed by Helmut Kiene (Kiene, 1989). None of the studies fit the format of a controlled, randomized, double-blind clinical trial (see app. F). Kiene points out that such studies would be difficult to do because visible local skin irritations appear early in mistletoe treatments; thus both patient and doctor would know about the treatment.[8]

Of 36 studies that Kiene decided were evaluable, he reported that 9 showed positive, statistically significant effects against diverse cancers, including ovarian, cervical, breast, stomach (postoperative), colorectal, and bronchial cancers and liver metastases. Usually the effect was to lengthen the survival time of the patient, commonly measured as median or average survival time; in one study, a significant reduction in the use of painkillers and psychopharmaceuticals was observed (see the glossary). The reviewer noted that the effect of mistletoe therapy tended to appear in situations involving patients with advanced stages of disease rather than patients with less advanced illness.

The antitumor effects observed in these studies with people are supported by studies with animal tumors. Furthermore, except for skin irritations, few uncomfortable side effects are reported by patients. This finding contrasts with the discomforts associated with more traditional anticancer radiation treatments and chemotherapy.

Much of the previous research was conducted in Germany, and the lead organization for a new study is also based there. NCI's Physicians' Data Query index identifies this study as a Phase III randomized trial of adjuvant treatment with INF–A (interferon alpha) versus INF–G (interferon gamma) versus mistletoe extract (iscador M) versus no further treatment following curative resection of high-risk stage I/IIB malignant melanoma.[9] A three-volume compendium of research papers on iscador, including translations of some from German, is available (Scharff, 1991).

---

[8]*However, such a study is not impossible. A control treatment could be used that also produced a (harmless) rash. In fact, this suggestion is made in the "Research Methodologies" chapter in a section discussing appropriate research designs. However, as Kiene (1989) cautions, local irritants are immunostimulatory; it would be necessary to make sure that their actions were strictly local.*

[9]*The protocol number is EORTC–DKG–80–1, and the NCI file entry was last modified in November 1993. The lead organization is the European Organization for Research on the Treatment of Cancer (EORTC) Melanoma Cooperative Group of Hamburg, Germany, with the first participant listed as U.R. Kleeberg of Haematologisch-Onkologische Praxis Altona. More than 20 European centers are involved in this trial, including hospitals in Germany, Austria, Belgium, Estonia, France, and Switzerland.*

Revici's Guided Chemotherapy

Emmanuel Revici, a Romanian-born physician, is still practicing in New York City in his late nineties. (His license was suspended in November 1993, but that is being challenged.) Revici has developed an approach to illness (particularly cancers) that he calls biologically guided chemotherapy (Lerner, 1994; Revici, 1961). The basis of Revici's approach is a concept that disease involves a biological dualism. While in a healthy body anabolism and catabolism balance, in a diseased body their imbalance results in diseases that are either anabolic (see the glossary) or catabolic. Correspondingly, the way the diseased body responds to treatment differs depending on the type of imbalance. In their choices of therapies, physicians must therefore be guided by which condition predominates.

Revici ascribes the effects of tumor cells to lipid imbalances. If fatty acids predominate—a catabolic condition—the tumor tissues are described as having an electrolytic imbalance and alkaline environment. If, instead, sterols predominate—an anabolic condition—there is a reduction in cell membrane permeability, according to Revici.

The patients Revici determines to have a predominance of fatty acids are treated with sterols and other agents with positive electrical charges that can theorectically counteract the negatively charged fatty acids. If sterols are predominant, treatment is with fatty acids and other agents that can increase the metabolic activity of fatty acids. The determination of anabolic (rich in sterols) or catabolic (rich in fatty acids) character is based on a series of medical tests and judgments about body type. For example, a lean individual would be more likely to have a catabolic condition, and a rounded individual, an anabolic one; Revici also considers females more likely to have an anabolic character, and males, a catabolic one. Based on the various tests, an individualized chemotherapy program is designed for each patient with cancer. (This individualization makes it harder to conduct controlled studies of treatment effectiveness.)

Along with Revici's choice of type of lipid to administer, he may incorporate other materials, such as selenium, in his lipid envelope. According to his theory, the additional agent will be delivered ("guided") directly to the tumor site because of the site's affinity for the selected lipid carrier. Because of this specificity, lower systemic drug toxicity is expected.

OAM has expressed interest in an evaluation of Revici's approach as a cancer treatment. Besides anecdotal reports concerning Revici's patients, one independent clinical trial was already conducted by Joseph Maisin, director of the Cancer Institute of the University of Louvain, Belgium. Although the results were never published, Maisin is reported to have written to Revici that dramatic improvements occurred in 75 percent of 12 terminal cancer patients. These improvements included tumor regression, disappearance of metastases, and cessation of hemorrhage.

Revici has applied his dualistic theory to other conditions besides cancer. He first developed therapies for different kinds of pain. Among the other conditions he is reported to have addressed are itching, insomnia, vertigo, migraine, radiation burns, osteoarthritis, rheumatoid arthritis, convulsions, postoperative bleeding, AIDS, ileitis, colitis, and drug addiction.

Future Research Opportunities

In general, alternative biological and pharmacological treatments are a rich area for investigation. At this time, further research would be helpful in the following specific approaches.

- *Antineoplastons.* These should have high priority. Antineoplastons could be investigated through best case series and patient outcome methodology.
- *Cartilage products.* Simone's offer to perform a prospective study on shark cartilage is now being followed up, aided by his receipt of IND approval from FDA in early 1994. In addition, an evaluation of bovine cartilage (Catrix) should be undertaken.
- *EDTA chelation therapy.* The study of EDTA as chelation therapy that was dropped in 1991 should be resumed. However, since it is unlikely that a sponsor can be found, as an alternative OAM should consider less costly ways of testing EDTA chelation therapy. One might be to assemble from the research of physicians currently using it a best case series (see Appendix F) of patients who have allegedly benefited from it for occlusive heart disease and related

conditions. A prospective outcomes study should be undertaken as well.

- *Ozone.* The data suggest that ozone may have some effectiveness with AIDS. Whether or not that is true, ozone should be evaluated for public health reasons because of its wide use among people with AIDS. Whether ozone has any anticancer effects, either in laboratory situations or in living organisms, should also be investigated.

- *Immunoaugmentative therapy.* Because of previous lack of documentation, a best case series (see app F.) should be assembled from cases treated, focusing on such intractable conditions as mesothelioma. An attempt should be made to document at least 10 indisputable successes. If these cases prove valid, a prospective patient outcomes study should be undertaken with self-selecting U.S. patients who are attending the immunoaugmentative therapy clinics in either Freeport (the Bahamas) or Germany.

- *714–X.* 714–X should be investigated through best case reviews, field investigations, and, if warranted, clinical trials.

- *Hoxsey method.* The Hoxsey treatment should be investigated both because of numerous anecdotal accounts attesting to its effectiveness and because the formula contains the poisonous substance pokeweed and is therefore a public health concern. Outcomes research should be conducted on patients at the Bio-Medical Center in Tijuana to determine what results, if any, are being achieved and what side effects may occur.

- *Essiac.* Essiac is widely used throughout North America. An observational study of patients taking this medication should be arranged.

- *Coley's toxins.* These should have high priority. Investigation could be done either by reactivating the Temple University study or by sending an observation team to China (Guo Zheren, Coley Hospital, Beijing Children's Hospital, People's Republic of China) or to Germany (Dr. Klaus F. Kölmel, Göttingen, Germany). H.C. Nauts and staff members at the Cancer Research Institute have indicated an interest in helping with any evaluation.

- *MTH–68.* This should have high priority. It shows promise as an innovative, nontoxic medication for various kinds of cancer and viral diseases. A possible approach is to join with the Hungarian scientists to initiate Phase III trials of MTH–68/N—trials that are now awaiting financial arrangements.

- *Neural therapy.* The literature should be studied, and a best case series should be assembled from cases treated. An attempt should be made to document at least 10 indisputable successes. If these cases prove valid, a prospective patient outcomes study should be undertaken with self-selecting patients.

- *Apitherapy.* Because of lack of documentation, a best case series should be assembled from cases treated. An attempt should be made to document at least 10 indisputable successes for each ailment treated. If these cases prove valid, a prospective patient outcomes study should be undertaken with self-selecting patients.

- *Iscador/mistletoe.* A best case series should be assembled from cases treated. An attempt should be made to document at least 10 indisputable successes. If these cases prove valid, a prospective patient outcomes study should be undertaken with self-selecting patients. The new multicenter European study should be monitored.

- *Revici's guided chemotherapy.* This should have high priority. A prospective clinical study of cancer patients should be evaluated.

Key Issues and Specific Recommendations

The following key issues and recommendations relate directly to the material in this chapter:

- Changes in regulations for FDA approval should be made if alternative pharmacological and biological treatments are to have a fair hearing.

- To prepare for innovative approaches, the director of OAM should work together with the FDA to develop a memorandum of understanding so that proposed trials that have been approved by OAM can proceed. FDA and State authorities should declare a moratorium on seizures, raids, import alerts, and licensing actions against physicians, researchers, and health care providers whose work has been chosen by OAM for evaluation. In 1992–93, the case of S.R. Burzynski was an urgent case in point (see the "Antineoplastons" section).

- In choosing specific treatments for testing, priority should be given to drugs and vaccines that address major causes of preventable death in the United States: cardiovascular disease, cancer, and AIDS. Priority should also be given to testing treatments that particularly show promise for safety and low costs. To gain public recognition and credibility, it is important that OAM achieve some clear successes.

References

Bedell, B. 1993. Alternative Medicine. Hearing before a subcommittee of the Committee on Appropriations, U.S. Senate, 103d Congress, First Session, ISBN 0-16-041294-3. U.S. Government Printing Office, Washington, D.C. pp. 67–101.

Belkin, M., and D. Fitzgerald. 1952. Tumor damaging capacity of plant materials. 1. Plants used as cathartics. J. Natl. Cancer Inst. 13:139–155.

Berkow, R., ed. 1992. The Merck Manual of Diagnosis and Therapy (16th ed.). Merck & Co., Rahway, N.J.

Bertelli, A., ed. 1990. "Antineoplastons: tissue culture and chemoprevention studies." Int. J. Tissue React, experimental and clinical aspects, Supplement to vol. XII, Bioscience Ediprint, Inc.

Bertelli, A., and G. Mathe, eds. 1985. Antineoplastons (1). Drugs Exp. Clin. Res. 12 (Suppl. 1).

Bertelli, A., and G. Mathe, eds. 1987. Antineoplastons (2). Drugs Exp. Clin. Res. 13 (Suppl. 1).

Bird, C. 1989. Galileo of the Microscope. H.J. Kramer, P.O. Box 1082, Tiburon, CA 94920.

Blumer, W., and E.M. Cranton. 1989. Ninety percent reduction in cancer mortality after chelation therapy with EDTA. Journal of Advancement in Medicine 2: 183–188.

Bocci, V., and L. Paulesu. 1991. Studies on the biological effects of ozone. 1. Induction of interferon gamma on human leukocytes. Haematologica 75:510–515.

Bodger, M.P., A.R. McGiven, and P.H. Fitzgerald. 1979a. Mitogenic proteins of pokeweed. I. Purification, characterization and mitogenic activity of two proteins from pokeweed [Phytolacca octandra]. Immunology 37:792.

Bodger, M.P., A.R. McGiven, and P.H. Fitzgerald. 1979b. Mitogenic proteins of pokeweed. II. The differentiation of human peripheral blood B lymphocytes stimulated with purified pokeweed mitogens (Po-2 and Po-6) from pokeweed [Phytolacca octandra]. Immunology 37:793–799.

Boyle, A.J., et al. 1963. Some in vivo effects of chelation—I. Rheumatoid arthritis. J. Chronic Dis. 16:325–328.

Brand, H. 1983. Neuraltherapie bei Tinnitus. Wein Med. Wochenschr. 133:545–547.

Brem, H., and J. Folkman. 1975. Inhibition of tumor angiogenesis mediated by cartilage. J. Exp. Med. 141:427–439.

Burzynski, S.R. 1973. Biologically active peptides in human urine: I. Isolation of a group of medium-sized peptides. Physiol. Chem. Phys. 5:437–447.

Burzynski, S.R. 1986. Antineoplastons: history of the research (I). Drugs Exp. Clin. Res. 12S:1–9.

Burzynski, S.R., and E. Kubove. 1986a. Toxicology studies on antineoplastons A-10 injections in cancer patients with five years follow-up. Drugs Exp. Clin. Res. 12S:47–55.

Burzynski, S.R., and E. Kubove. 1986b. Initial clinical study with antineoplaston A2 injections in cancer patients with five years follow-up. Drugs Exp. Clin. Res. 13S:1–12.

Burzynski, S.R., T.L. Loo, D.H. Ho, et al. 1976. Biologically active peptides in human urine: III. Inhibitors of the growth of human leukemia, osteosarcoma, and HeLa cells. Physiol. Chem. Phys. 8:13–22.

Carpendale, M., J. Freeberg, and J.M. Griffiss. 1993. Does ozone alleviate AIDS diarrhea? J. Clin. Gastroenterol. 17(2):142–145.

Casdorph, H.R. 1981. EDTA chelation therapy: efficacy in arteriosclerotic heart disease. Holistic Med. 3:101–117.

Chowka, P.B. 1985. Does Mildred Nelson have an herbal cure for cancer? In J. Moffet, ed. Points of Departure: An Anthology of Non-Fiction. New American Library, New York.

Clarke, N.E. 1960. Atherosclerosis, occlusive vascular disease and EDTA. Am. J. Cardiol. 6:233–236.

Clarke, N.E., et al. 1955. The "in vivo" dissolution of metastatic calcium: an approach to atherosclerosis. Am. J. Med. Sci. 229:142–149.

Clarke, N.E., et al. 1956. Treatment of angina pectoris with disodium ethylene diamine tetraacetic acid. Am. J. Med. Sci. 232:654–666.

Coley, W.B. 1894. Treatment of inoperable malignant tumors with toxins of erysipelas and the Bacillus prodigiosus. Trans. Am. Surg. Assoc. 12:183–212.

Cranton, E.M. 1985. The current status of EDTA chelation therapy (editorial). J. of Holistic Medicine 7:3–7.

Cranton, E.M., and J.P. Frackelton. 1982. Current status of EDTA chelation therapy in occlusive arterial disease. J. of Holistic Medicine 4:24–33.

Cranton, E.M., and J.P. Frackelton. 1989. Free radical pathology in age-associated diseases: treatment with EDTA chelation, nutrition, and antioxidants. J. of Advancement in Medicine 2:17–54.

Csatáry, L.K. 1971. Viruses in the treatment of cancer. Lancet 22 (728):825.

Csatáry, L.K. 1986. Biological response modifiers for cancer treatment. 14th International Cancer Congress. Budapest, Hungary, August 21–27.

Csatáry, L.K. 1989. Attenuated veterinary virus vaccines for the treatment of colorectal cancer, as biological response modifiers (Abstract). 2nd International Conference on Gastrointestinal Cancer, Jerusalem, Israel, August 27–September 1.

Csatáry, L.K., J.J. Romvary, B. Toth, et al., 1982. In vivo study of interference between herpes and influenza viruses. J. Med. 13:1–7.

Csatáry, L.K., et al. 1984. Interference between human hepatitis A virus and an attenuated pathogenic avian virus. Acta Microbiol. Hung. 31:153–158.

Csatáry, L.K., et al. 1985. In vivo interference between pathogenic and non-pathogenic viruses. J. Med. 16:563–573.

Csatáry, L.K., et al. 1990. Treatment of malignant tumors with attenuated Newcastle disease virus vaccine (strain MTH–68), a phase II trial. A poster abstract at the 15th International Cancer Congress, Hamburg, August 12–22. J. Cancer Res. Clin. Oncol. 116 (Suppl.).

Csatáry, L.K., S. Eckhart, I. Bukosza, et al. 1993. Attenuated veterinary virus vaccine for the treatment of cancer. Cancer Detection and Prevention 17:619–627.

Dombradi, C., and S. Foldeak. 1966. Screening report on the antitumor activity of purified Arctium lappa extracts. Tumori 52:173.

Dorman, T., and T. Raven. 1991. Diagnosis and Injection Techniques in Orthopedic Medicine. Williams and Wilkins, Baltimore.

Dosch, M. 1985. Illustrated Atlas of the Techniques of Neural Therapy with Local Anesthetics. Haug Publishers, Portland, Ore.

Dosch, P. 1984. Manual of Neural Therapy According to Huneke. Karl Haug Publishers, Heidelberg.

Fleckenstein, A. 1950. Die periphere Schmerzauslösung und Schmerzausschaltung. Steinkpoff, Frankfurt.

Foldeak, S., and C. Dombradi, 1964. Tumor-growth inhibiting substances of plant origin. I. Isolation of the active principle of Arctium lappa. Acta. Phys. Chem. 10:91–93.

Folkman, J. 1976. The vascularization of tumors. Sci. Am. 234:58–64.

Freeburg, J., and M. Carpendale. 1988. Ozone inactivates HIV at non-toxic concentration. IVth International Conference on AIDS, Abstract #3560, Stockholm.

Friedman, F., et al. 1962. The extraction and refinement of two antitumor substances. Trans. N.Y. Acad. Sci. Ser. II 25:29–32 (For related references, see Moss, 1992, pp. 481–482.)

Garber, G., et al. 1991 The use of ozone-treated blood in the therapy of HIV infection and immune disease: a pilot study for safety and efficacy. AIDS 5(9):981–984.

Glum, G.L. 1988. Calling for an Angel. Silent Walker Publishing, Los Angeles.

Green, S. 1992. Antineoplastons: an unproved cancer therapy. JAMA 267:2924–2928.

Hajto, T., K. Hostanska, M Formalski, et al. 1990a. The antitumoral activity of immunomodulatory beta-galactoside-specific mistletoe lectins in connection with the clinical use of mistletoe extracts (Iscador). Deutsch Zeitschrift fuer Onkologie 23:1–10 (translation)

Hajto, T., K. Hostanska, K. Frei, et al. 1990b. Increased secretion of tumor necrosis factor-alpha, interleukin 1 and interleukin 6 by human mononuclear cells exposed to beta-galactoside-specific lectin from clinically applied mistletoe extract. Cancer Res. 50:3322–3326.

Hajto, T., K. Hostanska, and H.J. Gabius. 1989. Modulatory potency of the beta-galactoside-specific lectin from mistletoe extract (Iscador) on the host defense system in vivo in rabbits and patients. Cancer Res. 49:4803–4808.

Havas, H., et al. 1958. Mixed bacterial toxins in the treatment of tumors. I. Methods of preparation and effects on normal or Sarcoma 37-bearing mice. Cancer Res. 18:141–148.

Havas, H., G. Schiffman, B. Bushnell, et al. 1990. The effect of a bacterial vaccine on tumors and the immune response of ICR/Ha mice. J. Biol. Response Mod. 9:194–204.

Hooker, M.H., and B.G. Gazzard. 1992. Ozone-treated blood in the treatment of HIV infection (letter). AIDS 6(1):131.

Huneke, F. 1950. in AG d.w.-dtsch. Aerztekammern. Meth. d . Herdnachw, Hippokrates Marquardt & Cie., Stuttgart.

Huneke, W. 1952. Impietoitherapie. Hippokrates Marquardt & Cie., Stuttgart.

Jung, M.L., S. Baudino, G. Ribereau-Gayon, et al. 1990. Characterization of cytotoxic proteins from mistletoe (Viscum album L.) Cancer Lett. 51:103–108.

Kiene, H. 1989. Clinical studies on mistletoe therapy for cancerous diseases, review. Therapeutikon 3(6):347–353.

Kim, C. 1992. Honey bee venom therapy for arthritis (RA, OA), fibromyositis (FM) and peripheral neuritis (PN). Pain, Journal of the Korean Pain Society 1:208–220.

Kim, C.M., ed. 1986. Managing Pain & Stress, I:4. Monmouth Pain Institute, Inc., Red Bank, N.J.

Klinghardt, D.K. 1990. Bee venom therapy for chronic pain. J. of Neurological & Orthopaedic Medicine & Surgery 11(3):195.

Klinghardt, D.K. 1991. Neural therapy (unpublished ms). Santa Fe, N.M.

Kölmel, K., et al. 1991. Treatment of advanced malignant melanoma by a pyrogenic bacterial lysate. A pilot study. Onkologie 14:411–417.

Kuemmerle, H.P., ed. 1988. Antineoplastons, Vols. I and II. In Advances in Experimental and Clinical Chemotherapy. Ecomedvertagsgesellschaft, Landsberg, Germany. (Vol. I is based on a workshop of the 15th International Congress of Chemotherapy, July 19–24, 1987.)

Kupchan, S.M., and A. Karim. 1976. Tumor inhibitors. 114. Aloe emodin: antileukemic principle isolated from rhamnus frangula L. Lloydia 39:223–224 (For related references, see Moss, 1992, p. 128.)

Langer, R., H. Brem, K. Falterman, et al. 1976. Isolations of a cartilage factor that inhibits tumor neovascularizations. Science 193:70–72.

Langham, M.E., and K.F. To'mey. 1978. A clinical procedure for the measurement of the ocular pulse-pressure relationship and the ophthalmic arterial pressure. Exp. Eye Res. 27:17–25.

Lerner, M. 1994. Choices in Cancer (working title). MIT Press, Cambridge, Mass.

Liotta, L.A. 1992. Cancer cell invasion and metastasis. Sc. Am. (February):54–63.

Lorence, R.M., P.A. Rood, and K.W. Kelley. 1988. Newcastle disease virus as an antineoplastic agent: induction of tumor necrosis factor-alpha and augmentation of its cytotoxicity. J. Natl. Cancer Inst. 80:1305–1312.

Mason, M. 1992. Body & Soul: Health Quest: Exploring unconventional medical therapies. The Washington Post, June 26, p. D5.

McDonagh, E.W., C.J. Rudolph, and E. Cheraskin. 1982. An oculocerebrovasculometric analysis of the improvement in arterial stenosis following EDTA chelation therapy. J. of Holistic Medicine 4(1):21–23.

Morita, K., T. Kada, and M. Namiki. 1984. A desmutagenic factor isolated from burdock [Arctium lappa Linne]. Mutat. Res. 129:25–31.

Moss, R. 1989. The Cancer Industry. Paragon House, New York.

Moss, R. 1992. Cancer Therapy: The Independent Consumer's Guide to Non-Toxic Treatment & Prevention. Equinox Press, New York. Note: for this report, this reference is generally used as a secondary source that cites primary references.

Nauts, H. 1976. Bacterial vaccine therapy of cancer. Dev. Biol. Stand. 38:487–494.

Nauts, H. 1982. Bacterial pyrogens: beneficial effects on cancer patients. Prog. Clin. Biol. Res. 107:687–696.

Nauts, H. 1989. Bacteria and cancer-antagonisms and benefits. Cancer Surv. 8:713–723.

Oettgen, H. 1980. Endotoxin-induced tumor necrosis factor. Recent Results Cancer Res. 75:207–212.

Office of Technology Assessment. 1990. Unconventional cancer treatments. U.S. Government Printing Office, Washington, D.C.

Old, L.J. 1987. Tumor necrosis factor. Another chapter in the long history of endotoxin. Nature 330:602–603.

Old, L.J. 1988. Tumor necrosis factor. Sci. Am. 258:59–60; 69–75.

Old, L.J., and E. Boyse. 1973. Current Enigmas in Cancer Research. The Harvey Lecture, Vol. 67. Academic Press, New York.

Olszewer, E., and J.P. Carter. 1989. EDTA chelation therapy: A retrospective study of 2,870 patients. Journal of Advancement in Medicine 2:197.

Olszewer, E., F.C. Sabbag, and J.P. Carter. 1990. A pilot double-blind study of sodium-magnesium EDTA in peripheral vascular disease. J. Nat. Med. Assoc. 82(3):173–177.

Peters, H.A. 1960. Chelation therapy in acute, chronic and mixed porphyria. In L.A. Johnson, ed. Metal Binding in Medicine. Lippincott, Philadelphia.

Pischinger, A. 1991. Matrix and matrix regulation: Basis for a holistic theory in medicine. Haug International, Brussels.

Prudden, J.F. 1985. The treatment of human cancer with agents prepared from bovine cartilage. J. of Bio. Response Mod. 4:551–584.

Prudden, J.F. 1993. A potent normalization. An interview. The Cancer Chronicles (No. 16, August).

Rao, C.V., D. Desai, B. Simi, et al. 1993. Inhibitory effect of caffeic acid esters on azoxymethane-induced biochemical changes and aberrant crypt foci formation in rat colon. Cancer Res. 53(18):4182–4188.

Revici, E. 1961. Research in Physiopathology as a Basis of Guided Chemotherapy with Special Application to Cancer. American Foundation for Cancer Research, New York.

Rudolph, C.J., E.W. McDonagh, and R.S. Barber. 1991. A nonsurgical approach to obstructive carotid stenosis using EDTA chelation. J. of Advancement in Medicine 4(3):157–166.

Scharff, P., ed. 1991. Iscador, Compendium of Research Papers (Vol. 1–3). Fellowship Community, 241 Hungry Hollow Road, Spring Valley, NY.

Schirrmacher, V., T. Ahlert, R. Heicappell, et al. 1986. Successful application of non-oncogenic virus for antimetastatic cancer immunotherapy. Cancer Rev. 5:19–32.

Schroeder, H.A., and H.M. Perry, Jr. 1955. Antihypertensive effects of metal binding agents. J. Lab. Clin. Med. 46:416.

Science News. 1993. Sweet route to heading off colon cancer. September 25, vol 144, p. 207.

Simone, C. 1993. Presentation at a hearing on alternative medicine before a subcommittee of the Committee on Appropriations, U.S. Senate, 103rd Congress, June 24.

Snow, S. 1993. The Essence of Essiac (self published). Box 396, Port Carling, Ontario, Canada POB 1J0.

Steigerwaldt, F., H. Mathies, and F. Damrau. 1966. Standardized bee venom (SBV) therapy of arthritis: controlled study of 50 cases with 84 percent benefit. IMS Ind. Med. Surg. 35:1045–1049.

Swanson, N. 1983. Moh's surgery. Arch. Dermatol. 119:761–773.

Trentham, D.E., R.A. Dynesius-Trentham, E.J. Orav, et al. 1993. Effects of oral administration of type II collagen on rheumatoid arthritis. Science 261:1727–1730.

Van Damme, J., M. Schaafsma, W.E. Fibbe, et al. 1989. Simultaneous production of interleukin 6, interferon-B and colony stimulating activity by fibroblasts after viral and bacterial infection. Eur. J. Immunol. 19:163–168.

Wagner, K., et al. 1988. Effect of ozone on HIV in experimentally infected human blood (abstract). 28th Interscience Conference on Antimicrobial Agents and Chemotherapy, Los Angeles.

Weeks, B. 1993. Letter from the president. Bee Well, the Quarterly Newsletter of the American Apitherapy Society, Inc., 3(2):1, 3.

Weeks, B. 1994. Personal communication, March 4.

Wells, K., et al. 1991. Inactivation of human immunodeficiency virus type 1 by ozone in vitro. Blood 78(7): 1882–1890.

Wheelock, F.E. 1966. Virus replication and high titered interferon production in human leukocyte cultures inoculated with Newcastle disease virus. J. Bacteriol. 92:1415–1421.

Wiewel, F. 1994. Personal communication to the editorial review board.

World Health Organization. 1989. In vitro screening of traditional medicine for anti-HIV activity: memorandum from a WHO meeting. Bull. World Health Organ. 67:613–618.

Wyngaarden, J.B., and Smith, L.H., eds. 1988. Cecil Textbook of Medicine (18th Ed.) W.B. Saunders Co., Philadelphia.

Zurier, R.B., et al. 1973. Effect of bee venom on experimental arthritis. Ann. Rheum. Dis. 32(5):466–70.

Herbal Medicine

PANEL MEMBERS

Jennifer Jacobs, M.D.—Cochair
John Reed, M.D.— Cochair

Michael Balick, Ph.D.
Steven Birch
Gerald Bodeker, Ed.D.
Carola Burroughs
Carlo Calabrese, N.D.
Edward Chapman, M.D.
Deepak Chopra, M.D.
Effie Chow, Ph.D.
Patricia D. Culliton, M.A. Dipl.Ac.
Robert Duggan
Peter Hindebergh, M.D.
Tori Hudson, N.D.
Ted Kaptchuk
Fredi Kronenberg, Ph.D.
Nancy Lonsdorf, M.D.
Kevin McNamee
Paul Ortega

CONTRIBUTING AUTHORS

Michael Balick, Ph.D.
James Duke, Ph.D.
Ted Kaptchuk
Robert S. McCaleb, Ph.D.
Richard Pavek
Cheryl Pellerin
John Reed, M.D.
James P. Swyers, M.A.

Overview

History of Herbal Medicine

Early humans recognized their dependence on nature in both health and illness. Led by instinct, taste, and experience, primitive men and women treated illness by using plants, animal parts, and minerals that were not part of their usual diet. Physical evidence of use of herbal remedies goes back some 60,000 years to a burial site of a Neanderthal man uncovered in 1960 (Solecki, 1975). In a cave in northern Iraq, scientists found what appeared to be ordinary human bones. An analysis of the soil around the bones revealed extraordinary quantities of plant pollen that could not have been introduced accidentally at the burial site. Someone in the small cave community had consciously gathered eight species of plants to surround the dead man. Seven of these are medicinal plants still used throughout the herbal world (Bensky and Gamble, 1993). All cultures have long folk medicine histories that include the use of plants. Even in ancient cultures, people methodically and scientifically collected information on herbs and developed well-defined herbal pharmacopoeias. Indeed, well into the 20th century much of the pharmacopoeia of scientific medicine was derived from the herbal lore of native peoples. Many drugs, including strychnine, aspirin, vincristine, taxol, curare, and ergot, are of herbal origin. About one-quarter of the prescription drugs dispensed by community pharmacies in the United States contain at least one active ingredient derived from plant material (Farnsworth and Morris, 1976).

Middle East medicine. The invention of writing was a focus around which herbal knowledge could accumulate and grow. The first written records detailing the use of herbs in the treatment of illness are the Mesopotamian clay tablet writings and the Egyptian papyrus. About 2000 B.C., King Assurbanipal of Sumeria ordered the compilation of the first known *materia medica*—an ancient form of today's *United States Pharmacopoeia*—containing 250 herbal drugs (including garlic, still a favorite of herbal doctors). The Ebers Papyrus, the most important of the preserved Egyptian manuscripts, was written around 1500

B.C. and includes much earlier information. It contains 876 prescriptions made up of more than 500 different substances, including many herbs (Ackerknecht, 1973).

Greece and Rome. One of the earliest materia medica was the *Rhizotomikon,* written by Diocles of Caryotos, a pupil of Aristotle. Unfortunately, the book is now lost. Other Greek and Roman compilations followed, but none was as important or influential as that written by Dioscorides in the 1st century A.D., better known by its Latin name *De Materia Medica.* This text contains 950 curative substances, of which 600 are plant products and the rest are of animal or mineral origin (Ackerknecht, 1973). Each entry includes a drawing, a description of the plant, an account of its medicinal qualities and method of preparation, and warnings about undesirable effects.

Muslim world. The Arabs preserved and built on the body of knowledge of the Greco-Roman period as they learned of new remedies from remote places. They even introduced to the West the Chinese technique of chemically preparing minerals. The principal storehouse of the Muslim materia medica is the text of Jami of Ibn Baiar (died 1248 A.D.), which lists more than 2,000 substances, including many plant products (Ackerknecht, 1973). Eventually this entire body of knowledge was reintroduced to Europe by Christian doctors traveling with the Crusaders. Indeed, during the Middle Ages, trade in herbs became a vast international commerce.

East India. India, located between China and the West, underwent a similar process in the development of its medicine. The healing that took place before India's Ayurvedic medical corpus was similar to that of ancient Egypt or China (i.e., sickness was viewed as a punishment from the gods for a particular sin). Ayurvedic medicine emerged during the rise of the philosophies of the Upanishads, Buddhism, and other schools of thought in India. Herbs played an important role in Ayurvedic medicine. The principal Ayurvedic book on internal medicine, the *Characka Samhita,* describes 582 herbs (Majno, 1975). The main book on surgery, the *Sushruta Samhita,* lists some 600 herbal remedies. Most experts agree that these books are at least 2,000 years old.

China and Japan. The earliest written evidence of the medicinal use of herbs in China consists of a corpus of 11 medical works recovered from a burial site in Hunan province. The burial itself is dated 168 B.C., and the texts (written on silk) appear to have been composed before the end of the 3rd century B.C. Some of the texts discuss exercise, diet, and channel therapy (in the form of moxibustion—see the "Alternative Systems of Medical Practice" chapter). The largest, clearest, and most important of these manuscripts, called by its discoverers *Prescriptions for Fifty-Two Ailments,* is predominantly a pharmacological work. More than 250 medicinal substances are named. Most are substances derived from herbs and wood; grains, legumes, fruits, vegetables, and animal parts are also mentioned. Underlying this entire text is the view that disease is the manifestation of evil spirits, ghosts, and demons that must be repelled by incantation, rituals, and spells in addition to herbal remedies.

By the Later Han Dynasty (25–220 A.D.), medicine had changed dramatically in China. People grew more confident of their ability to observe and understand the natural world and believed that health and disease were subject to the principles of natural order. However, herbs still played an important part in successive systems of medicine. The *Classic of the Materia Medica,* compiled no earlier than the 1st century A.D. by unknown authors, was the first Chinese book to focus on the description of individual herbs. It includes 252 botanical substances, 45 mineral substances, and 67 animal-derived substances. For each herb there is a description of its medicinal effect, usually in terms of symptoms. Reference is made to the proper method of preparation, and toxicities are noted (Bensky and Gamble, 1993).

Since the writing of the *Classic of the Materia Medica* almost 2,000 years ago, the traditional Chinese materia medica have been steadily increasing in number. This increase has resulted from the integration into the official tradition of substances from China's folk medicine as well as from other parts of the world. Many substances now used in traditional Chinese medicine originate in places such as Southeast Asia, India, the Middle East, and the Americas. The most recent compilation of Chinese materia medica was published in 1977. The *Encyclopedia of Traditional Chinese Medicine Substances* (*Zhong yao da ci dian*), the culmination of a 25-year research project conducted by the Jiangsu College of New Medicine, contains 5,767 entries and is the most definitive compilation of China's herbal tradition to date (Bensky and Gamble, 1993).

Traditional Chinese medicine was brought to Japan via Korea, and Chinese-influenced Korean medicine was adapted by the Japanese during the reign of Emperor Ingyo (411–453 A.D.). Medical envoys continued to arrive from Korea throughout the next century, and by the time of the Empress Suiko (592–628 A.D.), Japanese envoys were being sent directly to China to study medicine. Toward the end of the Muromachi period (1333–1573 A.D.) the Japanese began to develop their own form of traditional oriental medicine, called *kampo* medicine. As traditional Chinese medicine was modified and integrated into kampo medicine, herbal medicine was markedly simplified.

Herbal Medicine in the United States

In North America, early explorers traded knowledge with the Native American Indians. The tribes taught them which herbs to use to sharpen their senses for hunting, to build endurance, and to bait their traps. In 1716, French explorer Lafitau found a species of ginseng, *Panax quinquefolius L.*, growing in Iroquois territory in the New World. This American ginseng soon became an important item in world herb commerce (Duke, 1989). The Jesuits dug up the plentiful American ginseng, sold it to the Chinese, and used the money to build schools and churches. Even today, American ginseng is a sizable crude U.S. export.

As medicine evolved in the United States, plants continued as a mainstay of country medicine. Approaches to plant healing passed from physician to physician, family to family. Even in America's recent past, most families used home herbal remedies to control small medical emergencies and to keep minor ailments from turning into chronic problems. During this period there was a partnership between home folk medicine and the family doctor (Buchman, 1980). Physicians often used plant and herbal preparations to treat common ills. Until the 1940s, textbooks of pharmacognosy—books that characterize plants as proven-by-use prescription medicines—contained hundreds of medically useful comments on barks, roots, berries, leaves, resins, twigs, and flowers.

As 20th-century technology advanced and created a growing admiration for technology and technologists, simple plant-and-water remedies were gradually discarded. Today, many Americans have lost touch with their herbal heritage. Few Americans realize that many over-the-counter (OTC) and prescription drugs have their origins in medicinal herbs. Cough drops that contain menthol, mint, horehound, or lemon are herbal preparations; chamomile and mint teas taken for digestion or a nervous stomach are time-honored herbal remedies; and many simple but effective OTC ache- and pain-relieving preparations on every druggist's and grocer's shelf contain oils of camphor, menthol, or eucalyptus. Millions of Americans greet the morning with their favorite herbal stimulant—coffee.

Despite the importance of plant discoveries in the evolution of medicine, some regulatory bodies such as the U.S. Food and Drug Administration (FDA)—the main U.S. regulatory agency for food and drugs—consider herbal remedies to be worthless or potentially dangerous (Snider, 1991). Indeed, today in the United States, herbal products can be marketed only as food supplements. If a manufacturer or distributor makes specific health claims about a herbal product (i.e., indicates on the label the ailment or ailments for which the product might be used) without FDA approval, the product can be pulled from store shelves.

Despite FDA's skepticism about herbal remedies, a growing number of Americans are again becoming interested in herbal preparations. This surge in interest is fueled by factors that include the following:

- Traditional European and North American herbs are sold in most U.S. health food stores. The same is true for Chinese and, to a lesser extent, Japanese herbal medicinals. Ayurvedic herbals are available in most large U.S. cities, as are culinary and medicinal herb shops called *botanicas* that sell herbs from Central and South America and Mexico. The reemergence of Native American Indian cultural influences has increased interest in Native American Indian herbal medicines.

- Pharmaceutical drugs are seen increasingly as overprescribed, expensive, even dangerous. Herbal remedies are seen as less expensive and less toxic.

- Exposure to exotic foreign foods prepared with non-European culinary herbs has led many Euroethnic Americans to examine and often consider using medicinal herbs that were brought to the United States along with ethnic culinary herbs.
- People increasingly are willing to "self-doctor" their medical needs by investigating and using herbs and herbal preparations. Many Americans—especially those with chronic illnesses such as arthritis, diabetes, cancer, and AIDS—are turning to herbs as adjuncts to other treatments.

The next section discusses the regulatory status of herbal medicine in various countries around the world, particularly in Europe and Asia, as well as in less developed countries. It is followed by an overview of promising European and Asian herbal medicine research and recommendations for making herbal medicine a more viable health care alternative in this country.

Regulatory Status of Herbal Medicine Worldwide

The World Health Organization (WHO) estimates that 4 billion people—80 percent of the world population—use herbal medicine for some aspect of primary health care (Farnsworth et al., 1985). Herbal medicine is a major component in all indigenous peoples' traditional medicine and is a common element in Ayurvedic, homeopathic, naturopathic, traditional oriental, and Native American Indian medicine (see the "Alternative Systems of Medical Practice" chapter).

The sophistication of herbal remedies used around the world varies with the technological advancement of countries that produce and use them. These remedies range from medicinal teas and crude tablets used in traditional medicine to concentrated, standardized extracts produced in modern pharmaceutical facilities and used in modern medical systems under a physician's supervision.

Europe

Drug approval considerations for phytomedicines (medicines from plants) in Europe are the same as those for new drugs in the United States, where drugs are documented for safety, effectiveness, and quality. But two features of European drug regulation make that market more hospitable to natural remedies. First, in Europe it costs less and takes less time to approve medicines as safe and effective. This is especially true of substances that have a long history of use and can be approved under the "doctrine of reasonable certainty." According to this principle, once a remedy is shown to be safe, regulatory officials use a standard of evidence to decide with reasonable certainty that the drug will be effective. This procedure dramatically reduces the cost of approving drugs without compromising safety. Second, Europeans have no inherent prejudice against molecularly complex plant substances; rather, they regard them as single substances.

The European Economic Community (EEC), recognizing the need to standardize approval of herbal medicines, developed a series of guidelines, *The Quality of Herbal Remedies* (EEC Directive, undated). These guidelines outline standards for quality, quantity, and production of herbal remedies and provide labeling requirements that member countries must meet. The EEC guidelines are based on the principles of the WHO's *Guidelines for the Assessment of Herbal Medicines* (1991). According to these guidelines, a substance's historical use is a valid way to document safety and efficacy in the absence of scientific evidence to the contrary. (App. C contains the complete WHO guidelines.) The guidelines suggest the following as a basis for determining product safety:

> A guiding principle should be that if the product has been traditionally used without demonstrated harm, no specific restrictive regulatory action should be undertaken unless new evidence demands a revised risk-benefit assessment. . . . Prolonged and apparently uneventful use of a substance usually offers testimony of its safety.

With regard to efficacy, the guidelines state the following:

> For treatment of minor disorders and for nonspecific indications, some relaxation is justified in the requirements for proof of efficacy, taking into account the extent of traditional use; the same considerations may apply to prophylactic use (WHO, 1991).

The WHO guidelines give further advice for basing approval on existing monographs:

> If a pharmacopoeia monograph exists it should be sufficient to make reference to this monograph. If no such monograph is available, a monograph

must be supplied and should be set out in the same way as in an official pharmacopoeia.

To further the standardization effort and to increase European scientific support, the phytotherapy societies of Belgium, France, Germany, Switzerland, and the United Kingdom founded the European Societies' Cooperative of Phytotherapy (ESCOP). ESCOP's approach to eliminating problems of differing quality and therapeutic use within EEC is to build on the German scientific monograph system (below) to create "European" monographs.

In Europe, herbal remedies fall into three categories. The most rigorously controlled are prescription drugs, which include injectable forms of phytomedicines and those used to treat life-threatening diseases. The second category is OTC phytomedicines, similar to American OTC drugs. The third category is traditional herbal remedies, products that typically have not undergone extensive clinical testing but are judged safe on the basis of generations of use without serious incident.

The following brief overviews of phytomedicine's regulatory status in France, Germany, and England are representative of the regulatory status of herbal medicine in Europe.

France, where traditional medicines can be sold with labeling based on traditional use, requires licensing by the French Licensing Committee and approval by the French Pharmacopoeia Committee. These products are distinguished from approved pharmaceutical drugs by labels stating "Traditionally used for . . ." Consumers understand this to mean that indications are based on historical evidence and have not necessarily been confirmed by modern scientific experimentation (Artiges, 1991).

Germany considers whole herbal products as a single active ingredient; this makes it simpler to define and approve the product. The German Federal Health Office regulates such products as ginkgo and milk thistle extracts by using a *monograph system* that results in products whose potency and manufacturing processes are standardized. The monographs are compiled from scientific literature on a particular herb in a single report and are produced under the auspices of the Ministry of Health Committee for Herbal Remedies (Kommission E). Approval of such remedies requires more scientific documentation than traditional remedies, but less than new pharmaceutical drug approvals (Keller, 1991).

In Germany there is a further distinction between "prescription-only drugs" and "normal prescription drugs." The former are available only by prescription. The latter are covered by national health insurance if prescribed by a physician, but they can be purchased over the counter without a prescription if consumers want to pay the cost themselves (Keller, 1991). OTC phytomedicines—used for self-diagnosed, self-limiting conditions such as the common cold, or for simple symptomatic relief of chronic conditions—are not covered by the national health insurance plan.

England generally follows the rule of prior use, which says that hundreds of years of use with apparent positive effects and no evidence of detrimental side effects are enough evidence—in lieu of other scientific data—that the product is safe. To promote the safe use of herbal remedies, the Ministry of Agriculture, Fisheries, and Food and the Department of Health jointly established a database of adverse effects of nonconventional medicines at the National Poisons Unit.

Asia

In more developed Asian countries such as Japan, China, and India, "patent" herbal remedies are composed of dried and powdered whole herbs or herb extracts in liquid or tablet form. Liquid herb extracts are used directly in the form of medicinal syrups, tinctures, cordials, and wines.

In China, traditional herbal remedies are still the backbone of medicine. Use varies with region, but most herbs are available throughout China. Until 1984 there was virtually no regulation of pharmaceuticals or herbal preparations. In 1984, the People's Republic implemented the Drug Administration Law, which said that traditional herbal preparations were generally considered "old drugs" and, except for new uses, were exempt from testing for efficacy or side effects. The Chinese Ministry of Public Health would oversee the administration of new herbal products (Gilhooley, 1989).

Traditional Japanese medicine, called kampo, is similar to and historically derived from Chinese medicine but includes traditional medicines from Japanese folklore. Kampo declined when Western medicine was introduced between 1868 and 1912, but by 1928 it had begun to revive. Today 42.7 percent of Japan's Western-trained medical practitioners prescribe kampo medicines (Tsumura, 1991), and Japanese national health insurance pays for these medicines. In 1988, the Japanese herbal medicine industry established regulations to manufacture and control the quality of extract products in kampo medicine. Those regulations comply with the Japanese government's Regulations for Manufacturing Control and Quality Control of Drugs.

Developing Countries

Herbal medicines are the staple of medical treatment in many developing countries. Herbal preparations are used for virtually all minor ailments. Visits to Western-trained doctors or prescription pharmacists are reserved for life-threatening or hard-to-treat disorders.

Individual herbal medicines in developing regions vary considerably; healers in each region have learned over centuries which local herbs have medicinal worth. Although trade brings a few important herbs from other regions, these healers rely mainly on indigenous herbs. Some have extensive herbal materia medica. A few regions, such as Southeast Asia, import large amounts of Chinese herbal preparations. But the method and form of herb use are common to developing regions.

In the developing world, herbs used for medicinal purposes are "crude drugs." These are unprocessed herbs—plants or plant parts, dried and used in whole or cut form. Herbs are prepared as teas (sometimes as pills or capsules) for internal use and as salves and poultices for external use. Most developing countries have minimal regulation and oversight.

Research Base

The professional literature of Europe and Asia abounds with efficacy and safety studies of many herbal medicines. It is beyond this report's resources to investigate the validity of this vast literature. The following is an overview of some of the more promising research on herbal remedies around the world.

Europe

European phytomedicines, researched in leading European universities and hospitals, are among the world's best studied medicines. In some cases they have been in clinical use under medical supervision for more than 10 years, with tens of millions of documented cases. This form of botanical medicine most closely resembles American medicine. European phytomedicines are produced under strict quality control in sophisticated pharmaceutical factories, packaged and labeled like American medicines, and used in tablets or capsules.

Examples of well-studied European phytomedicines include *Silybum marianum* (milk thistle), *Ginkgo biloba* (ginkgo), *Vaccinium myrtillus* (bilberry extract), and *Ilex guayusa* (guayusa). Their efficacy is well documented. Herbs of American origin, such as *Echinacea* (purple coneflower) and *Serenoa repens* (saw palmetto), are better studied and marketed in Europe than in the United States. Below is an overview of recent research on these phytomedicines and American herbs.

- **Milk thistle *(Silybum marianum)*.** Milk thistle has been used as a liver remedy for 2,000 years. In 1970s studies, seed extracts protected against liver damage and helped regenerate liver cells damaged by toxins (alcohol) and by diseases such as hepatitis (Bode et al., 1977) and cirrhosis (Ferenci et al., 1989). More recently, a 6-month treatment of milk thistle significantly improved liver function in 36 patients with alcohol-induced liver disease (Feher et al., 1990). Animal studies show that it may protect against radiation damage caused by x rays (Flemming, 1971), and it gave "complete protection" to rats against brain damage caused by the potent nerve toxin triethyltin sulfate (Varkonyi et al., 1971). European hospital emergency rooms use intravenous milk thistle extract to counteract cases of liver poisoning from toxins such as those in the *Amanita phalloides* mushroom.
- **Bilberry extract *(Vaccinium myrtillus)*.** Bilberry extract is believed to help prevent or treat fragile capillaries. Capillary fragility can cause fluid or blood to leak into the tissues, causing hemorrhage, stroke, heart attack, or blindness. Less serious effects include a tendency to bruise easily, varicose veins, poor night vision, coldness, numbing, and leg cramping. Bilberry extract may protect capillaries and other small blood vessels by increasing the flexibility of red blood cell membranes.

This action allows capillaries to stretch, increasing blood flow, and red blood cells can deform into a shape that eases their way through narrow capillaries.

European clinical trials have shown the effectiveness of bilberry extract for venous insufficiency of the lower limbs in 18- to 75-year-old subjects (Corsi, 1987; Guerrini, 1987). It has been used to treat varicose veins in the legs, where it significantly improved symptoms of varicose syndrome such as cramps, heaviness, calf and ankle swelling, and numbness (Gatta, 1982). These trials revealed no significant side effects, even at 50 percent over the normal dose. In two clinical trials, a standardized bilberry extract was given to 115 women with venous insufficiency and hemorrhoids following pregnancy. Both studies documented improvements of symptoms, including pain, burning, and pruritus, all of which disappeared in most cases (Baisi, 1987; Teglio et al., 1987).

- ***Ginkgo biloba* extract.** Though this oriental herb has a different traditional use in Asia, *Ginkgo biloba* is one of Europe's most lucrative phytomedicines (Duke, 1988). In Europe, ginkgo is used mainly against symptoms of aging. It is believed to stimulate circulation and oxygen flow to the brain, which can improve problem solving and memory. It was shown to increase the brain's tolerance for oxygen deficiency and to increase blood flow in patients with cerebrovascular disease (Haas, 1981). No other known circulatory stimulant, natural or synthetic, has selectively increased blood flow to disease-damaged brain areas. In a French study, "the results confirmed the efficacy of [ginkgo extract] in cerebral disorders due to aging" (Taillandier et al., 1988). In another experiment, those given ginkgo showed consistent and significant improvement over the control group on all tests, including mobility, orientation, communication, mental alertness, recent memory, and other factors (Weitbrecht and Jansen, 1985). A "digit copying test" and a computerized classification test confirmed the improved cognitive function related to use of this herb (Rai et al., 1991).

Ginkgo extracts also stimulate circulation in the limbs, reducing coldness, numbness, and cramping. In elderly people, ginkgo improved pain-free walking distance by 30 percent to 100 percent (Foster, 1990). It also lowered high cholesterol levels in 86 percent of cases tested and prevented oxygen deprivation of the heart (Schaffler and Reeh, 1985). The extract seems to affect neurons directly, as shown by a recent French study (Yabe et al., 1992). Another French study proved protection against cell damage, this time by ultraviolet light (Dumont et al., 1992).

A German study documented benefits of long-term ginkgo use in reducing cardiovascular risks, including those associated with coronary heart disease, hypertension, hypercholesterolemia, and diabetes mellitus (Witte et al., 1992). By maintaining blood flow to the retina, ginkgo extracts inhibited deteriorating vision in the elderly. An adequate amount of extract may reverse damage from lengthy oxygen deprivation of the retina. The assessment by doctors and patients of the patients' general condition showed a significant improvement after therapy. These results show that visual field damage from chronic lack of blood flow is reversible (Raabe et al., 1991).

- ***Ilex guayusa* (guayusa).** In animal studies, a concentrated aqueous herbal preparation from guayusa leaves significantly reduced uncontrolled appetite, excessive thirst, and weight loss associated with diabetes (Swanston-Flatt et al., 1989). Although guayusa's active principles are not established, guayusa contains guanidine, a known hypoglycemic (blood sugar–lowering) substance (Duke, 1992b).

- ***Echinacea* (purple coneflower).** The subject of more than 350 scientific studies, most conducted in Europe, *Echinacea* seems to stimulate the immune system nonspecifically rather than against specific organisms. In laboratory tests, *Echinacea* increased the number of immune system cells and developing cells in bone marrow and lymphatic tissue, and it seemed to speed their development into immunocompetent cells (cells that can react to pathogens). It speeds their release into circulation, so more are present in blood and lymph, and increases their phagocytosis rate—the rate at which they can digest foreign bodies. *Echinacea* also inhibits the enzyme hyaluronidase, which bacteria use to enter tissues and cause infection. This inhibition helps wounds to heal by stimulating new tissue formation.

Echinacea exhibits interferonlike antiviral activity documented through extensive experiments in Germany. For example, in a double-blind, placebo-controlled study of 180 volunteers, *Echinacea*'s therapeutic effectiveness for treating flu-like symptoms was "good to very good" (Braunig et al., 1992). Another study showed that orally administered *Echinacea* extracts significantly enhanced phagocytosis in mice (Bauer et al., 1988). Water-soluble *Echinacea* components strongly activated macrophages (Stimpel et al., 1984), enhanced immune system cell motility, and increased these cells' ability to kill bacteria. Other immune system cells were stimulated to secrete the disease-fighting tumor necrosis factor and interleukins 1 and 6 (Roesler et al., 1991). Another study showed that *Echinacea* polysaccharides increased the number of immunocompetent cells in the spleen and bone marrow and the migration of those cells into the circulatory system. The authors said these effects resulted in excellent protection of mice against consequences of lethal listeria and candida infections (Coeugniet and Elek, 1987).

- **Saw palmetto *(Serenoa repens)*.** These berries have been used to treat benign prostatic hypertrophy (BPH). The standardized extract was clinically evaluated as effective, has no observed side effects, and costs 30 percent less than the main prescription drug marketed in the United States for BPH (Champpault et al., 1984).

  Another effective herbal drug for treating BPH is made from *Prunus africanum* and is widely prescribed in France. It is interesting to note that the U.S. government is funding a multicenter study on BPH treatment to find the most cost-effective criteria for surgical versus medical treatment. However, because the study includes neither saw palmetto nor *Prunus africanum*, it may not reflect the "state of the art" in clinical medicine worldwide.

China

Since the early 19th century, attempts have been made to understand the actions and properties of traditional Chinese medicine through scientific research. Nearly all of this work has been conducted during the past 60 years, primarily in laboratories in China, Korea, Japan, Russia, and Germany. It was also during this time that most of the drugs used in modern biomedicine were developed. It is therefore not surprising that most of the biomedical research into the effects and uses of traditional Chinese medicinal substances has attempted to isolate their active ingredients and to understand their effects on body tissues.

Several institutions and laboratories at the forefront of medicinal plant research in China are working to identify and study the active ingredients in traditional Chinese herbal remedies. Researchers at the Institute of Materia Medica in Beijing study the use of herbal remedies to prevent and treat the common cold, bronchitis, cancer, and cardiovascular disease and to prevent conception. The institute has isolated compounds such as bergenin from *Ardisia japonica*, traditionally used to treat chronic bronchitis, and monocrotaline from *Crotalaria sessiliflora*, used in folk medicine to treat skin cancer. Most of China's 5,000 medicinal plant species are represented in the institute's herbarium. Other Chinese research organizations with major programs on medicinal herbs are the Institute of Chinese Medicine, Beijing; the Institute of Materia Medica, Shanghai; the Institute of Organic Chemistry, Shanghai; the Municipal Hospital of Chinese Traditional Medicine, Beijing; the College of Pharmacy, Nanking; and the Department of Organic Chemistry and Biochemistry, Beijing University (Duke and Ayensu, 1985).

Many herbs in China have been extensively studied by using methods acceptable from a Western perspective. For example, a 1992 article in the *Journal of Ethnopharmacology* reported that during the preceding 10 years more than 300 original papers on *Panax ginseng* had been published in Chinese and English (Liu and Xiao, 1992). Ginseng is one of the world's most thoroughly researched herbs. Following is an overview of recent research on ginseng and other herbs in China. Unless otherwise indicated, the data on specific herbs are taken from *Chinese Herbal Medicine: Materia Medica*, revised edition, compiled and translated by Dan Bensky and Andrew Gamble (1993).

- **Ginseng root *(Panax ginseng [ren shen])*.** The Chinese first used oriental ginseng (*Panax ginseng*) more than 3,000 years ago as a tonic, a restorative, and a specific treatment for several ailments. By the 10th century, oriental ginseng had traveled the Silk Road to the Arabic countries (Kao, 1992), and during the next 4 centuries it spread to Europe, where the French, among others, used it to treat asthma and stomach troubles (Vogel, 1970).

In modern times, ginseng has been extensively studied in China, Japan, and Korea and, to a lesser degree, in the United States. In its various forms, ginseng or its compounds have various physiological effects. These include antistress capabilities (Cheng et al., 1986; Yuan et al., 1988), antihypoxia effects (Cheng et al., 1988; Han et al., 1979; Qu et al., 1988), alteration of circadian rhythms by modifying neurotransmitters (Lu et al., 1988; Zhang and Chen, 1987), cardiac performance effects (Chen et al., 1982), protection against myocardial infarction in animals (Chen, 1983; Fang et al., 1986), histamine response effects (Zhang et al., 1988), inhibition of platelet aggregation (Shen et al., 1987; Yang et al., 1988), alteration of circadian variation of plasma corticosterone (Li et al., 1988), modulation of immune functions (Qian et al., 1987; Wang et al., 1980), and delay of the effects of aging (Tong and Chao, 1980; Zhang, 1989).

- **Fresh ginger rhizome** ***(Zingiber officinale [sheng jiang]).*** In one study, preparations of sheng jiang and brown sugar were used to treat 50 patients with acute bacillary dysentery. A cure rate of 70 percent was achieved in 7 days. Abdominal pain and tenesmus (an urgent but ineffectual attempt to urinate or defecate) disappeared in 5 days, stool frequency returned to normal in 5 days, and stool cultures were negative within 4 days, with no side effects.

  In another study, 6 to 10 thin pieces of sheng jiang placed over the testes were used to treat acute orchitis (inflammation of the testicles). The ginger was changed daily or every other day. All participants felt a hot-to-numbing sensation in the scrotum, while a few reported local erythema and edema. Among 24 patients in the study, average cure time was 3 days. In a control group of four patients, average healing time was 8.5 days. This technique is not recommended for patients with scrotum lesions.

- **Chinese foxglove root** ***(Rehmannia glutinosa [sheng di huang]).*** A preparation of this herb and *Radix glycyrrhiza uralensis (gan cao)* was used to treat 50 cases of hepatitis in various stages. Within 10 days, 41 cases showed improved symptoms, reduced liver and spleen size, and improved liver function tests. Experiments from the 1930s seemed to show that sheng di huang, given to rats via gastric lavage or injection, lowered serum glucose levels. Later studies of this problem showed variable results. Work in Japan showed that the herb is useful in treating experimental hyperglycemia in rats. In other studies, decoctions of sheng di huang have been used to treat rheumatoid arthritis in adults and children. In one uncontrolled study, 12 subjects all showed reduced joint pain and swelling, increased function, improved nodules and rash, and lowered temperature. Followup over 3 to 6 months showed only one relapse, which was treated successfully with the same preparation.

- **Baical skullcap root** ***(Scutellaria baicalensis [huang qin]).*** Huang qin was shown to inhibit the skin reaction of guinea pigs to passive allergic and histamine tests. It has been shown to be effective in treating guinea pigs with allergic asthma. Huang qin also prevented pulmonary hemorrhage in mice subjected to very low pressure. Huang qin has an inhibitory effect against many kinds of bacteria in vitro, including *Staphylococcus aureus, Corynebacterium diphtheriae, Pseudomonas aeruginosa, Streptococcus pneumoniae,* and *Neisseria meningitidis.* In one report, one strain of bacteria (*Staph. aureus*) that was resistant to penicillin remained sensitive to this herb. According to one study, 100 patients with bacillary dysentery received a prescription composed mainly of huang qin. Mean recovery times were 2.5 days until symptoms disappeared, 3.3 days until normal stool examination, and 4.3 days until negative stool cultures.

- **Coptis rhizome, or yellow links** ***(Coptis chinensis [huang lian]).*** Huang lian and one of its active ingredients, berberine, have broad effects in vitro against many microbes. It strongly inhibits many bacteria that cause dysentery; it is more effective than sulfa drugs but less effective than streptomycin or chloramphenicol. Decoctions of huang lian have been effective against some bacteria that developed resistance to streptomycin and other antibiotics. The herb's antimicrobial ingredient is generally considered to be berberine. Experiments on chicken embryos show that huang lian has an inhibitory effect against flu viruses and the Newcastle virus.

Huang lian preparations have a strong inhibitory effect in vitro against many pathogenic fungi. Capsules of powdered huang lian were given to patients with typhoid fever, with good results. In one report, two cases that were resistant to antimicrobials responded to this herb. In another study, 30 cases of pulmonary tuberculosis were treated with huang lian for 3 months; all improved.

A 10-percent solution of huang lian also was used to treat 44 cases of scarlet fever. It was as effective as penicillin or a combination of penicillin and a sulfa drug. Huang lian also has been successfully used to treat diphtheria; in one study, the fever subsided in 1 to 3 days. Huang lian ointments or solutions promoted healing and reduced infections in first- and second-degree burns. It also has positive effects on blood pressure, smooth muscle, lipid metabolism, and the central nervous system; is effective as an anti-inflammatory; and has been used successfully in gynecology, ophthalmology, and dermatology patients.

- **Woad leaf *(Isatis tinctoria [da qing ye])*.** Da qing ye kills some kinds of bacteria, including some strains resistant to sulfa drugs. It was reported effective in hundreds of cases of encephalitis B, with cure rates of 93 percent to 98 percent. In most cases the fever subsided in 1 to 4 days, and symptoms disappeared 3 to 5 days later. Da qing ye has been effective by itself in mild and moderate cases; other herbs, acupuncture, and Western drugs should be added in severe cases.

  In a study of 100 subjects, only 10 percent of the group given a da qing ye decoction twice daily had upper respiratory infections during the study period versus 24 percent of the control group. When a mixture of decoctions of da qing ye and Herba taraxaci mongolici cum radice (*pu gong ying*) was given to 150 children with measles, signs and symptoms disappeared in 4 to 5 days. In 68 of 100 cases, da qing ye was used successfully to treat infectious hepatitis.

- **Wild chrysanthemum flower *(Chrysanthemum indicum [ye ju hua])*.** Ye ju hua has been used to treat hypertension, either alone as an infusion or with *Elos lonicerae japonicae* (jin yin hua) and *Herba taraxaci mongolici cum radice* (pu gong ying) in a decoction. Ye ju hua preparations have an inhibitory effect in vitro against some bacteria and viruses. Preparations given orally or as injections lowered blood pressure. Preparations made from the whole plant had more toxicity and less efficacy than those made from the flower alone.

  One study was performed with 1,000 subjects to see whether ye ju hua would prevent colds. The subjects were compared with their own histories and against a matched set of 261 controls. A ye ju hua decoction was taken once a month by people with histories of infrequent colds, twice a month by those with three to five colds a year, and weekly by those with frequent colds. Comparison with their own histories showed a 13.2-percent reduction in frequency, but a greater frequency in comparison with the controls. At the same time, another clinical series of 119 cases of chronic bronchitis was observed. Using the same preparation, this group experienced a 38-percent reduction in acute attacks in comparison with their seasonally adjusted rate for the previous year.

- **Bletilla rhizome *(Bletilla striata [bai ji])*.** Bai ji, in powdered form or in a powder made from starch and a decoction of bai ji, helped control bleeding in seven of eight cases of surgical wounds to dogs' livers. Pure starch was much less effective. Similar results have been achieved with sponges soaked in a sterile water-extraction solution of the herb. In anesthetized dogs with 1-mm-diameter stomach perforations, washing the perforations with 9 g of powdered bai ji through a tube closed the perforations in 15 minutes. Eight hours after the procedure the abdomens were opened, and no trace of gastric contents was found. When the dogs' stomachs were full or the perforations were larger, powdered bai ji had no effect.

  In another study, powdered bai ji was used to treat 69 cases of bleeding ulcers, and in all cases the bleeding stopped within 6.5 days. In another series of 29 perforated ulcer cases, the powdered herb was successful in 23 cases, 1 required surgery, and the other 4 died (1 went into hemorrhagic shock while under treatment, and the other 3 were in precarious condition on admission).

In other studies, powdered bai ji was given to 60 chronic tuberculosis patients who had not responded to normal therapy. After taking the herb for 3 months, 42 were clinically cured, 13 significantly improved, and 2 showed no change. A sterile ointment made from decocted bai ji and petroleum jelly was used in a local application to treat 48 cases of burns and trauma (less than 11 percent of total body area). Dressings were changed every 5 to 7 days, and all patients recovered within 1 to 3 weeks.

- **Salvia, or cinnabar root *(Salvia miltiorrhiza [dan shen]).*** Dan shen caused coronary arteries to dilate in guinea pig and rabbit heart specimens. In one study of 323 patients given a dan shen preparation for 1 to 9 months, there was marked improvement in 20.3 percent of clinical cases and general improvement in 62 percent of cases. Results were best when patients had coronary artery disease and no history of myocardial infarction. In a clinical series of more than 300 patients with angina pectoris, a combination of dan shen and *Lignum dalbergiae odoriferae (jiang xiang)* given intramuscularly or intravenously improved symptoms in 82 percent and electrocardiograms in 50 percent of cases.

- **Corydalis rhizome *(Corydalis yanhusuo [yan hu suo]).*** Yan hu suo is widely used to treat pain. Powdered yan hu suo is a very strong analgesic, about 1 percent the strength of opium. In one clinical study of 44 patients with painful or difficult menstruation, 50 mg of the yan hu suo active ingredient, dihydrocorydaline, given 3 times a day brought significant relief in 14 cases and reduced pain in another 18 cases. Side effects included reductions in menstrual flow, headaches, and fatigue.

- **Root of Szechuan aconite *(Aconitum carmichaeli [fu zi]).*** Fu zi's toxicity has always been a major concern. It is usually prepared with salt to reduce its toxicity. Anesthetized dogs or cats given fu zi preparations showed a sharp drop in blood pressure. In another experiment, fu zi caused blood vessels to dilate in lower extremities and coronary vessels. In normal dosage for humans, fu zi slightly lowers blood pressure, while a large overdose can cause rapid heartbeat or ventricular fibrillation. This herb seems to have some cardiotonic function and a regulatory effect on heart rhythm. Administered with herbs such as *Cortex cinnamomi cassiae (rou gui), Panax ginseng (ren shen), Rhizoma zingiberis officinalis (gan jiang),* and *Radix glycyrrhiza uralensis (gan cao),* fu zi raised blood pressure in animals with acute hemorrhage. In one study, patients with congestive heart failure were treated by intramuscular injections of a fu zi preparation. In all cases, including one of cardiogenic shock, the result was increased cardiac output as well as decreased breathing difficulty, liver swelling, and general edema. A few cases showed temporary side effects of flushing and slight tremors.

- **Licorice root *(Glycyrrhiza uralensis [gan cao]).*** Gan cao preparations have been used with common antituberculosis drugs in many large clinical studies among patients who did not respond to standard treatment. In most cases, symptoms improved or disappeared and x rays improved markedly. In many clinical studies using gan cao for ulcers with groups of 50 to 200 subjects, effectiveness was around 90 percent. It was especially useful to treat the pain, which disappeared or improved within 1 to 3 weeks. The more recent the onset of disease, the better the results. In almost all cases the powdered herb was most effective.

  In rats with experimentally induced atherosclerosis, gan cao lowered cholesterol levels and stopped progression of lesions. In several experiments, the herb reduced the toxicity of some substances, including cocaine, and moderately reduced the toxicity of others, including caffeine and nicotine. When decocted with fu zi, it sharply reduced fu zi's toxicity.

- **Dryopteris root, or shield fern *(Dryopteris crassirhizoma [guan zhong]).*** *Dryopteris crassirhizoma* is called *dong bei guan zhong* because it is found in northeastern (*dong bei*) China. In recent times this herb has been prescribed as a preventive measure during influenza epidemics. Guan zhong preparations strongly inhibit the flu virus in vitro. In one clinical trial, 306 people took twice-weekly doses of guan zhong and 340 served as controls. In the treatment group, 12 percent became ill versus 33 percent of the controls. Local versions of guan zhong from Guangdong, Hunan, and Jiangxi provinces have mildly inhibitory effects in vitro against many pathogenic bacteria. Guan zhong also is effective against pig roundworms in vitro, and it expels tapeworms and liver flukes in cattle.

In other studies, decoctions and alcohol extracts of dong bei guan zhong strongly stimulated the uterus of guinea pigs and rabbits. It increased the frequency and strength of contractions. Intramuscular injections of dong bei guan zhong preparations were used with more than 91-percent success to treat postpartum, postmiscarriage, and postsurgical bleeding.

- **Garlic bulb** ***(Allium sativum [da suan]).*** Da suan preparations have a strong inhibitory effect in vitro against amebae. In one study, concentrated da suan decoctions were used to treat 100 cases of amebic dysentery. The cure rate was 88 percent, and the average hospital stay was 7 days. In this clinical study, purple-skinned bulbs were more effective than white-skinned bulbs. Patients were discharged on a regimen that included purple-skinned da suan in the daily diet.

  When used with Chinese leek seeds, da suan juice and decoctions have a strong inhibitory effect in vitro against many pathogenic bacteria. Da suan can be effective against bacteria that resist penicillin, streptomycin, and chloramphenicol. In one clinical study, 130 patients with bacillary dysentery were given da suan enemas. Of the followup colonoscopies, 126 showed that pathological changes were resolved within 6.3 days. In other studies with hundreds of patients, da suan's effectiveness against bacillary dysentery was more than 95 percent. Again, purple-skinned garlic seemed more effective than white-skinned, and fresh bulbs were more effective than old ones. In one clinical study, 17 cases of encephalitis B were treated with an intravenous drip of da suan preparations and supportive care. Except for one fatality, all other cases recovered.

India

Ayurveda, the oldest existing medical system, is recognized by WHO and is widely practiced. The word comes from two Sanskrit roots: *ayus* means life or span; *veda* means knowledge or science. India recently increased research on traditional Ayurvedic herbal medicines after observations that they are effective for conditions to which they have traditionally been applied. For example, the ancient Sanskrit text on Ayurveda, the *Sushruta Samhita,* noted that *Commiphora mukul* was useful in treating obesity and conditions equivalent to hyperlipidemia, or increased concentrations of cholesterol in the body. The plant has been used by Ayurveda practitioners for at least 200 years and may have been in use since the writing of the *Sushruta Samhita* more than 2,000 years ago. In a recent study, the crude gum from *Commiphora mukul* significantly lowered serum cholesterol in rabbits with high cholesterol levels. The plant substance also protected rabbits from cholesterol-induced atherosclerosis (hardening of the arteries). This finding led to pharmacological and toxicological studies that showed this herbal remedy to be effective in humans, with no adverse side effects. Approval was obtained from the national regulatory authority in India for further clinical trials (Verma and Bordia, 1988). The drug is marketed in India and other countries for treatment of hyperlipidemia (Chaudhury, 1992).

The following other Ayurvedic herbs have recently been studied in India under modern scientific conditions:

- ***Eclipta alba.*** In Ayurvedic medicine, *Eclipta alba* is said to be the best drug for treating liver cirrhosis and infectious hepatitis. *Eclipta alba* and *Wedelia calendulacea* are widely used in India for jaundice and other liver and gall bladder ailments. One recent study showed that a liquid extract from fresh *Eclipta* leaves was effective in vivo in preventing acute carbon tetrachloride-induced liver damage in guinea pigs. Clinically, the powdered drug is effective against jaundice in children (Wagner et al., 1986).

- **Common teak tree** ***(Tectona grandis).*** Trunk wood and bark of the common teak tree are described in Ayurvedic medicine as a cure for chronic dyspepsia (indigestion) associated with burning pain. Teak bark forms an ingredient of several Ayurvedic preparations used to treat peptic ulcer. Pandey et al. (1982) experimentally screened teak bark and its effect on gastric secretory function and ulcers in albino rats and guinea pigs. The solution reduced gastric ulcers in restrained albino rats and significantly inhibited gastric and duodenal ulcers in guinea pigs.

- **Indian gooseberry** *(Emblica officinalis [amla]).* Jacob et al. (1988) studied the effect of total serum cholesterol by using amla to supplement the diets of normal and hypercholesterolemic men aged 35–55. The supplement was given for 28 days in raw form. Normal and hypercholesterolemic subjects showed decreased cholesterol levels. Two weeks after the supplement was withdrawn, total serum cholesterol levels of the hypercholesterolemic subjects rose almost to initial levels.

- ***Picrorhiza kurroa.*** *P. kurroa* rhizomes are main ingredients of a bitter tonic used in fever and dyspepsia (indigestion). This drug occupies a prestigious position in Ayurveda. It often substitutes for *Gentiana kurroo,* the Indian gentian. Powdered rhizomes also are used as a remedy for asthma, bronchitis, and liver diseases. Other researchers have reported that a *P. kurroa*-derived mixture called *kutkin* exhibits hepatoprotective activity; that *P. kurroa* acts as a bile enhancer; that it has antiasthmatic effects in patients with chronic asthma; and that it has immunomodulating activity in cell-mediated and humoral immunity. Another study (Bedi et al., 1989) shows that *P. kurroa* works to boost the immune system as a supplement to other treatments in patients with vitiligo, a skin disease that causes discolored spots.

- **Articulin-F.** This herbomineral formula contains roots of *Withania somnifera,* stem of *Boswellia serrata,* rhizomes of *Curcuma longa,* and a zinc complex. Kulkarni et al. (1991) performed a randomized, double-blind, placebo-controlled crossover study of articulin-F to treat osteoarthritis, a common progressive rheumatic disease characterized by degeneration and eventual loss of articular cartilage. Articulin-F treatment produced a significant drop in pain severity and disability score, whereas radiological assessment showed no significant changes.

- **Abortifacient plants.** Nath et al. (1992) organized a survey program in Lucknow and Farrukhabad, two towns in Uttar Pradesh, India, from March to July 1987. During the survey, they recorded the common folk medicine used by women and consulted Ayurvedic and Unani drug encyclopedias for the antireproductive potential of the following medicinal plants: leaves of *Adhatoda vasica,* leaves of *Moringa oleifera,* seeds of *Butea monosperma,* seeds of *Trachyspermum ammai,* flowers of *Hibiscus sinensis,* seeds of *Abrus precatorius,* seeds of *Apium petroselinium,* buds of *Bambusa arundensis,* leaves of *Aloe barbadensis,* seeds of *Anethum sowa,* seeds of *Lepidium sativum,* seeds of *Raphanus sativus,* seeds of *Mucuna pruriens,* seeds of *Sida cordifolia,* seeds of *Blepharis edulis,* flowers of *Acacia arabica,* and seeds of *Mesua ferrea.* Plant materials were collected, authenticated, chopped into small pieces, air dried in shade, and then ground to a 60-mesh powder. During the survey, female rats were given aqueous or 90-percent ethanol extracts of the plants orally for 10 days after insemination by males, with special attention to effects on fetal development. Leaf extracts of *Moringa oleifera* and *Adhatoda vasica* were 100-percent abortive at doses equivalent to 175 mg/kg of starting dry material.

- **Neem** *(Azadiractica indica)* and **turmeric** *(Curcuma longa).* In the Ayurveda and Sidha systems of medicine, neem and turmeric are used to heal chronic ulcers and scabies. Charles and Charles (1991) used neem and turmeric as a paste to treat scabies in 814 people. Ninety-seven percent of cases were cured within 3 to 15 days. The researchers found this to be a cheap, easily available, effective, acceptable mode of treatment for villagers in developing countries, with no adverse reactions.

- **Trikatu.** Trikatu is an Ayurvedic preparation containing black pepper, long pepper, and ginger. It is prescribed routinely for several diseases as part of a multidrug prescription. These herbs, along with piperine (alkaloid of peppers), have biological effects in mammals, including enhancement of other medicaments. Of 370 compounds listed in the *Handbook of Domestic Medicines and Common Ayurvedic Remedies* (Handbook, 1979), 210 contain trikatu or its ingredients. Trikatu is a major decoction used to restore the imbalance of *kapha, vata,* and *pitta,* the body's three humors (see the "Alternative Systems of Medical Practice" chapter). *Piper* species are used internally to treat fevers, gastric and abdominal disorders, and urinary difficulties. Externally they are used to treat rheumatism, neuralgia, and boils. *P. longum* and *P. nigrum* are folklore remedies for asthma, bronchitis, dysentery, pyrexia, and insomnia (Akamasu, 1970; Chopra and Chopra, 1959; Perry, 1980; Youngken, 1950). In Chinese folklore, *P. nigrum* is mentioned as a treatment for epilepsy (Pei, 1983). The efficacy of *P. longum* fruits in reducing asthma in adults (Upadhyaya et al., 1982) and children has been reported (Dahanukar et al., 1984). *P. nigrum* promoted digestive juice secretion (Shukla, 1984) and increased appetite (Sumathikutty et al., 1979). *P. longum* was reported useful in patients with gastric disorders accompanied by clinical symptoms of achlorhydria (Kishore et al., 1990).

Native American Indian Herbal Medicine

In 1977 and 1978, Croom (see Kirkland et al., 1992) spent 2 years documenting plant remedies among the Lumbee Indians, the largest group of Native American Indians east of the Mississippi River. Following are some often-used medicinal plant remedies of the Lumbee:

- **Rabbit tobacco *(Gnaphalium obtusifolium).*** These annual herbs reach a height of 1 to 3 feet and have erect stems with brown, shriveled leaves persisting into winter and stems covered with feltlike hairs in summer. The leaves are 1 to 3 inches long, and alternate. The flowers, minute in whitish heads, appear in late summer to fall. Fields, pastures, and disturbed areas are the sites of this common native plant of the eastern United States. It is used to treat colds, flu, neuritis, asthma, coughs, and pneumonia. This is one of the most popular plants used by the Lumbee. The decoction is drunk hot, like most medicinal teas, and is said to cause profuse sweating.

- **Poke *(Phytolacca americana).*** Also a common native plant of the eastern United States, poke is a robust, perennial herb that reaches a height of 9 feet. It has a large white root; a green, red, or purple stem; alternate leaves up to 1 foot long; and white flowers in a drooping raceme. The fruit is a dark purple to black berry, round, soft, and juicy. Poke is found in waste areas, road sides, disturbed habitats, fields, and pastures. It is used to treat asthma, spring tonic, boils (risings), sores, intestinal worms in people or chickens, cramps, and stomach ulcers. Poke is said to inhibit gram-positive and gram-negative bacteria and is listed as a parasiticide in the *British Herbal Pharmacopoeia.*

- **Pine *(Pinus echinata, P. palustris, P. virginiana).*** Pines are resinous evergreen trees with needlelike foliage leaves in bundles of two to five. The male and female reproductive structures are in separate cones on the same tree; the female cone matures to a large woody cone with winged seeds; pollen sheds in the spring. Pine is used to treat colds, flu, pneumonia, fever, heartburn, arthritis, neuritis, and kidney problems.

- **Oak *(Quercus laevis, Q. phellos).*** These deciduous trees have alternate, unlobed, or variously lobed leaves and minute flowers; the fruit is an acorn. Oak is used to treat kidney problems (including Bright's disease), bladder problems, virus, menstrual bleeding, diarrhea, sores, sprains, and swellings. It is also used as a booster for other remedies.

- **Sassafras *(Sassafras albidum).*** These deciduous, aromatic, small trees or shrubs have green twigs and—when mature—thick, furrowed bark. The leaves are 2.5 to 5 inches long; alternate; and either unlobed, lobed on one side, or three-lobed. Flowers are small and yellow in clusters at the end of twigs. The fruit is a dark blue, fleshy drupe on a bright red stalk and cup. This common native plant of fencerows, woodland borders, and old fields of the eastern United States is used to treat measles, chicken pox, colds, flu, and fever. It is also used as a "shotgun heart remedy," a blood purifier, and a spring tonic.

According to the *Handbook of Northeastern Indian Medicinal Plants* Native American Indians used about 25 percent of the flora of Maryland for medicinal purposes (Duke, 1986). A few examples of medicinal plant species in Maryland are as follows:

- **Sweetflag or calamus *(Acorus).*** The root has been used to treat flatulence, colds, coughs, heart disease, bowel problems, colic, cholera, suppressed menses, dropsy, gravel, headache, sore throat, spasms, swellings, and yellowish urine. Some tribes considered the root a panacea; others thought it had mystic powers.

- **Bloodroot *(Sanguinaria).*** This very poisonous plant is emetic, laxative, and emmenagogue. It has been used to treat chronic bronchitis, diphtheria, sore throat, uterine and other cancers, tetterworm, deafness, and dyspepsia; it has also been used as a pain reliever and sedative.

In Appalachia it is carried as a charm to ward off evil spirits.

- **Yellowdock.** Contains anthraquinones of value in the treatment of ringworm and some types of psoriasis. Rumicin from the roots reportedly destroys skin parasites. The anthraquinones are proven laxatives.
- **Coneflower *(Echinacea, Rudbeckia).*** *Echinacea* (purple coneflower) reportedly increases resistance to infection, bad coughs, dyspepsia, venereal disease, insect bites, fever, and blood poisoning.
- **Witch hazel.** A proven astringent and hemostat (to stop bleeding).
- ***Lobelia (Lobelia cardinalis).*** Cardinal flower was used to indurate ulcers and to treat stomachache, syphilis, and worms. The leaf tea was used for cold, croup, epistaxis (nosebleed), fever, headache, rheumatism, and syphilis. *Lobelia inflata* (Indian tobacco) yields lobeline sulfate, used in antitobacco therapy. It is used as an antiasthmatic, an expectorant, and a stimulant for bronchitis; it also is used to treat aches, asthma, boils, croup, colic, sore throat, stiff neck, and tuberculosis of the lungs. Some smoked the herb to break a tobacco habit.
- **Mayapple *(Podophyllum peltatum).*** Early Native American Indians used the roots as a strong purgative, liver cleanser, emetic, and worm expellant. A resin made from the plant has been used to treat venereal warts and exhibits antitumor activity; it also is used for snakebite and as an insecticide for potato bugs.
- **Wild cherry *(Prunus virginiana).*** The bark has been used to treat sores and wounds, diarrhea, cold and cough, tuberculosis, hemoptysis, scrofula, sore throat, stomach cramps, and piles. Native American Indians treated snow blindness by leaning over a kettle of boiling bark "tea." Some smoked the bark for headache and head cold.
- **White willow *(Salix alba).*** The bark is astringent, expectorant, hemostatic, and tonic. It is used to treat calluses, cancers, corns, tumors, and warts. Salicylic acid (used to make aspirin) is found in white willow. Leaves and bark of different willows are used in a tea to break a fever. Some Native American Indians burned willow stems and used the ashes to treat sore eyes.

Barriers to Herbal Medicine Research in the United States

The regulatory lockout of natural remedies has crippled natural products research in U.S. universities and hospitals. There is no dedicated level of support by the Federal Government for herbal medicine research. Herbalists may apply under existing guidelines for approval of new pharmaceutical drugs, but this burden is unrealistic because the total cost of bringing a new pharmaceutical drug to market in the United States is an estimated $140 million to $500 million (Wall Street Journal, 1993). Because botanicals are not patentable (although they can be patented for use), an herbal medicine manufacturer could never recover this expenditure. Therefore, herbal remedies are not viable candidates for the existing drug approval process: pharmaceutical companies will not risk a loss of this magnitude, and herb companies lack the financial resources even to consider seeking approval.

Another major barrier is that the academic infrastructure necessary for proper study of ethnomedical systems has seriously eroded in recent decades and must be reinvigorated to accommodate the newly recognized need for preserving traditional medical systems and biological diversity. Pharmacognosy and other academic studies of medicinal plants have declined alarmingly in the United States. North American scientists, once at the forefront of this research, lag behind their European and Japanese colleagues, reducing the likelihood that they will discover useful new medicines from plants. This problem is exacerbated by the fact that much of the discipline of botany has moved away from field studies and into molecular and laboratory approaches. Today only a handful of active full-time ethnobotanists are trained to catalog information on the medicinal properties of plants.

In contrast to the United States, many European and Asian countries have taken a more holistic approach to researching the efficacy of herbal remedies. In Germany, France, and Japan, the past 20 years have seen a rapid increase in research into and use of standardized, semipurified (still containing multiple individual chemicals) herbal extracts called phytomedicines. In Europe and Japan, phytomedicines treat conditions ranging from serious, life-threatening diseases such as heart disease and cancer to simple symptomatic relief of colds, aches and pains, and other conditions treated by OTC drugs in the United States. Phytomedicines include preventive medicines, an often-neglected area of medicine in the United States. The FDA has approved many plant-derived "heroic" cures, but never a plant-derived preventive medicine.

Research Needs and Opportunities

Much modern-day medicine is directly or indirectly derived from plant sources, so it would be foolish to conclude that plants offer no further potential for the treatment or cure of major diseases. Worldwide, the botanical pharmacopoeia contains tens of thousands of plants used for medicinal purposes. Hundreds, perhaps thousands, of definitive texts, monographs, and tomes on herbal remedies exist. But most of this information is outside current databases and remains unavailable to physicians, researchers, and consumers.

Globally, herbal remedies have been researched under rigorous controls and have been approved by the governments of technologically advanced nations. The scientific validation is good to excellent, and the history of clinical use is even stronger. Many phytomedicines have been used by thousands of physicians in their practices and are consumed under medical supervision by tens of millions of people.

A great deal of literature exists on the use of phytomedicines in Europe and within native medical systems in China, Japan, India, and North America. Much of this literature can be found in a unique database developed and maintained by the University of Illinois at Chicago, College of Pharmacy. The database, NAPRALERT (Natural Products Alert), holds references for more than 100,000 scientific articles and books on natural products (plant, microbial, and animal extracts). NAPRALERT includes considerable data on the chemistry and pharmacology (including human studies) of secondary metabolites of known structure, derived from natural sources. About 80 percent of the references are from post-1975 literature, the rest from pre-1975 literature (see the "Research Databases" chapter for more information on NAPRALERT).

In 1981 the U.S. Department of Agriculture (USDA), in conjunction with the National Cancer Institute, concluded a 25-year study of plants with possible anticancer properties. One result is published in the *Handbook of Medicinal Herbs* (Duke and Ayensu, 1985). This work lists 365 folk medicinal species and identifies more than 1,000 pharmacologically active phytochemicals. Toxicity estimates are given for many of these biologically active compounds. More recently, Dr. James Duke of USDA published databases on biologically active compounds of more than 1,000 species of plants with potential medicinal uses (Duke, 1992a, 1992b). Duke proposed to FDA a computer-calculated toxicity index to parallel the Ames Human Exposure Rodent Potency (HERP) index for carcinogenicity. He calls his index the Better Understanding of Relative Potency (BURP) index.

Much of the literature on traditional Chinese and other Asian countries' herbal medicine is only now beginning to be translated into English. While much of this information is in the form of folklore, there is a growing body of data from scientifically valid literature on herbal medicine research in China as well as India and Japan. In 1986, the book *Chinese Herbal Medicine: Materia Medica* was published by Dan Bensky and Andrew Gamble, both of whom are fluent in Chinese dialects and studied herbal medicine in Asia. Revised in 1993 (Bensky and Gamble, 1993), it presents an indepth study of 470 herbs used in traditional Chinese medicine. Each entry details the traditional properties, actions and indications, principal combinations, dosage, and contraindications of the herbs, as well as summaries of abstracts regarding pharmacological and clinical research conducted in Asia. The revised edition also provides a brief description of the appearance of each herb.

Although very little laboratory or clinical research has been performed on Native American Indian herbal remedies, extensive listings of herbs and their uses have been compiled by ethnobotanists for several tribes. One source, *American Indian Medicine* (Vogel, 1970), cites references in the professional ethnobotanical literature on herbal medicines for the following tribes: Alabama-Koasati, Arakara, Algonquian, Arapaho, Aztec, Catawba, Cheyenne, Chickasaw, Choctaw, Comanche, Congaree, Creek, Dakota, Delaware, Hoh, Hopi, Houma, Huron, Illinois-Miami, Iroquois, Kwakiutl, Lake St. John Montagnais, Mayan, Menomini, Mescalero Apache, Malecite, Meswaki, Michigan, Mohawk, Mohegan, Natchez, Navajo, Nebraska, Oglala Sioux,

Ojibwa, Omaka, Pawnee, Penobscot, Ponca, Potawatomi, Quileute, Rappahannock, San Carlos Apache, Seminole, Sioux, White Mountain Apache, Ute, Winnebago, Yuma, and Zuni. Moerman's database (Moerman, 1982) lists more than 2,000 species of Native American Indian medicinal plants, and Duke (1986) lists more than 700 eastern ones.

These sources—the NAPRALERT database, USDA laboratory research, the Bensky and Gamble book, and the Native American Indian herbal medicinal books—are the foundation on which the U.S. Government, particularly the National Institutes of Health (NIH), can begin substantial research into herbal medicines.

Much unwritten knowledge resides in the hands of healers in many societies where oral transmission of information is the rule. Unfortunately, in many regions this information is endangered because there are no young apprentices to whom elderly healers can pass on their unwritten wisdom; the knowledge that has been refined over thousands of years of experimentation with herbal medicine is being lost. A major research opportunity in this area would be to catalog information on herbal medicines from thousands of traditional healers in cultures where these skills are normally transmitted through an apprentice system. Some organizations have recently increased their efforts to catalog endangered herbal knowledge from traditional medical systems in Latin America, such as those practiced in the rain forests of Belize (Arvigo and Balick, 1993) and Peru (Duke and Martinez, in press).

Basic Research Priorities

Basic research into characterizing these plant products and compounds in terms of standardized content and potential toxicity is needed to allow safe and replicable research to document clinical efficacy. Basic science research should be conducted to evaluate research on the biochemical effects of traditional herbal prescriptions from Western, Ayurvedic, oriental, and other traditions (see the "Alternative Systems of Medical Practice" chapter).

Clinical Research Priorities

Research in phytomedicines in the United States could follow on the results of existing high-quality European and Asian research on plant medicines and should focus on replicating results of key studies or addressing weaknesses in those studies. Reviews of foreign literature and translations of non-English literature would be helpful. Current widespread use of herbal medications as "food supplements" in the United States provides a ready base of users, producers, and practitioners for clinical research in traditional and modern applications of botanical medicine.

Key Research Issues

Before a comprehensive research agenda is developed, several key issues must be addressed, including the following: the impending loss of knowledge about traditional healing in many societies; the impending loss of large numbers of plant species of potential medicinal value; impediments to the use of herbal remedies outside the cultures in which they originated; and determination of the conditions under which herbal medicines are most appropriate, safe, and effective. Additionally, several regulatory issues hamper research into herbal medicines.

Loss of Knowledge

The knowledge of traditional healers in remote Amazonian or Central American regions may have the potential to make a significant contribution to Western society. But few, if any, practitioners of these lesser known medical systems practice outside their native range, and those who still practice within these regions are elderly and often have not found younger disciples.

Loss of Plant Species of Potential Medicinal Value

This loss of knowledge from traditional healers comes at a time when native flora in many areas, especially tropical regions, are being destroyed at an alarming pace. In the United States alone, an estimated 10 percent of all species of flowering plants will be extinct by the year 2000, including an estimated 16 species of medicinally useful plants (Farnsworth et al., 1985).

One hopeful sign is that the U.S. Government recently formed a cooperative biodiversity group including representatives from NIH, the National Institute of Mental Health, the National Science Foundation (NSF), and the U.S. Agency for International Development. This group intends to fund research to locate and catalog medicinally active substances that can be analyzed and used for new pharmaceutical drug development, while working to preserve biological diversity in developing countries.

Use in Practice

Basic to the use of medicinal herbs in many societies is the practice of using whole, unrefined plant material. The material may be leaves, buds, flowers, bark, or roots, separately or in combination. In some cases an herbal remedy is a complex mixture of many plants. There is an age-old belief that whole-plant medicines have fewer dangerous side effects and provide a more balanced physiological action than plant-derived pharmaceutical drugs whose single ingredient has been isolated, concentrated, and packaged as a pill or liquid.

Herbs and herbal preparations generally are self-administered. Often they are purchased through native herbalists who prescribe one or more herbs or preparations on the basis of medical and health approaches that often include concepts of attaining balance in the client's body, psychology, and spirit (see the "Community-Based Medical Practices" section of the "Alternative Systems of Medical Practice" chapter). Consequently, it is often difficult to assess the relative value of herbal remedies versus prescription drugs on a one-to-one basis.

Indeed, herbal remedies of all types, including those from China, are composed of a multitude of ingredients whose interactions with the body are exceedingly complex. A high level of sophistication of research methodology is necessary to describe the interaction between the human body and substances as complex as those contained in many herbal remedies. Only recently has such a rigorous methodology begun to be developed. For example, the Chinese herb *Herba hedyotidis diffusae* (*bai hua she she cao*) has been shown clinically effective in the prevention and treatment of a variety of infectious diseases. However, it has not been demonstrated to have a significant inhibitory effect in vitro against any major pathogen. Only as techniques became available to test the immunological system did it become apparent that at least part of the herb's effect was due to its enhancement of the body's immune response (Bensky and Gamble, 1993).

Another complicating factor in researching traditional Chinese herbal medicine is the fact that Chinese medicine characteristically tries to treat the whole body to alleviate disease stemming from one body organ. Therefore, it rarely relies on a single herb to treat an illness. Instead, formulas usually contain 4 to 12 different herbs (Duke and Ayensu, 1985).

Beyond the problem of trying to test herbal preparations that may contain many active ingredients is the question of whether the research eventually will lead to the isolation of single active ingredients that can be packaged and sold separately. Intense debate surrounds the issue of how to conduct clinical trials of herbal medicines according to Western pharmaceutical clinical standards. Critics say there is an inherent problem with the single-active-ingredient approach preferred by pharmaceutical companies that are actively involved in herbal medicine research. The problem, they say, is that isolating a single compound may not be the most appropriate approach in situations where a plant's activity decreases on further fractionation (separation of active ingredients by using solvents) or where the plant contains two or three active ingredients that must be taken together to produce the full effect (Chaudhury, 1992). Beckstrom-Sternberg and Duke (1994) have documented several cases where synergy has been lost by using the single-ingredient approach to developing drugs from plants.

A good example of this single-active-ingredient versus whole-plant debate is illustrated by intense interest among pharmaceutical companies in the compound called genistein. Genistein is part of a class of compounds called flavonoids that occur naturally in plants such as kudzu, licorice, and red clover. Soybeans contain high concentrations of genistein, and lima beans reportedly are even higher in genistein than soybeans (Duke, 1993). There is increasing evidence that genistein may inhibit the growth of cancers of the stomach (Yanagihara et al., 1993), pancreas (Ura et al., 1993), liver (Mousavi and Adlercreutz, 1993), and prostate (Peterson and Barnes, 1993). Genistein is believed to inhibit the growth of cancers because of its antiangiogenetic properties (i.e., it prevents the growth of new blood vessels—a process known as angiogenesis—to tumors).

Genistein is being intensely studied as a possible preventive or treatment for breast cancer, which kills an estimated 44,000 women in the United States each year (Duke, 1993). Studies indicate a correlation between a high intake of foods containing genistein (soy products) and a low incidence of hormone-dependent cancers such as breast cancer (Hirayama, 1986) and prostate cancer (Baker, 1992). The growth of certain cancers, especially breast cancers, has been shown to depend on the female sex hormone estrogen. Genistein exhibits estrogenlike activity in plants and is often called a phytoestrogen. In humans it binds to estrogen receptors (Baker, 1992). It has been suggested that these phytoestrogens may compete with endogenous estrogen on the cellular level, further reducing the cellular proliferation and the potentially carcinogenic effects of estrogen (Tang and Adams, 1981). Thus, it may prevent the growth of estrogen-dependent cancer by competing for estrogen sites on the tumor cells.

If genistein is developed as an isolated pharmaceutical drug, it may have some action against cancer, but the purified compound may not be as potent as genistein in its natural state, and trials may give misleading results. The reason is that all plant species containing genistein also contain other flavonoid compounds, which may have synergistic effects when ingested with genistein. Formononetin—a precursor of equol, which also occurs with genistein—is said to be more active estrogenically than genistein (Spanu et al., 1993). Although genistein clearly inhibits angiogenesis, several other compounds are pseudoestrogens. With this in mind, the question arises: Is a mixture of genistein, formononetin, and other flavonoids, as occurs in many plants, more estrogenic (and antiangiogenic) than an equivalent quantity of any one of these components? If so, the herbal or dietary approach may make more sense than a genistein "silver bullet" approach.

Safety, Efficacy, and Appropriateness

Opinions about the safety, efficacy, and appropriateness of medicinal herbs vary widely among medical and health professionals in countries where herbal remedies are used. Some countries' professionals accept historical, empirical evidence as the only necessary criterion for herbal medicine's efficacy. Others would ban all herbal remedies as dangerous or of questionable value.

The problem is further complicated by the fact that many "patent medicines" available in world trade often are sold as herbal medicinal preparations when they include nonherbal substances. These nonherbal additives often include toxic metals (cinnabar, i.e., mercury) (Kang-Yum and Oransky, 1992), poisonous substances (powdered scorpion), or refined prescription drugs (Catlin et al., 1993). Usually labeled "Chinese herbal medicine," many of these products are manufactured in Thailand, Taiwan, or Hong Kong and exported to the United States, where they are sold in retail outlets. The California Department of Health Services, in conjunction with the Oriental Herbal Association, recently published a list of 20 popular Asian patent medicines (see app. E) that contain toxic ingredients.

Regulatory Issues

The increased use of plant medicines has potential for improving public health and lowering health care costs. Phytomedicines, if combined with the preventive model of medical practice, could be among the most cost-effective, practical ways to shift the focus of modern health care from disease treatment to prevention. But drug regulatory policy prevents the United States from taking advantage of these phytomedicines for two reasons. The first is the exorbitant expense involved in investigating each chemical compound in a given plant extract before it can be tested for clinical usefulness. Hence there is an urgent need to rework current research guidelines to allow the whole plant material or combination mixture (an herbal remedy containing more than one plant) to be evaluated instead of requiring separate evaluations of each chemical component of the therapeutic ingredients.

The second reason is that regulatory requirements for proof of safety and efficacy constitute an economic disincentive for private industry to conduct additional scientific studies. Relaxing regulatory requirements for efficacy for herbal products might make it economically feasible for more private companies to pursue research into issues of safety and quality control. Even with such regulatory change, some public funding of research is needed to confirm the remedies' validity. Public funds are needed because private industry has no incentive to develop an herbal product that might displace a patented drug from an approved treatment regime.

Recommendations

The Panel on Herbal Medicine recommends the following:

- OAM should hold a research organizational conference to facilitate planning in herbal medicine research. The conference would help to identify state-of-the-art questions in ethnomedical research, existing databases, and research personnel needed to support basic and clinical research needs in this area.
- Federal funding agencies such as NSF and NIH must begin to support the training of ethnobotanists—specifically in the field of ethnomedicine—and to offer funding opportunities to foster the rebirth of this field at U.S. universities and research institutions. This is a critical priority because much traditional knowledge in herbal remedies is in danger of disappearing, as are the plant species used in these systems of medicine.
- The bias against plant medicines must be eliminated by restructuring the requirements for proof of efficacy and concentrating on safety, and by removing the need for extensive analyses of chemically complex natural product medicines (thus eliminating the "monosubstance bias"). Several international regulatory models exist to guide the United States in this direction. For example, the German "Kommission E" (expert committee for herbal remedies) monographs give a good example of how the United States might simplify the approval of natural products without sacrificing safety or quality standards. (The "doctrine of reasonable certainty" that influences the approval of drugs under this system was previously mentioned.)

Adopting a more realistic standard of evidence for established plant medicines would eliminate much of the expense required for approval of new and unknown chemical drugs. Doing so would be similar to having standardized the crude drug senna leaf, used in the United States as an OTC laxative and documented for safety, effectiveness, and quality.

Another option might be to require pharmaceutical companies that are testing a plant-derived, single-ingredient pharmaceutical on a specific condition to demonstrate that it is more effective than the natural product. For example, before a patent could be issued to a pharmaceutical company for an isolated compound such as genistein, the company would first have to prove that the isolated compound is more effective than genistein consumed in context (as a food). But some market incentive, such as exclusive prescriptive marketing rights, might be needed to allow the pharmaceutical company to recoup its research costs.

- Legislative action may be required to restate FDA's mandate with respect to herbal products and traditional medications. The current regulatory mandate puts FDA in a difficult position. It is expected to "protect the public" but has no expertise or resources to evaluate the global herbal medicine inventory. If a crisis such as the contaminated tryptophan affair (see the "Diet and Nutrition" chapter) were to occur with a popular herbal product, FDA might attempt to prohibit the sale of medicinal herbs altogether. Instead of expecting FDA to be an omnipotent protector, Congress should legislate a more educational, informational role.

With respect to herbs used in popular health care, a proactive FDA role in establishing quality and safety standards would benefit the public and industry. A certification system for herbal content and potency of marketed products could be set up by FDA with USDA and the herbal industry. Such a system could draw on the existing global database and other countries' regulatory experiences. Participation in a voluntary product certification system would be a marketing advantage for ethical producers, allowing them, for example, to make a statement such as "This product meets U.S. government purity and potency standards." New statutory authority also would be necessary to establish a category that would allow traditional usages to be listed on labels according to criteria similar to WHO guidelines.

Finally, if herbal remedy producers were given the option to apply for specific health condition label indications based on new FDA phytomedicine standards, the United States would have the same three-tiered regulatory system adopted by other developed countries. Such a voluntary system would let consumers make intelligent personal choices about the use of medicinal herb products while mandating safety standards consistent with existing OTC practices for potentially toxic drugs such as aspirin and ibuprofen.

- OAM should review the TRAMIL approach, in which distinguished Caribbean botanists, chemists, ethnologists, and physicians review promising herbs and label them as reasonably safe and effective for people who cannot afford the prescription alternatives.

References

Ackerknecht, E.H. 1973. Therapeutics: from the Primitives to the Twentieth Century. Hafner Press, New York.

Akamasu, E. 1970. Modern Oriental Drugs. Yishiyakusha, Tokyo.

Artiges, A. 1991. What are the legal requirements for the use of phytopharmaceutical drugs in France? J. Ethnopharmacol. 32:231–234.

Arvigo, R., and M. Balick. 1993. Rainforest Remedies: 100 Healing Herbs of Belize. Lotus Press, Twin Lakes, Wis.

Baisi, F. 1987. Report on Clinical Trial of Bilberry Anthocyanocides in the Treatment of Venous Insufficiency in Pregnancy and of Postpartum Hemorrhoids. Presidio Ospedaliero di Livorno, Italy.

Baker, M.E. 1992. Evolution of regulation of steroid-mediated intercellular communication in vertebrates: insights from flavonoids, signals that mediate plant-rhizobia symbiosis. J. Steroid Biochem. Mol. Biol. 41(3–8):301–308.

Bauer, V., K. Jurcie, J. Puhlmann, and H. Wagner. 1988. Immunologische in-vivo und in-vitro untersuchungen mit echinacea-extrakten (Immunologic in vivo and in vitro studies on echinacea extracts). Arzneimittelforschung 38(2):276–281.

Beckstrom-Sternberg, S.M., and J.A. Duke. 1994. Potential for synergistic action of phytochemicals in spices. In G. Charalambous, ed. Spices, Herbs, and Edible Fungi. Elsevier Sciences B.V., New York.

Bedi, K.L., U. Zutshi, C.L. Chopra, and V. Amla. 1989. Picrorhiza kurroa, an Ayurvedic herb, may potentiate photochemotherapy in vitiligo. J. Ethnopharmacol. 27:347–352.

Bensky, D. and A. Gamble. 1993. Chinese Herbal Medicine: Materia Medica (revised edition). Eastland Press Inc., Seattle.

Bode, J.C., U. Schmidt, and H.K. Durr. 1977. Silymarin for the treatment of acute viral hepatitis? Med. Klin. 72:513–518.

Braunig, B., M. Dorn, Limburg, E. Knick, and Bausendorf. 1992. Echinacea purpureae radix for strengthening the immune response in flu-like infections. Zeitschrift für Phytotherapie 13:7–13.

Buchman, D.D. 1980. Herbal Medicine. Gramercy Publishing Company, New York.

Catlin, D.H., M. Sekera, and D.C. Adelman. 1993. Erythroderma associated with the ingestion of an herbal product. West. J. Med. 159:491–493.

Champpault, G., J.D. Patel, and A.M. Bonnard. 1984. A double-blind trial of an extract of the plant *Serenoo repens* in benign prostatic hyperplasia. Br. J. Clin. Pharmacol. 18(3):461–462.

Charles, V., and S.X. Charles. 1991. The use and efficacy of Adadirachta indica ADR (neem) and Curcuma longa (turmeric) in scabies. Tropical and Geographical Medicine (November):178–181.

Chaudhury, R.R. 1992. Herbal Medicine for Human Health. World Health Organization (SEARO, No. 20).

Chen, X. 1983. Protective and FFA metabolic effect of ginsenosides on myocardial ischemia. Journal of Medical Cell and Cardiology 25:121–123.

Chen, X., Q.Y. Zhu, L.Y. Li, and X.L. Tang. 1982. Effect of ginsenosides on cardiac performance and hemodynamics of dogs. Acta Pharmacologica Sinica 3:235–239.

Cheng, X.J., Y.L. Liu, G.F. Lin, and X.T. Luo. 1986. Comparison of action of Panax ginsenosides and Panax quinquonosides on anti-warm stress in mice. Journal of Shenyang College of Pharmacy 3(3):170–172.

Cheng, X.J., X.R. Shi, and B. Lin. 1988. Effects of ginseng root saponins on brain Ach and serum corticosterone in normobaric hypoxia stressed mice. Presented at the 5th Southeast Asian and Western Pacific Regional Meeting of Pharmacologists, Chinese Pharmacological Association, Beijing.

Chopra, R.N., and I.C. Chopra. 1959. A review of work on Indian medicinal plants. Indian Council of Medical Research Special Report Series No. 1, pp. 99, 107.

Coeugniet, E.G., and E. Elek. 1987. Immunomodulation with Viscum album and Echinacea purpurea extracts. Onkologie 10(3 Suppl.):27–33.

Corsi, S. 1987. Report on Trial of Bilberry Anthocyanosides (Tegens-inverni della beffa) in the Medical Treatment of Venous Insufficiency of the Lower Limbs. Casa di Cura S. Chiara, Florence, Italy.

Dahanukar, S.A., S.M. Karandikar, and M. Desai. 1984. Efficacy of Piper longum in childhood asthma. Indian Drugs 21:384–388.

Duke, J.A. 1986. Handbook of Northeastern Indian Medicinal Plants. Quarterman Press, Lincoln, Mass.

Duke, J.A. 1988. Handbook of Nuts. CRC Press, Inc., Boca Raton, Fla.

Duke, J.A. 1989. Ginseng: A Concise Handbook. Reference Publications Inc., Algonac, Mich.

Duke, J.A. 1992a. Handbook of Phytochemical Constituents of GRAS Herbs and Other Economic Plants. CRC Press, Inc., Boca Raton, Fla.

Duke, J.A. 1992b. Handbook of Biologically Active Phytochemicals and Their Activities. CRC Press, Inc., Boca Raton, Fla.

Duke, J. 1993. Lupinus perennis: hypotensive wildflower under hypertensive wires. Coltsfoot 14(6):4–5.

Duke, J.A., and E.S. Ayensu. 1985. Handbook of Medicinal Herbs. CRC Press, Inc., Boca Raton, Fla.

Duke, J.A., and R.V. Martinez. In press. Amazonian ethnobotanical dictionary. In Handbook of Ethnobotanicals (Peru). CRC Press, Inc., Boca Raton, Fla.

Dumont, E., E. Petit, T. Tarrade, and A. Nouvelot. 1992. UV-C irradiation-induced peroxidative degradation of microsomal fatty acids and proteins: protection by an extract of Ginkgo biloba (EGb 761). Free Radic. Biol. Med. 13(3):197–203.

EEC Directive 75/318/EEC as amended.

Fang, X., N. Shen, and B. Lin. 1986. Beneficial changes in prostacyclin and thromboxane A2 by ginsenosides in myocardial infarction and reperfusion of dogs. Acta Pharmacologica Sinica 7:226–230.

Farnsworth, N.R., O. Akerele, A.S. Bingel, D.D. Soejarta, and Z. Eno. 1985. Medicinal plants in therapy. Bull. World Health Organ. 63(6):965–981.

Farnsworth, N.R., and R.W. Morris. 1976. Higher plants: the sleeping giant of drug development. Am. J. Pharm. March/April:46.

Feher, H., et al. 1990. Hepaprotective activity of silymarin therapy in patients with chronic alcoholic liver disease. Orv. Hetil. 130:51.

Ferenci, P., B. Dragosics, H. Dittrick, et al. 1989. Randomized controlled trial of silymarin treatment in patients with cirrhosis of the liver. J. Hepatol. 9(1):105–113.

Flemming, K. 1971. Therapeutic effect of silymarin on x-irradiated mice. Arzneimittelforschung 21(9):1373–1375.

Foster, S. 1990. Ginkgo. American Botanical Council, Austin, Tex.

Gatta, L. 1982. Controlled Clinical Trial Among Patients Designed to Assess the Therapeutic Efficacy and Safety of Tegens 160. Ospedale Filippo del Ponte, Varese, Italy.

Gilhooley, M. 1989. Pharmaceutical drug regulation in China. Food Drug Cosmetic Law Journal 44:21–39.

Guerrini, M. 1987. Report on Clinical Trial of Bilberry Anthocyanosides in the Treatment of Venous Insufficiency of the Lower Limbs. Istituto di Patologia Speciale Medica e Metodologia Clinica, Universit de Siena, Italy.

Haas, H. 1981. Brain disorders and vasoactive substances of plant origin. Planta Med. (Suppl.):257–265.

Han, B.H., M.H. Park, L.K. Woo, W.S. Woo, and Y.N. Han. 1979. Studies on antioxidant components of Korean ginseng. Korean Biochemistry Journal 12(1):33.

Handbook of Domestic Medicine and Common Ayurvedic Remedies. 1979. Central Council for Research in Indian Medicine and Homeopathy, New Delhi, pp. 91–112.

Hirayama, T. 1986. Nutrition and cancer—a large scale cohort study. Prog. Clin. Biol. Res. 206:299–311.

Jacob, A., M. Pandey, S. Kapoor, and R. Saroja. 1988. Effect of the Indian gooseberry (amla) on serum cholesterol levels in men aged 35–55 years. Eur. J. Clin. Nutr. 42:939–944.

Kang-Yum, E., and S.H. Oransky. 1992. Chinese patent medicine as a source of mercury poisoning. Vet. Hum. Toxicol. 34(3):235–238.

Kao, F.F. 1992. The impact of Chinese medicine on America. Am. J. Chin. Med. 20(1):1–16.

Keller, K. 1991. Legal requirements for the use of phytopharmaceutical drugs in the Federal Republic of Germany. J. Ethnopharmacol. 32:225–229.

Kirkland, J., H.F. Mathews, C.W. Sullivan III, and K. Baldwin, eds. 1992. Herbal and Magic Medicine: Traditional Healing Today. Duke University Press, Durham, N.C., and London.

Kishore, P., P.N. Pandey, S.N. Pandey, and S. Dash. 1990. Preliminary trials of certain Ayurvedic drug formulation of Amalpitta. Sachitra Ayurved 33:40–45.

Kulkarni, R.R., P.S. Patki, V.P. Jog, S.G. Gandage, and B. Patwardhan. 1991. Treatment of osteoarthritis with a herbomineral formulation: a double-blind, placebo-controlled, cross-over study. J. Ethnopharmacol. 33:91–95.

Li, J.C., Y.P. Li, and L.S. Xue. 1988. Influence of ginseng saponins on the circadian rhythm in brain monoamine neurotransmitters. Presented at the 5th Southeast Asian and Western Pacific Regional Meeting of Pharmacologists, Chinese Pharmacological Association, Beijing.

Liu, C., and P. Xiao. 1992. Recent advances on ginseng research in China. J. Ethnopharmacol. 36:27–38.

Lu, G., X.J. Cheng, and W.X. Yuan. 1988. Effect of ginseng root saponins on serum corticosterene and neurotransmitters of hypobaric hypoxic mice. IRCS Med. Sc. Libr. Compend. 5(6):259.

Majno, G.M. 1975. Healing Hand: Man and Wound in the Ancient World. Harvard University Press, Cambridge, Mass.

Moerman, D.C. 1982. Geraniums for the Iroquois. A Field Guide to American Indian Medicinal Plants. Reference Publications, Algonac, Mich., 242 pp.

Mousavi, Y., and H. Adlercreutz. 1993. Genistein is an effective stimulator of sex hormone-binding globulin production in hepatocarcinoma human liver cancer cells and suppresses proliferation of these cells in culture. Steroids 58:301–304.

Nath, D., N. Sethi, R.K. Singh, and A.K. Jain. 1992. Commonly used Indian abortifacient plants with special reference to their teratologic effects in rats. J. Ethnopharmacol. 36:147–154.

Pandey, B.L., R.K. Goel, N.K.R. Pathak, M. Biswas, and P.K. Das. 1982. Effect of Tectona grandis linn. (common teak tree) on experimental ulcers and gastric secretion. Indian J. Med. Res. 76(Suppl.):89–94.

Pei, Y.Q. 1983. A review of pharmacology and clinical use of piperine and its derivatives. Epilepsia 24:177–181.

Perry, L.M. 1980. Medicinal Plants of East and Southeast Asia: Attributed Properties and Uses. MIT Press, Cambridge, Mass.

Peterson, G., and S. Barnes. 1993. Genistein and biochanin A inhibit the growth of human prostate cancer cells but not epidermal growth factor receptor tyrosine autophosphorylation. Prostate 22:335–345.

Qian, B.C., X.X. Zhang, B. Li, C.Y. Xu, and X.Y. Deng. 1987. Effects of ginseng polysaccharides on tumor and immunological function in tumor-bearing mice. Acta Pharmacologica Sinica 8:6–14.

Qu, J.B., Y.N. Cao, and X.Y. Ma. 1988. Effects of ginseng leaves and root saponins on animals in acute hypoxia due to negative air pressure. Presented at the 5th Southeast Asian and Western Pacific Regional Meeting of Pharmacologists, Chinese Pharmacological Association, Beijing.

Raabe, A., M. Raabe, and P. Ihm. 1991. Therapeutic follow-up using automatic perimetry in chronic cerebroretinal ischemia in elderly patients: prospective double-blind study with graduated dose Ginkgo biloba treatment (EGb 761). Klin. Monatsbl. Augenheilkd. 199(6):432–438.

Rai, G.S., C. Shovlin, and K.A. Wesnes. 1991. A double-blind, placebo-controlled study of Ginkgo biloba extract in elderly outpatients with mild to moderate memory impairment. Curr. Med. Res. Opin. 12(6):350–355.

Roesler, J., A. Emmendorffer, C. Stienmuller, B. Luettig, H. Wagner, and M.L. Lohmann-Matthes. 1991. Application of purified polysaccharides from cell cultures of the plant Echinacea purpurea to test subjects mediates activation of the phagocyte system. Int. J. Immunopharmacol. 13(7):931–941.

Schaffler, K., and P. Reeh. 1985. Long-term drug administration effects of Ginkgo biloba on the performance of healthy subjects exposed to hypoxia. In Effects of Ginkgo Biloba Extracts on Organic Cerebral Impairment. Eurotext Ltd., London.

Shen, J.J., Y.Y. Jin, Y.S. Wu, and X. Zhou. 1987. Effects of ginseng saponins on ^{14}C-arachidonic acid metabolism in rabbit platelets. Acta Pharmaceutica Sinica 22:166–169.

Shukla, A.K. 1984. Endocrine Response of Certain Species on Albino Rats (doctoral thesis). Banaras Hindu University, Varanasi, India.

Snider, S. 1991. Beware the unknown brew: herbal teas and toxicity. FDA Consumer (May):31–33.

Solecki, R.S. 1975. Shanidar IV, a Neanderthal flower burial of northern Iraq. Science 190:880.

Spanu, F., A. Tava, L. Pacetti, and E. Piano. 1993. Variability of oestrogenic isoflavone content in a collection of subterranean clover from Sicily. Journal of Genetics and Breeding 47:27–34.

Stimpel, M., A. Proksch, H. Wagner, and M.L. Lohmann-Matthes. 1984. Macrophage activation and induction of macrophage cytotoxicity by purified polysaccharide fractions from the plant Echinacea purpurea. Infect. Immun. 46(3):845–849.

Sumathikutty, M.A., K. Rajaraman, B. Sankarikutty, and A.G. Mathew. 1979. Chemical composition of pepper grades and products. Journal of Food Science and Technology 16:249–254.

Swanston-Flatt, S.K., C. Day, P.R. Flott, et al. 1989. Glycemic effects of traditional European plant treatments for diabetes: studies in normal and streptozotocin diabetic mice. Diabetes Res. 10(2):69–73.

Taillandier, J. 1988. Ginkgo biloba extract in the treatment of cerebral disorders due to aging. In E.W. Funfgeld, ed. Rokan (Ginkgo Biloba): Recent Results in Pharmacology and Clinic. Springer-Verlag, Berlin.

Tang, B.Y., and N.R. Adams. 1981. Oestrogen receptors and metabolic activity in the genital tract after ovariectomy of ewes with permanent infertility caused by exposure to phytoestrogens. J. Endocrinol. 89(3):365–370.

Teglio, L. 1987. Quad. Clin. Ostet. Ginecol. 42:221.

Tong, L.S., and C.Y. Chao. 1980. Effects of ginsengoside Rg1 of Panax ginseng on mitosis in human blood lymphocytes in vitro. Am. J. Chem. Med. 8(3):254.

Tsumura, A. 1991. Kampo, How the Japanese Updated Traditional Herbal Medicine. Japan Publications, Inc., Tokyo and New York.

Upadhyaya, S.D., C.M. Kansal, and N.N. Pandey. 1982. Clinical evaluation of Piper longum on patients of bronchial asthma—a preliminary study. Nagarjuna 25:256–258.

Ura, H., T. Obara, K. Okamura, and M. Namiki. 1993. Growth inhibition of pancreatic cancer cells by flavonoids. Gan To Kagaku Ryoho 20(13):2083–2085.

Varkonyi, T. 1971. Brain edema in the rat induced by triethyltin sulfate. 10 Effect of silymarin on the electron-microscopy picture. Arzneimittelforschung 21(1):148–149.

Verma, S.K., and A. Bordia. 1988. Effect of Commiphora mucul (gum guggul) in patients with hyperlipidemia with special reference to HDL cholesterol. Indian J. Med. Res. 87:356–360.

Vogel, V.L. 1970. American Indian Medicine. University of Oklahoma Press, Norman, Okla.

Wagner, H., B. Geyer, Y. Kiso, H. Hikino, and G.S. Rao. 1986. Coumestans as the main active principles of the liver drugs Eclipta alba and Wedelia calendulacea. Planta Med.:370–377.

Wall Street Journal. 1993. Vital statistics: disputed cost of creating a drug. November 9.

Wang, B.X., J.C. Cui, and A.J. Lui. 1980. The effect of polysaccharides of root of Panax ginseng on the immune function. Acta Pharmaceutica Sinica 17:312–320.

Weitbrecht, W.V., and W. Jansen. 1985. Doubleblind and comparative (Ginkgo biloba versus placebo) therapeutic study in geriatric patients with primary degenerative dementia—a preliminary evaluation. In A. Agnoli et al., eds. Effects of Ginkgo Biloba Extract on Organic Cerebral Impairment. John Libbey Eurotext Ltd., London.

Witte, S., I. Anadere, and E. Walitza. 1992. Improvement of hemorheology with Ginkgo biloba extract: decreasing a cardiovascular risk factor. Fortschr. Med. 110(13):247–250.

World Health Organization. 1991. Guidelines for the Assessment of Herbal Medicines. Programme on Traditional Medicines, Geneva.

Yabe, T., M. Chat, E. Malherbe, and P.P. Vidal. 1992. Effects of Ginkgo biloba extract (EGb 761) on the guinea pig vestibular system. Pharmacol. Biochem. Behav. 42(4):595–604.

Yanagihara, K., A. Ito, T. Toge, and M. Numoto. 1993. Antiproliferative effects of isoflavones on human cancer cell lines established from the gastrointestinal tract. Cancer Res. 53(23):5815–5821.

Yang, Y., Z. Chen, G. Luo, and Y. Zhang. 1988. The mechanism of inhibitory effects of panaxadiol saponin on rabbit platelet aggregation. Presented at the 5th Southeast Asian and Western Pacific Regional Meeting of Pharmacologists, Chinese Pharmacological Association, Beijing.

Youngken, H.W. 1950. A Textbook of Pharmacognosy. McGraw-Hill, New York.

Yuan, W.X., X.J. Wu, and F.X. Yang. 1988. Effects of ginseng root saponins on brain monoamine and serum corticosterone in heat stressed mice. Presented at the 5th Southeast Asian and Western Pacific Regional Meeting of Pharmacologists, Chinese Pharmacological Association, Beijing.

Zhang, F.L., and X. Chen. 1987. Effects of ginsenosides on sympathetic neurotransmitter release in pithed rats. Acta Pharmacologica Sinica 8:217–220.

Zhang, F.L., A.G. Meehan, and M.J. Rand. 1988. Effects of ginsenosides on noradrenergic transmission, histamine response and calcium influx in rabbit ear isolated artery. Presented at the 5th Southeast Asian and Western Pacific Regional Meeting of Pharmacologists, Chinese Pharmacological Association, Beijing.

Zhang, J.T. 1989. Progress of research on three kinds of anti-aging drugs. Information of the Chinese Pharmacological Society 6(3–4):4.

Diet and Nutrition in the Prevention and Treatment of Chronic Disease

PANEL MEMBERS

Gar Hildenbrand—Chair
Jonathan Collin, M.D.
Alan Gaby, M.D.
Marie Galbraith
Daniel Kanofsky, M.D., M.P.H.
Janet Smith
Jack Taylor, D.C.

CONTRIBUTING AUTHORS

Roberta Baer, Ph.D.
Claire Cassidy, Ph.D.
Lilian Cheung, Sc.D.
Harriett Harvey
Gar Hildenbrand
L. John Hoffer, M.D., C.M., Ph.D.
J. Daniel Kanofsky, M.D., M.P.H.
Lawrence H. Kushi, Sc.D.
Mildred Seelig, M.D., M.P.H.
James P. Swyers, M.A.
Walter Willett, M.D., Dr.P.H.

Introduction

Status of Diet and Nutrition Research in the United States

Diet and nutrition research goes on in almost every medical school, university, and pharmaceutical laboratory throughout the world. Thus, the knowledge of how to prevent illness and maintain health through nutrition grows every year. However, for such areas as reversing the effects of chronic disease through dietary or nutritional intervention or determining levels of nutrients required to achieve optimal metabolic or immune system functioning, there often is no critical mass of researchers or funds to follow up promising initial experimental results.

In fact, the history of nutrition research is marked by examples where, for one reason or another, preliminary reports of a positive therapeutic effect of a certain vitamin, mineral, or nutritional manipulation appear but are often not followed up by the overwhelming majority of the medical community. In cases where such therapies eventually are proven to be safe and effective, it is sometimes not until years or even decades after the initial reports. The result is that many individuals may die or suffer needlessly, while effective interventions are available but not yet validated.

For example, in the 1930s, Australian psychiatrist John Cade began a series of crude experiments on guinea pigs in which he injected them with the urine of psychiatric patients to test his hypothesis that mania—a mood disorder characterized by, among other things, periods of euphoria—might represent a state of intoxication resulting from an excess of some commonly occurring metabolite. Depression, on the other hand, might represent the effects of abnormally low levels of the same metabolite (Johnson, 1984). Although all the urine samples proved toxic to the guinea pigs—Cade traced the toxicity to the urea component of the urine—the urine from the manic patients was far more toxic than urine from the schizophrenic or depressive patients.

In his attempts to find out what was increasing the toxicity of the urea in the manic patients' urine, Cade happened upon the compound lithium citrate, which he eventually began injecting

Helpful Definitions for Reading This Chapter:

antioxidant: A compound that prevents oxidation of substances, particularly lipids, in food or in the body. Antioxidants are especially important in preventing the oxidation of polyunsaturated lipids in the membranes of cells. An antioxidant is able to donate electrons to electron-seeking compounds such as free radicals (see below). This in turn reduces electron capture and, thus, breakdown of unsaturated fatty acids and other cell components by oxidizing agents.

atherosclerosis: A buildup of fatty material in the arteries, including those in the heart.

carbohydrate: A compound containing carbon, hydrogen, and oxygen atoms; most are known as sugars, starches, and dietary fiber.

diet: All of the foods a person consumes either on a daily basis or on average over a period of time.

enzyme: A compound, usually a protein, that speeds the rate of a chemical reaction but is not altered by the chemical reaction.

epidemiology: The study of the occurrence, cause, and prevention of disease and death in human populations.

fatty acid: A principal component of fats and oils. A fatty acid is composed of a chain of carbon and hydrogen atoms with an acid group at one end. Examples include stearic acid (a saturated fatty acid), oleic acid (a monounsaturated fatty acid), and linoleic acid (a polyunsaturated fatty acid).

free radical: Short-lived form of compounds with an unpaired electron in the outer electron shell. Because free radicals have an electron-seeking nature, they can be very destructive to electron-dense areas of cells, such as DNA and cell membranes.

lipid: A compound containing an abundance of carbon and hydrogen, little oxygen, and sometimes other atoms. Lipids include fats, oils, and cholesterol.

lipoprotein: A compound found in the bloodstream containing a core of lipids with a shell of protein, phospholipid, and cholesterol.

macronutrients: Compounds, such as fats, proteins, and carbohydrates, that must be broken down or metabolized by the body to obtain energy or basic building material.

micronutrients: Minerals and vitamins that are required for proper functioning of the body. These often act as cofactors or coenzymes in enzymatic processes.

myocardial infarction: Death of part of the heart muscle due to a heart attack.

nutrients: Chemical substances in food that nourish the body by providing energy, building materials, and factors to regulate needed chemical reactions in the body.

nutrition: The biological science of nutrition includes the processes by which the organism ingests, digests, absorbs, transports, metabolizes, and excretes food substances. Nutrition as a science and discipline also includes areas such as food policy, dietary behaviors, agricultural practices, cultural and anthropological aspects of food, etc.

prospective studies: Studies in which subjects are enrolled prior to their having developed the endpoint (i.e., condition or disease) of interest, and they are often followed until they develop such endpoints. Examples of prospective studies include clinical trials, in which some study subjects are given an investigator-imposed intervention, and cohort or panel studies, which usually do not include investigator-imposed intervention.

retrospective studies: Studies undertaken to determine whether those with and without a particular disease or condition differ according to past exposures. Examples of such studies include case-control studies and retrospective cohort studies.

by itself into the guinea pigs to judge its effect. To his amazement, the guinea pigs became lethargic and unresponsive for several hours after receiving lithium, before fully recovering. In 1949, Cade published the results of a crude clinical trial, stating that lithium salts given to 10 manic patients resulted in a dramatic improvement in each one's condition (Cade, 1949). Unfortunately for Cade, just as his results were reaching the United States, a number of table salt substitutes containing lithium chloride had just been recalled by the Food and Drug Administration (FDA) due to toxic side effects and, in some cases, death with heavy use. So much publicity was given to the toxicity associated with these salt substitutes—which were marketed for use by people on salt-restricted diets—that for 5 years after Cade's original report, relatively little work with lithium was undertaken (Georgotas and Gershon, 1981).

According to medical historian Frederick Johnson (1984), "Cade's report of lithium treatment of mania might well have succumbed to the same fate as that suffered by many proposed therapeutic techniques before and after that time ... had lithium salts been at all expensive or hard to come by...." Instead, because canisters of lithium salts were to be found in most hospitals and pharmacies at the time, many psychiatrists in the mid-1950s, for lack of adequate treatments for manic disorders, simply started experimenting with lithium on their own. By the mid-1960s, a spate of reports appeared in the medical literature reporting on the effectiveness of lithium in the treatment of manic and other psychiatric disorders (Gershon and Yuwiler, 1960; Schlagenhauf et al., 1966). Today lithium, in some patients with bipolar disorders (i.e., mood swings), is the most successful therapeutic drug of the five major types of drugs currently used in psychiatry (Horrobin, 1990), often producing normalization in acute mania patients in 1 to 3 weeks.

A situation analogous to the lithium story occurred in the late 1980s in the United States. Just as reports were emerging that suggested the effectiveness of the amino acid L-tryptophan in treating mild depression (Boman, 1988), chronic insomnia (Demisch et al., 1987), and mood disorders (Maurizi, 1988), there was a severe outbreak of a sometimes deadly inflammatory disorder called eosinophilia myalgia syndrome (EMS). The cause of the EMS outbreak was linked by epidemiologists to the over-the-counter use of tryptophan (Varga et al., 1993). Although all cases of this disorder were eventually found to be caused by contaminants in batches of tryptophan produced by a single manufacturer in Japan (Barnhart et al., 1990) and not by the effects of tryptophan itself, this nutritional supplement was taken off the market by the FDA and is no longer available over the counter. Just as with lithium, the publicity about toxicities associated with tryptophan may have hindered rational scientific discourse about the effectiveness of this nutritional therapy for some time to come. In fact, FDA uses the tryptophan example to justify its efforts to regulate as drugs most dietary and nutritional supplements whose manufacturers make any health claims (U.S. Food and Drug Administration, 1992).

There have been numerous other instances in recent decades when individuals or groups of individuals have advocated nutritional interventions or alternative dietary lifestyles as a means of preventing or even treating disease and have met not only indifference but often hostility. This was especially true for those advocating vegetarianism or an extremely low-fat diet as a means of preventing or treating illnesses such as heart disease (see below). As was the case with John Cade and lithium, it took many decades for the facts to win out over misconceptions and biases.

The rest of this chapter discusses a number of areas of diet and nutrition research in which there is at least preliminary scientific evidence indicating the need for more in-depth studies, but for which there often is no critical mass of researchers or funds to follow up promising initial experimental results. However, it should be noted that only an overview of the field is presented, and it is by no means comprehensive. This field of research is so complex and diverse that no more than a few examples can be offered for each subsection.

First, however, it is instructive to discuss briefly the evolution of the modern affluent diet and evidence relating chronic disease with its excesses and micronutrient deficiencies. Also presented is a discussion of the evolution of present dietary guidelines and why some consider them inadequate.

Evolution of the Modern "Affluent" Diet

Over the course of evolution, human beings (and their primate predecessors) adapted gradually to a wide range of naturally occurring foods, but the types of food and mix of nutrients (in terms of carbohydrates, fats, and proteins) remained relatively constant. Food supplies were often precarious, and the threat of death from starvation was a constant preoccupation for most of the Earth's inhabitants.

About 12,000 years ago, an agricultural revolution brought profound dietary changes to many human populations. The ability to produce and store foods became widespread, and some foods, such as grains, were preferentially cultivated. These new techniques and the overabundance of some foods they produced presented novel challenges to the human digestive system.

The Industrial Revolution, which began about 200 years ago in Europe and soon spread to North America, introduced more radical changes in the human diet due to advances in food production, processing, storage, and distribution. Recent technological innovations, along with increased material well-being, or affluence, and lifestyles that have allowed people more freedom in deciding what and when they wish to eat (amplified by modern marketing techniques), have led to even further major dietary changes in developed countries. Indeed, such innovations as sugared breakfast cereals and a variety of snack items were unheard of before World War II; Hampe and Wittenberg (1964) estimated that 60 percent of the items on supermarket shelves in 1960 came into existence in the 15 years following World War II.

Health Consequences of the Modern Affluent Diet

Because changes in the dietary patterns of the more technologically developed countries, such as the United States, have been so dramatic and rapid, the people consuming these affluent diets have had little time to adapt biologically to the types and quantities of food available to them today. The longer term adverse health effects of the affluent diets prevailing in these countries—characterized by an excess of energy-dense foods rich in animal fat, partially hydrogenated vegetable oils, and refined carbohydrates but lacking in whole grains, fruits, and vegetables—have become apparent only in recent decades.

Comparisons of population groups have demonstrated a close and consistent relationship between the adoption of this affluent diet and the emergence of a range of chronic, noninfectious diseases, such as coronary heart disease, cerebrovascular disease, various cancers, diabetes mellitus, gallstones, dental caries (cavities), gastrointestinal disorders, and various bone and joint diseases (World Health Organization, 1990). Some nutrition and health experts believe that the relationship between rapid changes in a population's diet and rapidly changing disease and mortality profiles is reflected in many recently acculturated (i.e., adapted to the dominant culture) groups in the United States who are now eating a diet more akin to that of the northern European and U.S. general populations (see the sidebar on page 214).

For example, increasing rates of diabetes mellitus have been reported in Native American and other populations that suddenly switch from a traditional to a more modern lifestyle (West, 1974). This disease has only recently become a major health problem for Native Americans, who now often have rates much higher than those found in either U.S. Caucasian or African-American populations. Indeed, although the overall rate of diabetes in the general U.S. population is between 1 and 3 percent, and 5 to 6 percent for those over age 35, it ranges from 10 to 50 percent among Pima Indians 35 years of age and older (Bennett et al., 1979; Neel, 1976). Furthermore, in Hawaii, the incidence of breast cancer for Caucasians is similar to U.S. mainland rates, but the incidence among Hawaii's Japanese population is more than twice the rate in Japan and approaches the rate for Caucasians (Muir et al., 1987).

The reasons for these abnormally high disease rates in American Indian and other non-Caucasian populations are complex; however, they include obesity related to changes in activity patterns and, probably, the increased consumption of refined carbohydrates and sugar. Also, intake of dietary fiber has decreased dramatically. Excessive caloric consumption in some of these populations also may be a major contributor; one study found that obese American Indians consumed 250 to 1,600 more calories than were recommended for persons of their height, gender, age, and level of activity (Joos, 1984).

In one of the few studies of its kind, a group of Native Hawaiians with multiple risk factors for cardiovascular disease believed to be related to consuming a nontraditional diet were placed on a "pre-Western contact," or traditional, Hawaiian diet to assess its effect on obesity and cardiovascular risk factors. Twenty individuals were placed on a diet low in fat (7 percent), high in complex carbohydrates (78 percent), and moderate in protein (15 percent) for 21 days. The subjects were encouraged to eat as much as they wanted. At the end of the diet modification period, the average weight loss was 7.8 kilograms (approximately 17 lbs.), and the average serum cholesterol dropped by about 14 percent. Blood pressure decreased an average of 11.5 mm Hg systolic and 8.9 mm Hg diastolic (Shintani et al., 1991).

Evolution of Federal Dietary Guidelines

Due to the rapid rise in chronic illness related to diet in recent decades, the focus of nutrition research has shifted from eliminating nutritional deficiency resulting from undernutrition to dealing with chronic diseases caused by nutritional excess, or "overnutrition." Since the 1950s, researchers have identified a number of types of dietary excess that appear to influence the incidence and course of specific chronic diseases.

Another growing concern among nutrition researchers is the accumulation of evidence indicating that inadequate intakes of some micronutrients over a long time may increase the risk of developing a variety of disease conditions, including coronary heart disease, many cancers, cataracts, and birth defects. Earlier, many of these conditions were not even considered diet-related. Furthermore, many other components of foods, in addition to those traditionally considered nutrients, may be important in achieving optimal health. Unfortunately, the "standard" American diet, while rich in calories, contains processed foods deficient in many important micronutrients and other components of the original unrefined foods.

The Federal Government has been involved in developing nutrition guidelines for the American public since the mid-1800s, when the U.S. Department of Agriculture (USDA) was established. However, such guidelines traditionally had dealt with how to prevent nutritional deficiencies, as well as how to promote the consumption of U.S. agricultural products. Only in the past several decades, as the focus of public health policy has shifted from preventing disease caused by nutritional deficiencies to preventing disease caused by overnutrition or nutritional imbalances, have Federal dietary guidelines attempted to address the latter. Today, such guidelines are becoming more difficult to develop and often meet fierce resistance from various lobbying groups when they are disseminated (Nestle, 1993).

Nevertheless, since the early 1970s, USDA and other Federal agencies and advisory groups have periodically released diet and nutrition guidelines dealing with preventing chronic illness related to nutrition. This material typically targets public health policymakers, medical doctors, or the general public. Two of the better known current Federal dietary and nutritional guidelines, from which public health policy is made, are the recommended daily allowances (RDAs) and the Food Guide Pyramid.

RDAs are defined as the average daily amounts of essential nutrients estimated, on the basis of available scientific knowledge, as adequate to meet the physiological needs of practically all healthy persons (Monsen, 1990). (See figure 1.) To establish the standards for RDAs, which are updated periodically (most recently with the 10th edition in 1989; see Monsen, 1990), the Food and Nutrition Board of the National Academy of Sciences critically evaluates the literature on human requirements for each nutrient, examines the individual variability of requirements, and tries to estimate the efficiency with which the nutrients are biologically available and used from foods consumed. The RDAs are levels that should be reached as averages in a period of several days, not necessarily daily.

RDAs are *not* meant to be guidelines for consumers; they were initially designed to serve as standards for planning food supplies for population groups (National Research Council, 1989). However, they are used as a partial basis for the development of other guidelines that *are* intended for consumers, such as the Food Guide Pyramid, which was released by USDA in 1992 to replace the old "basic four" food groups. The Food Guide Pyramid is designed to give consumers information on how to eat a "balanced" diet that will provide them with the RDAs for essential nutrients while lowering their risks of chronic illness due to nutritional excesses (*Journal of the American Dietetic Association*, 1992). Sweets, fats, and oily foods are at the top of the pyramid, indicating that they should be consumed in small amounts. Dairy products such as milk, yogurt, and cheese, and meats, poultry, fish, dried beans, eggs, and nuts are just below, indicating they should be consumed in moderation. Fruits and vegetables follow; bread, cereal, rice, and pasta are at the bottom of the pyramid,

Figure 1. Food and Nutrition Board, National Academy of Sciences—National Research Council Recommended Dietary Allowances,[a] Revised 1989

Designed for the maintenance of good nutrition of practically all healthy people in the United States

							Fat-Soluble Vitamins				Water-Soluble Vitamins							Minerals						
Category	Age (years) or Condition	Weight[b] (kg)	Weight[b] (lb)	Height[b] (cm)	Height[b] (in)	Protein (g)	Vitamin A (μg RE)[c]	Vitamin D (μg)[d]	Vitamin E (mg α-TE)[e]	Vitamin K (μg)	Vitamin C (mg)	Thiamin (mg)	Riboflavin (mg)	Niacin (mg NE)[f]	Vitamin B_6 (mg)	Folate (μg)	Vitamin B_{12} (μg)	Calcium (mg)	Phosphorus (mg)	Magnesium (mg)	Iron (mg)	Zinc (mg)	Iodine (μg)	Selenium (μg)
Infants	0.0–0.5	6	13	60	24	13	375	7.5	3	5	30	0.3	0.4	5	0.3	25	0.3	400	300	40	6	5	40	10
	0.5–1.0	9	20	71	28	14	375	10	4	10	35	0.4	0.5	6	0.6	35	0.5	600	500	60	10	5	50	15
Children	1–3	13	29	90	35	16	400	10	6	15	40	0.7	0.8	9	1.0	50	0.7	800	800	80	10	10	70	20
	4–6	20	44	112	44	24	500	10	7	20	45	0.9	1.1	12	1.1	75	1.0	800	800	120	10	10	90	20
	7–10	28	62	132	52	28	700	10	7	30	45	1.0	1.2	13	1.4	100	1.4	800	800	170	10	10	120	30
Males	11–14	45	99	157	62	45	1,000	10	10	45	50	1.3	1.5	17	1.7	150	2.0	1,200	1,200	270	12	15	150	40
	15–18	66	145	176	69	59	1,000	10	10	65	60	1.5	1.8	20	2.0	200	2.0	1,200	1,200	400	12	15	150	50
	19–24	72	160	177	70	58	1,000	10	10	70	60	1.5	1.7	19	2.0	200	2.0	1,200	1,200	350	10	15	150	70
	25–50	79	174	176	70	63	1,000	5	10	80	60	1.5	1.7	19	2.0	200	2.0	800	800	350	10	15	150	70
	51+	77	170	173	68	63	1,000	5	10	80	60	1.2	1.4	15	2.0	200	2.0	800	800	350	10	15	150	70
Females	11–14	46	101	157	62	46	800	10	8	45	50	1.1	1.3	15	1.4	150	2.0	1,200	1,200	280	15	12	150	45
	15–18	55	120	163	64	44	800	10	8	55	60	1.1	1.3	15	1.5	180	2.0	1,200	1,200	300	15	12	150	50
	19–24	58	128	164	65	46	800	10	8	60	60	1.1	1.3	15	1.6	180	2.0	1,200	1,200	280	15	12	150	55
	25–50	63	138	163	64	50	800	5	8	65	60	1.1	1.3	15	1.6	180	2.0	800	800	280	15	12	150	55
	51+	65	143	160	63	50	800	5	8	65	60	1.0	1.2	13	1.6	180	2.0	800	800	280	10	12	150	55
Pregnant						60	800	10	10	65	70	1.5	1.6	17	2.2	400	2.2	1,200	1,200	320	30	15	175	65
Lactating	1st 6 months					65	1,300	10	12	65	95	1.6	1.8	20	2.1	280	2.6	1,200	1,200	355	15	19	200	75
	2nd 6 months					62	1,200	10	11	65	90	1.6	1.7	20	2.1	260	2.6	1,200	1,200	340	15	16	200	75

[a]The allowances, expressed as average daily intakes over time, are intended to provide for individual variations among most normal persons as they live in the United States under usual environmental stresses. Diets should be based on a variety of common foods in order to provide other nutrients for which human requirements have been less well defined. See text for detailed discussion of allowances and of nutrients not tabulated.

[b]Weights and heights of Reference Adults are actual medians for the U.S. population of the designated age, as reported by NHANES II. The median weights and heights of those under 19 years of age were taken from Hamill et al. (1979) (see pages 16–17). The use of these figures does not imply that the height-to-weight ratios are ideal.

[c]Retinol equivalents. 1 retinol equivalent = 1 μg retinol or 6 μg β-carotene. See text for calculation of vitamin A activity of diets as retinol equivalents.

[d]As cholecalciferol. 10 μg cholecalciferol = 400 IU of vitamin D.

[e]α-Tocopherol equivalents. 1 mg d-α tocopherol = 1 α-TE. See text for variation in allowances and calculation of vitamin E activity of the diet as α-tocopherol equivalents.

[f]1 NE (niacin equivalent) is equal to 1 mg of niacin or 60 mg of dietary tryptophan.

indicating that they should be consumed in rather large amounts in comparison with the foods at the top of the pyramid (see figure 2).

Guidelines such as the Food Guide Pyramid are intended to inform consumers, as well as public health policymakers, about what kinds and amounts of certain foods are best suited for maintaining health and lowering the risks of nutrition-related illnesses. Generally, this approach to affecting health through diet and nutrition interventions involves manipulating the "typical," or mainstream, diet so that foods with less nutritional value are eaten less and foods with more nutritional value are eaten more.

The Federal Government's approach to dietary intervention, which has been formulated over the years by boards composed of nutrition scientists, generally does not recommend supplementing this "typical" diet with vitamins or nutritional supplements (National Research Council, 1989). It also does not take a "good food" or "bad food" approach (Herron, 1991) or suggest that certain foods are "off limits" because of their propensity to cause chronic disease (Nestle, 1993).

However, this is only one approach to promoting health and preventing illness through dietary intervention. There are many "alternative" dietary approaches that contend that no matter how much one manipulates the typical American diet, it is not enough to promote *optimal* health or stave off eventual chronic illness. Alternative approaches represent a continuum of philosophies, from the idea that diet supplementation somewhat beyond RDAs is necessary to promote optimal health to the idea that supplementation well above RDAs is often required to treat some chronic disorders. Further along this continuum is the approach advocating drastic modification of patients' diets—either completely eliminating or adding certain types of foods—to treat specific types of conditions, such as cancer and cardiovascular disease. Finally, there is the approach that promotes eating a less refined,

Figure 2. The Food Guide Pyramid

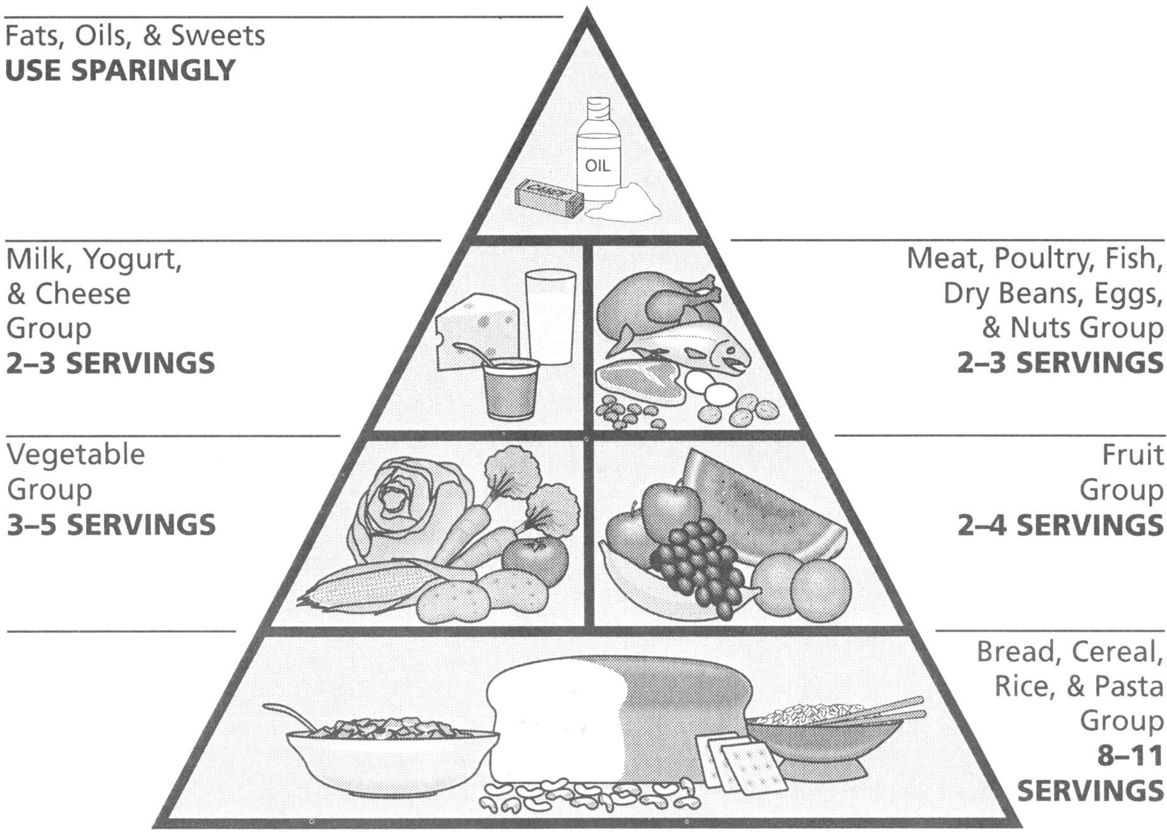

Source: U.S. Department of Agriculture and U.S. Department of Health and Human Services, 1990.

more "naturalistic" diet as the only way to promote optimal health and prevent illness. This last approach holds that staples of the typical American diet (e.g., meat and dairy products) are basically unhealthful and should be avoided altogether. The remainder of this chapter describes representative alternative therapies along this continuum.

Alternative Approaches to Diet and Nutrition That May Prevent or Control Chronic Illness as Well as Promote Health

The Use of Vitamins and Other Nutritional Supplements in the Prevention of Chronic Disease

Vitamins are organic substances required by all living organisms for healthy life and growth. Among their many properties, vitamins function as coenzymes (helpers to the primary enzyme) in metabolic reactions. Higher animals, particularly humans, cannot synthesize vitamins and therefore must ingest them as part of their diet. Deficiency in a particular vitamin results in a specific vitamin deficiency disease, such as rickets (a bone deformity from lack of vitamin D) and scurvy (the infamous sailors' deficiency disease of old, caused by lack of vitamin C-containing fruits and vegetables on sailing ships). Each type of deficiency disease is typically characterized by a "classic" set of symptoms.

Vitamins of the B complex and vitamin C are water soluble (i.e, they dissolve readily in water). The B complex vitamins are found in food sources such as whole wheat bread, fruits, green and yellow leafy plants, and animal sources such as eggs, dairy products, and liver. They include B_1 (thiamine), B_2 (riboflavin), B_3 (nicotinic acid, or niacin), pantothenic acid, B_6 (pyridoxine), biotin, folic acid, and B_{12}. Certain other substances, such as choline, also may be considered as belonging to the B complex. Vitamin C (ascorbic acid) is present in certain fruits and green vegetables.

All the remaining vitamins (A, D, E, and K) are fat, or lipid, soluble (i.e., they dissolve more readily in oil than in water). Vitamin A (in the form of carotenoids) occurs naturally in green leafy and yellow vegetables; spinach, collards, kale, chard, carrots, and sweet potatoes are particularly good sources. Vitamin E (tocopherol) is found in many plant oils, such as corn oil. In adults vitamin K is supplied by intestinal bacteria.

The Standard American Diet

The mainstream, or "standard," American diet, which is one of the world's most affluent diets, is derived primarily from the traditions of the British and German cultures. The British tradition emphasizes meat and bread. These staples traditionally form the core of the meal, with vegetables serving as side dishes and fruits either eaten as snacks between meals or mixed with wheat, milk, and eggs to form a sweet pudding, pie, or cake, which is called a "dessert" (Kittler and Sucher, 1989).

The German tradition emphasizes dairy foods, especially milk and cheese (Kittler and Sucher, 1989). Pork is a staple for Germans and is the second most important red meat for Americans, who like it in every form from roast to "lunchmeat" (cold cuts) to sausages and bacon. Two core American meat-and-grain foods are actually of German origin: hamburgers and frankfurters (or wieners) (Yoder, 1981).

A number of other minerals and nutrients, such as iron, calcium, magnesium, selenium, and zinc, have been found essential for preventing deficiency diseases. For example, magnesium, which is required for the activation of more than 300 enzymes in the body and for the use of some vitamins and minerals, is required for normal function and structure of the arteries, heart, kidneys, and bone (Seelig, 1980), and for the neuromuscular system (Durlach, 1988; Galland, 1991). There also are a number of "essential" amino acids and fats (that is, humans cannot synthesize them). Some other amino acids are considered "semiessential" because humans cannot synthesize them fast enough to meet metabolic needs.

Research base. The relatively few studies that have explicitly investigated the role of vitamin and mineral supplements in promoting health and preventing disease have generally found benefits from the supplements. In fact, evidence is increasing rapidly for a beneficial role of supplementation with a number of nutrients, including vitamins B_6, C, and E; beta-carotene and other carotenes; folic acid; calcium; magnesium; and other factors. Although there is little dispute about the importance and functions of many vitamins and nutrients, questions arise regarding the levels necessary to produce optimum health. Many contend that the optimal levels of these compounds can be obtained in a normal diet and that the effect of additional amounts is negligible (National Research Council, 1989). To answer such questions, it is first necessary to compare some nutrient levels in the typical American diet with current RDAs as well as with what some now consider to be optimal levels based on the most recent research. The following includes data from recent studies on the minerals calcium, iron, and magnesium as well as the vitamins C, D, E, beta-carotene, and folic acid.

Calcium. Some authorities have recommended that women (including young women) consume 1,000 to 1,500 milligrams (mg) of calcium per day to develop and maintain bone health and prevent osteoporosis (Office of Medical Applications of Research, 1984). Although it is technically feasible to achieve this level by diet alone, most people in the United States do not get that much calcium in their diet. In fact, the median intake among American women is only 600 mg per day, or around half the optimal level. Furthermore, 25 percent of women consume less than 400 mg per day (based on an average of 4 nonconsecutive days over 1 year) (U.S. Department of Agriculture, 1988).

Iron. Approximately 8 percent of low-income women and 10 to 20 percent of low-income children are believed to be iron deficient (Public Health Service, 1989). While the RDA for women is 15 mg per day, only slightly more than 10 percent of women achieve this goal from diet alone; less than 10 percent of low-income women achieve this level (Block and Abrams, 1993; U.S. Department of Agriculture, 1988). Iron deficiency is not an important public health problem among men; indeed, some evidence suggests that iron overload in men may be a source of illness, such as heart disease (Sullivan, 1992). Absorption of iron from supplements and plant sources is quite low if body stores of iron are adequate; however, iron from red meat continues to be absorbed even if body stores of iron are plentiful (Ascherio and Willett, 1994). Therefore, until this hypothesis can be more fully studied, it may be prudent for men to avoid daily consumption of red meat.

Magnesium. Extensive metabolic balance studies done by the USDA Research Service showed that the ratio of dietary calcium to magnesium that best maintained equilibrium (i.e., output equaling intake) was 2:1 (Hathaway, 1962). This ratio is achieved at the median magnesium intake of approximately 600 mg per day. However, dietary surveys taken in the last decade have found that most Americans' diets provide less than 300 mg/day (Lakshmanan et al., 1984; Morgan and Stampley, 1988; Spillman, 1987). Thus, like that of calcium, the median daily intake of magnesium in the United States appears to be inadequate.

Long-term magnesium deficiency causes damage to arteries and the heart in all species of animals tested—rodents, cats, dogs, cattle, and monkeys (Seelig, 1980; Seelig and Heggtveit, 1974). It also adversely affects fat metabolism, increasing the "bad" lipids—low-density lipoprotein (LDL) cholesterol and triglycerides, which are associated with atheromas (fat deposits in arteries)—and decreasing the levels of "good" lipids—high-density lipoprotein (HDL) cholesterol, which remove fat deposits from the arterial wall (Altura et al., 1990; Rayssiguier, 1981, 1984, 1986; Rayssiguier et al., 1993).

On the other hand, magnesium supplementation appears to be effective in reversing this process. For example in a double-blind, placebo-controlled study, 47 patients with coronary artery disease and heart attacks were treated with oral magnesium or placebo for 3 months. Those who received the magnesium experienced a 27-percent decrease in the "bad" lipids in contrast to a slight increase in the placebo group. There was also a tendency toward increased HDL in the magnesium group (Rasmussen et al., 1989a). The investigators observed that these findings support the assumption that magnesium deficiency might be involved in the causation of coronary artery disease. Oral magnesium preparations have also favorably influenced blood lipids in diabetes mellitus, lowering high levels of LDL and raising low levels of HDL (Corica et al., 1994).

In another study in which about half of 374 men at high risk for serious cardiovascular disease were put on a diet high in magnesium (a predominantly vegetarian diet containing 900 to more than 1,200 mg of magnesium daily) and half were put on a regular diet (containing about 300 to 500 mg of magnesium daily), sudden cardiac deaths were 1.5 times more common in the low-magnesium group. Total complications occurred in 60 percent of the low-magnesium group versus 28.6 percent of the high-magnesium group (Singh, 1990). Total mortality was 18 percent and 10.7 percent in the low- and high-magnesium groups, respectively. Furthermore, in a 6-week study of 206 non-insulin-dependent diabetic patients there was significant lowering of LDL levels and slight raising of HDL levels on a high-magnesium diet versus no change in 194 comparable patients on their usual diets (Singh et al., 1991).

Epidemiological evidence also supports the premise that magnesium protects against cardiovascular disease in humans. Areas of the world where the intake of magnesium is high from either drinking water or diet have low prevalence of cardiovascular disease (Anderson et al., 1980; Durlach et al., 1989; Eisenberg, 1992; Hopps, 1981; Leary, 1986; Marier, 1978). In the United States, the Southeast (where water is soft and is low in magnesium) is known as the heart attack-kidney stone belt, whereas the northern Midwest Plains states (where water is hard and is high in magnesium) have lower cardiovascular disease rates and longer life expectancies (Hopps, 1981; Hopps and Feder, 1986).

In Germany, large-scale retrospective studies of nearly 5,000 patients indicate that magnesium supplements added to drugs used to prevent preterm delivery resulted in improved weights of infants, reducing incidence of low birth weights (whether due to prematurity or intrauterine growth retardation), and decreased the incidence of toxemias of pregnancy, including pregnancy-induced hypertension, preeclampsia, and eclampsia (Conradt, 1984; Conradt and Weidinger, 1982; Conradt et al., 1984). Two randomized double-blind studies of a total of 1,500 pregnant women, half of whom received placebo and the other half a magnesium salt supplement, showed that significantly fewer of the magnesium group developed eclampsia; in addition, there were significantly fewer low birth weights among the infants of the magnesium group. The conclusion was that magnesium supplements during pregnancy improved the outcome (Kovacs et al., 1988; Spaetling and Spaetling, 1987). It has been suggested that magnesium deficiency is a contributory factor in these conditions (Conradt et al., 1984; Kontopoulos et al., 1980; Seelig, 1980; Weaver, 1988), a concept that has been proved in magnesium deficiency-induced hypertension of pregnancy and in low birth weight of lambs born to ewes fed low-magnesium diets (Weaver, 1986, 1988). That preeclamptic women retain more magnesium after a loading test (injection of magnesium salt solution) than normal women do is direct evidence of the magnesium deficit in toxemia of pregnancy (Kontopoulos et al., 1980; Valenzuela and Munson, 1987).

Vitamin C. Vitamin C is an important antioxidant nutrient that is synthesized by most animal species but not by humans. The current RDA is 60 mg, an amount easily obtainable in diet. Nevertheless, 25 percent of women consume less than 40 mg per day in their 4-day average (U.S. Department of Agriculture, 1988). The optimal level of vitamin C intake is unknown, but a diet rich in fruits and vegetables can provide 250 to 500 mg per day (Becker, 1993). Interestingly, estimates of nutrition during the Paleolithic Age (the Old Stone Age, roughly 1,000,000 to 9,000 B.C.) suggest that early humans may have consumed as much as 390 mg per day of vitamin C (Eaton and Konner, 1985). As with vitamin E (see below), there is evidence that intakes well above 60 mg per day may reduce the risks of cataracts. The potential therapeutic attributes of vitamin C are discussed in detail in the next section, Orthomolecular Medicine.

Vitamin D. The current RDA for adults is 200 international units (IUs). However, there are few studies in adults to verify that this is the optimal level (Gloth et al., 1991). Although this vitamin can be synthesized by humans by exposure to the sun, many elderly persons, for example, who are often inside much of the day get little or no sun. Since fortified milk is the principal dietary source of vitamin D, persons who obtain little calcium from milk or who have inadequate sun exposure may have inadequate vitamin D intake (Gloth et al., 1991).

Vitamin E. Vitamin E, or alpha-tocopherol, is another important antioxidant nutrient. The current RDA for vitamin E is 8 IU for women and 10 for men. This is a reduction from an earlier RDA of 30 IU for both men and women. A well-selected diet containing numerous servings of fruits and vegetables, nuts, whole-grain breads, and vegetable oils can achieve a diet containing 30 IU (Becker, 1993). However, few Americans consume such a diet.

Current median intake in the U.S. population is approximately 5 IU, with 10 percent of the population consuming little more than 3 IU. Levels of 100 IU or higher have been associated with significantly reduced risk of coronary heart disease in both men and women (Rimm et al., 1993; Stampfer et al., 1993). However, this effect has been seen at levels obtainable only from supplements. Indeed, the use of vitamin E supplements for 2 or more years was associated with a 41-percent decrease in risk of coronary disease among women (Stampfer et al., 1992) and a 37-percent decrease in men (Rimm et al., 1993). In addition, consumption of supplements containing vitamin E has been associated with significant reduction in risk of oral cancer (Gridley et al., 1992). This effect was seen even after controlling for factors such as smoking and alcohol consumption. Moreover, although persons with a high intake of fruits and vegetables had a 40-percent reduction in risk of oral cancer, those who used a vitamin E supplement in addition to high fruit and vegetable intake had an 80-percent reduction in risk.

Cataracts are a major cause of blindness worldwide and represent a significant fraction of health care costs in the United States. A number of studies have found that ingesting antioxidants, such as vitamin E, significantly reduced the risk of cataracts (Taylor, 1992). In one study, daily supplementation with 400 IU of vitamin E was associated with a 60-percent reduction in risk of cataracts, whereas daily use of 300 mg or more of vitamin C resulted in a 75-percent reduction in cataract risk (Robertson et al., 1989). Others have also found a high intake of dietary carotenoids associated with reduced cataract risk (Hankinson et al., 1992; Jacques et al., 1988).

Beta-carotene. This antioxidant is found in orange fruits and vegetables such as carrots, sweet potatoes, and squash, and in dark green leafy vegetables. As much as 20 to 30 mg can be obtained from just a few fresh carrots. This also is the level currently being used as the test dose in a number of intervention studies to determine whether it can reduce cancer risk (see below). However, current median intake is less than 2 mg per day, and approximately 25 percent of Americans consume 1 mg per day or less (U.S. Department of Agriculture, 1988). There also is evidence that other naturally occurring carotenoids, in addition to beta-carotene, may be important as antioxidants in reducing the risk of disease.

A number of recent studies have suggested that beta-carotene, among other antioxidants, may have a protective effect against certain cancers. For example, low blood levels of beta-carotene are consistently associated with the subsequent development of lung cancer (Ziegler, 1991).

Furthermore, in a recent prospective trial in China funded by the National Cancer Institute (NCI) and the Cancer Institute of the Chinese Academy of Medical Sciences, 29,584 adults were given several combinations of vitamin and mineral supplements. Linxian, a rural county in Henan province, northern China, has one of the highest rates of esophageal cancer in the world. Death rates for this cancer in Linxian are 10 times higher than the Chinese average and 100 times greater than for American whites.

During the period of the study, there were 2,127 deaths among study participants, with 32 percent of all deaths resulting from esophageal or stomach cancer. Only the combination of beta-carotene, vitamin E, and selenium significantly reduced death rates in the study population, and most of the reduction was due to lower cancer rates. This included not only a reduction in esophageal cancer and stomach cancer but also a 45-percent reduction in fatal lung cancer that did not reach statistical significance (Blot et al., 1994). The doses in the study were typically two to three times the U.S. RDA, and the risk reduction appeared to begin 1 to 2 years after vitamin and mineral supplementation began.

However, two other recent trials to assess the ability of beta-carotene to prevent cancer have not shown such positive results. A Finnish study in which almost 30,000 male smokers aged 50 to 59 were given daily supplements of vitamin E (alpha-tocopherol), beta-carotene, or both found no reduction in the incidence of lung cancer (Heinonen and Albanes, 1994). In fact, the study observed a higher incidence of lung cancer among men who received the beta-carotene than among those who did not. Nor was there any reduction in the formation of colon polyps—a precursor of colon cancer—in a study in which 864 individuals received placebo or beta-carotene (25 mg daily), vitamin C (1 g daily), and vitamin E (400 mg daily) for 4 years (Greenberg et al., 1994).

There are several problems with trying to compare these studies. Most important is whether a period of 4 to 6 years is sufficient to detect a beneficial effect of an agent that acts early in the development of cancer—which could be decades before the cancer is diagnosed. Also, it is possible that only persons with low levels of beta-carotene may benefit from supplementation. The *New England Journal of Medicine* managing editors warned in a recent editorial that consumers should not overinterpret the latest negative findings, just as they should not overinterpret the earlier positive findings (Angell and Kassirer, 1994).

Folic acid (folate). The current RDA for folate is 180 micrograms (µg) per day for women, but recent studies have shown that intake of 400 µg by pregnant women can greatly reduce the risk of neural tube defects (i.e., defects of the spinal cord tube) (Willett, 1992). Intake must be at this level in the earliest weeks after conception to be effective. Unfortunately, most women are not yet aware that they are pregnant then.

Researchers examining the role of folate in preventing cancer and cardiovascular disease have found that less than optional levels of folate may be linked to these diseases. For example, a recent study of almost 1,500 male physicians revealed that the risk of suffering a heart attack was elevated more than threefold by a common metabolic abnormality called homocysteinemia, which is correctable by consuming more folate. None of the study participants who suffered heart attacks would be considered folate deficient by current nutritional standards. However, the results of this study indicate that their intake of folate was clearly less than optimal for preventing cardiovascular disease (Stampfer et al., 1992). In addition, folic acid supplementation was associated with reduced risk of colorectal cancer (Giovannucci et al., 1993). In contrast, folate from food alone was not significantly related to reduced risk of colon cancer.

In another double-blind, placebo-controlled trial of 96 healthy persons over age 65, the consumption of vitamin and mineral supplements was associated with a significant reduction in illness from infections and improved immune function (Chandra, 1992). The vitamin used was a therapeutic-level, multiple vitamin containing, among other nutrients, 400 µg of folate and 16 mg of beta-carotene. Participants receiving the vitamin formulation experienced half as many days of infection-related illness over the treatment year as did persons receiving the placebo (i.e., 23 days for the treatment group compared with 48 days for the untreated group).

Thus, it may be that approximately 400 µg per day of folic acid is necessary for men and women of all ages. Although this level can be obtained from a well-chosen diet containing, for example, six servings of fruit or vegetables and fortified cereal per day (Block and Abrams, 1993), few in the United States consume such a diet. In fact, a recent study found that 25 percent of pregnant women who were surveyed consumed only 128 µg or less of folate and 10 percent consumed only 90 µg per day in their 4-day average (Johnson et al., 1994).

Risks associated with vitamin and mineral supplementation. All vitamins, as well as other substances, including water, can be toxic at some upper level. Under certain conditions or for particular subgroups, dangers may arise in taking large doses of some vitamins and minerals. For example, persons on anticoagulant (blood-thinning) therapy should avoid high doses of vitamin E, because prolonged bleeding can occur. Accidental poisonings of children have occurred with a number of vitamins, most notably with large doses of iron and vitamins A and D. Indeed, the accidental fatal poisoning of children by ingestion of their mothers' high-dose iron tablets is a health problem that deserves wider recognition. Childproof caps have been required on iron tablets for several years, but greater awareness among parents is needed to prevent children from removing such protective devices.

Nevertheless, evidence suggests that most vitamins are safe for long-term use at levels well above the RDAs for most adults. For example, Hathcock (1991) found a "possible adverse effect level" for vitamins C, E, B_6, and folate only with *long-term* ingestion at 10 times the RDA or greater and at 5 times the RDA for vitamin A. Minerals such as iron, zinc, and selenium, however, may be associated with greater risk of toxicity at levels of less than 10 times the RDA for long-term use.

The use of pharmacological doses (i.e., levels of intake substantially above those traditionally assumed necessary to prevent deficiency) of some vitamins and magnesium salts is an accepted practice in mainstream medicine for treatment of a few established conditions. However, such cases are relatively isolated, and the use of pharmacological doses of vitamins for many diseases remains controversial. This subject is discussed next.

Orthomolecular Medicine: Therapeutic Use of High-Dose Nutrient Therapy in Treatment of Chronic Disease

Varying the concentrations of substances normally present in the body may control mental disease.
—Linus Pauling

In theory, the concept behind orthomolecular medicine is quite simple. Orthomolecular medicine is the pursuit of good health and the treatment of disease with the optimal concentration of substances *normally* present in the body. Nobel laureate Linus Pauling first used the term *orthomolecular* in his 1968 article, "Orthomolecular Psychiatry," in the journal *Science* (Pauling, 1968). The prefix *ortho* implies correct or proper; in using the term *orthomolecular,* Pauling was calling for the "right molecules in the right amounts" (Huemer, 1986).

Pauling's *Science* article concentrated on the psychiatric implications of the concept. It referred to the work of two Canadian psychiatrists, Abram Hoffer and Humphrey Osmond, who had for several years been treating acute schizophrenia with large doses of nicotinic acid (vitamin B3) and vitamin C as enhancements to or replacements for the then state-of-the-art therapies, electroconvulsive therapy (ECT) and major tranquilizer therapy. Hoffer and Osmond first became interested in vitamin B3 as a therapeutic biochemical agent because of reports in the literature that patients with pellagra, a disease caused by a vitamin B3 deficiency, displayed many of the same psychiatric symptoms as did patients with schizophrenia.

In a series of double-blind, placebo-controlled clinical trials in the 1950s and early 1960s, Hoffer and Osmond began giving patients with schizophrenia up to 6 grams a day of vitamin B3, as well as large doses of vitamin C and other vitamins, in addition to the normal treatment regimen. They reportedly doubled the recovery rate, halved the rehospitalization rate, and practically eliminated the suicide rate among this patient group in comparison with the patients receiving only ECT or tranquilizers. These positive results were reported in 5-, 10-, and 15-year followups (Hoffer and Osmond, 1960, 1964; Osmond, 1969).

In his *Science* article, Pauling indicated some of the ways orthomolecular concepts could be usefully applied to many other areas of medicine. He then suggested that increasing the intake of such nutrients to levels well above those usually associated with prevention of overt deficiency disease could have previously unrecognized health benefits for some, but not all, people (Pauling, 1968).

One outcome of the increased attention focused on the megavitamin issue by Pauling's *Science* article was the publication of a report by the American Psychiatric Association's Task Force on Megavitamin Therapy in Psychiatry (Lipton et al., 1973), which roundly criticized the work of Hoffer and Osmond and declared megavitamin therapy to be of no value. Proponents of this new form of medical intervention criticized these reports as having numerous misstatements and inaccuracies. In particular, orthomolecular psychiatry proponents argued that the two reports had based their conclusions on flawed studies that attempted to replicate the use of niacin for the treatment of schizophrenia in chronically hospitalized psychotic patients. The treatment, according to proponents, had been shown effective only in acute schizophrenia of relatively recent onset (i.e., within a few months to a year or two), which meant that trials in chronically ill patients were doomed to failure (Hoffer, 1974; Pauling, 1974).

Concurrent with the studies of niacin in psychiatry in the early 1970s, Pauling began collaborating with Scottish surgeon Evan Cameron on a series of retrospective studies to determine whether vitamin C was effective in the treatment of cancer. In the late 1970s, Pauling and Cameron reported a significant prolongation of lifespan of vitamin C-treated patients over that of cancer patients who did not receive vitamin C therapy (Cameron and Pauling, 1976). These studies were undertaken as followups to a clinical trial conducted by Cameron with Alan Campbell, which reported complete cessation of tumor progression in 3 patients and complete tumor regression in 5 patients of 50 advanced-cancer patients treated intravenously for long periods with high doses of vitamin C (Cameron and Campbell, 1974).

The results of Pauling and Cameron's retrospective studies were published in the *Proceedings of the National Academy of Sciences (PNAS),* which took the unusual step of running an accompanying editorial along with the second *PNAS* paper criticizing its methodology and calling for better designed double-blind prospective studies to confirm or refute vitamin C's anticancer activity. Following this, the NCI funded two highly publicized clinical trials of vitamin C at the Mayo Clinic in Rochester, MN, both of which reported negative results for the use of vitamin C in the treatment of cancer (Creagan et al., 1979; Moertel et al., 1985). However, Pauling argued that the first Mayo Clinic study was flawed because almost all the patients had previously received chemotherapy, which may have affected their response to vitamin C. He contended that the second study was flawed as well, in part, because it did not use Cameron's protocol and vitamin C therapy was not carried out for long enough (Richards, 1986).

Despite the negative results of the Mayo Clinic studies, Pauling and others continued to promote vitamin C and other immune-modulating substances as important adjuvants to the treatment of cancer. They believed that neither surgery, radiation, nor chemotherapy could ever be completely effective in eliminating all the cancer cells from a patient's body. Thus it is necessary, they argued, to enhance the patient's immune defenses against cancer with large doses of vitamin C (Cameron and Pauling, 1976). The rationale for this is based on earlier observations that cancer patients tended to be significantly depleted of vitamin C (Baird and Cameron, 1973; Bodansky et al., 1951) and that those animals that have the ability to produce their own vitamin C significantly increased their own production of vitamin C—to an equivalent of 16 grams per day for the average human—when challenged with a potent carcinogen or when experimentally burdened with cancer (Burns et al., 1960; Schmidt et al., 1963). However, Cameron and Pauling never suggested that vitamin C (or other nutrients) should be used instead of conventional cancer therapy but rather as an adjunct to therapy (Cameron and Pauling, 1976). Pauling and others also have advocated high doses of vitamin C as a means of treating or preventing other diseases, including the common cold and influenza (Pauling, 1976).

Although the negative results from the Mayo Clinic studies as well as results from the American Psychiatric Association study managed to put a damper on claims made by the proponents of orthomolecular medicine for more than a decade, interest in this subject has been renewed recently. One reason is that in isolated instances, orthomolecular treatments have indeed proved effective in treating certain chronic illnesses. For example, megadose niacin is now routinely prescribed to treat hypercholesterolemia (i.e., abnormally high levels of LDL cholesterol in the blood) and has been shown to reduce cardiac mortality in large-scale trials (Vega and Grundy, 1994; Zhao et al., 1993). Likewise, vitamin A in dosages substantially higher than the RDA is a highly effective treatment for an uncommon form of leukemia (Bunce et al., 1994; Skrede et al., 1994), and the effectiveness of high-dose vitamin E in surgical wound healing and burn therapy has been recognized for years (Haberal et al., 1987; Zhang et al., 1992).

Finally, as the data have mounted on the role such antioxidants as vitamin C may play in preventing disease and maintaining health, younger investigators are increasingly being attracted to this field. These investigators are now equipped with more accurate and sensitive methods for exploring the validity of theories that were previously rejected outright but were never adequately tested (Barinaga, 1991).

Research base. The following are examples of orthomolecular treatments for which there is at least preliminary evidence suggesting their effectiveness in treating various chronic, debilitating illnesses but for which larger, more detailed studies are needed. This is by no means a comprehensive list. For the reader's convenience, these therapies are presented by type of conditions for which they are applied. These conditions include AIDS, cancer, a variety of heart and vascular conditions, lymphedema, and mental and neurological disorders.

Acquired immunodeficiency syndrome (AIDS). AIDS is a clinical disorder caused by a retrovirus infection (i.e, human immunodeficiency virus, or HIV), which is the end stage of a progressive sequence of immunosuppressive changes. The drawbacks of current pharmacological therapy for HIV infection, such as zidovudine (AZT), include deleterious toxic side effects, inability to improve the immune dysfunctions and undernutrition initiated by the retrovirus infection, and the occurrence of AZT-resistant HIV strains. These drawbacks necessitate new strategies for developing novel therapies to treat AIDS. Low toxicity nutritional agents with immuno-enhancing and antioxidant activities may help normalize retrovirus-induced immune dysfunctions, undernutrition, and other pathological symptoms, thereby retarding the progression of the disease to AIDS. Data on the immune-stimulating effects of vitamin A and beta-carotene in HIV-infected individuals are presented below.

Vitamin A. In the early 1980s, Seifter and colleagues showed through a series of experiments that vitamin A or beta-carotene (its precursor) decreases the immune deficiency that results when animals are exposed to a wide variety of immunocompromising conditions such as trauma, infection, irradiation, and treatment with cytotoxic agents (Seifter et al., 1982, 1983a, 1983b, 1984). Seifter and others also studied the effects of vitamin A supplementation in animals infected with the Moloney murine sarcoma virus, a retrovirus having many features in common with human immunodeficiency virus (HIV), the virus that causes AIDS (Kanofsky et al., 1987, 1990; Seifter et al., 1982, 1985, 1991). The vitamin A supplementation Seifter and his colleagues used in those experiments was approximately 10 to 15 times the recommended dietary allowance.

There is evidence suggesting that vitamin A supplementation in immune-compromised individuals may be necessary to correct a vitamin A deficiency caused by HIV infection. For example, Lack and colleagues (1993) found that approximately 50 percent of 120 HIV-positive patients, who were both symptomatic and asymptomatic, had a low serum vitamin A level. In another study, Semba and colleagues (1993) measured serum vitamin A levels in HIV-positive drug abusers and concluded that vitamin A deficiency may be common during HIV infection. Low vitamin A status was independently associated with decreased CD4 cells and a much greater mortality rate.

Beta-carotene. Alexander and colleagues (1985) reported that extremely large oral doses of beta-carotene (180 mg per day) can increase the number of CD4 cells in the blood of healthy humans, with no observable toxicity. The CD4 cell is the white blood cell that becomes markedly depressed in AIDS patients. According to these researchers, "Our data suggest that beta-carotene administration might be considered for patients with AIDS."

Coodley and colleagues (1993), in an 8-week, double-blind crossover study of 21 HIV-positive patients, compared 180 mg per day of beta-carotene with placebo. The results showed a statistically significant increase in total white blood cell count, percent change in CD4 count, and percent change in CD4:CD8 ratios. The CD4:CD8 ratio is often used as an indicator of whether a patient's status is getting worse, holding steady, or improving.

Watson and colleagues gave a much smaller dose of beta-carotene (60 mg per day) to 11 HIV-infected patients over 4 months. The authors saw no change in T-helper lymphocytes (CD4), T-suppressor lymphocytes (CD8), or total T-cell lymphocytes. However, they did see an increase in the number of cells with natural killer markers and markers of activation (IL-2R, transferrin receptors) (Garewal et al., 1992). This indicates that beta-carotene may be enhancing certain aspects of the immune response.

Furthermore, Fryburg and colleagues (1992) gave 120 mg per day of beta-carotene and 1 multivitamin tablet a day to seven AIDS patients for 4 weeks. The mean CD4 count at baseline (i.e., before treatment) was approximately 53 cells/mm^3. After 4 weeks of beta-carotene therapy, it rose to 76 cells/mm^3. However, it returned to approximately 53 cells/mm^3 6 weeks after treatment was stopped. A recommendation was made for beta-carotene to be tried in larger groups of patients.

Bianchi-Santamaria and colleagues (1993) gave 60 mg per day of beta-carotene 20 days of each month for 21 months to 64 patients with AIDS-related complex, which is the stage of HIV infection that occurs just before full-blown AIDS. This is the study with by far the longest duration and also is the largest and most recent. Mean CD4 count at baseline was approximately 451 cells/mm^3. After 21 months of beta-carotene treatment, the mean CD4 count rose to approximately 519 cells/mm^3, an increase of 15 percent. Normally, the mean CD4 count in these patients would be expected to drop. Furthermore, the authors suggested that the beta-carotene accounted for the apparent recovery of patients from asthenia, fever, nocturnal sweating, diarrhea, and weight loss. Unfortunately, this study did not have a control group.

Bronchial asthma. Asthma, better termed hyperactive airway disease, is an autoimmune disease characterized by increased responsiveness of the tracheobronchial tree to exogenous and endogenous stimuli. The hallmark of this illness is widespread inflammation and narrowing of the tracheobronchial tree. This is manifested clinically by dyspnea (shortness of breath), wheezing, and cough, which generally occur simultaneously.

Asthma is typically managed with bronchodilator therapy and/or anti-inflammatory drugs. However, currently used pharmaceutical formulations for bronchodilation, such as theophylline, have a narrow therapeutic margin because adverse effects often occur at concentrations high enough to be effective (Taburet and Schmit, 1994). In addition, prednisone, the most common anti-inflammatory drug used to treat asthma, is also associated with a variety of adverse side effects. Such limited effectiveness of presently available treatments has recently sparked research into less toxic, immune-enhancing nutritional approaches to treating asthma. Data on the efficacy of vitamin C and magnesium in the treatment of this condition are presented below.

Vitamin C. Bielory and Gandhi (1994) conducted a comprehensive literature search of relevant English-language papers pertaining to the use of vitamin C in in the treatment of asthma and allergy and analyzed the studies according to their design, inclusion and exclusion criteria, population studied, variables or factors tested, method of intervention or treatment with vitamin C, and results and conclusions. They found a number of studies that support the use of vitamin C in asthma and allergy. Significant results included positive effects of vitamin C on pulmonary function tests; bronchoprovocation challenges with methacholine, histamine, or allergens; improvement in white blood cell function and motility; and a decrease in respiratory infections. On the other hand, their review also revealed several studies that did not support a beneficial role for vitamin C in asthma and allergy. These studies did not report improvements in pulmonary function tests or bronchoprovocation challenges or on other reactivity or specific immunologic factors and levels.

From their review, the researchers concluded that the majority of the studies were too short-term and assessed immediate effects of vitamin C supplementation. Rather, long-term supplementation with vitamin C or delayed effects need to be examined for the studies to be valid. The researchers went on to note that although the current literature does not support a definite indication for the use of vitamin C in asthma and allergy, the promising and positive studies were worth following up. Furthermore, the researchers suggested, with a large portion of health care dollars being spent on alternative medicine and vitamin C in particular, further studies are needed to define its role, if any, in the treatment of this condition.

Magnesium. First reported almost 50 years ago (Haury, 1938), the efficacy of magnesium in the treatment of bronchial asthma has received considerably more attention in the past few years. Its bronchodilating effect was reported in patients with mild asthmatic attacks, and when that was found effective, applied to those with severe attacks (Okayama et al., 1988). Intravenous magnesium sulfate was found to relieve respiratory failure in asthmatic patients not responsive to standard drug therapy (Hauser and Braun, 1991; McNamara et al., 1989; Neves et al., 1991; Noppen et al., 1990; Okayama et al., 1991; Skobeloff et al., 1989) and has been considered lifesaving (Dellinger, 1991; Kuitert and Kletchko, 1991).

Not all published trials of magnesium treatment of bronchial asthma, however, have been successful (Green and Rothrock, 1992; Kufs, 1990). However, the protocols of those studies reporting no therapeutic benefit of magnesium in asthma patients have been criticized on the grounds that insufficient dosages were used, with the result that the serum levels found effective in the treatment of preeclampsia and eclampsia (see below) were not achieved (Fesmire, 1993). Another criticism leveled at the negative efficacy reports was that the study group was too small for significance; this was countered by pointing out that analysis of results from the first 40 patients indicated withholding magnesium from comparably compromised patients would be unethical, so the study was ended and the results were reported (Skobeloff and McNamara, 1993).

Cancer. The rationale for the use of high dosages of vitamins, particularly vitamin C, to treat cancer was discussed in the beginning of this section. The following is a review of more recent data that have emerged since the negative results of the Mayo Clinic studies for vitamin C, as well as quite intriguing data on the use of high dosages of coenzyme Q10 in the treatment of certain cancers.

Vitamin C. The possible value of vitamin C as an adjuvant in cancer therapy is supported in animal and human studies. Indeed, vitamin C, used in conjunction with other treatment modalities, has been shown to improve the effectiveness of those treatments (Meadows et al., 1991; Poydock, 1991; Tsao, 1991). Of equal interest, vitamin C supplementation has been shown to reduce the toxicity of conventional chemotherapeutic agents, such as adriamycin (Fujita et al., 1982), and to reduce the toxicity and improve therapeutic gain of radiation therapy (Okunieff, 1991). There also is evidence that some of the severe toxicity associated with interleukin-2/LAK cell therapy may result from the drastic reduction in plasma vitamin C levels that this therapy causes (Marcus et al., 1987). Thus, these examples suggest that the use of vitamin C or other nutrients as adjuncts to therapy may reduce toxicity and thereby permit the use of more effective doses of the therapeutic agent.

Coenzyme Q_{10}. Recently, Lockwood and colleagues (1994) treated 32 breast cancer patients with antioxidants, fatty acids, and 90 mg of coenzyme Q_{10} (CoQ_{10}) per day and reported partial tumor regression in six patients. In one of the cases, the dosage was increased to 390 mg per day and, reportedly, within 2 months the tumor was no longer detectable by mammography. Encouraged by this, Lockwood and colleagues treated another patient with a verified breast tumor with 300 mg per day, and after 3 months they could find no sign of remaining tumor. Folkers reported that administration of this enzyme increases levels of immunoglobulin G, an antibody that is known to participate in antibody-dependent cellular toxicity against virally infected cells and, possibly, against cancer cells (Folkers et al., 1982, 1993). The same studies also showed increases in T4 lymphocytes—the immune cells targeted and destroyed by HIV infection—when CoQ_{10} was given with pyridoxine to AIDS patients.

Arteriosclerosis, heart attacks, arrhythmias, sudden cardiac death, strokes, and toxemias of pregnancy. *Vitamin E.* Postoperative thromboembolism, a major complication of surgery, involves the formation of blood clots in the deep veins of an extremity. The clots can break off and travel to blood vessels in the lungs, causing a pulmonary embolism that can be fatal. This is often a major postoperative complication despite the use of various treatments that are partially effective in preventing it. As far back as the late 1940s, Alton Ochsner repeatedly advocated the administration of vitamin E to prevent postoperative thromboembolism. His vitamin E regimen consisted of 200 to 600 IU of alpha-tocopherol per day, administered intramuscularly or by mouth, beginning no later than the day of surgery and continuing through the postoperative period (Kay et al., 1950; Ochsner, 1964, 1968; Ochsner et al., 1950a, 1950b, 1951). As late as 1968 he wrote, "For 15 years I have used alpha-tocopherol (vitamin E) routinely in the treatment of patients who have been subjected to trauma of any magnitude. None of these patients have had pulmonary embolism" (Ochsner, 1968).

In 1981, Kanofsky and Kanofsky completed a search of the American and British literature, which disclosed six studies comparing a vitamin E-treated group with a control group (Coon and Whitrock, 1951; Coon et al., 1952; Crump and Heiskell, 1952; Ochsner et al., 1951; Kawahara, 1959; Moorman et al., 1953; Wilson and Parry, 1954). All these controlled studies were published between 1951 and 1959. That none of the studies used a double-blind design is unfortunate, since the diagnosis of deep-vein thrombosis or pulmonary embolism was primarily based on the observations of clinicians, which can be easily influenced by bias. However, Kanofsky and Kanofsky analyzed the data from the six studies and found a highly statistically significant effect from the vitamin E treatment. There was a twofold greater risk of deep vein thrombosis, a sixfold greater risk of all pulmonary embolism, and a ninefold greater risk of fatal pulmonary embolism in the control group than in the vitamin E-treated group (Kanofsky and Kanofsky, 1981). The authors postulated that the physiological mechanism that might explain these results involved the ability of vitamin E to inhibit platelet aggregation.

Magnesium. Magnesium also has anticoagulant activity, acting directly on the steps involved in blood coagulation, counteracting the procoagulant effect of calcium (Greville and Lehmann, 1944; Herrmann et al., 1970; Seelig, 1993), and decreasing platelet clumping. In the 1950s there were reports of use of magnesium to prevent and treat clinical thrombotic conditions (Hackethal, 1951; Heinrich, 1957, Schnitzler, 1957). Animal studies demonstrated that magnesium supplements prevented formation of coronary artery thromboses when the animals were fed a thrombogenic diet (Savoie et al., 1973; Szelenyi et al., 1967). Case reports have been published of patients with magnesium deficiency characterized by neuromuscular disorders and whose thromboemboli were prevented from recurring by magnesium supplements; when the supplements were discontinued, the thromboemboli recurred (Dupont et al., 1969; Durlach, 1967). Recent findings have demonstrated that magnesium inhibits blood coagulation and arterial constriction by increasing the production of factors with antithrombotic and vasodilating activities by the inner lining (endothelium) of blood vessels. These findings have shed light on magnesium's usefulness in both eclampsia and heart attacks.

The anticoagulant activity of magnesium has found practical application in microsurgery, in which local application during the surgical procedure prevented thrombotic and subsequent scarring lesions (Acland, 1972). When used intravenously in dogs and rabbits with partially constricted coronary arteries, magnesium prevented formation of microthrombi distal to the partial occlusion, a finding considered pertinent to human angina with and without blockage of coronary arteries (Gretz et al., 1987).

Since the 1920s, large doses of magnesium (producing blood levels as high as two to three times normal) had been shown to be effective in the treatment of preeclampsia (hypertension with proteinuria or edema, or both, due to the influence of pregnancy or recent pregnancy) (Lazard, 1925). Diuretics and anticonvulsants eventually replaced magnesium as the preferred treatment for this condition, until studies showed that magnesium treatment resulted in better outcomes, including more live births (Zuspan and Ward, 1965) and was the more appropriate treatment (Sibai, 1990).

It appears that adequate magnesium is necessary to maintain the integrity of the inner lining of the blood vessel and to increase its production of the vasodilating, anti-platelet-aggregating (antithrombosis) substance (Briel et al., 1987; Watson et al., 1986). This activity of magnesium in inhibiting thrombosis has provided the rationale for its use in patients who have had a heart attack. In a large, double-blind study of 2,300 patients, called the second Leicester Intravenous Magnesium Intervention Trial, half of the patients received an intravenous injection of magnesium within three hours of a heart attack. This was followed by a 24-hour magnesium infusion in a dose sufficient to raise the blood level of magnesium to twice that of normal levels. This treatment, which was given in conjunction with the standard treatment for a heart attack, reduced heart failure and mortality by 25 percent in comparison with patients who received only the standard treatment (Woods et al., 1992; Woods and Fletcher, 1994).

However, a much larger "megatrial" of magnesium therapy in heart attack victims failed to find such an effect (Casscells, 1994; Unsigned Commentary, 1994). It has been proposed that the failure of the megatrial (called ISIS-4) to find the lifesaving effect of magnesium in heart attack patients may have been due to the institution of magnesium treatment only after use of a clot-dissolving treatment. This resulted in a delay of almost 8 hours before the magnesium was given. In contrast, in the earlier study, the magnesium was given immediately upon hospitalization. Thus, in ISIS-4, the magnesium may have been given after the damage to the heart muscle was done (Casscells, 1994; Woods and Fletcher, 1994).

Lymphedema. Lymphedema, a swelling of the arms or legs resulting from pathology in the lymphatic system, often can be disabling or even crippling. It has been estimated that 32 to 75 percent of women who undergo surgery for breast cancer will have some chronic lymphedema of the arm on the affected side (Casley-Smith and Casley-Smith, 1986). Unfortunately, the treatment of this side effect of breast cancer surgery is often neglected (Farncombe et al., 1994). Recently, however, there has emerged an orthomolecular treatment for this condition using benzopyrones. An overview of the studies utilizing this compound for the treatment of lymphedema is presented below.

Benzopyrones. Since the mid-1980s, J.R. Casley-Smith has recommended the use of large doses of benzopyrones for the treatment of lymphedema. The benzopyrones, though now frequently synthesized, were originally derived from plants. The coumarins and flavonoids, such as rutin, are benzopyrones. Szent-Gyorgi, the Nobel prize winner who isolated vitamin C, discovered that a lack of benzopyrones caused greatly increased capillary fragility and permeability (Casley-Smith and Casley-Smith, 1986). Since then, benzopyrones have sometimes been called "vitamin P" or "P factors."

Casley-Smith and colleagues believe that large doses of benzopyrones alleviate lymphedema by stimulating macrophage cells to break down unwanted proteins in the edema fluid (Piller et al., 1988). Once excess protein is eliminated, the edema fluid that it causes is no longer retained. Thus, they believe that the benzopyrones safely change a slowly worsening condition into a slowly improving one. There now are at least six double-blind studies demonstrating that the benzopyrones are a safe and effective treatment for lymphedema (Casley-Smith et al., 1986, 1993; Cluzan and Pecking, 1989; Desprez-Curely et al., 1985; Piller et al., 1985, 1988).

Unfortunately, no benzopyrones are available as pharmaceuticals in the United States. Approval for drugs containing rutin and other bioflavonoids was withdrawn in 1970 by FDA on the grounds that there was no substantial evidence of the effect they were purported to have. However, Casley-Smith has argued that FDA used old, greatly outmoded data, which allegedly showed that these drugs could not be absorbed (Casley-Smith and Casley-Smith, 1986). He and others are emphatic that more recent data show that the benzopyrones are absorbed and are effective. Moreover, Casley-Smith and others believe that because benzopyrones possess specific immune-stimulating properties and can reduce every type of high-protein edema, they eventually will become extremely valuable therapeutic agents in a wide variety of clinical conditions (Casley-Smith and Casley-Smith, 1986).

Mental and neurological disorders. Despite continued widespread skepticism among mainstream psychiatric professionals about the effectiveness of vitamin therapy in the treatment of neurological disorders, a small but growing number of researchers persist in studying the use of vitamins for such conditions. In fact, reports continue to surface on the effectiveness of vitamins such as folic acid as well as a variety of antioxidant vitamins in treating various mental and neurological disorders.

Folic acid. Low serum folate has been reported in 10 to 33 percent of psychiatric patients. In one retrospective survey, psychiatric patients treated with folic acid spent less time in the hospital and made significantly better social recoveries than those in whom low serum folates were not treated (Carney and Sheffield, 1970). Godfrey and colleagues recently demonstrated that 41 (33 percent) of 123 patients with depression or schizophrenia had borderline or definite folate deficiency. These patients took part in a double-blind, placebo-controlled trial of methylfolate (the actively transported form of folate), taking 15 mg daily for 6 months in addition to standard psychotropic medication. Among both depressed and schizophrenic patients, methylfolate significantly improved clinical and social recovery (Godfrey et al., 1990). These researchers speculate that folate or methylfolate may have a direct pharmacological action irrespective of whether the subjects were folate deficient.

Antioxidant therapy. Antioxidant therapy with nutrients such as vitamin C, vitamin E, and beta-carotene has been hypothesized as a treatment for schizophrenia (Lohr, 1991). The hypothesis is based on evidence that the serum of schizophrenics has high levels of lipid peroxides and the enzyme superoxide dismutase. Both these substances are indicators of unwanted oxidative products (mainly free radicals).

Just focusing on vitamin C, there is a substantial body of animal and clinical data that ascorbic acid may have an antipsychotic effect (Beauclair et al., 1987; Giannini et al., 1987; Heikkila et al., 1983; Kanofsky et al., 1988, 1989a; Milner, 1963; Rebec et al., 1984; Thomas and Zemp, 1977; Tolbert et al., 1979a, 1979b), which seems to be most apparent when ascorbic acid is given in combination with antipsychotic medication. A double-blind study showed that vitamin C increases the antipsychotic effects of haloperidol in treating PCP psychoses (Giannini et al., 1987). Observational studies and one double-blind study have indicated a similar adjunctive role for vitamin C in treating schizophrenia (Beauclair et al., 1987; Kanofsky et al., 1989a, 1989b; Milner, 1963). No one has studied the simultaneous use of several antioxidants in the treatment of schizophrenia, which seems a worthwhile avenue of research (Kanofsky and Sandyk, 1992; Lohr, 1991).

Double-blind studies have shown that tardive dyskinesia (a late-occurring, movement-disorder side effect of antipsychotic medication) can be treated with vitamin E supplementation. The therapeutic effect of vitamin E seems most likely when it is introduced within several years after the onset of the disorder (Adler et al., 1993; Egan et al., 1992; Elkashef et al., 1990). Several studies of patients with Alzheimer's disease have been performed in which brain tissue at autopsy showed evidence of increased brain lipid peroxidation (Farooqui et al., 1988; Hajimohammadreza and Brammer, 1990; Subbarao et al., 1990). Conceivably, antioxidants such as vitamin C and vitamin E might prevent this increase; however, much more research needs to be done before this treatment could be seriously considered (Lohr, 1991). In view of current evidence that vitamin E, either alone or in combination with deprenyl (an inhibitor of monoamine oxidase in the brain), fails to delay continued neurological deterioration in Parkinson's disease (Parkinson Study Group, 1993), it is also possible that to be most effective, antioxidant therapy must be introduced very early in the development of neurological and psychiatric disorders—prior to the point at which irreversible cell damage has occurred. A similar argument can be made with regard to the effectiveness of orthomolecular therapy in schizophrenia itself.

Magnesium. A condition known as "latent tetany" syndrome, which is seen in some patients with slight magnesium deficiency, is characterized by depressive anxiety, weakness, irritability, fatigue, and many ill-defined complaints (Durlach, 1988; Fehlinger et al., 1987; Galland, 1991–1992). This syndrome has characteristics that resemble premenstrual syndrome as well as chronic fatigue syndrome, both of which have responded favorably to supplementation with magnesium compounds alone or with other nutritional supplements (Abraham and Lubran, 1981; Stewart and Howard, 1986; London et al., 1991; Facchinetti et al., 1981).

There is evidence suggesting that magnesium deficiency participates in the abnormalities of migraine headaches and that migraines will respond to treatment with magnesium (Swanson, 1988; Weaver, 1990). Transient ischemic attacks, another disorder which like migraine is associated with cerebral arterial spasms, has also been found to respond to magnesium (Fauk et al. 1991). These clinical findings of magnesium's protective effects against ischemia (loss of blood flow) and hypoxia (oxygen deprivation) make it worthwhile to examine the considerable animal evidence that magnesium deficiency increases susceptibility to brain damage caused by cerebral arterial spasm, arterial blockage (i.e., stroke), or trauma (McIntosh et al., 1988; Blair et al., 1989; Okawa, 1992) and that magnesium treatments offer the potential for minimizing such brain damage (McIntosh et al., 1989; Vink, 1991–1992; Smith et al., 1983).

Clinicians in Japan have shown in a small pilot study that intravenous magnesium infusions improved the cerebral flow of stroke victims (who before treatment had low magnesium levels in their cerebrospinal fluid) (Iwasaki et al., 1989). Indeed, 10 patients who received magnesium therapy had a better return of normal cerebral functioning than did ten control patients who did not receive magnesium after a stroke. Whether prompt magnesium treatment after a stroke and/or after brain trauma will improve the prognosis of such patient deserves further investigation.

Selenium. In certain regions of the world, including Great Britain and parts of the United States and Canada, selenium levels in food are so low that the possibility of subclinical deficiency (and a possibly related adverse effect on mood) exists. Benton and Cook (1991) conducted a double-blind, crossover trial of 50 subjects in ostensibly good health. They were randomly assigned to receive a 100-microgram selenium tablet or placebo each day for 5 weeks. After a 6-month washout, they received the alternate treatment for 5 weeks. Benton and Cook concluded that the intake of selenium tablets was associated with an elevation of mood, particularly in subjects whose diets were relatively deficient in the trace element.

Amino acids. A double-blind, randomized study showed S-adenosylmethionine—the physiologically active form of the amino acid methionine—to be a more rapidly acting antidepressant than the pharmaceutical drug imipramine in treating major depression (Bell et al., 1988). At the end of this 2-week study, 66 percent of the S-adenosylmethionine patients had a clinically significant improvement in depressive symptoms versus 22 percent of the imipramine patients. If S-adenosylmethionine does turn out to be a more rapidly acting drug—taking days rather than weeks to achieve results—this characteristic may offer a considerable advantage in light of the known risk of suicide during the early nonresponding phase of treatment with most, if not all, other antidepressants.

Clinical trials of the amino acid glycine given orally to schizophrenic patients have yielded conflicting results. However, in the most recent double-blind study, Javitt and colleagues (1994) showed a statistically significant improvement in negative symptoms of schizophrenia when glycine was added to conventional antipsychotic drug regimens. This suggests that glycine may serve as a distinctive and valuable adjunctive treatment for schizophrenia.

Essential fatty acids. Vaddadi and colleagues (1989) reported the results of a double-blind crossover trial of essential fatty acid supplementation in 48 predominantly schizophrenic psychiatric patients. Active treatment produced highly significant improvements in total psychopathology scores and a significant improvement in memory.

Food and Macronutrient Modification Diets as a Method for Controlling and Treating Chronic Illnesses

This section is an overview of the theoretical basis and available research on a variety of diets that are advocated for the treatment of chronic conditions such as cancer, cardiovascular disease, and food allergies. Virtually all of these dietary interventions emphasize the intake of much more produce (fresh and freshly prepared vegetables, fruits, whole grains, and legumes), providing high nutrient density while at the same time restricting such "empty" calories as those provided by sweets, fats, and overprocessed foods. In these diets, moreover, overall caloric intake tends to be lower than that of the general U.S. population.

Nutrient modification for the treatment of cancer. Cancer accounts for one of every five deaths in the United States (American Cancer Society, 1990). More than 1 million cases of new cancers are diagnosed every year, and about 75 million, or one in three Americans now living, will eventually have cancer (Public Health Service, 1990). Cancer is not one disease but a constellation of more than 100 different diseases, each characterized by the uncontrolled growth and spread of abnormal cells. Cancer may strike at any age, though it does so more frequently with advancing age. Although corroborative intervention data are not yet available, it is estimated that 35 percent of cancer deaths may be related to diet (Eddy, 1986).

The rationale behind most dietary regimens for the treatment of cancer—and for vegetarian, low-fat, high-fiber dietary regimens in particular—is that if dietary excesses can lead to the development of certain cancers, then such cancers may be susceptible to dietary manipulation as well. These diets, for the most part, share certain characteristics with the kinds of foods currently recommended by mainstream groups, such as the American Cancer Society (ACS), for lowering the risk of developing cancer and heart disease. Recent ACS guidelines for cancer prevention suggest reducing the intake of fat, alcohol, and salt-cured and smoked foods while increasing the intake of fruits, vegetables, and whole grains (Nixon, 1990). One way these alternative dietary regimens for cancer differ, however, from mainstream preventive recommendations is that they may emphasize a few particular foods and limit or totally eliminate others.

In September 1990 the U.S. Congress Office of Technology Assessment (OTA) completed a study of a number of unconventional cancer treatments. Among these was a variety of dietary regimens developed for the treatment of cancer and/or the support of patients undergoing conventional cancer therapy. This report, *Unconventional Cancer Treatments,* focused on three of the most well-known dietary interventions for cancer: the Gerson therapy, the Kelley regimen, and the macrobiotic diet. These three regimens and a few others are reviewed below. Findings from the OTA report as well as studies done since that report was released are covered.

Gerson therapy. The Gerson therapy was developed by physician Max Gerson in the early part of this century. Gerson was born in Germany in 1881 and immigrated to the United States in 1936. He received his New York medical license in 1938 and his U.S. citizenship in 1944. He opened a private medical practice in New York City and in 1946 also began treating patients at nearby Gotham Hospital.

He gained renown in Germany through his success in treating tuberculosis of the skin through low-salt dietary management (Gerson,

1929). He then began testing modifications of this regimen in other conditions, including pulmonary tuberculosis (Gerson, 1934). He first used his diet for cancer in 1928, reportedly after a woman with a bile duct cancer that had spread to her liver insisted that he put her on his diet despite his reluctance to do so (Lerner, 1994). Much to his surprise, Gerson wrote, the woman recovered (Gerson, 1958). Afterward, Gerson tried variations and combinations of foods and other agents on his patients, noted the ones who reacted favorably, and adjusted subsequent patients' regimens accordingly (Gerson, 1978). By the time he came to America, he was focusing on treating cancer patients.

In 1946 Gerson testified before a subcommittee of the Senate Committee on Foreign Relations, which was holding a hearing on a proposed bill to authorize increased Federal spending for cancer research. Gerson reported to the Senate committee that he had developed a dietary regimen that was effective for the treatment of advanced cancer. According to the historian Patricia Spain Ward, Gerson's testimony was supported by the director of the Gotham Hospital, with which Gerson was affiliated, as well as others in attendance (Ward, 1988). Gerson described five patients in clinical detail and submitted written case histories of those and five more patients who had been treated with his regimen, in whom he had observed improvements in "general body health" and, in some cases, tumor reduction. In a later publication, Gerson noted that in six additional patients his treatment appeared to reduce inflammation around the tumors, relieve pain, improve psychological condition, and provide at least temporary tumor regression (Gerson, 1949). In the mid-1950s, Gerson first published explanations of the components of his regimen and the rationale for their use, along with some of the clinical outcomes he observed.

Gerson believed that his treatment regimen reversed the conditions he thought necessary to sustain the growth of malignant cells. He attached great importance to the elimination of "toxins" from the body and the role of a healthy liver in recovery from cancer. Gerson noted that if the liver was damaged (e.g., by cancer or cirrhosis) the patient had little chance of recovery on his or her treatment regimen (Gerson, 1949, 1986). He observed that cancer patients who died during treatment showed a marked degeneration of the liver, which he presumed was due to the release of unspecified toxic factors into the bloodstream by the process of tumor regression. He believed that these toxic tumor-breakdown products poisoned the liver and other vital organs (Cope, 1978).

Another central point of Gerson's approach concerned the balance of potassium and sodium in the body. He believed that an imbalance in the concentration of these substances contributes to cancer-induced edema, a condition in which cellular damage leads to infiltration by excess sodium and water, failure of cellular transport mechanisms, subsequent failure of cellular energy production, and, finally, loss of resistance to cancer. Therefore, he sought to eliminate sodium in patients' diets, supplement it with potassium, and thereby alter the internal environment supporting the tumor (Gerson, 1954a, 1954b, 1954c).

At present, the Gerson therapy is an integrated set of treatments that include the restriction of salt in combination with potassium supplementation of the diet. Thyroid supplements also are given to stimulate metabolism and cell energy production. Hourly feedings of fresh, raw juices of vegetables and fruits are given in addition to a basically vegetarian diet. Fat intake is restricted (to lower intake of potential tumor promotors), and protein is temporarily restricted (to promote nonspecific, cell-mediated immunities). Coffee enemas are provided to manage pain and to stimulate bowel and liver enzymes that may increase the release of toxins (Gerson Institute, undated-a). Other treatments beyond the ones specified by Gerson have been added to the current protocol in recent years. Gerson gave patients raw liver juice several times daily, but the practice has been abandoned by current practitioners because of bacteria in the liver juice that caused major infections in some patients (Office of Technology Assessment, 1990).

Critics of the Gerson therapy point to the fact that it is based on the beliefs of a physician who practiced many years ago and whose knowledge of the cause of cancer was rudimentary (Green, 1992). Proponents of the therapy argue, rather, that Gerson was far ahead of his time; however, they also note that many of Gerson's original assumptions and therapies have been updated to take into account the latest scientific evidence (Hildenbrand, 1986).

Because of such misconceptions about Gerson and how his therapy is currently administered, proponents contend that it has never been given a fair evaluation by mainstream science. Furthermore, they argue that such myths and misconceptions about the Gerson therapy are perpetuated by major medical journals that routinely publish articles attacking the basic tenets of the therapy while refusing to publish rebuttals to such attacks (Lechner and Hildenbrand, 1994).

Research base. There have been several attempts by a number of groups and individuals to assess the clinical effects of the Gerson regimen. However, none have yet offered any definitive results (Office of Technology Assessment, 1990). The following is an overview of early and more recent cases.

In 1959, NCI reviewed 50 case histories presented in Gerson's book, *A Cancer Therapy: Results of Fifty Cases.* NCI concluded that in the majority of cases a number of basic criteria were not met. NCI also concluded overall that Gerson's data provided no demonstration of benefit (Avery, 1982; U.S. Department of Health and Human Services, 1987). The Gerson Institute, however, disputed NCI's findings and charged that NCI had dismissed legitimate evidence on the basis of technicalities. In addition, the Gerson Institute claimed that even though NCI had indicated six cases were acceptable for further review and another 20 needed further documentation, NCI's own records indicate that such reviews were never done (Gerson Institute, undated-b).

More recently, an exploratory study of the clinical effects of some components of the Gerson regimen was conducted by Peter Lechner, M.D., at the University Hospital of Graz, Austria. This study used a modified Gerson therapy (i.e., liver juice and thyroid supplements were omitted, the number of coffee enemas was limited, and a high-calorie beverage was added to double energy consumption) as an adjunctive treatment. Lechner reported that patients following the modified Gerson regimen showed no side effects attributable to the treatment and did not become malnourished. One of the patients with inoperable liver metastases who followed the Gerson treatment showed a temporary regression. In Lechner's opinion, there were subjective benefits from the modified Gerson regimen: patients needed less pain medication, were in better psychological condition, and experienced less severe side effects from chemotherapy than did control patients (Lechner and Kronberger, 1990).

Lechner's study also suggested that a modified Gerson regimen might be effective in lowering rates of postsurgical complications and secondary infections, increasing tolerance of conventional radiotherapy and chemotherapy, reducing reliance on analgesics, providing for an improved overall psychological profile, retarding progress of liver metastases, and improving the state of malignant effusions (Lechner and Kronberger, 1990).

A research team from the University of London that visited the Mexican clinic offering the Gerson therapy (see below) in 1989 on behalf of a British insurance company studied 27 cases in detail. Of those cases, 20 were considered not assessible. Of the 7 assessible cases, 3 showed progressive disease, 1 showed stable disease, and 3 (43 percent of the accessible cases) were in regression. Moreover, the therapy clearly provided a subjective benefit for the patients and their families. In light of the poor prognosis of most of the patients they observed at the clinic, the British team concluded that the example of the Gerson therapy demonstrated a "way forward" for the treatment of cancer (Sikora et al., 1990).

The Gerson Research Organization of San Diego is currently conducting large retrospective reviews of treatment outcomes of more than 5,400 patient charts, including 5-year survival rates by stage (Hildenbrand et al., 1993), for patients treated by the Mexican medical group Centro Hospitalario Internacional del Pacifico, S.A. This facility, a semi-intensive care hospital, has offered Gerson's treatment since 1976. The review will include patients who either had no previous treatment or failed previous treatment as well as patients who received complementary conventional treatments.

Kelley regimen for cancer. In the 1960s, William Donald Kelley, an orthodontist by training, developed and publicized a nutritional program for cancer after reportedly being told by his doctor that he had metastatic pancreatic cancer and had only 2 months to live (Office of Technology Assessment, 1990). By trial and error, he self-administered doses of enzymes, vitamins, and minerals to treat his cancer. After his recovery, he applied his dietary program to his family; he also believed that his wife and two of his three children had developed cancer (Kelley, 1969). The Kelley regimen clearly derives from Gerson's. Common elements include carrot juice, a basically vegetarian diet, coffee enemas, and pancreatic enzymes, although pancreatic enzymes play a more emphatic role in the Kelley treatment. The Kelley regimen for cancer became one of the most widely known unconventional cancer treatments. Although Kelley is no longer practicing his treatment, the regimen has been continued in a variety of forms by his followers.

One of the people who adopted the Kelley regimen for the treatment of cancer patients was New York physician Nicholas Gonzalez, M.D. Gonzalez has examined the Kelley regimen and provided his own analysis of Kelley's individual metabolic profiles. According to Gonzalez, Kelley believed that human beings are of three genetically based types: sympathetic dominants, parasympathetic dominants, and balanced types. Sympathetic dominants, who have highly efficient and developed sympathetic nervous systems but inefficient parasympathetic nervous systems, evolved in tropical and subtropical ecosystems, eating plant-based diets. Parasympathetic dominants, in which the opposite is the case, evolved in colder regions, eating meat-based diets. Balanced types, whose nervous systems are equally developed, evolved in intermediate regions, eating mixed diets (Office of Technology Assessment, 1990).

Kelley developed a diet for each type according to the type's hypothesized historical origins. He had also traced a characteristic path of "metabolic decline" for each group when it consumed the wrong diet. He associated "hard tumors" with severely compromised sympathetic dominants, and "soft tumors" (cancers of the white blood cells and lymph system) with severely compromised parasympathetic dominants (Office of Technology Assessment, 1990).

As offered by Gonzalez, the Kelley program stresses biodiversity, tailoring diets to individual needs and ranging from purely vegetarian to diets requiring fatty red meat several times daily. Patients consume many supplements—vitamins, minerals, and trace elements—in 130 to 160 capsules daily.

Research base. In his 1987 manuscript *One Man Alone: An Investigation of Nutrition, Cancer, and William Donald Kelley,* Gonzalez presented case histories of 50 patients he selected from his files (Gonzalez, 1987). This case series has been singled out by proponents as one of the most convincing in support of an unconventional cancer treatment (Office of Technology Assessment, 1990).

In 1990, OTA attempted to find out whether the information presented in these cases would be convincing to the medical community by asking six physicians on its advisory panel to review the cases; three of the physicians supported some unconventional treatments, though none was associated with Kelley or Gonzalez, and the other three were mainstream oncologists. Fifteen cases were judged by the reviewers generally supportive of some unconventional medicine as *definitely* showing a positive effect from the Kelley program; in contrast, the mainstream oncologists found that 13 of these 15 were unconvincing and that 2 were unusual (Office of Technology Assessment, 1990).

Another nine cases were judged unusual or suggestive by the supportive group, and unconvincing by the mainstream group. Another 14 cases were judged by the supportive physicians as having been helped by a combination of the Kelley regimen and mainstream cancer therapy; the mainstream group found 12 of these cases unconvincing and 2 unusual. Finally, 12 cases were considered unconvincing by both groups of physicians. The different interpretations of these cases by physicians who are open to unconventional medicine and those who are not illustrates the difficulty in evaluating therapies that fall outside the bounds of conventional medical wisdom.

Gonzalez recently submitted to NCI a meticulously documented best case series (Friedman, 1993). At least 6 of the 24 cases reportedly document complete remissions of cancers, 5 of them metastatic to various sites including liver, pleura, brain, and bone. Two additional cases reportedly document partial remissions.

Macrobiotic diet for cancer. The philosophy and general components of the "standard macrobiotic diet" are described below in the "Alternative Dietary Lifestyles and Cultural Diets" section of this chapter. In the area of cancer management and treatment, the macrobiotic philosophy holds that the development of cancer is determined by dietary, environmental, social, and personal factors; by extension, existing cancers may be influenced by the same factors. The development of cancer is described as a long-term, multistep process that begins well in advance of actual tumor formation (Kushi and Jack, 1983).

According to macrobiotic teachings, accumulated toxins result from overconsumption of milk, cheese, meat, eggs, and other fatty, oily, or greasy foods. Also included in this list are foods with a cooling or freezing effect, such as ice cream, soft drinks, and orange juice (Kushi and Jack, 1983). Macrobiotics uses the traditional oriental concepts of yin (expansive) and yang (contractive) to devise a framework for explaining and formulating a set of dietary recommendations to treat each type of cancer.

A macrobiotic approach to treating cancer would first classify each patient's illness as predominantly yin or yang, or sometimes a combination of both, partly on the basis of the location of the primary tumor in the body and the location of the tumor in the particular organ. In general, tumors in peripheral or upper parts of the body or in hollow, expanded organs are considered yin; examples include lymphoma, leukemia, Hodgkin's disease, and tumors of the mouth (except tongue), esophagus, upper stomach, breast, skin, and outer regions of the brain. Tumors in lower or deeper parts of the body or in more compact organs are considered yang; examples include cancers of the colon, rectum, prostate, ovaries, bone, pancreas, and inner regions of the brain. Cancers thought to result from a combination of yin and yang forces include melanoma (skin cancer) and cancers of the lung, bladder, kidney, lower stomach, uterus, spleen, liver, and tongue (Kushi and Jack, 1983).

For cancers classified as predominantly yang, the standard macrobiotic diet is recommended, with slight emphasis on yin foods. The same diet is recommended for yin-classified cancers, with a slight emphasis on yang foods. Patients with cancers resulting from both yin and yang imbalances are advised to follow "a central way of eating," as suggested in the standard macrobiotic diet. Different cooking styles also are recommended on the basis of this disease classification (Kushi and Jack, 1983).

Research base. The available information on the effectiveness of the macrobiotic diet for treating cancer comes from retrospective case reviews and anecdotal reports, some of which come from the popular literature, and two unpublished retrospective studies (Office of Technology Assessment, 1990). A number of individual accounts of patients who attributed their recovery from cancer to their adherence to a macrobiotic diet have been written in recent years.

In one unpublished retrospective study, Carter and colleagues (1990) compared survival times between 23 pancreatic cancer patients maintained on a macrobiotic diet and similar patients who received conventional cancer therapy. The authors reported that the mean survival (the average) and the median survival (the point in time after diagnosis by which half the group died) was significantly longer for the macrobiotically maintained patients. A followup study by Carter also showed improved survival time for 11 patients with prostate cancer on a macrobiotic diet. However, OTA pointed out that the studies had design flaws that may have overstated the effect (Office of Technology Assessment, 1990).

In another unpublished manuscript, Newbold (undated) presented six case histories of patients with advanced cancer who adopted a macrobiotic diet in addition to using mainstream treatment. These cases were well described medically, including references to appropriate diagnostic tests (all but one case was definitely biopsy proven) and followup scans and tests (Office of Technology Assessment, 1990).

As in the review of the Kelley regimen, when OTA asked its independent advisory panel of six physicians to review Newbold's cases the three mainstream reviewers did not find any of the cases compelling, while two physicians who were open to unconventional therapies were more positive about the outcomes. One concluded that five of the six cases (all except the one without the biopsy-proven diagnosis) showed positive effects from the macrobiotic diet. The remaining physician found two cases that seemed "legitimate," two "highly suggestive," one "suggestive," and one not convincing (Office of Technology Assessment, 1990).

The retrospective studies presented by Carter and Newbold's case histories were later combined and published in the *Journal of the American*

College of Nutrition (Carter et al., 1993). Although the design flaws noted by OTA were still extant in the study, an accompanying editorial suggested that these findings may provide clues to a new approach to the dietary management of cancer (Weisburger, 1993). The editorial stated that the macrobiotic diet has "been construed by classical nutritionists as inadequate. . . . Yet, the application to control the growth of cancer may actually be based on the fact that it is an inadequate diet." The editorial continued by stating that "Perhaps the time has come to teach nutritionists that, in some instances, a nutritional regimen clearly deficient in growth promoting substances might actually be helpful in controlling otherwise untreatable diseases."

Additional cancer diets. Additional cancer diets reviewed by the Office of Technology Assessment included the Livingston/Wheeler regimen and the Wigmore treatment.

Livingston/Wheeler regimen. This regimen is mentioned here because its practitioners advocate diet as a means of potentiating antitumor immunity. Based on Dr. Virginia Livingston's observation of a putative cancer-causing microorganism, the treatment combines vaccines, bacterial reagents, a patented retinoic acid, intravenously administered vitamins, long-term use of antibiotics, and a modified Gerson diet with coffee enemas. Her San Diego-based clinic has continued, after her death, to offer her treatment.

Wigmore treatment. This treatment is an empirically developed dietary regimen (Wigmore, 1985) that uses seed sprouts, wheat grass juice, and uncooked vegetables and fruits. The available literature contains accounts of positive outcomes in cancer, but they are presented without conventional documentation, making it impossible to confirm or deny them. Although advocates have gone to considerable lengths to present supportive literature for their practices (Wigmore, 1993), formal clinical testing has been limited to studies of the reversible, short-term effects of the diet on serum lipids, lipoprotein, and apolipoprotein (W. Ling et al., 1992), which findings are consistent with, if less extensive than, those of similar fat-restricted, basically vegetarian diets (Walford et al., 1992).

Fat-modified diets for treatment of cardiovascular disease and diabetes. Coronary artery disease is the leading cause of death and disability in the United States. Seven million people, nearly 3 percent of the U.S. population, have clinical coronary heart disease. Every year, 1.5 million Americans have acute heart attacks, which kill approximately 520,000 persons, 247,000 of whom are women (American Heart Association, 1991). In fact, cardiovascular diseases—primarily coronary heart disease and stroke—kill nearly as many Americans each year as all other diseases combined (National Center for Health Statistics, 1990). Furthermore, more than 60 million Americans, or 30 percent of the adult population, currently have high blood pressure (National Heart, Lung, and Blood Institute, 1985), which makes them prime candidates for stroke and heart or kidney disease.

Balloon angioplasty (inserting a tiny balloon into the circulatory system and inflating it to open up a plaque-blocked artery) is performed approximately 300,000 times a year in the United States. Although angioplasty provides immediate and possibly lifesaving relief for many patients, it is not a long-term solution. There is no evidence that angioplasty does anything to prevent future angina (severe chest pain) or heart attacks, and about 30 to 40 percent of all angioplasty-treated vessels block up again within 6 months, meaning another angioplasty must be performed (Becker, 1991). Each angioplasty procedure costs about $20,000.

For the most severe cases of heart disease, surgeons remove veins (usually from the legs) and use them to "detour," or bypass, around the clogged arteries of the heart. Even though people who undergo bypass operations experience a reduction in chest pain, the benefits of this surgery, which costs approximately $30,000, often wear off (Myrmel, 1993).

Researchers have known for several decades that a proper diet may prevent the onset of cardiovascular disease. However, once an individual develops this chronic condition, surgery and drugs have been considered the only available methods in mainstream medicine for trying to reverse its effects (Califf et al., 1989). Only recently has diet been considered an alternative to drugs and surgery for treating cardiovascular disease. In the mid-1970s, Nathan Pritikin began using an extremely low-fat, high-fiber diet along with exercise to treat heart disease patients and showed that he could lessen their clinical symptoms. Then in the late 1980s, San Francisco physician Dean Ornish set out to do the same. However, Ornish was armed with a powerful new tool: the angiogram, which is an interior picture of patients' blood vessels. Using "before" and "after" angiograms, Ornish was able to see how changes in diet and lifestyle affected the status of the blockage, or plaque, in the artery. The Pritikin and Ornish diets are described below.

Pritikin diet. The diet is named after the man who developed it, Nathan Pritikin, who had been told by his cardiologist that he was at great risk of death from myocardial infarction. Therefore, he patterned for himself a diet modeled after a vegetarian diet followed by the people of Uganda, who were shown to be essentially free from death by heart attacks (Martin, 1991). In the late 1960s, after a few years on this diet, Pritikin decided that it had saved his life and founded his clinic in Santa Monica to treat cardiac patents.

The Pritikin diet is basically vegetarian, high in complex carbohydrates and fiber, low in cholesterol, and extremely low in fat (less than 10 percent of daily calories). The Pritikin diet also requires 45 minutes of walking daily. Although this diet and exercise program can be followed completely on an outpatient basis, the Pritikin Longevity Center in Santa Monica recommends that patients attend a 26-day program to learn how to prepare their new type of meals and practice new daily exercise and living habits.

Ornish diet. This diet was developed by Dean Ornish, M.D., an assistant clinical professor of medicine at the University of California, San Francisco. The Ornish diet is basically vegetarian, allowing no meat, poultry, or fish, and permitting only the white of eggs. Also, no nuts, caffeine, or dairy products, except a cup a day of nonfat milk or yogurt, are allowed, and no oil or fat is permitted—not even for cooking. Two ounces of alcohol a day are allowed. Providing an average of about 1,800 calories a day, the diet provides 75 percent of its calories from carbohydrates and less than 10 percent from fat (Ornish, 1990). The American Heart Association's recommended adult "prudent diet" calls for total fat of less than 30 percent, which Ornish feels is not really low enough, even for healthy adults, but especially not for people trying to reverse atherosclerosis (Ornish, 1990). Ornish provides his patients all their lunch and dinner meals, precooked, packed in Tupperware, and handed out a week's worth at a time.

In many ways, the Ornish diet is similar to the Pritikin diet. Both are basically vegetarian (although Pritikin does allow 85 grams of chicken or fish per week), high in complex carbohydrates, high in fiber, low in cholesterol, and extremely low in fat (less than 10 percent of daily calories). However, Ornish's program—run on an outpatient basis—calls for stress reduction practices in addition to the diet and emphasizes emotional social support systems, particularly between members of the group. It also requires daily stretching and an hour's walk three times a week.

Research base. The following is an overview of the available research on these two ultra-low-fat dietary regimens.

Pritikin diet. In a study of men taking the Pritikin 26-day course, all 21 participants reduced their cholesterol level, 19 reduced their triglyceride level, and 16 had a reduction in their estradiol level (Rosenthal et al., 1985).

In another study assessing the effectiveness of the Pritikin diet and exercise program on cardiovascular hemodynamics, 20 subjects were divided in two groups (active/treatment and control). These data were compared to a group of 10 healthy individuals not involved in the program. Hemodynamic parameters were collected at admission and at the end of the 26-day program. In obese and hypertensive subjects not on medication who followed the Pritikin program, the cardiac index increased by 10 percent, mean arterial pressure decreased by 5 percent, and the systemic vascular resistance index decreased by 18 percent. Little change was seen in controls. There also was an improvement in ventricular performance (Mattar et al., 1990).

The Pritikin diet has also been studied in connection with adult-onset diabetes mellitus and peripheral vascular disease. Studies suggest that it may show promise in controlling newly diagnosed cases of adult-onset diabetes without drugs. One study (Barnard et al., 1982) evaluated 60 patients who had completed the Pritikin 26-day program. Of the 23 who were taking oral hypoglycemic agents upon entry, all but 2 were off medication by the end of the program. Of the

17 patients who were taking insulin, all but 4 were off medication at discharge. Two of those 4 had their insulin reduced by 50 percent, while the remaining 2 had no major change in their insulin dosage. Fasting blood glucose levels were significantly reduced in all patients; serum cholesterol levels were similarly reduced, as were triglyceride levels. The group as a whole lost an average of 4.3 kg of body weight and achieved 40.5 percent of their desired weight loss. Maximum work capacity increased significantly, while daily walking increased from approximately 11.7 minutes a day to approximately 103 minutes.

In another study, University of California, Los Angeles (UCLA) investigator Dr. James R. Barnard put 650 diabetic patients on the Pritikin diet. After 3 weeks, some 76 percent of the newly diagnosed diabetics, along with 70 percent of those on oral agents, had normal glucose levels (Barnard et al., 1992). However, only 40 percent of those already receiving insulin responded to the diet. According to Barnard, muscles, which may become severely insulin resistant during drug treatment, respond to exercise and a low-fat diet In contrast, drugs may eventually weaken the pancreas while failing to reduce physically and financially devastating vascular complications (e.g., deterioration of eyes and kidneys).

Ornish diet. In what is now known as the Lifestyle Heart Trial, in the late 1970s and early 1980s Ornish conducted a series of trials in which patients with confirmed heart disease were placed on a diet and lifestyle modification program. In the first study, after 30 days people reported a substantial reduction in frequency of angina (heart pain), and many were pain free. Cholesterol levels were down about 20 percent, and high blood pressure was reduced (Ornish et al., 1979). In a followup study in the early 1980s, Ornish reported that 30 days of his regimen were enough to improve blood flow to the heart in some patients and that patients could exercise almost 50 percent more, on average, than they could before beginning the treatment (Ornish et al., 1983).

Finally, in a prospective, randomized, controlled trial to determine the effectiveness of his program over a longer time, Ornish and his colleagues put 28 men and women whose arteries were partially blocked on his program for a full year. Twenty other patients were assigned to a "usual care" group. After 1 year, without the use of lipid-lowering drugs, patients in the experimental group (i.e., receiving the Ornish treatment) reported a 91-percent reduction in the frequency of angina, a 42-percent reduction in the duration of angina, and a 28-percent reduction in the severity of angina. In contrast, control group patients reported a 165-percent rise in frequency, a 95-percent rise in duration, and a 39-percent rise in severity of angina (Ornish et al., 1990).

Patients in the experimental group also showed a significant overall regression, or reduction, of coronary atherosclerosis (blocked arteries) as measured by angiograms. In contrast, patients in the usual care group had a significant overall progression, or worsening, of their coronary atherosclerosis. This finding led Ornish to conclude that the conventional recommendations for patients with heart disease, such as a 30-percent fat diet, are not sufficient to bring about an improvement in many patients.

Ornish has never tested separately each component of his multifaceted program, so it is impossible to be sure which component contributed most to the improvements. If it was the dietary regimen that led to the improvements, it is a regimen that most Americans would have a hard time following, admits Ornish (Schardt, 1993). However, some researchers believe that it does not take such a radically restricted diet to start reversing the effects of heart disease. In a study in Germany, 56 men suffering from angina caused by partially blocked arteries were placed on a reduced-fat diet (less than 20 percent of calories from fat, 7 percent of calories from saturated fat, and 200 mg of cholesterol a day). As in the Ornish program, they also participated in an exercise program. After a year, angiograms showed that the blockages in 32 percent of the men on the low-fat diet had improved, compared with just 17 percent in the control group (Schuler et al., 1992).

In addition, in the late 1980s, researchers in Britain placed 26 men with partially blocked arteries and elevated blood cholesterol on carefully monitored diets and reduced their fat intake to 27 percent of calories—about three-fourths of what the average American eats. The diet's saturated fat and cholesterol amounts also were substantially less than most Americans eat, while its fiber content was slightly higher. Over the next 3 years, the men on the fat-restricted diet suffered only one-third as many deaths, heart attacks, and strokes as men in the control group—who were not told what to eat, and whose diets were not monitored (Watts et al., 1992). Furthermore, angiograms showed that the openings in the arteries of 38 percent of the men who changed their diets became slightly larger.

Food elimination diets for treatment of food allergies. Allergies to food, or food intolerance, have become a major area of research in recent years. Many of the researchers involved in this research specialize in environmental medicine (see the "Alternative Systems of Medical Practice" chapter), which is the science of assessing the impact of such environmental factors as chemicals, foods, and inhalants on health. It provides an understanding of the interface between the external environment and the biological function of the individual.

Dietary management of food allergies is based on avoidance of food antigens and the 4-day rotary diversified diet. With the rotary diet and avoidance of repetitive food exposures, it is possible to reduce sensitivity to foods and hasten recovery from food allergies. Nutritional supplements are prescribed as indicated by objective nutritional testing and the symptoms of the patient.

Research base. Miller (1977) studied eight chronically ill food-sensitive patients who were tested with provocation-neutralization techniques. The patients were treated with injections of allergy extracts and compared to those treated with placebos. In a rigidly controlled study, King (1988) showed a correlation between oral food challenge and provocation-neutralization testing. Treatment using results from this testing showed significant symptom relief. Using neutralization therapy, Rea and colleagues (1984) found significant improvement in 20 patients with known food sensitivity in signs and symptoms of allergy reactions to certain foods.

Food intolerance is also being studied as a causal or contributing factor in rheumatoid arthritis. In a clinical trial in Norway, Kjeldsen-Kragh and colleagues (1991) found that fasting followed by dietary restriction could relieve the symptoms of rheumatoid arthritis on a long-term basis. They subjected 27 rheumatoid arthritis patients to a 7- to 10-day fast (except for herbal teas, garlic, vegetable broth, a decoction of potatoes and parsley, and extracts from carrots, beets, and celery) followed by 1 year of an individually adjusted vegetarian diet. The diet-restricted patients stayed on a Norwegian health farm the first 4 weeks of the study. A control group of 26 patients stayed in a convalescent home for 4 weeks but ate an ordinary diet throughout the trial.

After 4 weeks, the diet group showed a decrease in pain score; a significant decrease in pain, morning stiffness, and the number of tender and swollen joints; and improved grip strength and ability to articulate the joints. There was also a significant improvement in a number of biochemical markers associated with inflammation. These improvements were maintained throughout the year. In contrast, the control group showed a decrease in pain score after its stay in the convalescent home, but none of the other indices improved. At the end of the study the conditions of the control patients had deteriorated.

This study suggests that there is a food allergy component to rheumatoid arthritis and that food restriction appears to be a useful supplement to the conventional medical treatment of rheumatoid arthritis. Darlington and colleagues (1986) and Beri and colleagues (1988) obtained similar results, but their studies lasted only 3 months.

There is also evidence that food elimination diets may benefit many children with hyperactivity (Kanofsky, 1986). Several research teams have used double-blind designs to demonstrate this point. The Institute of Child Health and Hospital for Sick Children in London undertook a randomized, crossover, placebo-controlled trial to evaluate the effect of diet on the development of hyperactivity (Egger et al., 1985). The first phase of the study consisted of placing 76 hyperactive children on a food elimination diet. The presupposition was that individuals can be sensitive to a food or food additive in their diet and that improvement occurs when the offending foods or food additives are removed from the diet. At the end of the first phase of the study, 62 of the 76 children (82 percent) improved on the diet, and a normal range of behavior was achieved in 21 (29 percent) of them. In addition to overactivity, other symptoms such as headaches, abdominal pain, antisocial behavior, and fits were also often alleviated.

In all, 48 foods were implicated as contributing to hyperactivity in the young patients. However,

34 of the 50 children for whom full data are available reacted to fewer than 7 foods. Two reacted to 30 foods. Five patients were also noted with symptoms from such inhalants as pollen, perfume, and house dust. Foods that frequently caused problems included cow's milk (64 percent of subjects tested), chocolate (59 percent), wheat (49 percent), and oranges (45 percent).

The second phase of the study included 28 children from the original group, who entered into a double-blind, crossover, placebo-controlled trial that reintroduced one incriminated food. Symptoms returned or were exacerbated much more often when patients were on active material than on placebo. One of the most interesting findings of the study is that the artificial food coloring tartrazine and the preservative benzoic acid were the commonest food items causing a reaction. The behavior of 79 percent of the 34 children tested deteriorated when tartrazine or benzoic acid was reintroduced into their diet. These findings are compatible with the work of Dr. Benjamin Feingold, the San Francisco allergist who implicated tartrazine and other artificial food additives in children's diets as contributors to hyperactivity. It is worth noting that the same London group also published a study stating that 93 percent of 88 children with severe, frequent migraines recovered on a diet that eliminated foods and food additives that had been shown to cause symptoms (Egger et al., 1983).

Some confirmation for the food elimination treatment for hyperkinesis was provided by Kaplan and colleagues (1989). In their study, 10 of 24 hyperactive children exhibited approximately a 50-percent improvement in behavior when placed on an elimination diet that was not as restrictive as the London diet.

Alternative Dietary Lifestyles in Prevention and Treatment of Chronic Illness

A number of alternative dietary lifestyles throughout the United States and the world are believed to increase resistance to illness. Although some diets, such as macrobiotics, have been intentionally developed in the past half-century, others have evolved more naturally over the centuries.

An "alternative lifestyle" diet can be described as any diet that differs from the mainstream American diet. Such diets include various forms of vegetarianism and diets with emphasis on "natural," "organic," "unrefined," "unprocessed," and/or other health foods in varying degrees. Others are drawn from other societies around the world, such as the "Mediterranean" diet.

Historically, there has been much skepticism among some health professionals about such diets. For example, when the vegetarian movement started in the United States about 50 years ago, people questioned whether adults subsisting on such diets could even do a full day's work and still survive (Krey, 1982). However, generations of people around the world have now grown up on these diets, helping to dispel such myths. Furthermore, many individuals and population groups have practiced vegetarianism on a long-term basis and have demonstrated excellent health (American Academy of Pediatrics, 1977). Indeed, the case against such diets has been largely cultural and economic (see the section "Barriers and Key Issues Related to Diet and Nutrition" in this chapter).

Vegetarian diets. Vegetarian diets are among the most common of alternative diets in the United States today. The degree of vegetarianism can vary widely, ranging from those who eat red meat infrequently to those who totally exclude any animal-derived foods, such as dairy products or eggs, from their diet. Vegetarianism is often categorized according to the extent of these restrictions. For example, people who consume dairy products and eggs but not other animal foods are referred to as *lacto-ovo-vegetarians,* while people who avoid all animal products are referred to as *vegans.* Studies of vegetarians in the United States and other industrialized nations probably provide the most extensive support for the idea that alternative dietary habits can favorably influence the incidence and pathology of disease.

This section focuses on the nutritional aspects of the two most widely studied variations on the vegetarian diet: the one followed by adherents of the Seventh-Day Adventist Church, and the macrobiotic diet. The health-related data from people eating these diets are compared with data taken from individuals in the general U.S. population.

Seventh-Day Adventists. The Seventh-Day Adventists are a Protestant sect that among other things preaches a clean, wholesome lifestyle and admonishes against eating animal flesh (i.e., red meat, poultry, fish). Thus, Seventh-Day Adventists are for the most part lacto-ovo-vegetarians. They also abstain from alcohol, tobacco, and caffeine-containing beverages, such as coffee and tea. Even though they avoid meat, Seventh-Day Adventists' diets are not substantially lower in fat intake than the typical American diet. For example, in one survey of lacto-ovo-vegetarian Seventh-Day Adventists, total fat intake averaged 36 percent of energy versus 37 percent for the average American (Phillips et al., 1983).

Macrobiotic diet. Along with Seventh-Day Adventists, people who consume a macrobiotic diet have been studied extensively to examine associations with disease risk factors. In addition, macrobiotic diets are among the most popular alternative dietary therapies for cancer and other chronic diseases (Cassileth et al., 1984).

The earliest version of the macrobiotic diet, termed the "zen macrobiotic diet," originated with the lecturer-philosopher Georges Ohsawa (1893–1966), the pen name for Yukikaza Sakurazawa, a Japanese teacher who studied the writings of Japanese physician Sagen Ishikuzuka (1850–1910). Ohsawa is said to have cured himself of serious illness by changing from the modern refined diet then sweeping Japan to a simple diet of brown rice, miso soup, sea vegetables, and other traditional foods. He initiated the development of macrobiotic philosophy, reportedly integrating elements of Eastern and Western perspectives with "holistic" perspectives on science and medicine. Ohsawa made his first of several visits to the United States in 1959.

Ohsawa outlined 10 stages of diet (designated by numbers –3 to +7). Diet –3 consists of 10 percent cereal grains, 30 percent vegetables, 10 percent soups, 30 percent animal products, 15 percent salads and fruits, 5 percent desserts, and beverages "as little as possible." With each higher number diet, Ohsawa reduced the percentages of foods from some categories or eliminated the category entirely and increased others, so that in the +3 diet, for example, 60 percent was cereals, 30 percent was vegetables, and 10 percent was soups.

Since the early 1970s, the macrobiotic movement in the United States has been under the leadership of Michio Kushi. Kushi, who studied with Ohsawa and came to the United States from Japan in 1949, preserved elements of Ohsawa's philosophy while incorporating a variety of broader and more complex components into macrobiotic philosophy and practice. Most notably, Ohsawa's 10-phase dietary levels were replaced with the general "standard macrobiotic diet," which Kushi described in detail in his 1983 book, *The Cancer Prevention Diet* (Kushi and Jack, 1983).

Unlike Seventh-Day Adventists, whose vegetarian diets usually include dairy products and eggs, the standard macrobiotic diet as practiced today tends to minimize consumption of all animal products except fish (M. Kushi, 1977, 1983). Thus the macrobiotic diet is predominantly *vegan*, with an emphasis on whole cereal grains and vegetables, preferably organically grown. As a result, it tends to be relatively high in complex carbohydrates and low in fat content (and, therefore, calories) in comparison with the standard American diet. One survey of 50 adults consuming a macrobiotic diet demonstrated that fat intake averaged 23 percent of energy, saturated fat intake averaged 9 percent of energy, and carbohydrate intake averaged 65 percent of energy (L. Kushi et al., 1988).

Research base. The following is an overview of the available research on the health-promoting and disease-preventing effects of the Seventh-Day Adventist and macrobiotic diets.

Seventh-Day Adventist diet. Despite their relatively high fat intake, Seventh-Day Adventists have less heart disease and incidence of some cancers than occurs in the general U.S. population. For example, Seventh-Day Adventists who eat little or no red meat have a lower death rate from heart disease than the general U.S. population (Phillips et al., 1978; Snowdon et al., 1984a). Indeed, studies on Seventh-Day Adventist males have shown that their serum cholesterol levels were lower and that the first heart attack occurred almost a decade later than average. The incidence of heart disease was only 60 percent as high as that of a control group in California (Register and Sonnenberg, 1973). Abstinence from tobacco and alcohol also may have contributed to this effect.

Studies comparing Seventh-Day Adventists with non-Adventists demonstrate that the former tend to have lower blood pressure levels as well. For example, in one study in which age, sex, and body size were taken into account, blood pressure levels for vegetarian Seventh-Day Adventists averaged 128.7 mm Hg systolic and 76.2 mm Hg diastolic versus nonvegetarians' average levels of 139.3 mm Hg systolic and 84.5 mm Hg diastolic (Armstrong et al., 1977). Similar findings were seen in other studies comparing vegetarian and nonvegetarian Seventh-Day Adventists (Melby et al., 1989).

Another study comparing blood pressure levels of vegetarian Seventh-Day Adventists with nonvegetarian Mormons, who similarly avoid tobacco and alcohol, demonstrated that the Seventh-Day Adventists still had lower blood pressure levels (Rouse et al., 1982). Comparisons of California Seventh-Day Adventists with their non-Adventist neighbors also demonstrated that the Adventists had lower LDL cholesterol levels (Fraser, 1988).

The overall cancer death rate of male Seventh-Day Adventists is only about half that of the overall cancer death rate of the U.S. general population, and the overall cancer death rate of female Seventh-Day Adventists is about 70 percent of that of the general population (Phillips et al., 1980). The lower death rates apply not only to those cancer sites known to be associated with cigarette smoking (e.g., lungs), but also to other sites such as the breast. In fact, Adventists have 80 to 90 percent of the general population's breast cancer death rate and only 50 to 60 percent of the colon and rectal cancer death rate (Phillips et al., 1980). These observations suggest that smoking habits alone cannot explain the difference between cancer death rates of Seventh-Day Adventists and those of the general population.

The results of other prospective dietary studies among Seventh-Day Adventists are mixed when vegetarians are compared with nonvegetarians. For instance, there appears to be little relationship between such dietary variables as total fat or animal fat intake with risk of breast cancer (Mills et al., 1988, 1989a). However, in two prospective cohort studies, Seventh-Day Adventists who rarely consumed meat, poultry, or fish appeared to have a lower risk of breast cancer than those who consumed these foods at least once a week (Mills et al., 1989a; Phillips and Snowdon, 1983). In neither of these studies was this association statistically significant.

However, a study of 35,000 California Seventh-Day Adventists, covering a followup period from 1976 to 1982, *did* indicate an increased risk of colon cancer with increasing animal fat intake (Morgan et al., 1988). Indeed, those individuals in the highest third of animal fat intake rates had a risk of developing colon cancer that was 1.8 times that of individuals in the lowest third of animal fat intake rates; people with intermediate animal fat intakes were intermediate in their risk (Morgan et al., 1988).

In another study of cancer among 25,000 California Seventh-Day Adventists covering 20 years (1960–80), men who consumed meat at least four times a week experienced a prostate cancer death rate of 41.9 deaths per 100,000 person-years versus 29.7 deaths per 100,000 person-years for men who did not consume meat (Phillips and Snowdon, 1983). In the study begun in 1976, daily consumption of meat was associated with a risk of developing prostate cancer 1.41 times greater than that of men who never ate meat (Mills et al., 1989b). In the earlier study, meat intake was also associated with increased risk of prostate cancer (Snowdon et al., 1984b).

On the other hand, increased consumption of beans and lentils appeared to decrease the risk of colon cancer in the Seventh-Day Adventist population (Morgan et al., 1988). In fact, among the people who ate the highest amounts of these foods, the risk of developing colon cancer was one-third that of people who ate the lowest amounts (Morgan et al., 1988). Furthermore, consumption of beans and lentils at least three times per week was associated with approximately 50 percent lower risk of developing prostate cancer than consumption of beans and lentils less than once a month (Mills et al., 1989b).

The association of vegetarianism with decreased risk of certain cancers appears to have correlates with biological parameters in Seventh-Day Adventists. Vegetarian Seventh-Day Adventists appear to have less colonic mucosal cell turnover than nonvegetarians and those at increased risk of colon cancer (Lipkin et al., 1985). This point is significant, because it is believed that decreased cell proliferation of the colonic mucosa may be a hallmark of decreased risk of colon cancer (Lipkin, 1974).

Macrobiotic diet. No studies to date have examined directly the role of a macrobiotic diet in chronic disease prevention. However, a number of studies have examined associations between macrobiotic diets and biological risk parameters such as blood pressure, cholesterol levels, and estrogen metabolism. The earliest of these studies were surveys of blood pressure and blood lipid levels, which were conducted in the Boston macrobiotic community. One of these studies showed that young adults eating a macrobiotic diet had blood pressure levels of 106 mm Hg systolic and 60 mm Hg diastolic, which was significantly lower than would be expected in the general population (Sacks et al., 1974). In fact, in comparison with people of similar age and sex in Framingham, MA, the subjects' systolic blood pressure was an average of 11 mm Hg lower and diastolic blood pressure 14 mm Hg lower (Sacks et al., 1975). In addition, those in the macrobiotic community who ate some animal food tended to have higher blood pressures than others in the macrobiotic community who did not (Sacks et al., 1974).

Blood lipid levels, a general indicator of coronary heart disease risk, also were substantially lower among the people eating macrobiotically than in the Framingham comparison group. In fact, average plasma total cholesterol levels among the macrobiotic vegetarians was 126 mg/dL versus a total average plasma cholesterol level of 184 mg/dL in the age- and sex-matched controls in the Framingham population (Sacks et al., 1975). Levels of low-density lipoprotein (LDL) cholesterol—the type of cholesterol that promotes heart disease—also were substantially lower in those eating a macrobiotic diet, averaging 73 mg/dL in the macrobiotic vegetarians and 118 mg/dL in the controls (Sacks et al., 1975). Although levels of high-density lipoprotein (HDL) cholesterol—the type of cholesterol that protects against heart disease—were also lower in the macrobiotic vegetarians (43 mg/dL vs. 49 mg/dL), the ratio of total to HDL cholesterol, a measure of the relative atherogenicity (i.e., ability to form plaques) of the blood lipid profile, was substantially lower among the macrobiotic vegetarians than in the comparison group (2.9 vs. 3.8). These differences persisted even when adjusted for weight differences. The relatively favorable blood cholesterol profile of macrobiotic vegetarians has been confirmed in several other surveys (Bergan and Brown, 1980; Knuiman and West, 1982; L. Kushi et al., 1988; Sacks et al., 1985).

In recent years, there has been increasing interest in the role of fat-soluble antioxidants in atherogenesis. It has been hypothesized that oxidation of LDL particles may be a critical step in the uptake of LDL by macrophages, as well as for some other mechanisms that increase the atherogenicity of LDL cholesterol (Steinberg and Witztum, 1990). The relative proportion of antioxidants to circulating LDL has been suggested as an additional measure of the atherogenicity of blood lipid levels (Berry, 1992). A study of macrobiotic vegetarians demonstrated that they had not only lower LDL levels but also higher plasma levels of antioxidants relative to cholesterol compared to nonvegetarians (Pronczuk et al., 1992).

The favorable cardiovascular disease profile of macrobiotic vegetarians is likely to be largely due to the relative avoidance of meat and dairy products. Indeed, when the diet of macrobiotic vegetarians was supplemented with 250 grams of beef per day, plasma total cholesterol increased by about 19 percent after 4 weeks, from an average of 140 mg/dL to 166 mg/dL (Sacks et al., 1981). Comparisons of macrobiotic vegetarians with lactovegetarians and nonvegetarians also indicate a direct relationship between average blood total cholesterol levels and dairy product intake (Sacks et al., 1985).

In the context of cancer risk, studies comparing women eating a macrobiotic diet with women eating a typical American diet demonstrate substantial differences in estrogen metabolism (Goldin et al., 1981, 1982). In fact, women eating a macrobiotic diet had substantially higher fecal excretion and lower urinary excretion of estrogens, with somewhat lower serum levels of estradiol. This point is significant because many cancers, especially breast cancer, are growth dependent on hormones such as estrogen. The altered estrogen metabolism profile of women eating macrobiotically may reflect a lower risk of breast cancer (Goldin et al., 1981, 1982).

Furthermore, in subsequent studies it was demonstrated that women eating macrobiotically had dramatically higher urinary excretion of lignans, such as enterolactone and enterodiol, and of isoflavonoids, such as daidzein and equol, than women consuming a lacto-ovo-vegetarian diet or an omnivorous diet. Women with breast cancer had the lowest levels of these phytoestrogens (Adlercreutz et al., 1986, 1987). These differences appeared to be related to greater intake of whole grains, legumes, and vegetables by the macrobiotic women.

It has been hypothesized that such a fiber-rich diet may, by the presence of these lignans and other weak estrogens (i.e., phytoestrogens) in the intestinal tract, stimulate the synthesis of sex hormone binding globulin in the liver and may thus decrease levels of free estradiol in the plasma (Adlercreutz et al., 1987). This may, in turn, reduce the risk of breast as well as other hormone-dependent cancers. It has also been suggested that these phytoestrogens (see the "Herbal Medicine" chapter) may actually compete with endogenous estradiol on the cellular level, further reducing the cellular proliferation and, hence, the potentially carcinogenic effects of estradiol (Price and Fenwick, 1985; Tang and Adams, 1980).

In addition to the general macronutrient differences (lower fat, higher complex carbohydrate intake) between macrobiotic diets and the standard American diet, certain foods in the standard macrobiotic diet may have specific anticancer effects. Examples of such foods, which are absent in the typical American diet, include various soyfoods, such as miso and tofu, and sea vegetables (see the "Diets of Other Cultures" section for a discussion of the health benefits of these foods).

Health risks associated with strict vegetarian diets. Except for vitamin B12 deficiency, diets that exclude meat or animal products do not produce deficiencies in adults if they are correctly followed. Nevertheless, there are reports in the literature that have associated some forms of vegetarianism with high risks of deficiencies in children and pregnant women (Debry, 1991). The nutrition of children on a vegetarian diet is considered to be adequate and well balanced when the diet contains dairy products and eggs. It has been suggested that a severe or strict vegetarian diet is not suitable for infants or toddlers. For example, serious deficiency states (e.g., rickets, osteoporosis, anemia, growth retardation) have been described in children subsisting on such regimens (Lentze, 1992). However, it is interesting to note that in a study that examined the maternity care records of 775 vegan mothers living on a commune in southern Tennessee, there was only one case of preeclampsia (Carter et al., 1987). The authors concluded that it is possible to sustain a normal pregnancy on a vegan diet, and the source of protein (i.e., animal or vegetable) does not seem to affect birth weight, as long as vegan mothers receive continuous prenatal care, supplement their diets with prenatal vitamins, calcium, and iron, and apply "protein-complementing" nutritional principles.

Diets of other cultures. A cultural diet is defined as the diet of any group of people who share beliefs and customs. By this definition, everyone in the United States is a member of some cultural group. For many cultural groups, food plays an important role in maintenance of both spiritual and physical health. The following is a brief overview of several cultural diets—Asian, Mediterranean, and traditional Native American Indian—that are thought to provide some protection against many of the nutritionally related chronic illnesses prevalent among users of the mainstream diet in the United States today. Although there are many more cultural diets than are covered here, solid scientific research has not yet been collected to establish whether they provide any particular health benefits.

Asian diet. This diet is consumed predominantly by people living in China, Southeast Asia, Korea, and Japan. Rice is a staple and the center of the meal, and there is little or no use of dairy products. Soybean products are important sources of protein and calcium. Dishes incorporate many different ingredients and may be stir-fried or steamed. This diet, in its traditional form, is low in fat and high in carbohydrates and sodium (Kittler and Sucher, 1989).

Mediterranean diet. The Mediterranean Basin is geographically defined as an inland sea that touches three continents—Europe, Asia, and Africa—and is surrounded by 15 almost contiguous countries: Spain, France, Italy, the former Yugoslavia, Albania, Greece, Turkey, Syria, Lebanon, Israel, Egypt, Libya, Tunisia, Algeria, and Morocco. Divided by language and, historically, by political and religious conflict, the Mediterranean countries have for centuries been joined by a similar diet of daily staples.

The Mediterranean diet consists of a daily intake of grains, potatoes, pasta, greens and other vegetables, fruit, beans and other legumes (e.g., lentils, split peas), nuts, cheese, and yogurt. Fish, poultry, eggs, sweets, and red meat are eaten less frequently. However, olive oil and garlic are almost always consumed in abundance (Spiller, 1991). In the case of Spain, France, and Italy, it is their southernmost parts that are considered Mediterranean, defined by their use of olive oil.

Another important aspect of the Mediterranean diet is its emphasis on less refined complex carbohydrates (e.g., pasta) in place of sugar and the highly refined starches generally consumed in the United States, even though direct evidence for benefit in reducing disease risk is limited. Anticipated reductions in colon cancer by diets high in grain fiber diets have been difficult to document epidemiologically, although inverse associations with vegetables have been seen repeatedly. However, reduced constipation and reduced risk of colonic diverticular disease are clear benefits (Willett et al., 1990).

It is interesting to note that in the northern areas of many of the European Mediterranean countries, where there is more use of butter, other animal fats, and meat, there is also a higher incidence of cancer (La Vecchia, 1993).

Traditional Native American Indian diet. Many foods used throughout the world today were probably first used by Indians of North, Central, and South America—for example, beans, corn, cranberries, peanuts, peppers, potatoes, pumpkin, squash, and tomatoes. Today, Native American Indians live in areas that are vastly different from one another, so there is no single typical diet. In fact, traditional diets are prepared infrequently except for ceremonial occasions. This is true even for the Arizona Hopi, who still live in old villages that their ancient ancestors inhabited (Kuhnlein and Calloway, 1977). Nevertheless, in many American Indian diets, corn is the staple food. It is eaten fresh roasted or boiled, as hominy, or as cornmeal in a variety of dishes. Meat is eaten when it can be obtained by hunting or fishing, but because it is so expensive to buy, it is used sparingly. Milk and dairy products are not used often because of a high incidence of lactose intolerance (lactose is the primary sugar in milk). Berries, wild plants, and roots are used when available (Robinson and Lawler, 1982).

Research base. The following provides an overview of research on the effectiveness of some components of the Asian, Mediterranean, and traditional Native American Indian diets in lowering some risk factors for disease.

Asian diet. In a cohort study of 265,000 people in Japan, consumption of miso soup (a food made from soybeans) appeared to reduce the risk of breast cancer (Hirayama, 1986) and stomach cancer (Hirayama, 1981). A similar inverse association was seen between stomach cancer and tofu intake (Hirayama, 1971). Furthermore, miso has been observed to inhibit formation of mammary tumors in rodents (Baggott et al., 1990) and may have antioxidant properties as well (Santiago et al., 1992).

Antioxidant properties have been proposed as a principal mechanism by which dietary compounds such as beta-carotene, vitamin E, indoles, and others exert cancer-preventive effects (Steinmetz and Potter, 1991a, 1991b). It has also been suggested that sea vegetables, perhaps through their high concentration of alginic acid, a type of dietary fiber, may decrease the risk of breast cancer (Teas et al., 1984; Yamamoto et al., 1987). Beans and bean products, especially those derived from soybeans (e.g., miso, tofu, tempeh), also contain protease inhibitors (Messina and Barnes, 1991), isoflavonoids (Adlercreutz et al., 1987), and other compounds that may play roles in cancer prevention (Axelson et al., 1984).

Mediterranean diet. The high consumption of olive oil is considered a major contributor to the disease-preventive aspects of this diet. Olive oil is a monounsaturated fat, meaning that somewhere along the fat, or fatty acid, molecule there is a single site not completely "saturated" with hydrogen atoms. Substituting monounsaturated fats, such as olive oil, for saturated fat in the diet has been shown to reduce LDL cholesterol without affecting HDL cholesterol, thus providing an improved ratio (Mensink and Katan, 1992). In addition, monounsaturated fats in the diet have been found to reduce blood sugar and triglycerides in adult-onset diabetics (Garg et al., 1992).

In one of the first studies of its kind, researchers in France placed approximately 300 patients who had recently had a heart attack (myocardial infarction) on a Mediterranean type of diet and compared their incidence of having a second myocardial infarction with that of a control group of patients who were placed on the standard therapeutic diet. The experimental group consumed significantly more bread and fruit, a margarine with a fatty acid composition

The Trouble With Margarine

Margarine starts out as a liquid vegetable oil. However, it is converted to a form that will remain solid at room temperature, and thus resemble butter in texture, by a process called hydrogenation. The hydrogenation of vegetable oils changes the three dimensional structure of the fatty acids that make up the oil, converting the naturally occurring *cis* fatty acids to *trans* fatty acids. Oils composed primarily of *hydrogenated* fats typically "melt" at higher temperatures than those composed of nonhydrogenated (polyunsaturated) fats.

Over the past few decades many American physicians and nutrition experts have advised people to eat margarine in place of butter and lard, which contain "saturated" animal fats and are associated with an increased risk of developing coronary heart disease (CHD). However, recent evidence suggests that consuming significant amounts of margarine may pose health risks of its own, unrelated to problems caused by saturated animal fats. This is because *trans* fatty acids have been found to increase blood levels of low-density lipoprotein cholesterol, which is associated with an increased risk of developing CHD. At the same time, *trans* fatty acids also lower blood levels of high-density lipoprotein cholesterol, which has a protective effect against CHD. In addition, recent epidemiological studies have found a positive association between the consumption of *trans* fatty acids and CHD. Thus, it now appears that consuming margarine may not offer any health advantages over consuming butter (Willett and Ascherio, 1994).

In fact, because the average American takes in approximately 4–7 grams of these *trans* fatty acids daily by eating margarine and processed foods containing partially hydrogenated vegetable oils, the number of excess deaths in the United States attributed to the consumption of such food products is likely to be substantial.

comparable to that of olive oil, and significantly less butter, cream, and meat than the control group. After a followup of about 27 months, there were only 3 cardiac deaths and 5 nonfatal myocardial infarctions in the experimental group versus 16 cardiac deaths and 17 nonfatal myocardial infarctions in the control group (de Lorgeril et al., 1994). It is interesting to note that the patients on the Mediterranean type of diet had increases in blood levels of vitamin E and C while controls did not.

Garlic, a staple of the Mediterranean diet, also has been implicated as a major disease-preventive food. A growing number of reports in the medical literature suggest that garlic supplementation may be effective in decreasing serum cholesterol levels by as much as 15 to 20 percent and thus may have a protective effect against cardiovascular disease (Kleijnen et al., 1989; Turner, 1990). Many of these studies have been faulted for having methodological problems, although a recent meta-analysis of the various studies reporting a cholesterol-lowering effect found that garlic *did* appear to significantly reduce total serum cholesterol (Silagy and Neil, 1994).

There are also reports suggesting that garlic may prevent the development of cancer in humans (Dorant et al., 1993). Lin and colleagues (1994) reported that processed garlic effectively reduced the amount of DNA damage caused by N-nitroso compounds, which are found in many foods such as cooked meat and have been implicated as carcinogens (cancer-causing compounds).

Traditional Native American Indian diet. In the case of the Hopi and Papago tribes, studies have shown that traditional foods have mineral content superior to federally provided commodity foods (Calloway et al., 1974). Followers of traditional Native American diets have found ways of maximizing available nutrients; an example is in the techniques of processing the corn used in tortillas, a staple in diets derived from the Mexican and Central American tradition. The corn is soaked in lime, which softens the skin of the corn kernels as well as increasing the calcium content of the resulting tortillas (Katz, 1987). Traditional lime soaking also liberates bound niacin in the corn. Because milled corn has been substituted for lime-soaked corn in Native American Indian diets, niacin deficiency has become a problem, and incidences of niacin-deficiency-induced pellagra have increased. Although few studies have been done on the possible disease-preventive aspects of the traditional Native American Indian diet, health surveys have found that heart disease and cancer, two diet-related diseases, are virtually nonexistent in some Indian populations, such as the Navajo (Reese, 1972).

Barriers and Key Issues Related to Alternative Diet and Nutrition Research

This chapter has so far dealt primarily with basic and clinical research relating to diet and nutrition interventions either for preventing or treating illness. However, to discuss such research without mentioning outside factors that will affect how research results are evaluated or disseminated to the public provides only a small part of the overall picture. Because nutritional and diet-otherapy interventions affect an array of biochemical and physiological processes in the body, evaluating the interventions' effectiveness requires equally complex methodologies. Also of concern to those who work in this field is to research and develop "alternatives" to institutionalized nutrition and feeding programs that directly contribute to diet- and nutrition-related chronic disease. Finally, there is the issue of dissemination; no matter how good the research, it is valuable only if it reaches those who will benefit from it. Research data should be disseminated not only to the doctors or other health personnel who may prescribe such therapies, but also to the eventual target audience (i.e., the patients). Some of these issues are discussed below.

Study Design

In most instances, it is virtually impossible to conduct a double-blind study of a dietary regimen. Patients obviously will know whether they are being fed a normal diet or a modified diet. Therefore, a single-blind design (in which the evaluator of the data is "blind" to who receives which treatment) is more appropriate for most dietary studies. However, in some instances a double-blind study is appropriate, such as when all subjects are given a tasteless, colorless pill. Also, investigators must consider the possibility of a negative placebo ("nocebo") effect in the control group as well as a placebo effect in the treatment group. In other words, patients who think they are not getting the therapy may not get better because of this knowledge—just as patients who think they are receiving an effective treatment may get better spontaneously, independent of the therapy. (See the "Mind-Body Interventions" chapter for a discussion of placebo and nocebo effects.)

The recommendation of the recent OTA report *Unconventional Cancer Treatments* offers an example of one possible methodological approach to evaluating many nutritional interventions. As a practical approach to evaluating the treatments they had examined, the OTA report's authors proposed a "best case review" conceptually similar to approaches used by NCI for evaluating biological response modifiers (BRMs) (Office of Technology Assessment, 1990). Best case reviews are discussed in detail in appendix F.

BRMs are agents that exert anticancer effects in a novel manner. Unlike conventional cytoxic therapy, which kills tumor cells with slightly less chemical toxicity than chemotherapy, BRMs stimulate, or potentiate, the body's immune system to overcome or at least restrain the invading tumor. Most BRMs currently being investigated are genetically engineered copies of peptides found naturally in the human body; among them are tumor necrosis factor, interleukins, and interferons. At an early stage in this clinical research, NCI researchers recognized that because BRMs act biologically and not chemically, they had to be evaluated using a procedure that is significantly different from the one used for standard cytotoxic agents (Oldham, 1982). With this in mind, in 1978 NCI created a special Biological Response Modifiers Program to coordinate research to identify, study, and clinically evaluate BRMs.

Clinical evaluation of BRMs is difficult because determining the optimal dose or dosing schedule for the agent is critically important. Also important is the identification of responsive tumor types and even of the stage of disease and metabolic condition of patients who are treated (Creekmore et al., 1991; Hawkins et al., 1986; Oldham, 1985). Consequently, experts in BRM research advise against testing BRMs in large, controlled clinical trials (Phase III trials) until after these parameters have been optimized in careful individual tests of the proposed therapy in patients believed to be the most likely to show a favorable response (Creekmore et al., 1991; Hawkins et al., 1986; Oldham, 1985). This type of evaluation is inherently exploratory and observational; therefore, it cannot be conducted in the same rigidly stipulated way as a Phase III trial.

Because such studies demand the continual application of good clinical and scientific judgment, they are demanding of the time and energy of investigators, who typically are experts keenly interested in the therapy under evaluation. This time-consuming process is necessary because the consequence of proceeding prematurely to a Phase III trial is an inconclusive or falsely negative result. Since dietary and nutritional interventions often affect biology in ways at least as complicated as the anticancer BRMs currently being evaluated by NCI, recommendations concerning the evaluation of BRMs should apply to the evaluation of many diet and nutrition interventions.

Furthermore, careful scientific judgment is needed as to when sufficient *evaluation* has gone on and *confirmation* is in order. For example, there is general agreement in the scientific community that the time is now at hand to "confirm" the efficacy of megadose antioxidants in the prevention of coronary artery disease progression in a large Phase III trial (Steinberg, 1993). This assessment is correct even though such trials are costly, and there is always a risk of a false negative result if all the relevant parameters have not yet been fully optimized. The interaction of a variety of factors in producing a therapeutic outcome would be expected to be of particular importance in biological or nutritional therapies (Christensen, 1993; Weglicki et al., 1993).

An excellent example of the superiority of good scientific judgment over the premature use of the controlled clinical trial is the discovery by George C. Cotzias that L-dopa is an effective treatment for Parkinson's disease (Cotzias et al., 1967). When Cotzias began his studies, L-dopa was regarded as an interesting therapeutic idea that had been determined to be without utility in a series of careful clinical trials that included controlled double-blind, Phase III methodology (Fehling, 1966; Lasagna, 1972). Had Cotzias not used good scientific judgment and persistent curiosity by testing L-dopa in careful, uncontrolled protocols that included larger doses than in the earlier, methodologically flawed trials, it is entirely possible that recognition of L-dopa's enormous value would have been delayed for decades or never recognized at all.

Phase III trials of orthomolecular therapy, for example, may also require a similarly innovative approach. One possibility, after preliminary, dose-optimization studies have been completed, is to randomly allocate suitable patients to conventional or orthomolecular programs. Much of the evaluation would have to be "open"; however, symptom-rating scales could be scored by observers unaware, or "blinded," to which patients received which treatment.

First and foremost, however, is the requirement for an openminded approach by intelligent and skeptical clinical investigators whose effort is respected by their peers. Such studies also will require good-faith cooperation from academic medical units and the support provided by adequate research funding. Evaluation of the research will have to include a recognition that initially negative results do not prove a therapy valueless: the therapy may merely have been incorrectly tested. Investigators should strive to develop hypotheses that can be objectively tested. Even when testing mechanisms are novel, they must be rigorous and reproducible by independent investigators, and their results must be convincing to openminded but skeptical reviewers. These objectives can and must be achieved. The cost of not achieving them may be the unnecessary delay or, worse, the complete dismissal of an effective treatment for a previously untreatable debilitating illness.

Alternatives to Federal and Other "Institutionalized" Programs That Influence Diet and Contribute to Chronic Disease

Not even increased openmindedness in mainstream research or increased Federal funds for research may be enough to get effective alternative diet and nutrition prophylactic and therapeutic treatments into more general use. Indeed, without some significant changes in Americans' beliefs and expectations about food and nutrition, promising research results—whether alternative or conventional—will have little impact. For example, studies indicate that Americans are quite aware of the relationship between nutrition and health (Cotugna et al., 1992). However, during the past two decades they have made little apparent progress toward meeting the RDAs (U.S. Department of Agriculture and U.S. Department of Health and Human Services, 1990), which recent research indicates may already be too low for many vitamins and nutrients. Although there has been an increase in consumption of low-fat milk and a decrease in the consumption of meat and eggs during the past decade, USDA's 1987–88 national food consumption survey (U.S. Department of Agriculture, 1988) indicated that Americans, on average, eat only one serving of fruit or fruit juice and two servings of vegetables per day. This amounts to roughly half the recommended Federal Government minimum (Patterson et al., 1990) and much less than the minimum advocated by many others. Furthermore, the consumption of saturated fat by women has consistently remained around 13 percent of total calories (Welsh, 1991).

Numerous Government programs and information dissemination channels exist that potentially could have a major positive influence on American dietary habits. Unfortunately, many, if not most, are having a negative rather than a positive impact on Americans' dietary knowledge, beliefs, and practices. These programs and channels include

- Government feeding and food support programs,
- Public education and the mass media,
- School-based and worksite programs, and
- Health care provider settings.

Government feeding and food support programs. The Food and Nutrition Service of USDA administers 14 food assistance programs that aim to "provide needy people with access to a more nutritious diet, to improve the eating habits of the Nation's children, and to stabilize farm prices through the distribution of surplus foods" (U.S. Department of Agriculture, 1993a). More than 25.4 million people participated in the Food Stamp Program in 1992, and more than 5.6 million participated in the Special Supplemental Food Program for Women, Infants, and Children (WIC). In addition, approximately 25 million children participate in the National School Lunch Program (NSLP) each day, and an average of 900,000 people participate daily in the Nutrition Program for the Elderly.

Studies have reported that participation in the Food Stamp Program or the size of the food stamp benefits, or both, have had a positive impact on the availability of nutrients. However, the effect of these programs on nutrient intake is negligible. Only WIC was found to increase intake of numerous nutrients, including iron, calcium, and vitamin C, among pregnant women (Rush et al., 1988) and preschool children (Rush et al., 1988). Moreover, when participants in NSLP were compared to nonparticipants, increased nutrient intakes of vitamin A, vitamin B_6, calcium, and magnesium (Hanes et al., 1984)—vitamins typically deficient in the school-aged population (Nelson et al., 1981)—were observed in the NSLP participant population.

Whether these various feeding programs provide adequate nutrition for Americans deserves critical analysis. For example, NSLP has been criticized for maintaining its outdated purpose of preventing nutritional deficiencies without including food patterns that would prevent such prevailing chronic diseases as heart disease, hypertension, cancer, and atherosclerosis (American School Food Service Association, 1991; Citizens' Commission, 1990). In light of the findings on the positive effects of fruits and vegetables (Steinmetz and Potter, 1991a, 1991b) and the negative effects of saturated fats (Willett, 1990) on health and chronic disease, it may be necessary to modify NSLP to at least meet the Dietary Guidelines for Americans (U.S. Department of Agriculture and U.S. Department of Health and Human Services, 1990).

In September 1993, assistant secretary of agriculture Ellen Haas announced plans to improve NSLP by doubling the amount of fresh fruits and vegetables supplied to schools and reducing the amount of fat in commodity foods (U.S. Department of Agriculture, 1993b). This modification is urgently needed to update NSLP so that it will be in line with the current scientific findings on diet and disease. Similar modifications should be made across all USDA feeding and food assistance programs to help Americans consume a better diet.

Furthermore, for the agricultural system to meet even the current USDA dietary guidelines, adjustments are required in the mix and output of farm products. Appropriate new food policies need to be in place to support such changes. For example, in the commodity area, the price and income support programs put a premium on milk fat, and surplus disposal operations are designed to increase the supply of high-fat butter and cheese on the market at artificially low prices. This system runs counter to encouraging better diet and nutrition in the population.

Public education and role of the mass media. The primary goal of public nutrition education is to bring about behavioral changes in individuals', groups', and populations' dietary patterns presumed to be detrimental to health. The educational program is designed to provide enough knowledge so that healthy choices in nutrition can be made. The mass media, including magazines, newspapers, and television, are a major source of nutrition information for the public (American Dietetic Association and International Food Information Council, 1990). An analysis of mass initiatives in the area of promoting healthy diet and nutrition choices indicates that such campaigns can be useful in setting the stage for behavior change (DeJong and Winsten, 1990). One example is a joint NCI-Kellogg (the cereal manufacturer) initiative that promoted consumption of a high-fiber diet through advertising and food labeling on cereal boxes. On the basis of purchase data from supermarkets in the Baltimore and Washington, DC, metropolitan area, the purchase of high-fiber cereals increased 37 percent in the 48 weeks of the initiative (Levy and Stokes, 1987).

Mass media-based education programs not only affect the intermediary steps to behavior change but also have proved to have a more direct influence on health, such as affecting changes in eating patterns and disease risk factors. For instance, the Finnish North Karelia Project showed that education programs using mass media strategies can markedly reduce certain coronary heart disease risk factors (Vartiainnen et al., 1991).

In recent years, the social marketing approach, which draws marketing techniques from the private sector and focuses on the thorough understanding of consumer needs and opinions, has been used increasingly in health promotion campaigns (J. Ling, 1992). This approach can yield promising new insights into consumer behavior and into product and strategy design (Walsh et al., 1993), thereby enhancing the efficacy of a health promotion initiative.

The National Heart, Lung, and Blood Institute's (NHLBI's) National High Blood Pressure Education Program (NHBPEP) and National Cholesterol Education Program are examples of Federal public education programs that extensively use mass media and social marketing strategies to convey health messages to the public. Both programs employ the strategy of focusing on raising knowledge and awareness on two tiers: among the public and among health care professionals. From NHBPEP's inception in 1972, awareness, treatment, and control rates for high blood pressure have increased dramatically (Rocella and Lenfant, 1992), and age-adjusted stroke mortality has fallen nearly 57 percent (Rocella and Horan, 1988).

Unfortunately, few nutrition messages in the mass media promote a healthy diet. Indeed, advertisements for foods that are high in sodium, fat, or sugar often compete directly against nutrition messages designed to help people make better food choices. For example, breakfast cereals, snacks, and fast foods are among the most heavily advertised products on television programs aimed at children (Cotugna, 1988), and the television "diet" consists of foods primarily of low nutritional value (Story and Faulkner, 1990). Television viewing also appears to affect food consumption. Studies have reported, for instance, that the amount of time spent watching television directly correlates with the request, purchase, and consumption of foods advertised on television (Clancy-Hepburn et al., 1974; Gorn and Goldberg, 1982; Taras et al., 1989). Consequently, the mass media, the food industry, the Government, and health professionals should collaborate to broadcast health promotion messages more extensively. One such example is the airing of public service announcements on Saturday morning children's television by a major fruit-processing company, which was prompted by the "Five-a-Day for Better Health" campaign initiated by NCI and the Produce for Better Health Foundation.

School-based and worksite programs. Schools are an ideal setting in which to model and encourage healthy lifestyle behaviors. More than 95 percent of American youth aged 5 to 17 are enrolled in schools (U.S. Department of Education, 1990). School-based nutrition education and physical activity programs appear to be ideal venues for effecting change in lifestyle-related risk factors for heart disease, cancer, and obesity. Children eat one to two meals per day in school, and the cafeteria can be a learning laboratory where students can practice and experience positive nutrition habits they learn from the school curriculum. Previous studies in school-based cardiovascular research, including the "Know Your Body" program (Walter et al., 1988), have shown that health promotion in schools can have a favorable impact on nutrition knowledge and diet-related skills (Contento et al., 1992) as well as on specific outcomes, such as blood cholesterol level, carbohydrate intake, fitness, blood pressure, and smoking status (Stone et al., 1989). In addition, school-based health promotion programs have had positive impacts on obesity (Resnicow, 1993).

Additional research of longer duration that includes multiple components (school food service, curriculum, family outreach) is needed to determine the degree to which schools can affect the exercise and diet habits of children. These studies could be similar to the ongoing NHLBI-funded "Child and Adolescent Trial for Cardiovascular Health" and the "Eat Well and Keep Moving" project at the Tesseract schools in Baltimore, MD.

Worksites are another important channel for promoting nutrition. Nearly 70 percent of adults between the ages of 18 and 65 are employed (U.S. Bureau of the Census, 1986). Thus worksites provide access to large numbers of people and offer the opportunity to make environmental and social norm changes that support healthy eating (Sorensen et al., 1986). Indeed, worksite educational programs have been shown effective in weight control (Sherman et al., 1989), cardiovascular risk reduction (O'Brien and Dedmon, 1990), smoking cessation (Windsor and Lowe, 1989), and cancer screening (Heimendinger et al., 1990). By modifying cafeteria menus and policy for meals served at corporate functions to support healthier choices and allowing time at work for nutrition education activity, worksites can be promising vehicles in modifying employees' eating habits. However, efforts should be made to overcome low participation rates and high dropout rates in worksite programs (American Dietetic Association, 1986).

Education of health care providers and patient counseling. Patients place a great deal of credibility in the nutrition advice given to them by their physicians (American Dietetic Association, 1990). Many physicians, however, fail to provide such advice to their patients. A study by the University of Minnesota found that only 10 percent of surveyed physicians gave nutrition advice to more than 80 percent of their patients (Kottke et al., 1988). Although many physicians view nutrition as an effective tool that should be used in medical practice, there are significant barriers that keep physicians from adequately counseling their patients on issues of diet and nutrition. These barriers include lack of time, adequate staffs, and insufficient insurance coverage (Glanz and Gilboy, 1992). In addition, physicians' perceived inability to effectively alter their patients' lifestyle practices contributes to this problem (Wechsler et al., 1983). Another major contributor to physicians failing to give their patients nutrition counseling may be their own lack of nutrition knowledge. More than one study of practicing physicians has found that only about half of those surveyed felt prepared to provide dietary counseling to their patients (Kimm et al., 1990).

This lack of adequate nutrition knowledge among physicians may be partly due to a deficient nutrition curriculum in U.S. medical schools. In fact, a survey of 45 U.S. medical schools by the National Academy of Sciences found the state of nutrition education in medical schools to be largely inadequate to meet the needs of patients and the medical profession (National Research Council, 1985). Improved standards for nutrition education in U.S. medical schools appear to be necessary if the vast preventive and therapeutic role of nutrition in health care is to be exploited to the fullest.

In the context of alternative diets or therapies, an additional barrier to effective counseling by conventional health care providers is the sometimes outright hostility toward alternative therapies held by these providers. For example, surveys have indicated that many cancer patients do not tell conventional providers that they are pursuing alternative therapies, in part, because the conventional health care provider is often unsupportive or skeptical of such therapies (Eisenberg et al., 1993). In extreme cases, some conventional providers will refuse to treat a patient whom the provider knows is seeing an alternative practitioner for the same condition. Such attitudes are substantial hurdles to overcome for both the adequate and objective evaluation and dissemination of effective alternative therapies.

Another problem physicians may encounter when trying to give nutrition counseling to patients is that American society is becoming increasingly multicultural. Health professionals often have difficulty communicating with clients whose cultural heritage is different from their own. This problem is particularly acute when a physician is dealing with someone who comes from a cultural group or society where health and religion are intertwined (Kittler and Sucher, 1989). For example, "looking good" is a common goal in many technologically developed societies, but various cultural groups have a different view. Mexican Americans, African Americans, and other ethnic groups do not share the typical American concepts of appropriate body size, particularly for adult women (Massara, 1980; Schreiber and Homiak, 1981; Stern et al., 1982). It has been suggested that the "mainstream" standards for weight in adult women are, in fact, based more on the value of thinness—which is related to youth and higher socioeconomic status (Cassidy, 1991; Sobal, 1991)—than on science or epidemiology (Ritenbaugh, 1982).

Therefore, successful nutritional counseling depends on culturally sensitive communication strategies; health care practitioners must be both knowledgeable about general ethnic, regional, and religious food habits and aware of individual practices and preferences. Health care professionals can improve cross-cultural counseling through a four-step process of self-evaluation, preinterview research, indepth interviewing, and unbiased data analysis. A detailed description of the rationale for these steps can be found in Kittler and Sucher (1990).

However, the success of cross-cultural counseling cannot always be measured by a patient's adherence to a diet. Differences in worldview, traditional food habits, and factors that influence dietary adaptation may be of greater consequence to a client than the health implications of the diet. The best chances of compliance occur when the health care practitioner is aware of personal cultural assumptions and is knowledgeable about the cultural heritage of a patient and its specific influences on the patient's food habits, and when diet modifications are made with consideration for individual cultural and personal preferences.

There are some examples of successful intervention programs that have been based on indepth studies of the total context of ethnic food consumption. Hall (1987) noted that materials designed for Mexican-American diabetics not only had to be translated into Spanish but also had to be redesigned, incorporating culturally relevant concepts, methods, meal plans, and activities, to be effective. The same study also found it advisable to incorporate recommendations for traditional home remedies that have been shown scientifically to be of value in the treatment of diabetes. For example, a diabetes intervention directed toward Mexican Americans may include the use of cooked prickly pear cactus (*nopales*), which has long been used in Mexican folk medicine to control diabetes (Frati-Munari et al., 1983). Traditional remedies, however, are encouraged only as complements to biomedical treatments; the Hall program suggests that prescribed diabetes medications be taken with traditional herbal teas (Hall, 1987).

Another excellent intervention program is a physician-based system of dietary risk assessment and intervention, designed for use with low-literacy, low-income southern populations (Ammerman et al., 1991, 1992). This program focuses on the top 20 contributors of saturated fat and cholesterol that, based on the National Health and Nutrition Examination Survey II (NHANES II) data, are commonly found in the diets of African-American populations in the South. Attention is also given to traditional southern food preparation practices, such as baking with lard, frying with vegetable shortening, and seasoning vegetables with meat fat (Ammerman et al., 1991). All assessment and intervention materials are based on food rather than on nutrients. Diet change recommendations are linked with recipes in a southern-style cookbook.

For those who do little cooking at home (a growing population), information is provided on how to eat sensibly at fast-food restaurants. Low-cost dietary alternatives and southern food preferences are emphasized throughout the materials, which are written at the fifth- to sixth-grade reading level. The goal of the program is to reduce saturated fat and cholesterol intake while preserving ethnic eating patterns—that is, to adapt the traditional diet rather than introduce a radical transformation of eating patterns (Ammerman et al., 1992). Evaluation of the program shows promising results, both in the physicians' administration of the program and in changes in patients' attitudes. Currently underway is a 5-year, randomized clinical trial of the effectiveness of the program in lowering cholesterol among patients in rural Virginia and North Carolina (Ammerman et al., 1992). In addition, a "northern" version of this approach and these materials is being tested.

Programs of the type described by Hall and Ammerman cannot be developed in the absence of the necessary data specific to the ethnic group being targeted. Multidisciplinary research with a nutritional-anthropological focus is necessary to explore these issues further.

Research Needs and Opportunities in Diet and Nutrition

It is virtually impossible to list all of the research opportunities in diet and nutrition that should be pursued more extensively and vigorously. Rather, this section presents broad areas where the data indicate that more intense efforts might yield significant results.

Optimal Levels of Vitamins, Minerals, and Other Nutritional Supplements

Although there have been many studies to determine the effect of a single vitamin deficiency, few studies have attempted to determine the *optimal* dietary requirement for most vitamins and minerals. There is increasing evidence that the consumption of nutrients at RDA levels is not adequate for promoting optimal health. Thus, nutritional supplementation above the RDAs for many vitamins and minerals may be indicated. The following areas of research in vitamin and nutritional supplementation are likely to yield significant results:

- Research is needed to determine how and at what levels such antioxidants as vitamins E and C and beta-carotene provide optimal immune enhancement.
- There is growing evidence that some carotenoids can directly affect cancer cells. Mechanisms may include free radical and other charged particle quenching, which would result in less damage to DNA; decreased adenylate cyclase activity, which would decrease proliferation of the cancer; generation of regulatory proteins that could alter cell cycles and metabolism; and other mechanisms as yet unknown (Bendich, 1991). Carotenoids have been shown to protect cells from mutagens. Further, research into the direct effects of antioxidants on cancer cells and on DNA repair mechanism is needed.
- Research is needed into the role that many vitamins play aside from being enzyme cofactors. In view of the interest in free radicals or reactive molecular intermediates in the pathogenesis of a variety of medical and neurological diseases, there is a wealth of opportunities for research on the ability of vitamins and other nutritional supplements to prevent or reverse the effects of these types of molecules.
- Research is needed in the United States to provide data from controlled studies to verify mostly European work on the clinical efficacy of minerals such as magnesium and selenium in the treatment of disease. More extensive intervention studies are needed to determine whether adding mineral supplements will improve the preventive effects of other dietary interventions (e.g., salt and fat restriction) against cardiovascular disease, and to verify the promising effects from Europe in prevention of abnormalities in pregnancy. In particular, the extended study of magnesium treatment of bronchial asthma is also indicated. There are already many clues on magnesium's mechanisms of action, and there are many data on clinical efficacy in a number of clinical diseases or complaints. It would be more feasible—not to mention less expensive—to set up double-blind intervention studies supplementing subjects' existing diets with magnesium or selenium, rather than try to get them to completely change their diet to include more foods containing these minerals.
- A recent National Institutes of Health (NIH) report (1994) on calcium recommended that optimal levels of intake by women to prevent osteoporosis should be 1,500 mg per day. Because the usual American intake of magnesium is no more than 300 mg per day, such a level of calcium intake would constitute a calcium-magnesium ratio of 5:1. It is noteworthy that in Finland, where the prevalence of osteoporosis is high (Simonen, 1991), the average calcium-magnesium intake ratio is 4:1, a ratio that has been associated with the highest death rate in young to middle-aged men from ischemic heart disease in the world (Karppanen et al., 1978). An NIH consensus development conference on magnesium, similar to the one held recently on calcium, would provide a much-needed forum for elucidating other avenues of research that may be warranted on this important mineral.

Alternative Dietary Lifestyles and Cultural Diets

Studies of Seventh-Day Adventists, macrobiotic vegetarians, and populations eating Asian and Mediterranean types of diets indicate that these groups are at lower risk of heart disease and some cancers. Likewise, studies usually demonstrate that blood pressure and blood lipid levels fall when participants follow a vegetarian diet (Cooper et al., 1982; Kestin et al., 1989; Margetts et al., 1986; Rouse et al., 1986). Prospective studies of vegetarian groups other than California Seventh-Day Adventists have found a decreased risk of heart disease and cancer as well as a decreased risk of death from all causes (Burr and Butland, 1988; Burr and Sweetnam, 1982; Chang-Claude et al., 1992; Frentzel-Beyme et al., 1988). Vegetarian populations, including Seventh-Day Adventists, also appear to be at decreased risk of other diseases such as gallbladder disease (Pixley et al., 1985) and diabetes mellitus (Snowdon and Phillips, 1985). Furthermore, such vegetarian diets as advocated under the Pritikin program appear to improve control of diabetes (Barnard et al., 1983).

Accordingly, studies of populations eating vegetarian and some cultural diets provide evidence that alternative dietary patterns may have a major impact on disease risk. Specifically, such studies show evidence of potentially profound implications for the risk of developing heart disease, certain cancers (such as colon or prostate cancer), and other chronic illnesses, such as diabetes. For example, in addition to containing large amounts of antioxidants, beans, leafy green vegetables, whole grains, many fruits, and fish are very rich in magnesium (Seelig, 1980). The Pritikin, Mediterranean, Seventh-Day Adventist, and macrobiotic diets are, thus, rich in magnesium. Studies have shown that magnesium supplementation of animals on atherosclerosis-inducing diets protects against arterial damage. Animal studies also have shown that magnesium deficiency increases hypercholesterolemia (especially the LDLs) and increases vulnerability to oxidative damage (Rayssiguier et al., 1989, 1993). It has recently been shown that magnesium repletion and vitamin E are mutually enhancing in protecting against magnesium deficiency- and stress hormone-induced cardiac necrosis (Freedman et al., 1990, 1991; Guenther et al., 1992, 1994a; Weglicki et al., 1992), and that vitamin E and magnesium deficiency shortens the time needed to induce atherosclerosis (Guenther et al., 1994b).

There is experimental evidence that magnesium deficiency (at least in very young rodents) can cause leukemias and lymphomas (Averdunk and Guenther, 1985; Battifora et al., 1968, 1969; Bois, 1968; Bois and Beaulnes, 1966; Bois et al., 1969; Hass et al., 1981a, 1981b; Jasmin, 1963; McCreary et al., 1967), especially when there is also deficiency in such antioxidants as vitamins C and E, and in selenium (Aleksandrowicz, 1975). The protective role of magnesium against certain diseases may be supported by epidemiological findings about geographic areas low in magnesium where there is a high prevalence of human and cattle lymphoid neoplasms, leukemias, and gastric cancers (Aleksandrowicz, 1973; Aleksandrowicz and Skotnicki, 1982; Seelig, 1979, 1993).

The studies of vegetarian groups and Asian and Mediterranean populations are congruent with the growing body of studies in other populations that indicate a potentially profound role for dietary factors in the etiology of various chronic illnesses. These include growing evidence of the undesirable health effects of meat and high-fat dairy intake and the health promotion effects of abundant consumption of vegetables, fruits, monounsaturated fats, garlic, and whole cereal grains.

The translation of the findings of these animal and human studies into therapeutic approaches may alleviate the burden of some of these diseases. Equally important are measures that are being taken by industry and the Federal Government to support healthful dietary habits. Studies need to be undertaken on a wide *variety* of alternative diets that have been found to be beneficial, including

- vegetarian diets,
- ultra-low-fat diets,
- high-polyunsaturated-fat diets,
- Mediterranean-type diets, and
- diets rich in soy foods, such as East Asian diets.

Initiatives also are needed along the following lines:

- There is a need for a more critical examination of dairy products on health, especially regarding fractures.
- There is a need for a more critical look at the effects of meat consumption on health—for example, on coronary heart disease, colon cancer, and fractures.
- More detailed data are needed on the effects of fruits, vegetables, monounsaturated fats, and garlic on cancer, coronary heart disease, cataracts, stroke, and so forth.
- There is a need for more information on the long-term effects of overrefined carbohydrates (e.g., sugar) on the human metabolism and immune functioning.

Qualitative research is needed on various aspects of cultural diets and the effects of cultural beliefs on health and illnesses. Such studies might include the following:

- Qualitative research on ethnic concepts of appropriate body shape and size by gender, age, and socioeconomic status.
- Qualitative research on ethnic definitions of health and approaches to health.
- Qualitative research on ethnic attitudes and approaches to dieting.
- Research on how the types of programs described by Hall and Ammerman can be adapted for use with other ethnic populations, and evaluation of such programs in meeting biomedical and nutritional goals (e.g., reduction of cholesterol levels).

The goal in all this research should be to elucidate categories and concepts of importance to members of the public and to determine which of their traditions should be encouraged. These data are critical in achieving the larger biomedical nutritional goal of a well-nourished and healthy population by using terms that can be understood by the lay public, especially members of minorities.

Studies on the Relationship Between Energy Consumption and Disease

Data that have been accumulating since the early part of this century indicate that overconsumption of energy may contribute to chronic illness, while restriction of energy may promote health and prolong life. Moreschi (1909) demonstrated that underfeeding could impede the growth of tumors. Rous (1914) confirmed and expanded those findings, but no further progress occurred until 1935 when McKay demonstrated a broad disease preventive effect, as well as extension of lifespan, as a result of caloric restriction (McKay et al., 1935).

In 1940, Albert Tannenbaum demonstrated that energy restriction *per se* in rodents can inhibit tumor initiation and growth, that increased caloric use stimulated by exogenous thyroid may inhibit certain cancers and metastases, and that fats can promote the growth, in many circumstances, of already initiated tumors (Tannenbaum, 1940, 1942a, 1942b, 1945a, 1945b). Later, Jose reported that Australian Aborigines who became malnourished upon weaning, and who regularly developed a decreased ability to produce antibodies, unexpectedly showed increased proliferative responses of T lymphocytes upon stimulation with certain phytomitogens (Jose et al., 1969).

As research progressed, it was demonstrated that protein-energy restriction could cause in animals the same enhanced response to phytomitogens seen in Australian Aborigines. In addition, experiments revealed that even at presumably dangerously low protein levels (3 to 5 percent), cell-mediated immunity remained intact and in some cases appeared to be greatly increased, as in the development of cell-mediated responsiveness to stimulation with minute doses of antigen. Additional effects were augmentation of delayed allergic reactions, increased capacity for lymphoid cells to initiate graft-versus-host reactions, up-regulated cellular immune responses against syngeneic and allogeneic tumor cells, and increased capacity to resist certain types of viral infections (Good et al., 1977, 1980).

A direct attempt to follow a high-quality energy-restricted diet as a health measure has been advocated for a number of years by R.L. Walford, M.D. at UCLA (Walford and Crew, 1989). Recently Walford participated in a 2-year experiment in which he monitored the health of eight humans growing and recycling all food in the 3.15-acre hermetically sealed experimental ecological enclosure called Biosphere 2 in Oracle, AZ. The eight Biosphere 2 subjects underwent 24 months of moderate caloric restriction (1,700 to 2,400 kcal per day, despite a heavy work load) with a very high quality semi-vegetarian diet in rigidly controlled circumstances. Physiologic changes in the eight volunteers over the 2-year stay were dramatic, with blood glucose dropping 15 percent, cholesterol dropping to an average of 125 mg/dL, and blood pressure dropping to low normal (Walford et al., 1992). Blood white cell counts also decreased, which, along with the decrease in glucose, mirrored changes seen in restricted monkeys and restricted rodents. Further tests are ongoing, but preliminary results thus suggest that humans respond, at least initially, much like all other mammals tested on dietary energy restriction. A great deal more study is needed to see if the immune-enhancing, life-prolonging effect of an energy-restricted diet in lower animals also is manifest in humans.

Patient Education Issues

Research shows that physicians can have a beneficial impact on their patients' lifestyle practices (Inui et al., 1976; Leon et al., 1987; Russell et al., 1979). For example, brief antismoking advice given to patients by general practitioners has been shown to reduce patients' smoking rates by as much as 7 percent (Russell et al., 1979), which is a potentially huge public health impact given the prevalence of smoking. Similar changes in populations' eating patterns, such as reduction in saturated fat intake, could also have a huge impact on decreasing the rates of diseases, such as coronary heart disease and certain cancers, where diet has been implicated in causation. What is lacking, however, are incisive screening questions that physicians can use to quickly assess a patient's nutritional risk within the time constraints of a visit to or by a physician. Research is necessary into this issue to determine what screening questions would be both timely and effective in identifying points of dietary intervention to reduce risk.

Broadening the Database on Intervention Information

Something that became apparent during the development of this chapter was the wealth of diet and nutrition information outside the regular electronic databases, such as MEDLINE. There is a great deal of social science and agriculture literature relating to diet and nutrition, as well as in the world literature, that is often overlooked. Furthermore, literature from before 1965 is not routinely stored in electronic databases; if it is, abstracts are not included. For example, dietary modification and the use of vitamins to prevent and affect disease was the subject of intense research in pre-World War II Germany (Gerson, 1929, 1935; Sauerbruch and Herrmannsdorfer, 1928) and, to a lesser extent, in the rest of Europe (Hval, 1932) and even in the United States (Banyai, 1931; Emerson, 1929; Mayer and Kugelmass, 1929). However, much of this information has been lost to many contemporary nutrition researchers because it is not cataloged in present-day electronic databases.

Much of this older information, as well as information from such countries as China, India, and Japan, is university-based clinical research that, if made more widely available, might be of enormous value to researchers investigating similar phenomena today. A fruitful research project could be to screen the older data, the social science and agricultural data, and the world data that are available in foreign databases to develop a bibliography of references that might be added to nationwide databases such as MEDLINE. The World Health Organization literature, for example, would be a good starting point in looking for information relating to databases on diet and nutrition research in other countries.

Attention should be given to examining many of the widespread popular and folk dietary suggestions for maintaining health or controlling illness. For example, cranberry juice has long been known as a folk remedy for controlling or curing bladder infections in women. Recent analyses of this popular treatment show that it actually is effective (Walsh, 1992). As noted previously, the prickly pear has long been used by Mexican Americans as a treatment for diabetes. Biochemical studies have shown that it does have a mild glucose-lowering effect, which is due to its content of glucose-6-phosphate isomerase (Frati-Munari et al., 1983; Ibanez-Camacho and Roman-Ramos, 1979). Laboratory testing of the efficacy of ethnic foods used as remedies, as was done with the prickly pear cactus, might provide interesting results.

Moreover, there are literally hundreds of popular folk sayings that might warrant serious scrutiny, first with literature, then with appropriate laboratory and clinical tests. Some examples are "When people feel weak, they should eat meat"; "People with lung disorders should avoid dairy products" (especially common in traditional medical systems such as Ayurveda); "An apple a day keeps the doctor away."

Such research should be supplemented by in-depth qualitative research on how and when these remedies are used.

Specific Disease Areas

AIDS. AIDS is a chronic disease characterized by progressive decline in immunocompetence. Because many vitamins and nutritional supplements are biological response modifiers that have been shown to stimulate or enhance immune response, the potential areas of fruitful research in this area are limitless.

There is at least preliminary evidence that vitamin A or beta-carotene (its precursor) decreases the immune deficiency that results when animals are exposed to a wide variety of immunocompromising conditions such as trauma, infection, irradiation, and treatment with cytotoxic agents (Seifter et al., 1982, 1983a, 1983b, 1984). There is evidence suggesting that vitamin A supplementation in immune-compromised individuals may be necessary to replace a vitamin A deficiency caused by HIV infection (Lack et al., 1993; Semba et al., 1993). Many other vitamins and nutritional supplements that have been shown to affect immune status also may be potentially potent tools for fighting this deadly infection. This area is ripe for intensive research.

Cancer. It is well accepted that cancer and its treatment can cause malnutrition and that malnutrition itself predicts a poor outcome (DeWys et al., 1980). In general, however, oral dietary treatments for cancer have not been evaluated by mainstream medicine for the possible prevention of malnutrition or for the possible effect on the course of the disease in cancer patients. There are no nutritional recommendations per se for the cancer patient in mainstream oncology (Office of Technology Assessment, 1990), and no diet is currently recommended publicly by NCI or the American Cancer Society for use in cancer treatment. Those nutritional support measures that are offered usually come only after patients have reached advanced stages of cancer and have become malnourished, often as a result of side effects of their treatment (e.g., chemotherapy) (American College of Physicians, 1989; Shike and Brennan, 1989).

Little is understood about the nutritional requirements of cancers. However, there is growing evidence that many types of tumors have an increased need for iron in order to grow (Elliott et al., 1993; Weinberg, 1992). Red meat is one of the best sources of iron, and iron from red meat continues to be absorbed even if body stores of iron are plentiful (Ascherio and Willett, 1994). Therefore, there is at least a theoretical basis for proposing that cancer patients eat a primarily vegetarian diet to slow the growth of their tumors. Furthermore, although the epidemiological data provide solid support for recommendations to consume an abundance of vegetables and fruits or vitamin supplements to prevent cancer, there is a need for research on the effects of such nutritional interventions on individuals who already have cancer. Immunological parameters such as certain immune cell activity or levels of certain cytokines (immune-cell-activating compounds) would provide information about whether such diets do or do not increase the body's ability to attack cancer cells.

The 1990 OTA report *Unconventional Cancer Treatments* suggested that at least certain aspects of most of the unconventional dietary regimens for cancer it reviewed (e.g., intake of fresh fruits and vegetables and reduction or elimination of sodium and fat) are consistent with current Federal dietary recommendations about reducing the risk of *contracting* certain types of cancer and other illnesses (Office of Technology Assessment, 1990). The controversial aspects of these therapies, according to OTA, is the idea that dietary treatment can cause the *regression* of cancer. It is possible that the earlier such dietary regimens are begun, the more effective they are. It would be informative to look at various aspects of some of these regimens to determine whether they conform to basic biochemical and immunological research relating micronutrient manipulation to improving immune function or the inhibition of cancer cell growth. For example, Simone (1983) suggested that coffee enemas may increase absorption of vitamin A. There is evidence that vitamin A may play a vital role in boosting immune function (see the section on orthomolecular medicine in this chapter). The Gerson diet is estimated to provide approximately 100,000 IU of vitamin A daily (Seifter,

1988). Further studies are needed to confirm the ability of such measures to increase the absorption of micronutrients.

Heart disease and diabetes. Studies such as those using fat-restricted or fat-modified diets (i.e., intake of greater amounts of monounsaturated fats) have produced quite credible evidence suggesting not only that cardiovascular disease may be stabilized through such methods, but also that death rates from cardiovascular disease can be greatly reduced. Dietary intervention for coronary heart disease may find broader application if attempts are made to further both clinical research and use. A systematic review of the literature, broader clinical evaluations, and the development of clinical guidelines could lead to general acceptance. Efforts to disseminate information and transfer technology may be essential. Cost comparisons with conventional treatments may be instructive.

The following are specific areas that are likely to yield fruitful results:

- Sufficient evidence now exists to compel larger scale, multicenter, randomized clinical trials of modified diets such as the Ornish regimen, the Mediterranean-type diet, and high-soy-content diets.
- Dean Ornish's program relies heavily on relaxation techniques as well as fat restriction. It would be informative to know which aspect of his regimen contributes most to the regression of heart disease. If the relaxation component turns out to be a significant factor, this knowledge could potentially save the overall health care system billions of dollars.
- The Pritikin diet and other diets that require low fat, low cholesterol, high fiber, and high complex carbohydrate consumption should be tested and evaluated (in terms of all their components) for the treatment of adult-onset diabetes. Even if a small percentage of the nation's 11 million diabetics could control their disease with diet, the savings—in health improvement, delayed mortality, and financial costs—would be enormous.

Food allergies. Despite the large body of literature on food allergies, there is still a need to further study the approach taken by environmental medicine in a variety of other conditions commonly encountered. A mechanism similar to that proposed for arthritis has been proposed in asthma, ulcerative colitis, migraines, hyperactivity, recurrent infections, and other common conditions. The testing techniques need further validation, as does treatment with immunotherapy, environmental control units, and basic biochemical understanding of the causes of chemical hypersensitivity and other "20th century" diseases.

More work needs to be done in the area of food intolerance and neuropsychiatric disorders. Egger and colleagues (1992) have recently implicated an immune system effect as being the mechanism by which incriminated foods produce hyperactivity. Work from other investigators is sorely needed.

Conclusion

This chapter has demonstrated that the more we learn about the potential influences of dietary factors on health, the more we must realize the need for maintaining an open mind. There are numerous examples where medical consensus—even when it represents the honest opinions of the most knowledgeable, leading scientists in the field—has clearly been wrong. For example, not long ago, the medical community strongly advised pregnant women to avoid taking vitamin supplements. Today pregnant women are advised to do exactly the opposite, especially with regard to taking folic acid to prevent neural tube defects. Another widespread erroneous consensus medical recommendation was the use of margarine rather than butter to reduce risk of coronary heart disease. It now seems, that at least some margarines, which are made from partially hydrogenated vegetable oils, are no better, if not worse, than butter in reducing the risk of heart disease.

Each of these cases was based on limited or no direct evidence. Further, many of the most promising research topics of today, such as the role of dietary antioxidants or alternative dietary lifestyles in preventing coronary heart disease and specific cancers, were topics dismissed by most nutritionists only a few years ago as practices of misguided vitamin and food faddists. Given the extreme complexities of the interrelationships between diet and human health and the relatively meager directly relevant data, an element of humility is appropriate in evaluating "alternative" dietary practices. Lack of data, such as from randomized trials, should *not* be confused with evidence of no benefit. However, a willingness to consider possible benefits of alternative diets does not imply blind acceptance of them, but rather should foster a rigorous scientific evaluation of potentially beneficial practices.

Unfortunately, nutritional therapies or dietary practices that do not readily fit into the "norm" previously have too often been routinely dismissed without such a rigorous examination. An ample investigation of a diet or nutritional intervention should test it in an appropriate model, under the appropriate conditions, and using appropriate research methodologies. In particular, potential study subjects must be selected with extreme care; that is, they should be individuals in which the dietary or nutritional modification, if truly beneficial, is likely to produce an effect. Moreover, if a study involves a micronutrient or vitamin or mineral supplementation, the dosage must be optimized to ensure that the intervention will have the opportunity to display an effect. Also, any evaluation of an alternative diet or nutrition research experiment will have to include a recognition that initially negative results do not prove any therapy is valueless; rather, the therapy may merely have been incorrectly tested. Thus, going the extra step is an imperative in conducting this type of research.

Finally, more efforts are needed in translating findings related to specific micro- and macronutrients to whole foods and practical, attractive diets. Only by doing this can physicians and public health officials adequately disseminate important diet and nutrition information to all sectors of the public.

References

Abraham, G.E., M.M. Lubran. 1981. Serum and red cell magnesium levels in patients with premenstrual tension. Am. J. Clin. Nutr. 34(11):2364–2366.

Acland, R. 1972. Prevention of thrombosis in microvascular surgery by use of magnesium sulphate. Brit. J. Plastic Surg. 25:292–299.

Adler, L.A., E. Peselow, J. Rotrosen, et al. 1993. Vitamin E treatment of tardive dyskinesia. Am. J. Psychiatry 150:1405–1407.

Adlercreutz, H., T. Fotsis, C. Bannwart, et al. 1986. Determination of urinary lignans and phytoestrogen metabolites, potential antiestrogens and anticarcinogens, in urine of women on various habitual diets. J. Steroid Biochem. 25:791–797.

Adlercreutz, H., K. Höckerstedt, C. Bannwart, et al. 1987. Effect of dietary components, including lignans and phytoestrogens, on enterohepatic circulation and liver metabolism of estrogens and on sex hormone binding globulin (SHBG). J. Steroid Biochem. 27:1135–1144.

Aleksandrowicz, J. 1973. Natural environment and health in protection of man's natural environment. Polish Sci. Publ., 518–528.

Aleksandrowicz, J. 1975. [Mycotoxins, bioelements, and perspectives in prophylaxis in the ecology of leukemia.] Rev. Esp. Oncologia 22:311–334. (in Spanish)

Aleksandrowicz, J., and A.B. Skotnicki. 1982. Leukemia Ecology: Ecological Prophylaxis of Leukemia (E. Nowak, trans.). (Available from National Technical Information Service, U.S. Department of Commerce, Springfield, VA 22161.)

Alexander, M., H. Newmark, and R.G. Miller. 1985. Oral beta-carotene can increase the number of OKT4 cells in human blood. Immunol. Lett. 9:221–224.

Altura, B.T., M. Brust, S. Bloom, et al. 1990. Magnesium dietary intake modulates blood lipid levels and atherogenesis. Proc. Natl. Acad. Sci. U.S.A. 87:1840–1844.

American Academy of Pediatrics, Committee on Nutrition. 1977. Nutritional aspects of vegetarianism, health foods, and fad diets. Pediatrics 59(3):460–464.

American Cancer Society. 1990. Cancer Facts and Figures—1989. American Cancer Society, New York.

American College of Physicians. 1989. Parenteral nutrition in patients receiving cancer chemotherapy. Ann. Intern. Med. 110(9):734–736.

American Dietetic Association, Society for Nutrition Education, Office of Disease Prevention and Health Promotion. 1986. Worksite Nutrition: A Decision-Maker's Guide. American Dietetic Association, Chicago.

American Dietetic Association and International Food Information Council. 1990. How Are Americans Making Food Choices?

American Heart Association. 1991. 1991 Heart and Stroke Facts. American Heart Association, Dallas.

American School Food Service Association. 1991. 1991 ASFSA legislative issue paper. Invest in our children: toward a national nutrition policy. School Food Service Journal 45(2):18–22.

Ammerman, A.S., B.M. DeVellis, P.S. Haines, et al. 1992. Nutrition education for cardiovascular disease prevention among low-income populations—description and pilot evaluation of a physician-based model. Patient Educ. Couns. 19(1):5–18.

Ammerman, A.S., P.S. Haines, R.F. DeVellis, et al. 1991. A brief dietary assessment to guide cholesterol reduction in low-income individuals: design and validation. J. Am. Diet. Assoc. 91(11):1385–1399.

Anderson, T.W., W.H. Leriche, D. Hewitt, and L.C. Neri. 1980. Magnesium, water hardness, and heart disease. In M. Cantin and M.S. Seelig, eds. Magnesium in Health and Disease. Spectrum, New York.

Angell, M., and J.P. Kassirer. 1994. Clinical research: what should the public believe? [editorial]. N. Engl. J. Med. 331(3):189–190.

Armstrong, B., A.J. van Merwyk, and H. Coates. 1977. Blood pressure in Seventh-Day Adventist vegetarians. Am. J. Epidemiol. 105:444–449.

Ascherio, A., and W.C. Willett. 1994. Are body iron stores related to the risk of coronary heart disease? N. Engl. J. Med. 330(16):1152–1154.

Averdunk, R., and T. Guenther. 1985. Phospholipid metabolism and concanavalin A stimulation of thymocytes from magnesium-deficient rats and magnesium-deficiency-induced T-cell lymphoma. Magnesium Bulletin 7:11–15.

Avery, R.J. 1982. Letter to G. Dego, University of London. Office of Cancer Communications, National Cancer Institute, August 24.

Axelson, M., J. Sjövall, G.E. Gustafsson, and K.D.R. Setchell. 1984. Soya—a dietary source of the non-steroidal oestrogen equol in man and animals. J. Endocrinol. 102:49–56.

Baggott, J.E., T. Ha, W.H. Vaughn, M.M. Juliana, J.M. Hardin, and C.J. Grubbs. 1990. Effect of miso (Japanese soybean paste) and NaCl on DMBA-induced rat mammary tumors. Nutr. Cancer 14:103–109.

Baird, G., and E. Cameron. 1973. Unpublished observations.

Banyai, A.L. 1931. The dietary treatment of tuberculosis. Am. Rev. Tuberculosis 23:546–575.

Barinaga, M. 1991. Vitamin C gets a little respect. Science 254:374–376.

Barnard, R.J., L. Lattimore, R.G. Holly, S. Cherny, and N. Pritikin. 1982. Response of non-insulin-dependent diabetic patients to an intensive program of diet and exercise. Diabetes Care 5:370–374.

Barnard, R.J., D.A. Martin, E.J. Ugianskis, and S.B. Inkeles. 1992. The role of diet and exercise in the management of hyperinsulinemia and associated atherosclerosis risk factors. Am. J. Cardiol. 69:440–444.

Barnard, R.J., M.R. Massey, S. Cherny, L.T. O'Brien, and N. Pritikin. 1983. Long-term use of high-complex-carbohydrate, high-fiber, low-fat diet and exercise in the treatment of NIDDM patients. Diabetes Care 6:268–273.

Barnhart, E.R., V.L. Maggio, L.R. Alexander, et al. 1990. Bacitracin-associated peptides and contaminated L-tryptophan. Lancet 336(8717):742.

Battifora, H.A., P.A. McCreary, B.M. Hahneman, and G.H. Laing. 1968. Chronic magnesium deficiency in the rat: studies of chronic myelogenous leukemia. Arch. Path. 122:610–620.

Battifora, H.A., P.A. McCreary, G.H. Laing, and G.M. Hass. 1969. Chronic granulocytic leukemia and malignant lymphoma in magnesium-deficient rats. Am. J. Path. 55:11a.

Beauclair, L., S. Vinogrodov, S.J. Riney, J.G. Csernansky, and L.E. Hollister. 1987. An adjunctive role for ascorbic acid in the treatment of schizophrenia? J. Clin. Psychopharmacol. 7:282–283.

Becker, G.J. 1991. Intravascular stents: general principles and status of lower-extremity arterial applications. Circulation 83(2 Suppl.):I122–I136.

Becker, G.L. 1993. The Antioxidant Pocket Counter: A Guide to the Essential Nutrients that Help Fight Cancer and Heart Disease. Times Books/Random House, New York.

Bell, K.M., L. Plon, W.E. Bunney, and S.G. Potkin. 1988. S-adenosylmethionine treatment of depression: a controlled clinical trial. Am. J. Psychiatry 145(9):1110–1114.

Bendich, A. 1991. Beta-carotene and the immune response. Proc. Nutr. Soc. 50:263–274.

Bennett, P.H., W.C. Knowles, N.B. Rushforth, R.F. Hammon, and P.J. Savage. 1979. The role of obesity in the development of diabetes of the Pima Indians. In J. Vague and P.H. Vague, eds. Diabetes and Obesity. Excerpta Medica, Amsterdam.

Benton, D., and R. Cook. 1991. The impact of selenium supplementation on mood. Biol. Psychiatry 29:1092–1098.

Bergan, J.G., and P.T. Brown. 1980. Nutritional status of "new" vegetarians. J. Am. Diet. Assoc. 76:151–155.

Beri, D., A.N. Malaviya, R. Shandilya, and R.R. Singh. 1988. Effect of dietary restrictions on disease activity in rheumatoid arthritis. Ann. Rheum. Dis. 47(1):69–72.

Berry, E.M. 1992. The effects of nutrients on lipoprotein susceptibility to oxidation. Current Opinion in Lipidology 3:5–11.

Bianchi-Santamaria, A., S. Fedeli, and L. Santamaria. 1993. Possible activity of beta-carotene in patients with the AIDS related complex (ARC). Presented at the IXth International Conference on AIDS, June 6–11, Berlin.

Bielory, L. and R. Gandi. 1994. Asthma and vitamin C. Ann. Allergy 73(2):89-96.

Blair, J.L., D.S. Warner, and M.M. Todd. 1989. Effects of elevated plasma magnesium versus calcium on cerebral ischemic injury in rats. Stroke 20:507–512.

Block, G., and B. Abrams. 1993. Vitamin and mineral status of women of childbearing potential. Ann. N. Y. Acad. Sci. 678:244–254.

Blot, W.J., J.-Y. Li, P.R. Taylor, et al. 1994. Lung cancer and vitamin supplementation. [letter to the editor]. N. Engl. J. Med. 331:614.

Blot, W.J., J.-Y. Li, P.R. Taylor, et al. 1993. Nutritional intervention trials in Linxian, China: supplementation with specific vitamin/mineral combinations, cancer incidence, and disease-specific mortality in the general population. J. Natl. Cancer Inst. 85:1483–1492.

Bodansky, O., F. Wroblewski, and B. Markhardt. 1951. Concentrations of ascorbic acid in plasma and white blood cells of patients with cancer and non-cancerous diseases. Cancer Res. 11:238–242.

Bois, P. 1968. Peripheral vasodilation and thymic tumors in magnesium-deficient rats. In G. Jasmin, ed. Endocrine Aspects of Disease Processes. W.H. Greene Inc., St. Louis.

Bois, P., and A. Beaulnes. 1966. Histamine, magnesium deficiency, and thymic tumors in rats. Can. J. Physiol. Pharmacol. 44:373–377.

Bois, P., E.B. Sandborn, and P.E. Messier. 1969. A study of thymic lymphosarcoma developing in magnesium-deficient rats. Cancer Res. 29:763–775.

Boman, B. 1988. L-tryptophan: a rational anti-depressant and a natural hypnotic? Aust. N. Z. J. Psychiatry 22(1):83–97.

Briel, R.C., T.H. Lippert, and H.P. Zahradnik. 1987. Changes in blood coagulation, thrombocyte function and vascular prostacyclin synthesis caused by magnesium sulfate. Geburtshilfe Frauenheilkd. 47:332–336.

Bunce, C.M., P.J. French, J. Durham, R.A. Stockley, R.H. Michell, and G. Brown. 1994. Indomethacin potentiates the induction of HL60 differentiation to neutrophils, by retinoic acid and granulocyte colony-stimulating factor, and to monocytes, by vitamin D_3. Leukemia 8(4):595–604.

Burns, J.J., A.H. Conney, G.D. Peter, et al. 1960. Observations on the drug-induced synthesis of D-glucuronic, L-gluconic, and L-ascorbic acids in rats. J. Pharmacol. Exp. Therap. 129:132–138.

Burr, M.L., and B.K. Butland. 1988. Heart disease in British vegetarians. Am. J. Clin. Nutr. 48:830–832.

Burr, M.L., and P.M. Sweetnam. 1982. Vegetarianism, dietary fiber, and mortality. Am. J. Clin. Nutr. 36:873–877.

Cade, J.F.J. 1949. Lithium salts in the treatment of psychotic excitement. Med. J. Aust. 36:349–352.

Califf, R.M., F.E. Harrell, Jr., K.L. Lee, et al. 1989. The evolution of medical and surgical therapy for coronary artery disease: a 15-year perspective. JAMA 261(14):2077–2086.

Calloway, D.H., et al. 1974. The Superior Mineral Content of Some American Indian Foods in Comparison to Federally Donated Counterpart Commodities.

Cameron, E., and A. Campbell. 1974. The orthomolecular treatment of cancer. II: Clinical trial of high-dose ascorbic acid supplements in advanced human cancer. Chem. Biol. Interact. 9:285–318.

Cameron, E., and L. Pauling. 1976. Supplemental ascorbate in the supportive treatment of cancer: prolongation of survival times in terminal human cancer. Proc. Natl. Acad. Sci. 73:3685–3689.

Carney, M.W.P., and B.F. Sheffield. 1970. Associations of subnormal serum folate and vitamin B_{12} and effects of replacement therapy. J. Nerv. Ment. Dis. 150:404–412.

Carter, J.P., G.P. Saxe, V. Newbold, et al. 1990. Cancers with Suspected Nutritional Links: Dietary Management (typescript). Nutrition Section, Tulane University School of Public Health and Tropical Medicine, New Orleans.

Carter, J.P., G.P. Saxe, V. Newbold, et. al. 1993. Hypothesis: dietary management may improve survival from nutritionally linked cancers based on analysis of representative cases. J. Am. Coll. Nutr. 12:209–226.

Casley-Smith, J.R., and Casley-Smith, R.J. 1986. High-Protein Edemas and the Benzopyrones. Lippincott, Sydney.

Casley-Smith, J.R., R.G. Morgan, and N.B. Piller. 1993. Treatment of lymphedema of the arms and legs with 5,6-benzo-alpha-pyrone. N. Engl. J. Med. 329:1158–1163.

Casley-Smith, J.R., N.B. Piller, and R.G. Morgan. 1986. Behandlung chronischer lymphedeme der Arme und Beine mit 5,6-Benzo-(alpha)-pyron: placebokontrollierte Doppelblind-cross-over Studie über die Dauer von einem Jahr. Therapiewoche 36:1068–1076.

Casscells, W. 1994. Magnesium and myocardial infarction. Lancet 343:807–809.

Cassidy, C. 1991. The good body: when big is better. Med. Anthropol. 13:181–213.

Cassileth, B.R., E.J. Lusk, T.B. Strouse, and B.J. Bodenheimer. 1984. Contemporary unorthodox treatments in cancer medicine: a study of patients, treatments, and practitioners. Ann. Intern. Med. 101:105–112.

Chandra, R.K. 1992. Effect of vitamin and trace-element supplementation on immune responses and infection in elderly subjects. Lancet 340:1124–1127.

Chang-Claude, J., R. Frentzel-Beyme, and U. Eilber. 1992. Mortality pattern of German vegetarians after 11 years of follow-up. Epidemiology 3:395–401.

Christensen, H.N. 1993. Riboflavin can protect tissues from oxidative injury. Nutr. Rev. 51:149–150.

Citizens' Commission on School Nutrition. 1990. White Paper on School Lunch Nutrition. Center for Science in the Public Interest, Washington, D.C.

Clancy-Hepburn, K., A.A. Hickey, and G. Nevill. 1974. Children's behavior responses to TV food advertisements. J. Nutr. Ed. 6:93–96.

Cluzan, R., and A. Pecking. 1989. Benzopyrone (Lysedem) double-blind cross-over study in patients with secondary upper limb edemas. In M. Nishi, S. Uchino, and S. Yabuki, eds. Progress in Lymphology—XII: Proceedings of the XIIth International Congress of Lymphology, Tokyo/Kyoto. [Excerpta Medica 1990:453–454.]

Conradt, A. 1984. [Current concepts in the pathogenesis of gestosis with special reference to magnesium deficiency.] Z. Geburtshilfe Perinatol. 188:49–58. (in German)

Conradt, A., and H. Weidinger. 1982. [The central position of magnesium in the management of fetal hypotrophy—a contribution to the pathomechanism of utero-placental insufficiency, prematurity and poor intrauterine fetal growth as well as preeclampsia.] Magnesium Bulletin 4:103–124. (in German, English abstract)

Conradt, A., H. Weidinger, and H. Algayer. 1984. On the role of magnesium in fetal hypotrophy, pregnancy-induced hypertension, and preeclampsia. Magnesium Bulletin 6:68–76.

Contento, I.R., A.D. Manning, and B. Shannon. 1992. Research perspective on school-based nutrition education. JNE 24:247–260.

Coodley, G.O., H.D. Nelson, M.D. Loveless, and C. Folk. 1993. Beta-carotene in HIV infection. J. Acquir. Immune Defic. Syndr. 6:272–276.

Coon, W.W., K.D. Miller, and R.M. Whitrock. 1952. Post-operative thromboembolism: an evaluation of true plasma antithrombin titers with particular reference to the Kay test and alpha-tocopherol-calcium gluconate prophylaxis. Surg. Forum 3:536–542.

Coon, W.W., and R.M. Whitrock. 1951. Post-operative thromboembolism: clinical evaluation of the efficacy of several laboratory tests and of prophylaxis afforded by alpha-tocopherol-calcium gluconate medication. Surg. Forum 2:310–316.

Cooper, R.S., R.B. Goldberg, M. Trevisan, et al. 1982. The selective lipid-lowering effect of vegetarianism on low-density lipoproteins in a cross-over experiment. Atherosclerosis 44:293–305.

Cope, F.W. 1978. A medical application of the Ling association-induction hypothesis: the high-potassium, low-sodium diet of the Gerson cancer therapy. Physiol. Chem. Phys. Med. NMR 10(5):465–468.

Corica, F., A. Allegra, A. Di Benedetto, et al. 1994. Effects of oral magnesium supplementation on plasma lipid concentrations in patients with non-insulin-dependent diabetes mellitus. Magnes. Res. 7:43–46.

Cotugna, N. 1988. TV ads on Saturday morning children's programming—what's new? J. Nutr. Ed. 20:125–127.

Cotugna, N., A.F. Subar, J. Heimendinger, and L. Kahle. 1992. Nutrition and cancer prevention knowledge, beliefs, attitudes and practices: the 1987 National Health Interview Survey. J. Am. Diet. Assoc. 92(8):963–968.

Cotzias, G.C., M.H. Van Woert, and L.M. Schiffer. 1967. Aromatic amino acids and modification of parkinsonism. N. Engl. J. Med. 276:374–379.

Creagan, E.T., C.G. Moertel, J.R. O'Fallon, et al. 1979. Failure of high-dose vitamin C (ascorbic acid) therapy to benefit patients with advanced cancer. A controlled trial. N. Engl. J. Med. 301(13):687–690.

Creekmore, S.P., W.J. Urba, and D.L. Longo. 1991. Principles of the clinical evaluation of biologic agents. In V.T. DeVita, Jr., S. Hellman, and S.A. Rosenberg, eds. Biologic Therapy of Cancer. Lippincott, Philadelphia.

Crump, W.E., and E.F. Heiskell. 1952. Alpha-tocopherol and calcium gluconate in the prevention of thromboembolism. Texas J. Med. 48:11–14.

Darlington, L.G., N.W. Ramsey, and J.R. Mansfield. 1986. Placebo-controlled, blind study of dietary manipulation therapy in rheumatoid arthritis. Lancet 1(8475):236–238.

de Lorgeril, M., S. Renaud, N. Mamelle, et al. 1994. Mediterranean alpha-linolenic acid-rich diet in secondary prevention of coronary heart disease. Lancet 343:1454–1459.

Debry, G. 1991. Diet peculiarities. Vegetarianism, veganism, crudivorism, macrobiotism. Rev. Prat. 41(11):967–972.

DeJong, W., and A. Winsten. 1990. The use of mass media in substance abuse prevention. Health Aff. 9:30–46.

Dellinger, R.P. 1991. Acute life-threatening asthma. Postgrad. Med. 90:63–66, 69–72, 77.

Demisch, K., J. Bauer, and K. Georgi. 1987. Treatment of severe chronic insomnia with L-tryptophan and varying sleeping times. Pharmacopsychiatry 20(6):245–248.

Desprez-Curely, J.P., R. Cluzan, and A. Pecking. 1985. Benzopyrones and post-mastectomy lymphedemas. Double-blind trial placebo versus sustained-release coumarin with trioxyethylrutin (TER). In J.R. Casley-Smith and N.B. Piller, eds. Progress in Lymphology, X. University of Adelaide Press, Adelaide.

DeWys, W., C. Begg, P. Lavin, et al. 1980. Prognostic effect of weight loss prior to chemotherapy in cancer patients. Am. J. Med. 69:491–497.

Dorant, E., P.A. van den Brandt, R.A. Goldbohm, R.J.J. Hermus, and F. Sturmans. 1993. Garlic and its significance for the prevention of cancer in humans: a critical review. Br. J. Cancer 67:424–429.

Dupont, B., J.C. Pony, G. LeBihan, and P. Leborgne. 1969. [Phlebothrombotic disease and magnesium.] Sem. Hop. Paris 45:3048–3054. (in French)

Durlach, J. 1967. [Physiologic antithrombotic role of magnesium. About a phlebothrombotic patient with magnesium deficiency.] Coeur Med. Interne 6:213–232. (in French)

Durlach, J. 1988. Magnesium in Clinical Practice. John Libbey, London.

Durlach, J., M. Bara, and A. Guiet-Bara. 1989. Magnesium level in drinking water: its importance in cardiovascular risk. In Y. Itokawa and J. Durlach, eds. Magnesium in Health and Disease. John Libbey, London.

Eaton, B.S., and M. Konner. 1985. Paleolithic nutrition: a consideration of its nature and current implications. N. Engl. J. Med. 312(5):283–289.

Eddy, D.M. 1986. Setting priorities for cancer control programs. J. Natl. Cancer Inst. 76:187–199.

Egan, M.F., R.M. Hyde, G.W. Alberts, et al. 1992. Treatment of tardive dyskinesia with vitamin E. Am. J. Psychiatry 149:773–777.

Egger, J., C.M. Carter, P.J. Graham, D. Gumley, and J.F. Soothill. 1985. A controlled trial of oligoantigenic diet treatment in the hyperkinetic syndrome. Lancet 1(8428):540–545.

Egger, J., A. Stolla, and L.M. McEwen. 1992. Controlled trial of hyposensitization in children with food-induced hyperkinetic syndrome. Lancet 339:1150–1153.

Egger, J., J. Wilson, C.M. Carter, M.W. Turner, and J. Soothill. 1983. Is migraine food allergy? A double-blind controlled trial of oligoantigenic diet treatment. Lancet 2(8355):865–869.

Eisenberg, D.M., R.C. Kessler, C. Foster, et al. 1993. Unconventional medicine in the United States: prevalence, costs, and patterns of use. N. Engl. J. Med. 328:246–252.

Eisenberg, M.J. 1992. Magnesium deficiency and sudden death [editorial]. Am. Heart J. 124:544–549.

Elkashef, A.M., P.E. Ruskin, N. Bacher, and D. Barrett. 1990. Vitamin E in the treatment of tardive dyskinesia. Am. J. Psychiatry 147(4):505–506.

Elliott, R.L., M.C. Elliott, F. Wang, and J.F. Head. 1993. Breast carcinoma and the role of iron metabolism. A cytochemical, tissue culture, and ultrastructural study. Ann. N. Y. Acad. Sci. 698:159–166.

Emerson, C. 1929. Treatment of tuberculosis by altering metabolism through dietary management (Gerson-Sauerbruch method). Nebr. State Med. J. 14(3):104–107.

Facchinetti, F., G. Sances, P. Borella, et al. 1991. Magnesium prophylaxis of menstrual migraine: effects on intracellular magnesium. Headache 31:298–301.

Farncombe, M., G. Daniels, and L. Cross. 1994. Lymphedema: the seemingly forgotten complication. J. Pain. Symptom. Manage. 9(4):269-276.

Farooqui, A.A., L. Liss, and L.A. Horrocks. 1988. Stimulation of lipolytic enzymes in Alzheimer's disease. Ann. Neurol. 23:306–308.

Fauk, D., R. Fehlinger, R. Becker, et al. 1991. Transient cerebral ischemic attack and calcium-magnesium imbalance: clinical and paraclinical findings in 106 patients under 50 years of age. Magnes. Res. 4:53–58.

Fehling, C. 1966. Treatment of Parkinson's syndrome with L-dopa: a double-blind study. Acta Neurol. Scand. 42:367–372.

Fehlinger, R., C. Kemnitz, K. Seidel, and T. Guenther. 1987. Electrolyte contents of serum and erythrocytes of patients with tetanic syndrome before and after treatment with magnesium. Magnesium Bull. 9:115–117.

Fesmire, F.M. 1993. Intravenous magnesium for acute asthma. Ann. Emerg. Med. 22:616–617.

Folkers, K., M. Morita, and J. McRee, Jr. 1993. The activities of coenzyme Q_{10} and vitamin B_6 for immune responses. Biochem. Biophys. Res. Commun. 193(1):88–92.

Folkers, K., S. Shizukuishi, K. Takemura, et al. 1982. Increase in levels of IgG in serum of patients treated with coenzyme Q_{10}. Res. Commun. Chem. Pathol. Pharmacol. 38(2):335–338.

Fraser, G.E. 1988. Determinants of ischemic heart disease in Seventh-Day Adventists: a review. Am. J. Clin. Nutr. 48:833–836.

Frati-Munari, A.C., J.A. Fernandez-Harp, H. de la Riva, R. Ariza-Andraca, and M. del Carmen Torres. 1983. Effects of nopal (Opuntia Sp.) on serum lipids, glycemia and body weight. Arch. Invest. Med. (Mex.) 14:117–125.

Freedman, A.M., A.H. Atrakchi, M.M. Cassidy, and W.B. Weglicki. 1990. Magnesium deficiency-induced cardiomyopathy: protection by vitamin E. Biochem. Biophys. Res. Commun. 170:1102–1106.

Freedman, A.M., M.M. Cassidy, and W.B. Weglicki. 1991. Magnesium-deficient myocardium demonstrates an increased susceptibility to an in vivo oxidative stress. Magnes. Res. 4:185–189.

Frentzel-Beyme, R., J. Claude, and U. Eilber. 1988. Mortality among German vegetarians: first results after five years of follow-up. Nutr. Cancer 11:117–126.

Friedman, M. 1993. Speech to the ad hoc advisory panel of the Office of Alternative Medicine, National Institutes of Health, July.

Fryburg, D.A., R. Mark, P.W. Askenase, and T.F. Patterson. 1992. The immunostimulatory effects and safety of beta-carotene in patients with AIDS. Presented at the VIIIth International Conference on AIDS, July 19–24, Amsterdam.

Fujita, K., K. Shimpo, and K. Yamada. 1982. Reduction of adriamycin toxicity by ascorbate in mice and guinea pigs. Cancer Res. 42:309–316.

Galland, L. 1991–1992. Magnesium, stress and neuropsychiatric disorders. Magnes. Trace Elem. 10:287–301.

Garewal, H.S., N.M. Ampel, R.R. Watson, R.H. Prabhala, and C.L. Dols. 1992. A preliminary trial of beta carotene in subjects infected with the human immunodeficiency virus. J. Nutr. 122:728–732.

Garg, A., S.M. Grundy, and M. Koffler. 1992. Effect of high carbohydrate intake on hyperglycemia, islet cell function, and plasma lipoproteins in NIDDM. Diabetes Care 15:1572–1580.

Georgotas, N., and S. Gershon. 1981. Historical perspectives and current highlights on lithium treatment in manic-depressive illness. J. Clin. Psychopharmacol. 1(1):27–31.

Gershon, S., and A. Yuwiler. 1960. Lithium ion: a specific psychopharmacological approach to the treatment of mania. J. Neuropsychiatry 1:229–241.

Gerson Institute. Undated-a. Gerson Therapy Center Opens. When Cancer Becomes Incurable by Orthodox Methods, Perhaps Gerson Therapy Is the Answer (flyer).

Gerson Institute. Undated-b. Gerson Therapy (information brochure).

Gerson, M.B. 1929. The origin and rationales of dietary treatment of tuberculosis. Med. Welt 3:1313–1317.

Gerson, M.B. 1934. Diet therapy for lung tuberculosis. Franz Deuticke, Leipzig/Vienna.

Gerson, M.B. 1935. Fluid-rich potassium diet as treatment for cardiorenal insufficiency. Münch. Med. Wochenschr. 82:571–574.

Gerson, M.B. 1949. Effects of a combined dietary regimen on patients with malignant tumors. Exp. Med. Surg. 7(4):299–317.

Gerson, M.B. 1954a. No cancer in normal metabolism. Med. Klin. 49(5):175–179.

Gerson, M.B. 1954b. Cancer, a problem of metabolism. Med. Klin. 49(26):1028–1032.

Gerson, M.B. 1954c. On the medications of cancer management in the manner of Gerson. Med. Klin. 49(49):1977–1978.

Gerson, M.B. 1958. A Cancer Therapy: Results of Fifty Cases. Gerson Institute, Bonita, Calif.

Gerson, M.B. 1978. The cure of advanced cancer by diet therapy: a summary of 30 years of clinical experimentation. Physiol. Chem. Phys. 10:449–464.

Gerson, M.B. 1986. A Cancer Therapy: Results of Fifty Cases (5th ed.). Gerson Institute, Bonita, Calif.

Gertz, S.D., R.S. Wajnberg, A. Kurgon, and G. Uretzky. 1987. Effect of magnesium sulfate on the thrombus formation following partial arterial constriction: implications for coronary vasospasm. Magnesium 6:225–235.

Giannini, A.J., R.H. Loiselle, L.R. DiMarzio, and J.D. Giannini. 1987. Augmentation of haloperidol by ascorbic acid in phencyclidine intoxication. Am. J. Psychiatry 144:1207–1209.

Giovannucci, E., M.J. Stampfer, G.A. Colditz, et al. 1993. Folate, methionine, and alcohol intake and risk of colorectal adenoma. J. Natl. Cancer Inst. 85:875–884.

Glanz, K., and M.B. Gilboy. 1992. Physicians, preventive care, and applied nutrition: selected literature. Acad. Med. 67(11):776–781.

Gloth, F.M., J.D. Tobin, S.S. Sherman, and B.W. Hollis. 1991. Is the recommended daily allowance for vitamin D too low for the homebound elderly? J. Am. Geriatr. Soc. 39:137–141.

Godfrey, P.S.A., B.K. Toone, M.W.P. Carney, et al. 1990. Enhancement of recovery from psychiatric illness by methylfolate. Lancet 336:392–395.

Goldin, B.R., H. Adlercreutz, J.T. Dwyer, L. Swenson, J.H. Warram, and S.L. Gorbach. 1981. Effect of diet on excretion of estrogens in pre- and postmenopausal incidence of breast cancer in vegetarian women. Cancer Res. 41:3771–3773.

Goldin, B.R., H. Adlercreutz, S.L. Gorbach, et al. 1982. Estrogen excretion patterns and plasma levels in vegetarian and omnivorous women. N. Engl. J. Med. 307:1542–1547.

Gonzalez, N.J. 1987. One Man Alone: An Investigation of Nutrition, Cancer, and William Donald Kelley (unpublished manuscript).

Good, R.A., D.G. Jose, W.C. Cooper, G. Fernandes, T. Kramer, and E.J. Yunis. 1977. Influence of nutrition on antibody production and cellular immune responses in man, rats, mice, and guinea pigs. In Suskind, ed. Malnutrition and the Immune Response. Raven, New York.

Good, R.A., A. West, and G. Fernandes. 1980. Nutritional modulation of immune responses. Fedn. Proc. 39:3089–3104.

Gorn, G., and M. Goldberg. 1982. Behavioral evidence of the effects of televised food messages on children. J. Consumer Res. 9:200–205.

Green, S. 1992. A critique of the rationale for cancer treatment with coffee enemas and diet. JAMA 268(22):3224–3227.

Green, S.M., and S.G. Rothrock. 1992. Intravenous magnesium for acute asthma: failure to decrease emergency treatment duration or need for hospitalization. Ann. Emerg. Med. 21:260–265.

Greenberg, E.R., J.A. Baron, T.D. Tosteson, et al. 1994. A clinical trial of antioxidant vitamins to prevent colorectal adenoma. N. Engl. J. Med. 331(3):141–147.

Greville, G.D., and H. Lehmann. 1944. Cation antagonism in blood coagulation. J. Physiol. 103:175–184.

Gridley, G., J.K. McLaughlin, G. Block, W.J. Blot, M. Gluch, and J.F. Fraumeni. 1992. Vitamin supplement use and reduced risk of oral and pharyngeal cancer. Am. J. Epidemiol. 135:1083–1092.

Guenther, T., V. Hoellriegl, J. Vormann, J. Bubeck, and H.G. Classen. 1994. Increased lipid peroxidation in rat tissues by magnesium deficiency and vitamin E depletion. Magnesium Bulletin 16:38–43.

Guenther, T., H.J. Merker, V. Hoellriegl, J. Vormann, J. Bubeck, and H.G. Classen. 1994. Role of magnesium deficiency and lipid peroxidation in atherosclerosis. Magnesium Bulletin 16:44–49.

Guenther, T., J. Vormann, V. Hoellriegl, G. Disch, and H.G. Classen. 1992. Role of lipid peroxidation and vitamin E in magnesium deficiency. Magnesium Bulletin 14:57–66.

Haberal, M., V. Mavi, and G. Oner. 1987. The stabilizing effect of vitamin E, selenium and zinc on leucocyte membrane permeability: a study in vitro. Burns Incl. Therm. Inj. 13(2):118–122.

Hackethal, K.H. 1951. [Magnesium prophylaxis and treatment of thrombosis and embolism.] Chirurgie 270:35–36. (in German)

Hajimohammadreza, I., and M. Brammer. 1990. Brain membrane fluidity and lipid peroxidation in Alzheimer's disease. Neurosci. Lett. 112:333–337.

Hall, T. 1987. Designing culturally relevant educational materials for Mexican American clients. The Diabetes Educator 13(3):281–285.

Hampe, E.C., and M. Wittenberg. 1964. The Lifeline of America: Development of the Food Industry. McGraw–Hill, New York.

Hanes, S.D., J. Vermeersch, and S. Gale. 1984. The national evaluation of school nutrition programs: program impact on dietary intake. Am. J. Clin. Nutr. 40:390–413.

Hankinson, S.E., M.J. Stampfer, J.M. Seddon, et al. 1992. Nutrient intake and cataract extraction in women: a prospective study. BMJ 305:335–339.

Hass, G.M., G.H. Laing, R.M. Galt, and P.A. McCreary. 1981a. Recent advances: immunopathology of magnesium deficiency in rats—induction of tumors; incidence, transmission and prevention of lymphoma-leukemia. Magnesium Bulletin 3(1a):217–228.

Hass, G.M., G.H. Laing, R.M. Galt, and P.A. McCreary. 1981b. Role of magnesium deficiency in immunity to neoplasia in the rat. Magnesium Bulletin 3:5–11.

Hathaway, M.L. 1962. Magnesium in Human Nutrition (Home Economics Research Report #19). USDA Agricultural Research Service, Washington, D.C.

Hathcock, J.N. 1991. Safety of vitamin and mineral supplements. In A. Bendich and C.E. Butterworth, Jr., eds. Micronutrients in Health and in Disease Prevention. Marcel Dekker, New York.

Haury, V.G. 1938. The bronchodilator action of magnesium and its antagonistic action (dilator action) against pilocarpine, histamine, and barium chloride. J. Pharmacol. 64:58–64.

Hauser, S.P., and P.H. Braun. 1991. Intravenous magnesium in asthmatic patients. A clinical trial and review of the literature. In B. Lasserre and J. Durlach, eds. Magnesium—A Relevant Ion. John Libbey, London.

Hawkins, M.J., D.F. Hoth, and R.E. Wittes. 1986. Clinical development of biological response modifiers: comparison with cytotoxic drugs. Semin. Oncol. 13:132–140.

Healing Newsletter. 1990. Critics assail OTA: "Unconventional Cancer Treatments" project director and staff taken to task. 6(1–2):17–19 (Gerson Research Organization, San Diego, Calif.).

Heikkila, R.E., L. Manzino, F.S. Cabbat, and J.G. Hanly. 1983. Ascorbic acid and the binding of DA agonists to neostriatal membrane preparations. Neuropharmacology 22:135–137.

Heimendinger, J., B. Thompson, J. Ockene, et al. 1990. Reducing the risk of cancer through worksite intervention. Occup. Med. 5(4):707–723.

Heinonen, O.P., and D. Albanes. 1994. The effect of vitamin E and beta carotene on the incidence of lung cancer in male smokers. N. Engl. J. Med. 330(15):1029–1034.

Heinrich, H.G. 1957. [Magnesium prophylaxis and therapy of thrombotic conditions.] Z. Gesell. Inn. Med. 12:777–779. (in German)

Herrmann, R.G., W.B. Lacefield, and V.G. Crowe. 1970. Effect of ionic calcium and magnesium on human platelet aggregation. Proc. Soc. Exp. Biol. Med. 135:100–103.

Herron, D.G. 1991. Strategies of promoting a healthy dietary intake. Nurs. Clin. North Am. 26(4):875–884.

Hildenbrand, C., K. Bradford, and G. Hildenbrand. 1993. Melanoma Retrospective Best-Case Review: Tabular Report—A Review in Progress (typescript). Gerson Research Organization, San Diego, Calif.

Hildenbrand, G. 1986. Let's set the record straight: A survey of the U.S. peer-reviewed medical literature regarding the developmental Gerson diet therapy (Parts I–II). Healing Newsletter 14–15 (Gerson Research Organization, San Diego, Calif.).

Hirayama, T. 1971. Epidemiology of stomach cancer. In T. Murakami, ed. Early Gastric Cancer (Gann Monograph on Cancer Research No. 11). University of Tokyo Press, Tokyo.

Hirayama, T. 1981. Relationship of soybean paste soup intake to gastric cancer risk. Nutr. Cancer 3:223–233.

Hirayama, T. 1986. Nutrition and cancer—a large-scale cohort study. Prog. Clin. Biol. Res. 206:299–311.

Hoffer, A., and H. Osmond. 1960. The Chemical Basis of Clinical Psychiatry. Charles C. Thomas, Springfield, Ill.

Hoffer, A., and H. Osmond. 1964. Treatment of schizophrenia with nicotinic acid: a ten-year follow-up. Acta Psychiatr. Scand. 40:171–189.

Hoffer, L.J. 1974. The controversy over orthomolecular therapy. J. Orthomolecular Psychiatry 3:167–185.

Hopps, H.C. 1981. How might geochemical factors affect senescence and age-associated pathology? In Aging and the Geochemical Environment (Report of Panel, National Research Council, National Academy of Sciences). National Academy Press, Washington, D.C.

Hopps, H.C., and G.L. Feder. 1986. Chemical qualities of water that contribute to human health in a positive way. Sci. Tot. Environm. 54:207–216.

Horrobin, D.F. 1990. The philosophical basis of peer review and the suppression of innovation. JAMA 263(10):1438–1441.

Huemer, R.P., ed. 1986. The Roots of Molecular Medicine: A Tribute to Linus Pauling. W.H. Freeman, New York.

Hval, E. 1932. Microscopic study of the capillaries of patients on the Gerson-Sauerbruch-Herrmannsdorfer diet. Acta Derm. Venereol. 13:593–600.

Ibanez-Camacho, R., and R. Roman-Ramos. 1979. Hypoglycemic effect of opuntia cactus. Arch. Invest. Med. (Mex.) 10:223–230.

Inui, T.S., E.L. Yourtee, and J.W. Williamson. 1976. Improved outcomes in hypertension physician tutorials. Ann. Intern. Med. 84:646–651.

Iwasaki, M., Y. Fukuo, Y. Kobayashi, et al. 1988. The use of magnesium in medical practice for cerebrovascular disease. Magnesium Res. 1:113.

Jacques, P.F., S.C. Hartz, L.T. Chylack, R.B. McGandy, and J.A. Sadowski. 1988. Nutritional status in persons with and without senile cataract: blood vitamin and mineral levels. Am. J. Clin. Nutr. 48:152–158.

Jasmin, G. 1963. [Lymphedema, hyperplasia, tumefaction of lymphatic tissue of the rat kept on a magnesium-deficient diet.] Rev. Can. Biol. 22:383–390. (in French)

Javitt, D.C., I. Zylberman, S.R. Zukin, et al. 1994. Amelioration of negative symptoms of schizophrenia by glycine. Am. J. Psychiatry 151:1234–1236.

Johnson, A.A., E.M. Knight, C.H. Edwards, et al. 1994. Dietary intakes, anthropometric measurements and pregnancy outcomes. J. Nutr. 124(6):936S–942S.

Johnson, F.N. 1984. The History of Lithium Therapy. Macmillan, London.

Joos, S. 1984. Economic, social, and cultural factors in the analysis of disease: dietary change and diabetes mellitus among the Florida Seminole Indians. In L. Brown and K. Mussell, eds. Ethnic and Regional Foodways in the United States. University of Tennessee Press, Knoxville.

Jose, D.G., J.S. Welch, and R.L. Doherty. 1969. Humoral and cellular immune responses to streptococci, influenza, and other antigens in Australian aboriginal school children. Aust. Pediatr. J. 5:209–218.

Journal of the American Dietetic Association. 1992. Pyramid power is here to stay: behind the new food guide. 92(8):925.

Kanofsky, J.D. 1986. Biochemical individuality and hyperkinesis. Medical Tribune. April 23, p. 37.

Kanofsky, J.D., and P.B. Kanofsky. 1981. Prevention of thromboembolic disease by vitamin E. N. Engl. J. Med. 305:173–174.

Kanofsky, J.D., S.R. Kay, J.P. Lindenmayer, and E. Seifter. 1988. Ascorbic acid and dopamine activity. Am. J. Psychiatry 145:904–905.

Kanofsky, J.D., S.R. Kay, J.P. Lindenmayer, and E. Seifter. 1989a. Ascorbic acid action in neuroleptic-associated amenorrhea. J. Clin. Psychopharmacol. 9(5):388–389.

Kanofsky, J.D., S.R. Kay, J.P. Lindenmayer, and E. Seifter. 1989b. Ascorbate: An adjunctive treatment for schizophrenia. J. Am. Coll. Nutr. 9:388–389.

Kanofsky, J.D., J. Padawer, J. Mendecki, and E. Seifter. 1990. Is there a role for vitamin A or beta-carotene in HIV therapy? J. Am. Coll. Nutr. 9:551.

Kanofsky, J.D., J. Padawer, and E. Seifter. 1987. Vitamin A and AIDS: an hypothesis and cautionary note. Medical Tribune, April 22, p. 26.

Kanofsky, J.D., and R. Sandyk. 1992. Antioxidants in the treatment of schizophrenia. Int. J. Neurosci. 62:97–100.

Kaplan, B.J., J. McNicol, R.A. Conte, and H.K. Moghadam. 1989. Dietary replacement in preschool-age hyperactive boys. Pediatrics 83(1):7–17.

Karppanen, H., R. Pennanen, and L. Passinen. 1978. Minerals, coronary heart disease and sudden coronary death. Adv. Cardiol. 25:9–24.

Katz, S. 1987. Food and biocultural evolution: a model for the investigation of modern nutritional problems. In Nutritional Anthropology. Alan R. Liss, Inc., New York.

Kawahara, H. 1959. Alpha-tocopherol in prophylaxis and treatment of venous thromboses. Surgery 46:768–774.

Kay, J.H., S.B. Hutton, G.N. Weiss, and A. Ochsner. 1950. Studies on an antithrombin. Surgery 28:24–28.

Kelley, W.D. 1969. One Answer to Cancer: An Ecological Approach to the Successful Treatment of Malignancy. Wedgestone Press, Winfield, Kan.

Kestin, M., I.L. Rouse, R.A. Correll, and P.J. Nestel. 1989. Cardiovascular disease risk factors in free-living men: comparison of two prudent diets, one based on lacto-ovovegetarianism and the other allowing lean meat. Am. J. Clin. Nutr. 50:280–287.

Kimm, S.Y., G.H. Payne, E. Lakatos, et al. 1990. Management of cardiovascular disease risk factors in children. A national survey of primary care physicians. Am. J. Dis. Child. 144(9):967–972.

King, W.P. 1988. Provocation neutralization: a two-part study. Otolaryngol. Head Neck Surg. 99:263–277.

Kittler, P., and K. Sucher. 1989. Food and Culture in America: A Nutrition Handbook. Van Nostrand Reinhold, New York.

Kittler, P., and K. Sucher. 1990. Diet counseling in a multicultural society. The Diabetes Educator 16(2):127–131.

Kjeldsen-Kragh, J., M. Haugen, C.F. Borchgrevink, et al. 1991. Controlled trial of fasting and 1-year vegetarian diet in rheumatoid arthritis. Lancet 338(8772):899–902.

Kleijnen, J., P. Knipschild, and G. ter Riet. 1989. Garlic, onions and cardiovascular risk factors. A review of the evidence from human experiments with emphasis on commercially available preparations. Br. J. Clin. Pharmacol. 28(5):535–544.

Knuiman, J.T., and C.E. West. 1982. The concentration of cholesterol in serum and in various serum lipoproteins in macrobiotic, vegetarian and non-vegetarian men and boys. Atherosclerosis 43:71–82.

Kontopoulos, V., M.S. Seelig, J. Dolan, A.R. Berger, and R.S. Ross. 1980. Influence of parenteral administration of magnesium sulfate to normal pregnant and to pre-eclamptic women. In M. Cantin and M.S. Seelig, eds. Magnesium in Health and Disease. Spectrum, New York.

Kottke, T.E., R.N. Battista, G.H. Defriese, and M.L. Brekke. 1988. Attributes of successful smoking cessation interventions in medical practice. A meta-analysis of 39 controlled trials. JAMA 259:2883–2889.

Kovacs, L., B.G. Molnar, E. Huhn, and L. Bodis. 1988. [Magnesium substitution in pregnancy: a prospective, randomized double-blind study.] Geburtshilfe Frauenheilkd. 48:595–600. (in German)

Krey, S.H. 1982. Alternate dietary lifestyles. Primary Care 9(3):595–603.

Kufs, W.M. 1990. Intravenous magnesium sulfate in acute asthma. JAMA 263:516–517.

Kuhnlein, H.V., and D.H. Calloway. 1977. Contemporary Hopi food pattern intakes. Ecol. Food Nutr. 6:159–173.

Kuitert, L.M., and S.L. Kletchko. 1991. Intravenous magnesium sulfate in acute, life-threatening asthma. Ann. Emerg. Med. 21:1243–1245.

Kushi, L.H. 1988. Foreword. In E. Esko, ed. Doctors Look at Macrobiotics. Japan Publications, New York.

Kushi, L.H. 1988. Letter to H. Sheehan, American Cancer Society, March 3.

Kushi, M. 1977. The Book of Macrobiotics. Japan Publications, Inc., New York.

Kushi, M. 1983. A Nutritional Overview of the Macrobiotic Diet. Typescript, December 19.

Kushi, M. 1988. Introduction. In E. Esko, ed. Doctors Look at Macrobiotics. Japan Publications, New York.

Kushi, M., and A. Jack. 1983. The Cancer Prevention Diet: Michio Kushi's Nutritional Blueprint for the Relief and Prevention of Disease. St. Martin's Press, New York.

La Vecchia, C. 1993. Dietary fat and cancer in Italy. Eur. J. Clin. Nutr. 47(Suppl. 1):S35–S38.

Lack, P., J.M. Livrozet, M. Bourgeay-Causse, V. Fayol, T. Saint-Marc, and J.L. Touraine. 1993. Vitamin status at the first blood test analysis in 120 HIV-seropositive patients. Presented at the IXth International Conference on AIDS, June 6–11, Berlin.

Lakshmanan, F.L., R.B. Rao, W.W. Kim, and J.L. Kelsay. 1984. Magnesium intakes, balances, and blood levels of adults consuming self-selected diets. Am. J. Clin. Nutr. 40:1380–1389.

Lasagna, L. 1972. The impact of scientific models on clinical psychopharmacology: a pharmacologist's view. Semin. Psychiatry 4:271–282.

Lazard, E.M. 1925. A preliminary report on the intravenous use of magnesium sulphate in puerperal eclampsia. Am. J. Obstet. Gynecol. 9:178–188.

Leary, A.W.P. 1986. Content of magnesium in drinking water and deaths from ischaemic heart disease in white South Africans. Magnesium 5:150–153.

Lechner, P., and G. Hildenbrand. 1994. A reply to Saul Green's critique of the rationale for cancer treatment with coffee enemas and diet: cafestol derived from beverage coffee increases bile production in rats; and coffee enemas and diet ameliorate human cancer pain in stages I and II. Townsend Letter for Doctors (May):526–530.

Lechner, P., and I. Kronberger. 1990. Experiences with the use of dietary therapy in surgical oncology. Aktuelle Ernährungsmedizin 2(15).

Lentze, M.J. 1992. Vegetarian and outsider diets in childhood. Schweiz Rundsch. Med. Prax. 81(9):254–258.

Leon, A.S., J. Connett, D.R. Jacobs, Jr., and R. Rauramaa. 1987. Leisure-time physical activity levels and risk of coronary heart disease and death: the multiple risk factor intervention trial. JAMA 258:2388–2395.

Lerner, M. 1994. Choices in Healing: Integrating the Best of Conventional and Complementary Approaches to Cancer. MIT Press, Cambridge, Mass.

Levy, A.S., and R.C. Stokes. 1987. Effects of a health promotion advertising campaign on sales of ready-to-eat cereals. Public Health Rep. 102:398–404.

Lin, X., J. Liu, and J.A. Milner. 1994. Dietary garlic suppresses DNA adducts caused by N-nitroso compounds. Carcinogenesis 15(2):349–352.

Ling, J.C., B.A. Franklin, J.F. Lindsteadt, and S.A. Gearon. 1992. Social marketing: its place in public health. Ann. Rev. Public Health 13:341–362.

Ling, W.H., M. Laitinen, and O. Haenninen. 1992. Shifting from conventional diet to an uncooked vegan diet reversibly alters serum lipid and apolipoprotein levels. Nutr. Res. 12:1431–1440.

Lipkin, M. 1974. Phase 1 and 2 proliferative lesions of colonic epithelial cells in diseases leading to colon cancer. Cancer 34:878–888.

Lipkin, M., K. Uehara, S. Winawer, et al. 1985. Seventh-Day Adventist vegetarians have a quiescent proliferative activity in colonic mucosa. Cancer Lett. 26:139–144.

Lipton, M.A., T.A. Ban, F.J. Kane, J. Levine, L.R. Mosher, and R. Wittenborn. 1973. Megavitamin and Orthomolecular Therapy in Psychiatry. American Psychiatric Association, Washington, D.C.

Lockwood, K., S. Moesgaard, and K. Folkers. 1994. Partial and complete remission of breast cancer in patients in relation to dosage of coenzyme Q_{10}. Biochem. Biophys. Res. Commun. 199(3):1504–1508.

Lohr, J.B. 1991. Oxygen radicals and neuropsychiatric illness: some speculations. Arch. Gen. Psychiatry 48:1097–1106.

London, R.S., L. Bradley, and N.Y. Chiamori. 1991. Effect of a nutritional supplement on premenstrual symptomatology in women with premenstrual syndrome: a double-blind longitudinal study. J. Am. Coll. Nutr. 10:494–499.

Marcus, S.L., J.P. Dutcher, E. Paietta, et al. 1987. Severe hypovitaminosis C occurring as the result of adoptive immunotherapy with high-dose Interleukin 2 and lymphokine-activated killer cells. Cancer Res. 47:4208–4212.

Margetts, B.M., L.J. Beilin, R. Vandongen, and B.K. Armstrong. 1986. Vegetarian diet in mild hypertension: a randomized controlled trial. BMJ 293:1468–1471.

Marier, J.R. 1978. Cardioprotective contribution of hard water to magnesium intake. Rev. Can. Biol. 37:115–125.

Martin, W. 1991. Nathan Pritikin and atheroma. Med. Hypotheses 36:181–182.

Massara, E. 1980. Obesity and cultural weight valuations: a Puerto Rican case. Appetite 1:291–298.

Mattar, J.A., C.E. Salas, D.P. Bernstein, D. Lehr, and R. Bauer. 1990. Hemodynamic changes after an intensive short-term exercise and nutrition program in hypertensive and obese patients with and without coronary artery disease. Arq. Bras. Cardiol. 54(5):307–312.

Maurizi, C.P. 1988. Why not treat melancholia with melatonin and tryptophan and treat seasonal affective disorders with bright light? Med. Hypotheses 27(4):271–276.

Mayer, E., and I.N. Kugelmass. 1929. Basic (vitamin) feeding in tuberculosis. JAMA 93(24):1856–1862.

McCreary, P.A., H.A. Battifora, B.M. Hahneman, G.H. Laing, and G.M. Hass. 1967. Leukocytosis, bone marrow hyperplasia and leukemia in chronic magnesium deficiency in the rat. Blood 29:683–690.

McIntosh, T.K., A.I. Faden, I. Yamakami, and R. Vink. 1988. Magnesium deficiency exacerbates and pretreatment improves outcome following traumatic brain injury in rats. J. Neurotrauma 5:17–31.

McIntosh, T.K., R. Vink, I. Yamakami, and A.I. Faden. 1989. Magnesium protects against neurological deficit after brain injury. Brain Res. 482:252–260.

McKay, C.M., M.F. Cromwell, and L.A. Maynard. 1935. The effect of retarded growth upon the length of the life span and upon the ultimate body size. J. Nutr. 10:63–79.

McNamara, R.M., W.H. Spivey, E. Skobeloff, and S. Jacubowitz. 1989. Intravenous magnesium sulfate in the management of acute respiratory failure complicating asthma. Ann. Emerg. Med. 18:197–199.

Meadows, G.G., H.F. Pierson, and R.M. Abdallah. 1991. Ascorbate in the treatment of experimental transplanted melanoma. Am. J. Clin. Nutr. 54:1284S–1291S.

Melby, L.C., D.G. Goldflies, G.C. Hyner, and R.M. Lyle. 1989. Relation between vegetarian/nonvegetarian diets and blood pressure in black and white adults. Am. J. Public Health 79:1283–1288.

Mensink, R.P., and M.B. Katan. 1992. Effect of dietary fatty acids on serum lipids and lipoproteins. Arteriosclerosis and Thrombosis 12:911–919.

Messina, M., and S. Barnes. 1991. The role of soy products in reducing risk of cancer. J. Natl. Cancer Inst. 83:541–546.

Miller, J.B. 1977. A double-blind study of food extract therapy. Ann. Allergy 38:185–191.

Mills, P.K., J.F. Annegers, and R.L. Phillips. 1988. Animal product consumption and subsequent fatal breast cancer risk among Seventh-Day Adventists. Am. J. Epidemiol. 127:440–453.

Mills, P.K., W.L. Beeson, R.L. Phillips, and G.E. Fraser. 1989a. Dietary habits and breast cancer incidence among Seventh-Day Adventists. Cancer 64:582–590.

Mills, P.K., W.L. Beeson, R.L. Phillips, and G.E. Fraser. 1989b. Cohort study of diet, lifestyle, and prostate cancer in Adventist men. Cancer 64:598–604.

Milner, G. 1963. Ascorbic acid in chronic psychiatric patients—a controlled trial. Br. J. Psychiatry 109:294–299.

Moertel, C.G., T.R. Fleming, E.T. Creagan, J. Rubin, M.J. O'Connell, and M.M. Ames. 1985. High-dose vitamin C versus placebo in the treatment of patients with advanced cancer who have had no prior chemotherapy: a randomized double-blind comparison. N. Engl. J. Med. 312:137–141.

Monsen, E. 1990. The 10th edition of the Recommended Dietary Allowances: what's new in the 1989 RDAs? J. Am. Diet. Assoc. 89:1748.

Moorman, R.H., H.E. Snyder, C.D. Snyder, and W.A. Grosjean. 1953. Alpha-tocopherol and alpha-tocopherol phosphate in the prophylaxis of thromboembolism. Arch. Surg. 67:137–141.

Moreschi, C. 1909. The connection between nutrition and tumor promotion. Z. Immunitätsforsch. 2:651–675.

Morgan, J.W., G.E. Fraser, R.L. Phillips, and M.H. Andress. 1988. Dietary factors and colon cancer incidence among Seventh-Day Adventists (abstract). Am. J. Epidemiol. 128:918.

Morgan, K.J., and G.L. Stampley. 1988. Dietary intake levels and food sources of magnesium and calcium for selected segments of the U.S. population. Magnesium 7:225–233.

Muir, C., J. Waterhouse, T. Mack, J. Powell, and S. Whelan. 1987. Cancer Incidence in Five Continents. International Agency for Research on Cancer, Lyon.

Myrmel, T. 1993. Treatment of ischemic heart disease—coronary surgery or angioplasty? An evaluation based on clinical and experimental data. Tidsskr. Nor. Laegeforen. 113(15):1873–1876.

National Center for Health Statistics. 1990. Health United States, 1989 (DHHS Pub. No. PHS-90-1232). U.S. Department of Health and Human Services, Hyattsville, Md.

National Heart, Lung, and Blood Institute. 1985. Hypertension prevalence and the status of awareness, treatment, and control in the United States: final report of the subcommittee on definition and prevalence of the 1984 joint national committee. Hypertension 7(3):457–468.

National Institutes of Health. 1994. NIH Consensus Development Conference on Optimal Calcium Intake. Bethesda, Md., June 6–8.

National Research Council, Committee on Nutrition in Medical Education, Food and Nutrition Board, Commission on Life Sciences. 1985. Nutrition Education in U.S. Medical Schools. National Academy Press, Washington, D.C.

National Research Council. 1989. Diet and Health: Implications for Reducing Chronic Disease Risk. National Academy Press, Washington, D.C.

Neel, J. 1976. Diabetes mellitus—a geneticist's nightmare. In W. Creutzfeld et al., eds. The Genetics of Diabetes Mellitus. Springer-Verlag, Heidelberg.

Nelson, K., J. Vermeersch, L. Jordan, J. Wellisch, and S. Gale. 1981. The national evaluation of school nutrition programs, review of research. Vol. II. System Development Corp., Santa Monica, Calif.

Nestle, M. 1993. Food lobbies, the Food Pyramid, and U.S. nutrition policy. Int. J. Health Serv. 23(3):483–496.

Neves, M.C., U. Brito, M.J.P. Miguel, O. Vivente, F. Barros, and J.R. Silva. 1991. Evaluation of Mg^{2+} aspartate HCl in asthmatic crises. Magnesium Bulletin 13:88–93.

Newbold, V. Undated. Remission of Cancer in Patients on a Macrobiotic Diet (unpublished manuscript).

Nixon, D.W. 1990. Nutrition and cancer: American Cancer Society guidelines, programs, and initiatives. CA 40(2):71–75.

Noppen, M., L. Vanmaele, N. Impens, and W. Schandevyl. 1990. Bronchodilating effect of intravenous magnesium sulfate in acute severe bronchial asthma. Chest 97:373–376.

O'Brien, S., and R.E. Dedmon. 1990. Cholesterol education at the worksite. AAOHN J. 38(5):216–221.

Ochsner, A. 1964. Thromboembolism. N. Engl. J. Med. 271:211.

Ochsner, A. 1968. Prevention and treating venous thrombosis. Postgrad. Med. 44:91–95.

Ochsner, A., M.E. DeBakey, and P.T. DeCamp. 1950. Venous thrombosis. JAMA 144:831–834.

Ochsner, A., M.E. DeBakey, P.T. DeCamp, and E. Rochs. 1951. Thromboembolism. Ann. Surg. 134:405–419.

Ochsner, A., J.H. Kay, P.T. DeCamp, S.B. Gutton, and G.A. Balla. 1950. Newer concepts of blood coagulation, with particular reference to postoperative thromboses. Ann. Surg. 131:652–659.

Office of Medical Applications of Research, National Institutes of Health. 1984. Osteoporosis. JAMA 252:799.

Office of Technology Assessment. 1990. Unconventional Cancer Treatments (OTA-H-405). U.S. Government Printing Office, Washington, D.C.

Okawa, M. 1992. [Effects of magnesium sulfate on brain damage by complete global brain ischemia]. Masui 41:341–355.

Okayama, H., T. Aikawa, M. Okayama, H. Sasaki, S. Mue, and T. Takishima. 1988. Bronchodilating effect of magnesium sulfate in bronchial asthma. JAMA 257:1076–1078.

Okayama, H., M. Okayama, T. Aikawa, M. Sasaki, and T. Takishima. 1991. Treatment of status asthmaticus with intravenous magnesium sulfate. J. Asthma 28:11–17.

Okunieff, P. 1991. Interactions between ascorbic acid and the radiation of bone marrow, skin, and tumor. Am. J. Clin. Nutr. 54:1281S–1283S.

Oldham, R.K. 1982. Biological response modifiers program. J. Biol. Response Mod. 1:81–100.

Oldham, R.K. 1985. Biologicals and biological response modifiers: design of clinical trials. J. Biol. Response Mod. 4:117–128.

Ornish, D.M. 1990. Dr. Dean Ornish's Program for Reversing Heart Disease. Random House, New York.

Ornish, D.M., S.E. Brown, L.W. Scherwitz, et al. 1990. Can lifestyle changes reverse coronary heart disease? Lancet 336:129–133.

Ornish, D.M., A.M. Gotto, R.R. Miller, et al. 1979. Effects of a vegetarian diet and selected yoga techniques in the treatment of coronary heart disease. Clin. Res. 27:720A.

Ornish, D.M., L.W. Scherwitz, R.D. Doody, et al. 1983. Effects of stress-management training and dietary changes in treatment of ischemic heart disease. JAMA 249:54–59.

Osmond, H. 1969. The background to the niacin treatment. Schizophrenia 1:4.

Parkinson Study Group. 1993. Effects of tocopherol and deprenyl on the progression of disability in early Parkinson's disease. N. Engl. J. Med. 328:176–183.

Patterson, B.H., G. Block, W.R. Rosenberger, D. Pee, and L.L. Kahle. 1990. Fruits and vegetables in the American diet: data from the NHANES II survey. Am. J. Public Health 80:1443.

Pauling, L. 1968. Orthomolecular psychiatry. Science 160:265–271.

Pauling, L. 1974. Dr. Pauling comments on the comments [letter to the editor]. Am. J. Psychiatry 131(12):1405–1406.

Pauling, L. 1976. Vitamin C, the Common Cold, and the Flu. Freeman, San Francisco.

Phillips, R.L., L. Garfinkel, J.W. Kuzma, W.L. Beeson, T.L. Lotz, and B. Brin. 1980. Mortality among California Seventh-Day Adventists for selected cancer sites. J. Natl. Cancer Inst. 65:1097–1107.

Phillips, R.L., F.R. Lemon, W.L. Beeson, and J.W. Kuzma. 1978. Coronary heart disease mortality among Seventh-Day Adventists with differing dietary habits: a preliminary report. Am. J. Clin. Nutr. 31:S191–S198.

Phillips, R.L., and D.A. Snowdon. 1983. Association of meat and coffee use with cancers of the large bowel, breast, and prostate among Seventh-Day Adventists: preliminary results. Cancer Res. 43(Suppl.):2403–2408.

Phillips, R.L., D.A. Snowdon, and B.N. Brin. 1983. Cancer in vegetarians. In E.L. Wynder, G.A. Leveille, J.H. Weisburger, et al., eds. Environmental Aspects of Cancer: The Role of Macro and Micro Components of Foods. Food & Nutrition Press, Westport, Conn.

Piller, N.B., R.G. Morgan, and J.R. Casley-Smith. 1985. A double-blind trial of 5,6-benzo-alpha-pyrone in human lymphedema. In J.R. Casley-Smith and N.B. Piller, eds. Progress in Lymphology, X. University of Adelaide Press, Adelaide.

Piller, N.B., R.G. Morgan, and J.R. Casley-Smith. 1988. A double-blind cross-over trial of O-(B-hydroxyethyl)-cutosides (benzo-pyrones) in the treatment of lymphedema of the arms and legs. Br. J. Plast. Surg. 41:20–27.

Pixley, F., D. Wilson, K. McPherson, and J. Mann. 1985. Effect of vegetarianism on development of gallstones in women. BMJ 291:11–12.

Poydock, E.M. 1991. Effect of combined ascorbic acid and B-12 on survival of mice with implanted Ehrlich carcinoma and L1210 leukemia. Am. J. Clin. Nutr. 54:1261S–1265S.

Price, K.R., and G.R. Fenwick. 1985. Naturally occurring estrogens in foods: a review. Food Addit. Contam. 2:73.

Pronczuk, A., Y. Kipervarg, and K.C. Hayes. 1992. Vegetarians have higher plasma alpha-tocopherol relative to cholesterol than do nonvegetarians. J. Am. Coll. Nutr. 11:50–55.

Public Health Service. 1989. Promoting Health/Preventing Disease: Year 2000 Objectives for the Nation. U.S. Department of Health and Human Services, Washington, D.C.

Public Health Service. 1990. Healthy People 2000: National Health Promotion and Disease Prevention Objectives. Full Report, with Commentary. U.S. Department of Health and Human Services, Washington, D.C.

Rasmussen, H.S., P. Aurup, K. Goldstein, et al. 1989a. Influence of magnesium substitution therapy on blood lipid composition in patients with ischemic heart disease: a double-blind, placebo-controlled study. Arch. Intern. Med. 149(5):1050–1053.

Rayssiguier, Y. 1981. Magnesium and lipid interrelationships in the pathogenesis of vascular diseases. Magnesium Bulletin 3:165–177.

Rayssiguier, Y. 1984. Role of magnesium and potassium in the pathogenesis of arteriosclerosis. Magnesium 3:226–238.

Rayssiguier, Y. 1986. Magnesium, lipids and vascular diseases: experimental evidence in animal models. Magnesium 5:182–190.

Rayssiguier, Y., E. Gueux, L. Bussiere, J. Durlach, and A. Mazur. 1993. Dietary magnesium affects susceptibility of lipoproteins and tissues to peroxidation in rats. J. Am. Coll. Nutr. 12:133–137.

Rayssiguier, Y., A. Mazur, P. Cardot, and E. Gueux. 1989. Effects of magnesium on lipid metabolism and cardiovascular disease. In Y. Itokawa and J. Durlach, eds. Magnesium in Health and Disease. John Libbey, London.

Rea, W.J., R.N. Podell, M.L. Williams, E. Fenyves, D.E. Sprague, and A.R. Johnson. 1984. Elimination of oral food challenge reaction by injection of food extracts: a double-blind evaluation. Arch. Otolaryngol. 110(4):248–252.

Rebec, G.V., J.M. Centore, L.K. White, and K.D. Alloway. 1984. Ascorbic acid and the behavioral response to haloperidol: implication for the action of antipsychotic drugs. Science 227:438–440.

Reese, F.G. 1972. Incidence of disease in the Navajo Indian. In D. Rabin, B. Anthony, S. Harrison, et al., eds. Health Problems of U.S. and North American Indian Populations. MSS Information Corp., New York.

Register, U.D., and L.M. Sonnenberg. 1973. The vegetarian diet. J. Am. Diet. Assoc. 62:253–261.

Resnicow, K. 1993. School-based obesity prevention. Proc. N. Y. Acad. Sci.

Richards, E. 1986. Vitamin C suffers a dose of politics. New Scientist, February 27, pp. 46–49.

Rimm, E.B., M.J. Stampfer, A. Ascherio, E. Giovannucci, G.A. Colditz, and W.C. Willett. 1993. Vitamin E consumption and the risk of coronary heart disease in men. N. Engl. J. Med. 328:1450–1456.

Ritenbaugh, C. 1982. New solutions to old problems: interaction of culture and nutrition. In N. Chrisman and T. Maretzki, eds. Clinically Applied Anthropology. Reidel, Dordrecht, Netherlands.

Robertson, J.M., A.P. Donner, and J.R. Trivithick. 1989. Vitamin E intake and risk of cataracts in humans. Ann. N. Y. Acad. Sci. 570:372–382.

Robinson, C.H., and M.R. Lawler. 1982. Normal and Therapeutic Nutrition. Macmillan, New York.

Rocella, E.J., and M.J. Horan. 1988. The National High Blood Pressure Education Program: measuring progress and assessing its impact. Health Psychol. 7(Suppl.):297–303.

Rocella, E.J., and C. Lenfant. 1992. Considerations regarding the cost and effectiveness of public and patient education programmes. J. Hum. Hypertens. 6(6):463–467.

Rosenthal, M.B., R.J. Barnard, D.P. Rose, S. Inkeles, J. Hall, and N. Pritikin. 1985. Effects of a high-complex-carbohydrate, low-fat, low-cholesterol diet on levels of serum lipids and estradiol. Am. J. Med. 78(1):23–27.

Rous, P. 1914. The influence of diet on transplanted and spontaneous mouse tumors. J. Exp. Med. 20:433–451.

Rouse, I.L., B.K. Armstrong, and L.J. Beilin. 1982. Vegetarian diet, lifestyle and blood pressure in two religious populations. Clin. Exp. Pharmacol. Physiol. 9:327–330.

Rouse, I.L., L.J. Beilin, D.P. Mahoney, et al. 1986. Nutrient intake, blood pressure, serum and urinary prostaglandins and serum thromboxane B_2 in a controlled trial with a lacto-ovo-vegetarian diet. J. Hypertens. 4:241–250.

Rush, D., J. Leighton, N.L. Sloan, et al. 1988. The National WIC Evaluation: evaluation of the Special Supplemental Food Program for Women, Infants, and Children. VI. Study of infants and children. Am. J. Clin. Nutr. 48(2 Suppl.):484–511.

Rush, D., N.L. Sloan, J. Leighton, et al. 1988. The National WIC Evaluation: evaluation of the Special Supplemental Food Program for Women, Infants, and Children. V. Longitudinal study of pregnant women. Am. J. Clin. Nutr. 48(2 Suppl.):439–483.

Russell, M.A.H., C. Wilson, C. Taylor, and C.D. Baker. 1979. Effect of general practitioners' advice against smoking. BMJ 2:231–235.

Sacks, F.M., W.P. Castelli, A. Donner, and E.H. Kass. 1975. Plasma lipids and lipoproteins in vegetarians and controls. N. Engl. J. Med. 292:1148–1151.

Sacks, F.M., A. Donner, W.P. Castelli, et al. 1981. Effect of ingestion of meat on plasma cholesterol of vegetarians. JAMA 246(6):640–644.

Sacks, F.M., D. Ornish, B. Rosner, S. McLanahan, W.P. Castelli, and E.H. Kass. 1985. Plasma lipoprotein levels in vegetarians: the effect of ingestion of fats from dairy products. JAMA 254:1337–1341.

Sacks, F.M., B. Rosner, and E.H. Kass. 1974. Blood pressure in vegetarians. Am. J. Epidemiol. 100:390–398.

Santiago, L.A., M. Hiramatsu, and A. Mori. 1992. Japanese soybean paste miso scavenges free radicals and inhibits lipid peroxidation. J. Nutr. Sci. Vitaminol. 38:297–304.

Sauerbruch, F., and A. Herrmannsdorfer. 1928. Outcomes and value of a dietary treatment for tuberculosis. Münch. Med. Wochenschr. 75:35–38.

Savoie, L.L., M. LePage, S. Moorjani, and P.J. Lupien. 1973. [Lipid modifications during development of cardiac necrosis in rats on a thrombogenic regimen.] Le Union Med. Canada 102:1457–1464.

Schardt, D. 1993. Do or diet: treating disease with food. In Nutrition Action. Center for Science in the Public Interest, Washington, D.C.

Schlagenhauf, G., J.P. Tupin, and R. White. 1966. The use of lithium carbonate in the treatment of manic psychosis. Am. J. Psychiatry 123:201–206.

Schmidt, F., H. Schmandte, and B. Gassman. 1963. Vitamin C und Krebs. Z. Arztl. Fortbild. 57:1315–1324.

Schnitzler, B. 1957. Thromboseprophylaxe mit Magnesium. Münch. Med. Wochenschr. 99:81–84.

Schreiber, J., and J. Homiak. 1981. Mexican Americans. In A. Harwood, ed. Ethnicity and Health Care. Harvard University Press, Cambridge, Mass.

Schuler, G., R. Hambrecht, G. Schlierf, et al. 1992. Regular physical exercise and low-fat diet. Effects on progression of coronary artery disease. Circulation 86(1):1–11.

Seelig, M.S. 1979. Magnesium (and trace substance) deficiencies in the pathogenesis of cancer. Biol. Trace Elem. Res. 1:273–297.

Seelig, M.S. 1980. Magnesium Deficiency in the Pathogenesis of Disease: Early Roots of Cardiovascular, Skeletal, and Renal Abnormalities. Plenum, New York.

Seelig, M.S. 1993. Magnesium in oncogenesis and in anticancer treatment; interaction with minerals and vitamins. In P. Quillan and R.M. Williams, eds. Adjuvant Nutrition in Cancer. Cancer Research Foundation, Arlington Heights, Ill.

Seelig, M.S., and H.A. Heggtveit. 1974. Magnesium interrelationships in ischemic heart disease: a review. Am. J. Clin. Nutr. 27(1):59–79.

Seifter, E. 1988. Personal communication to Patricia Spain Ward.

Seifter, E., J. Padawer, and J.D. Kanofsky. 1991. Vitamin A supplements and the AIDS vaccines. J. Am. Coll. Nutr. 10:548.

Seifter, E., G. Rettura, J. Padawer, A.A. Demetriou, and S.M. Levenson. 1983. A new approach to tumor therapy. In K.H. Spitzy and K. Karrer, eds. Proceedings of the 13th International Congress of Chemotherapy, Vienna, Austria, August 28–September 2. Concepts in Cancer Chemotherapy. Vienna: Verlag H. Egerman (between 1983 and 1984), volume 13, part 258.

Seifter, E., G. Rettura, J. Padawer, D. Fryburg, and S.M. Levenson. 1983. Nutritional and other agents modify the stress component of tumor growth. Advances 1:12–17.

Seifter, E., G. Rettura, J. Padawer, and S.M. Levenson. 1982. Moloney murine sarcoma virus tumors in CBA/J mice: chemopreventive and chemotherapeutic actions of supplemental beta-carotene. J. Natl. Cancer Inst. 68:835–840.

Seifter, E., G. Rettura, J. Padawer, et al. 1984. Morbidity and mortality reduction by supplemental vitamin A or beta-carotene in CBA mice given total-body gamma radiation. J. Natl. Cancer Inst. 73:1167–1177.

Seifter, E., B.A. Weinzweig, A.A. Demetriou, and J. Padawer. 1985. Supplemental vitamin A (VA): probable utility as adjunctive therapy in AIDS. Cancer Detection and Prevention 8, Abstract 27:084.

Semba, R.D., N.M. Graham, W.T. Caiaffa, J.B. Margolick, L. Clement, and D. Vlahov. 1993. Increased mortality associated with vitamin A deficiency during HIV-1 infection. Arch. Intern. Med. 153(18):2149–2154.

Sherman, J.B., L. Clark, and M.M. McEwen. 1989. Evaluation of a worksite wellness program: impact on exercise, weight, smoking, and stress. Public Health Nurs. 6(3):114–119.

Shike, M., and M.F. Brennan. 1989. Supportive care of the cancer patient. In V.T. DeVita, Jr., S. Hellman, and S.A. Rosenberg, eds. Cancer: Principles and Practice of Oncology (3rd ed.). Lippincott, Philadelphia.

Shintani, T.T., C.K. Hughes, S. Bechlam, and H.K. O'Connor. 1991. Obesity and cardiovascular risk intervention through the ad libitum feeding of a traditional Hawaiian diet. Am. J. Clin. Nutr. 53:1647s–1651s.

Sibai, B.M. 1990. Magnesium sulfate is the ideal anticonvulsant in preeclampsia-eclampsia. Am. J. Obstet. Gynecol. 162:1141–1145.

Sikora, K., N. James, and A. Reed. 1990. Juices, coffee enemas, and cancer. Lancet 336(8716):677–678.

Silagy, C., and A. Neil. 1994. Garlic as a lipid lowering agent—a meta-analysis. Journal of the Royal College of Physicians of London 28(1):349–352.

Simone, C.B. 1983. Cancer and Nutrition. McGraw-Hill, New York.

Simonen, O. 1991. Incidence of femoral neck fractures, senile osteoporosis in Finland. Calcif. Tiss. Intl. (Suppl.)49:58-510.

Singh, R.B. 1990. Effect of dietary magnesium supplementation in the prevention of coronary heart disease and sudden cardiac death. Magnes. Trace Elem. 9:143–151.

Singh, R.B., S.S. Rastogi, U.V. Mani, J. Seth, and L. Devi. 1991. Does dietary magnesium modulate blood lipids? Biol. Trace Elem. Res. 30:59–64.

Skobeloff, E.M., and R.M. McNamara. 1993. Intravenous magnesium for acute asthma. Ann. Emerg. Med. 22:617–618.

Skobeloff, E.M., W.H. Spivey, R.M. McNamara, and L. Greenspan. 1989. Intravenous magnesium sulfate for the treatment of acute asthma in the emergency department. JAMA 262:1210–1213.

Skrede, B., S.O. Lie, R. Blomhoff, and K.R. Norum. 1994. Uptake and storage of retinol and retinyl esters in bone marrow of children with acute myeloid leukemia treated with high-dose retinyl palmitate. Eur. J. Haematol. 52(3):140–144.

Smith, D.H., K. Okiyama, T.A. Gennarelli, and T.K. McIntosh. 1993. Magnesium and ketamine attenuate cognitive dysfunction following experimental brain injury. Neurosci. Lett. 157:211–214.

Snowdon, D.A., and R.L. Phillips. 1985. Does a vegetarian diet reduce the occurrence of diabetes? Am. J. Public Health 75:507–512.

Snowdon, D.A., R.L. Phillips, and W. Choi. 1984. Diet, obesity, and risk of fatal prostate cancer. Am. J. Epidemiol. 120:244–250.

Snowdon, D.A., R.L. Phillips, and G.E. Fraser. 1984. Meat consumption and fatal ischemic heart disease. Prev. Med. 13:490–500.

Sobal, J. 1991. Obesity and socioeconomic status: a framework for examining relationships between physical and social variables. Med. Anthropol. 13:231–247.

Sorensen, G., T. Pechacek, and U. Pallonen. 1986. Occupational and worksite norms and attitudes about smoking cessation. Am. J. Public Health 76:544–549.

Spaetling, L., and G. Spaetling. 1987. Magnesium supplementation in pregnancy: a double-blind study after treatment with intravenous magnesium sulfate—a preliminary report. Magnesium Bulletin 9:49–50.

Spiller, G.A. 1991. The Mediterranean Diets in Health and Disease. Van Nostrand Reinhold, New York.

Spillman, D.M. 1987. Calcium, magnesium and calorie intake and activity levels of healthy adult women. J. Am. Coll. Nutr. 6:454.

Stampfer, M.J., C.H. Hennekens, J.E. Manson, G.A. Colditz, B. Rosner, and W.C. Willett. 1993. Vitamin E consumption and the risk of coronary disease in women. N. Engl. J. Med. 328:1444–1449.

Stampfer, M.J., R. Malinow, W.C. Willett, et al. 1992. A prospective study of plasma homocyst(e)ine and risk of myocardial infarction in U.S. physicians. JAMA 268:877–881.

Steinberg, D. 1993. Antioxidant vitamins and coronary heart disease. N. Engl. J. Med. 328:1487–1489.

Steinberg, D., and J.L. Witztum. 1990. Lipoproteins and atherogenesis: current concepts. JAMA 264:3047–3052.

Steinmetz, K.A., and J.D. Potter. 1991a. Vegetables, fruits, and cancer. I. Epidemiology. Cancer Causes and Control 2:325–357.

Steinmetz, K.A., and J.D. Potter. 1991b. Vegetables, fruits, and cancer. II. Mechanisms. Cancer Causes and Control 2:427–442.

Stern, M., J.A. Pugh, S.P. Gaskill, and H.P. Hazuda. 1982. Knowledge, attitudes, and behavior related to obesity and dieting in Mexican Americans and Anglos: the San Antonio Heart Study. Am. J. Epidemiol. 115(6):917–928.

Stewart, A., and J. Howard. 1986. Magnesium and potassium deficiencies in women with pre-menstrual syndrome. Magnesium Bull. 8:314–316.

Stone, E.J., C.L. Perry, and R.V. Luepker. 1989. Synthesis of cardiovascular behavioral research for youth health promotion. Health Educ. Q. 16(2):155–169.

Story, M., and P. Faulkner. 1990. The prime time diet: a content analysis of eating behavior and food messages in television program content and commercials. Am. J. Public Health 80:738–740.

Subbarao, K.V., J.S. Richardson, and L.C. Ang. 1990. Autopsy samples of Alzheimer's cortex show increased peroxidation in vitro. J. Neurochem. 55:342–345.

Sullivan, J.L. 1992. Stored iron as a risk factor for ischemic heart disease. In R.B. Lauffer, ed. Iron and Human Disease. CRC Press, Ann Arbor, Mich.

Swanson, D.R. 1988. Migraine and magnesium: eleven neglected connections. Perspectives Biol. Med. 31:526–557.

Szelenyi, I., J. Rigo, B.O. Ahmed, and J. Sos. 1967. The role of magnesium in blood coagulation. Thromb. Diath. Haemorrh. 18:626–633.

Taburet, A.M. and B. Schmit. 1994. Pharmacokinetic optimisation of asthma treatment. Clin. Pharmacokinet. 26(5):396-418.

Tang, B.Y., and N.R. Adams. 1980. Effect of equol on oestrogen receptors and on synthesis of DNA and protein in the immature rat uterus. J. Endocrinol. 85:291–297.

Tannenbaum, A. 1940. The initiation and growth of tumors. Introduction. 1. Effects of underfeeding. Am. J. Cancer 38(3):335–350.

Tannenbaum, A. 1942a. The genesis and growth of tumors. 2. Effects of caloric restriction per se. Cancer Res. 2:460–467.

Tannenbaum, A. 1942b. The genesis and growth of tumors. 3. Effects of a high-fat diet. Cancer Res. 2:468–475.

Tannenbaum, A. 1945a. The dependence of tumor formation on the degree of caloric restriction. Cancer Res. 5(11):609–615.

Tannenbaum, A. 1945b. The dependence of tumor formation on the composition of the calorie-restricted diet as well as on the degree of restriction. Cancer Res. 5(11):616–625.

Taras, H.L., J.F. Sallis, T.L. Patterson, et al. 1989. Television's influence on children's diet and physical activity. J. Dev. Behav. Pediatr. 10:176–180.

Taylor, A. 1992. Role of nutrients in delaying cataracts. Ann. N. Y. Acad. Sci. 669:111–123.

Teas, J., M.L. Harbison, and R.S. Gelman. 1984. Dietary seaweed (laminaria) and mammary carcinogenesis in rats. Cancer Res. 44:2758–2761.

Thomas, T.N., and J.W. Zemp. 1977. Inhibition of dopamine-sensitive adenylate cyclase from rat brain striatal homogenates by ascorbic acid. J. Neurochem. 28:663–665.

Tolbert, L.C., T.N. Thomas, L.D. Middaugh, and J.W. Zemp. 1979a. Ascorbate blocks amphetamine-induced turning behavior in rats with unilateral nigro-striatal lesions. Brain Res. Bull. 4:43–48.

Tolbert, L.C., T.N. Thomas, L.D. Middaugh, and J.W. Zemp. 1979b. Effect of ascorbic acid on neurochemical, behavioral, and physiological systems mediated by catecholamines. Life Sci. 25:2189–2195.

Tsao, C.S. 1991. Inhibiting effect of ascorbic acid on the growth of human mammary tumor xenografts. Am. J. Clin. Nutr. 54:1274S–1280S.

Turner, M. 1990. Garlic and circulatory disorders. J. R. Social Health 110(3):90–93.

U.S. Bureau of the Census. 1986. Statistical Abstract of the United States: 1986. U.S. Government Printing Office, Washington, D.C.

U.S. Department of Agriculture, Human Nutrition Information Service. 1988. Nationwide Food Consumption Survey, Continuing Survey of Food Intakes by Individuals. Women 19–50 and Their Children 1–5 Years, 4 Days (NFCS, CSFII 86–3). Washington, D.C.

U.S. Department of Agriculture. 1993a. Food Assistance Programs.

U.S. Department of Agriculture. 1993b. USDA News. Espy launches fresh start for school meals program. Release No. C749.93. Washington, D.C. September.

U.S. Department of Agriculture and U.S. Department of Health and Human Services. 1990. Nutrition and Your Health: Dietary Guidelines for Americans (3rd ed.). U.S. Government Printing Office, Washington, D.C.

U.S. Department of Education, National Center for Educational Statistics. 1990. Digest of Educational Statistics (NCES 91-660).

U.S. Department of Health and Human Services. 1987. Unproven Methods: The Gerson Therapy. National Cancer Institute statement, February 5.

U.S. Food and Drug Administration. 1992. Dietary Supplements Task Force—Final Report. National Technical Information Service, U.S. Department of Commerce, Springfield, Va.

Unsigned Commentary. 1994. Teething problems for two innovations. Science 264:1540.

Vaddadi, K.S., P. Courtney, C.J. Gilleard, M.S. Manku, and D.F. Horrobin. 1989. A double-blind trial of essential fatty acid supplementation in patients with tardive dyskinesia. Psychiatry Res. 27:313–323.

Valenzuela, G.J., and L.A. Munson. 1987. Magnesium and pregnancy. Magnesium 6:128–135.

Varga, J., S.A. Jimenez, and J. Uitto. 1993. L-tryptophan and the eosinophilia-myalgia syndrome: current understanding of the etiology and pathogenesis. J. Invest. Dermatol. 100(1):97S–105S.

Vartiainnen, E., H. Korhonen, P. Pietinen, et al. 1991. Fifteen-year trends in coronary risk factors in Finland, with special reference to North Karelia. Int. J. Epidemiol. 20(3):651–662.

Vega, G.L., and S.M. Grundy. 1994. Lipoprotein responses to treatment with lovastatin, gemfibrozil, and nicotinic acid in normolipidemic patients with hypoalphalipoproteinemia. Arch. Intern. Med. 154(1):73–82.

Vink, R. 1991–1992. Magnesium and brain trauma. Magnes. Trace Elem. 10:1–10.

Walford, R.L., and M. Crew. 1989. How dietary restriction retards aging: an integrative hypothesis. Growth Develop. Aging 53:139–140.

Walford, R.L., S.B. Harris, and M.W. Gunion. 1992. The calorically restricted, low-fat, nutrient-dense diet in Biosphere 2 significantly lowers blood glucose, total leukocyte count, cholesterol, and blood pressure in humans. Proc. Natl. Acad. Sci. U. S. A. 89:11533–11537.

Walsh, B.A. 1992. Urostomy and urinary pH. J. ET. Nurs. 19(4):110–113.

Walsh, D.C., R.E. Rudd, B.A. Moeykens, and T.W. Moloney. 1993. Social marketing for public health. Health Aff. 12(2):104–119.

Walter, H.J., A. Hofman, R.D. Vaughan, and F.L. Wynder. 1988. Modification of risk factors for coronary heart disease: five-year results of a school-based intervention trial. N. Engl. J. Med. 318:1093–1100.

Ward, P.S. 1988. History of Gerson Therapy. A contract report for the U.S. Congress Office of Technology Assessment. Revised June 1988.

Watson, K.V., C.F. Moldow, P.L. Ogburn, and H.S. Jacob. 1986. Magnesium sulfate: rationale for its use in preeclampsia. Proc. Natl. Acad. Sci. U. S. A. 83:1075–1078.

Watts, G.F., B. Lewis, J.N.H. Brunt, et al. 1992. Effects on coronary artery disease of lipid-lowering diet, or diet plus cholestyramine, in the St. Thomas' Artherosclerosis Regression Study (STARS). Lancet 339:563–569.

Weaver, K. 1986. Pregnancy-induced hypertension and low birth weight in magnesium-deficient ewes. Magnesium 5:191–200.

Weaver, K. 1988. Magnesium and fetal growth. Tr. Subst. in Environmental Med. 22:136–142.

Weaver, K. 1990. Magnesium and migraine. Headache 30:168.

Wechsler, H., S. Levine, R.K. Idelson, M. Rohman, and J.O. Taylor. 1983. The physician's role in health promotion: a survey of primary-care practitioners. N. Engl. J. Med. 308:97–100.

Weglicki, W.B., A.M. Freedman, S. Bloom, et al. 1992. Antioxidants and the cardiomyopathy of Mg deficiency. Am. J. Cardiovasc. Pathol. 4:210–215.

Weglicki, W.B., R.E. Stafford, A.M. Freedman, M.M. Cassidy, and T.M. Phillips. 1993. Modulation of cytokines and myocardial lesions by vitamin E and chloroquine in a Mg-deficient rat model. Am. J. Physiol. 264:C723–C726.

Weinberg, E.D. 1992. Roles of iron in neoplasia: promotion, prevention, and therapy. Biol. Trace Elem. Res. 34(2):123–140.

Weisburger, J.H. 1993. Guest editorial: a new nutritional approach in cancer therapy in light of mechanistic understanding of cancer causation and development. J. Am. Coll. Nutr. 12:205-208.

Welsh, S., and J.F. Guthrie. 1991. The Changing American diets. In: A. Bendich and C. Butterworth, eds. Preventive Nutrition: The Role of Micronutrients in Health and Disease. Marcel Dekker: New York.

West, K.M. 1974. Diabetes in American Indians and other native populations of the New World. Diabetes 23(10):841–855.

Wigmore, A. 1985. Why Suffer? Avery Publishing, Wayne, N.J.

Wigmore, A. 1993. Scientific Appraisal of Dr. Ann Wigmore's Living Foods Lifestyle. Ann Wigmore Press, Boston.

Willett, W.C. 1990. Nutritional Epidemiology. Oxford University Press, New York.

Willett, W.C. 1992. Folic acid and neural tube defect: can't we come to closure? Am. J. Public Health 82:666–668.

Willett, W.C., and A. Ascherio. 1994. Trans fatty acids: are the effects only marginal? Am. J. Public Health 84(5):722–724.

Willett, W.C., M.J. Stampfer, G.A. Colditz, B.A. Rosner, and F.E. Speizer. 1990. Relation of meat, fat, and fiber intake to the risk of colon cancer in a prospective study among women. N. Engl. J. Med. 323:1664–1672.

Wilson, M.G., and E.W. Parry. 1954. Alpha-tocopherol in the prophylaxis of thromboembolism. Lancet 1:486–488.

Windsor, R.A., and J.B. Lowe. 1989. Behavioral impact and cost analysis of a worksite self-help smoking cessation program. Prog. Clin. Biol. Res. 293:231–242.

Woods, K.L., and S. Fletcher. 1994. Long-term outcome after intravenous magnesium sulphate in suspected acute myocardial infarction: the second Leicester Intravenous Magnesium Intervention Trial (LIMIT-2). Lancet 343:816–819.

Woods, K.L., S. Fletcher, C. Roffe, and Y. Haider. 1992. Intravenous magnesium sulphate in suspected acute myocardial infarction: results of the second Leicester Intravenous Magnesium Intervention Trial (LIMIT-2). Lancet 339:1553–1558.

World Health Organization. 1990. Diet, Nutrition, and the Prevention of Chronic Diseases: Report of a WHO Study Group (World Health Organization Technical Report Series 979). WHO, Geneva.

Yamamoto, I., H. Maruyama, and M. Moriguchi. 1987. The effect of dietary seaweeds on 7,12-dimethylbenz[a]-anthracene-induced mammary tumorigenesis in rats. Cancer Lett. 35:109–118.

Yoder, D. 1981. The sausage culture of the Pennsylvania Germans. In A. Fenton and R. Owen, eds. Food in Perspective. John Donald, Edinburgh.

Zhang, M.J., Q.F. Wang, L.X. Gao, H. Jin, and Z.Y. Wang. 1992. Comparative observation of the changes in serum lipid peroxides influenced by the supplementation of vitamin E in burn patients and healthy controls. Burns 18(1):19–21.

Zhao, X.Q., B.G. Brown, L. Hillger, et al. 1993. Effects of intensive lipid-lowering therapy on the coronary arteries of asymptomatic subjects with elevated apolipoprotein B. Circulation 88(6):2744–2753.

Ziegler, R.G. 1991. Vegetables, fruits, and carotenoids and the risk of cancer. Am. J. Clin. Nutr. 53(1 Suppl.):251S–259S.

Zuspan, F.P., and M.C. Ward. 1965. Improved fetal salvage in eclampsia. Obstet. Gynecol. 26:893–897.

Part II
Conducting and Disseminating Research

Introduction

This part of the report discusses issues that confront all the alternative medical systems and practices, particularly those whose efficacy is under investigation. Although alternative medicine does not differ from mainstream medicine in the need for reasonable, responsible research and validation of safety and effectiveness, there are some issues unique to this branch of medicine:

- Lack of dedicated alternative medical research facilities.
- Lack of adequate funding for alternative medical research.
- Lack of training for alternative medical researchers.
- Lack of an adequate, centrally located research database.
- Difficulties in matching appropriate research methods to subjects being researched.
- Difficulties in obtaining appropriate National Institutes of Health (NIH) peer review of alternative medical grant applications.
- Difficulties in data collection related to various legal and regulatory constraints.

Consumers and clinicians have a definite and immediate need for access to the best and latest information about alternative medical practices, and NIH needs to be able to hear from health care consumers about their experiences with alternative practices.

Research Infrastructure: Institutions and Investigators

PANEL MEMBERS AND CONTRIBUTING AUTHORS

David Eisenberg, M.D.—Chair

Barbara A. Brennen, M.S.	*Norma Jennings*
Seymour Brenner, M.D.	*Abraham R. Liboff, Ph.D.*
Deepak Chopra, M.D.	*Nancy Lonsdorf, M.D.*
Serafina Corsello, M.D.	*Laura Nader, Ph.D.*
Michael L. Culbert, D.Sc.	*Richard Pavek*
Jonathan Davidson, M.D.	*Kenneth Pittaway, N.D., Ph.D.*
Patrick M. Donovan, N.D.	*Nelda Samarel, Ed.D.*
Robert Duggan	*Paul Scharff, M.D.*
Judy Epstein	*Oscar Carl Simonton, M.D.*
Thomas E. Harries, Ph.D.	*James P. Swyers, M.A.*
Tori Hudson, N.D.	*Marvin C. Ziskin*

Introduction

This chapter reviews and discusses separately the following issues: the status of alternative medical research at conventional and nonconventional research institutions, the availability of properly trained investigators who can adequately and professionally investigate and validate potentially promising alternative medical treatments and systems, and the degree of exposure that conventionally trained medical students and researchers have to alternative medical principles. Recommendations are offered for revising the present-day research infrastructure to create opportunities for alternative medical research.

Status of Alternative Medical Research in the United States

Conventional Research Institutions

Although there are pockets of alternative medical research going on at many conventional scientific research institutions across the United States, including the National Institutes of Health (NIH), by far most alternative medical research is being conducted outside such institutions. A major factor that promotes conventional research over novel research at most institutions in this country is the peer review process, which is intended to prevent poor research from being funded or disseminated.

Peer reviewers have a major role in shaping the general direction of all research. If peer reviewers favor conventional research, they may be inclined to fund research proposals that stay within the bounds of the conventional. Thus, in this country, which prides itself on innovation and discovery, there is an increasing tendency to do only "safe" research. Researchers who cannot get their results published and/or funded because of peer review bias can have only limited careers in the research sciences. To be an unpublished investigator is to be isolated; to be published is to obtain status. An investigator in academia who does not publish enough original research within a certain time likely will not be tenured and may be terminated altogether. Furthermore, once published, the investigator must continue to publish regularly to remain employed and employable. The pressure to publish breeds a tendency to perform research that builds logically and in small steps upon generally known or suspected phenomena, rather than research on novel ideas (see the "Peer Review" chapter for more details on the shortcomings of the peer review process).

Therefore, investigators wanting to pursue novel research projects often hesitate to step far outside the conventional path. If they do try to pursue something revolutionary, they may find it hard to obtain funding or may be advised by their peers that pursuing "offbeat" ideas can lead to lost status, unpublished work, lack of funding for even conventional projects, or being shunned by other researchers who fear disapproval by association (Sherrill and Larson, 1993).

Favoring the conventional is also a factor in funding researchers because many funding sources use peer review committees of researchers as grant reviewers. Although funding for research projects and investigators comes from many sources, Government funds are the largest source in this country (U.S. Department of Commerce, 1989). Foundations, universities, colleges, and private sources are lesser but highly important sources, especially for alternative medicine investigators. How NIH, a large dispenser of biomedical research funds, approaches the evaluation of alternative medical research proposals is likely to have a major influence on attitudes toward alternative medical research in the United States.

Nonconventional Research Institutions

Several alternative medical colleges have research departments and are actively engaged in research. Their approach to research usually differs from that of conventional medical institutions because of different emphasis and less exposure to methodological training. First, what is alternative to the conventional institution is normal to the alternative institution. Second, research that would be considered basic at a conventional institution—such as that which asks whether something works at all—is frequently not an issue for the alternative institution. Researchers at unconventional institutions are much more likely to be interested in determining dosages or conducting outcomes studies than in investigating whether or how something works. In contrast, the interest of conventional researchers in dosages and outcome studies is more likely later in the research process than near the beginning.

Most of the 16 chiropractic colleges and all of the osteopathic medical colleges have research facilities. Other institutions with research capacities in the United States include Bastyr University (Seattle), National College of Naturopathic Medicine (Portland, OR), Southwest College of Naturopathic Medicine and Health Sciences (Scottsdale, AZ), and the Traditional Acupuncture Institute (Columbia, MD). Many current research efforts at these institutions are in long-term health issues, the very issues that are of current concern for conventional medicine and the public health system.[1]

However, funding is precarious for these institutions. Almost without exception, NIH funding has not been available. Limited funding is available from private sources but is inadequate for current needs. Because of the limited funding, research departments at such institutions have had only minimal development of infrastructure and faculty. Further, at present there is little communication between these research facilities and their conventional counterparts, even though increased communication may benefit this country's health care.

Alternative Medical Investigator Training

Today, alternative medical researchers represent a spectrum of disciplines and training. Many of these researchers are conventionally trained investigators who see in alternative medical practices and approaches to health a means of addressing some shortcomings of conventional biomedicine. Others are trained by and conduct research at nonconventional colleges and institutions devoted to systems of health that derive from nonconventional perspectives. In addition, there are disciplined investigators in the social sciences who see strong connections between their daily work and healing disease. Still others are less formally trained but believe they have developed the ability to heal others through various direct, personal means; these individuals may have little or no formal academic training but may spend time in clinical investigation.

The disparate groups in alternative medicine need training to become accomplished alternative medical investigators. Some require training in proper and acceptable research methods, and others need exposure to alternative medical practices so as to be better prepared to evaluate those

[1] *Such issues are more difficult to solve than acute illness, as was mentioned in the introduction to this report.*

practices properly. Indeed, the basic contention here is that individuals conducting research in alternative medicine are more likely to be successful if they have some level of dual training in conventional medical research methodology and a field of alternative medicine. Further, alternative medicine practitioners have suggested that research in alternative medicine should be performed by individuals and teams trained in as wide as possible an array of research methodologies.

Exposure to Alternative Medical Principles in Conventional Medical Schools

Training of medical and health investigators in colleges and universities begins at the undergraduate level. Currently, most undergraduate institutions and conventional medical schools and teaching hospitals do not offer exposure to alternative medical practices or views. This omission from the standard medical curriculum adversely affects the use of alternative medicine in the clinic and the nature and extent of biomedical research.

Nevertheless, several mainstream medical institutions have recently begun or are developing basic academic medical courses to introduce medical students and physicians in training to the history, theory, and practice of alternative medical therapies. Currently, there are courses or programs at the following universities: Arizona, Columbia, Georgetown, Harvard, Louisville, Maryland, Michigan State University, Stanford, Tufts, the University of California at San Francisco, and Virginia. The courses are potentially the foundation for future systematic exploration of alternative medicine practices at these schools.

A few other conventional institutions integrate alternative medicine in at least a limited way into their curriculums. For example, several nursing colleges, universities, and teaching hospitals are currently providing practical courses in one or more of the biofield therapies and in biofeedback, yoga, or meditation. It is likely that additional opportunities exist to train in alternative medical practices in some departments of psychology, anthropology, and social sciences.

If they are properly designed, courses like these will not only provide information on the utility of specific therapeutic approaches but also develop a larger framework for understanding the strengths and limitations of Western medicine. They also will promote recognition of the contributions that theoretical and research models in alternative medicine may make to enlarging conventional research methodology.

Recommendations

The following are specific recommendations relating to improving the research infrastructure so that there are fewer inherent barriers to those interested in pursuing research into topics that do not necessarily fall into predefined categories.

Improving Research Infrastructure

The Office of Alternative Medicine (OAM) should make it a priority to survey the basic needs of alternative medical research institutions and help arrange funding and other support. In addition, it should look for ways to encourage the ongoing work in alternative medicine being conducted at conventional institutions. Bringing these alternative and conventional facilities into the same arena could create new dialog to enhance all medical research efforts.

However, it is not enough to increase the funding for alternative medical research at existing institutions; a genuine atmosphere of collaboration must be fostered. In order for alternative medicine research to proceed with reasonable speed, there must be dedicated alternative medicine research centers with support facilities. The following are all viable approaches that should be considered:

- First, it is recommended that OAM be upgraded to become the Center for Alternative Medicine (CAM) similar to NIH's current National Center for Research Resources (see sidebar). With CAM as a freestanding unit, NIH would be able to fund, as well as investigate, systems and processes that fall outside the normal purview of other freestanding NIH units.

  Unlike current institutes at NIH where alternative medicine research is required to compete for priority with many other subjects, the proposed CAM could concentrate on alternative medicine, serving as both a grant-funding agency and an "in-house" evaluator of alternative medical practices.

  If NIH were to lead the way in this fashion, universities and medical colleges would be encouraged to begin their own alternative

National Center for Research Resources

The National Center for Research Resources (NCRR) develops and provides the shared resources essential for biomedical research funded by NIH: research project and resource grant support are used to develop cutting-edge biomedical research technologies and sophisticated instrumentation; to locate and characterize the most appropriate models for the study of human disease; to establish and maintain clinical environments in which technology can be transferred from the laboratory to the bedside; and to develop research capability in minorities and minority institutions. NCRR funds the following programs and research centers:

- Biological Models and Materials Research Program
- Biomedical Engineering and Instrumentation Program
- Biomedical Research Support Program
- Biomedical Research Technology Program
- Comparative Medicine Program
- General Clinical Research Centers Program
- Research Centers in Minority Institutions Program

medical research programs. Researchers funded by CAM would gain experience in alternative medical research and could use their new expertise to become the core faculty of research facilities in independent medical institutions.

- It is recommended that existing research centers be enhanced and new ones installed at alternative medical institutions throughout the United States. Here, also, expert faculty from various disciplines would join to evaluate efficacy, safety, cost-effectiveness, and mechanisms of action of alternative medicine through basic and clinical research.
- It is recommended that new research centers devoted primarily to the assessment of alternative medicine be founded at leading universities and conventional medical institutions throughout the United States. Expert faculty members from various disciplines would evaluate efficacy, safety, cost-effectiveness, and mechanisms of action of alternative medicine through basic and clinical research. Where appropriate, they would also compare different methodologies for conducting these evaluations. (This concept has received considerable support from proponents of alternative medicine.)

  Ideally, these centers would create an academic "critical mass" that would begin to bring the conventional and alternative medical communities together. This approach may be an effective way of generating authoritative, dispassionate investigations of alternative medicine. The establishment of research centers of this type would complement, not replace, the proposed CAM or intramural or extramural investigations of existing NIH institutes.

At the new and enhanced centers, highly trained research investigators and alternative medicine practitioners would collaborate to conduct interdisciplinary research, developing protocols and implementing clinical investigations. Core faculties at the centers would develop protocols for initial review by an institutional research advisory board, which would be responsible for critical review of each protocol for clinical importance, methodological soundness, and administrative feasibility. Advisory boards could include the OAM director, ex officio, thus ensuring ongoing collaboration with NIH.

Although each center would receive sufficient funding for protocol development and the implementation of small feasibility or pilot studies, larger trials (such as those requiring hundreds of patients randomized to a variety of experimental or control conditions) would likely require additional funding from NIH, the Agency for Health Care Policy and Research (AHCPR), or other public or private sources. Larger outcome studies and surveys could use multiple research centers as individual sites for ongoing studies.

These centers would need sufficient funding for a core faculty, support of a research board, a modest fellowship program, and a library database. Funding of specific projects would be determined competitively.

The research centers could take different forms; for example, they might be modeled after the comprehensive cancer centers established and funded by the National Cancer Institute (NCI). The programs of these NCI-funded centers must include several key elements: basic laboratory research, clinical research, and linkages between basic and clinical research; high-priority clinical trials research; research on prevention and control; education and training of researchers and health care professionals; public information services; and community service and outreach.

Development and Funding of Research Projects

Should funding become more widely available for alternative medical researchers, a natural offshoot would be more institutions taking an interest in conducting alternative medical research, which would necessarily attract more trained investigators. The following are recommended as ways to support research projects:

- OAM's current competitive request for applications (RFA) program (see the "Peer Review" chapter) should be continued and expanded. In its first round of 30 research grants, OAM encouraged collaborations between medical researchers and practitioners of alternative medicine; proposals were reviewed on a competitive basis and funded accordingly. (NIH reported that the first RFA elicited more than 800 inquiries and 463 grant applications.)
- In addition to its current RFA program, OAM should initiate RFAs to perform selected clinical trials and certain critical experiments, specifically with the aim of validating previously reported results, resolving apparent conflicts, and testing new approaches.
- OAM should also assemble one or more patient outcomes research teams (PORTs) based on the AHCPR model. The PORTs could conduct multiple field investigations. In addition, or alternatively, OAM should hire several full-time field investigators, as has been recommended by two U.S. senators and the office's first advisory committee, the 1993 Ad Hoc Advisory Panel to the Office of Alternative Medicine.
- OAM should investigate ways to provide joint public-private funding of its research and educational programs. Expansion of the funding base would increase opportunities for alternative medical research. Individual foundations and philanthropists may be interested in providing cofunding for a variety of initiatives concerning alternative medicine research and training.

Incentive Activities

- RFAs should be generated by individual institutes at NIH seeking clinical and basic research projects from investigators who are receptive to researching alternative medical practices relevant to the missions of those institutes.
- Some incentive process should be developed to encourage experienced, previously funded investigators to add experts in alternative medical practices to their investigation teams and to add study arms involving aspects of alternative medical practices to their existing research foci. The incentive process could provide for earmarked funds or special scoring during the rating of proposals.
- RFAs should be generated by AHCPR, a Public Health Service agency within the Department of Health and Human Services, for conducting alternative medical research relevant to the outcomes research this agency sponsors for the determination of appropriate clinical practices.
- A similar funding or rating incentive scheme could be used to encourage broadening AHCPR-sponsored research designs and clinical care studies to include alternative medical practices.

A vigorous, broadly based peer review system with participation by experts in alternative medical practices will be necessary to ensure that any such affirmative research incentives are awarded to studies where the research really does test appropriately designed alternative interventions.

Establishment of an OAM Research Project Database

To address its research project needs, it is recommended that OAM do the following:

- Establish a database of ongoing research projects and project proposals on alternative medicine that is readily available to researchers. Such a listing of both existing and proposed research projects could enhance alternative medical research by preventing redundancy and fostering joint efforts by several researchers. The database could include OAM-funded research, other NIH-funded research (many institutes currently have ongoing alternative medical research projects),[2] and all other identifiable alternative medical research that has been approved by an institutional review board.

- OAM should also develop a clearinghouse function within OAM for planned projects so that unnecessary duplicate studies can be avoided and appropriate collaborations encouraged.

In addition, OAM should do the following:

- Facilitate access to information and guidance concerning all aspects of methodology from study planning through conduct, analysis, and development of reports or manuscripts for publication. (See app. F.)
- Develop a list or network of experienced investigators willing to help with such designated areas as project development, conduct, and analysis; link alternative and conventional researchers; provide methodology seminars and workshops; and offer other services on a volunteer or consultant basis. OAM should organize the network and maintain responsibility for planning and hosting seminars.

Fostering Collaboration on Existing Studies Within the Federal Government

For collaboration on such existing studies, OAM should perform the following:

- Identify ongoing randomized controlled trials supported by NIH that could allow for the simultaneous testing of alternative medical therapies as adjuncts or additional experimental conditions. For example, a controlled trial assessing the efficacy of chemotherapy for a particular cancer could allow for patients to be randomized to chemotherapy alone or to a group receiving chemotherapy and an alternative medical practice such as herbal treatment or visualization.
- Include alternative medical practices among the procedures under study when AHCPR conducts outcomes research. This could be accomplished by including in the planning process a spectrum of alternative medical practice researchers to help create study protocols of alternative methods to compare with the conventional methods, focused on specific outcomes (e.g., optimal recovery from acute back pain, optimal recovery from surgical intervention, or optimal management of conditions for which both medical and surgical options are under consideration, including heart disease and prostate disease).

Interactions Within the Public Health Service

Enacting the following recommendations could strengthen alternative medical research and training in the United States:

- OAM should develop and maintain a close working relationship with the Food and Drug Administration (FDA) and with NIH's Office of Protection for Research Risks to ensure that the highest standards of protection of human subjects are applied to all aspects of alternative medical research.
- OAM should establish and maintain a working relationship with FDA to better assist alternative practitioners with the drug development and regulatory processes. OAM and FDA should also ensure that protocols for testing alternative treatments and regulating relevant devices are commensurate (that is, neither unduly restrictive nor unduly lenient) with the risks involved in their use and are based on appropriate scientific principles.

---

[2]*Current projects related to alternative medicine supported by the various NIH institute include the following: National Heart, Lung, and Blood Institute: transcendental meditation in the control of hypertension, research by Dean Ornish (see the "Diet and Nutrition" chapter) in cardiac rehabilitation. National Institute of Arthritis and Musculoskeletal and Skin Diseases: refocus of the research agenda for treating fibromyalgia to include alternative clinical treatments. Division of Cancer Prevention of the National Cancer Institute: nutritional approaches to cancer prevention. National Institute on Drug Abuse: acupuncture in the treatment of substance abuse. National Institute on Allergy and Infectious Diseases: acupuncture for peripheral neuropathy in AIDS. National Institute on Aging: use of tai chi for movement disorders in the elderly. National Institute of Mental Health: biofeedback, hypnosis, and Navajo spirituality. There are also 43 projects listed in the NIH grants and contracts database related to spirituality and religion.*

- Since many questions relating to alternative medicine involve outcomes studies, OAM should investigate areas of mutual interest with AHCPR, which presently does such studies.

Interactions With Other Countries

In pursuit of international collaboration, OAM should explore the following:

- Learn about alternative medical practices in other countries and establish collaborations with their alternative medical practitioners. For example, it is well known that Great Britain has considerable clinical experience and government interest in "complementary medicine." Extensive professional and government interest in alternative medicine have also been shown in other European nations (e.g., Germany), as well as in China, Japan, India, and the former Soviet Union.
- Explore areas of mutual interest with appropriate government agencies from other countries with interests in alternative medicine and encourage collaborations with NIH's Fogarty International Center.

Upgrading Medical Education

It is recommended that comprehensive programs be developed and disseminated as soon as possible to bring an understanding of alternative medicine and its practices into conventional medical education. These programs should include both theoretical presentations and practical approaches in alternative medicine. OAM could speed the process greatly by hosting a conference of interested institutional administrators and helping to develop an implementation plan.

Theoretical courses in such a plan should include the following:

- The history of medicine, including alternative medicine and medical education.
- Perspectives on how alternative medicine may enrich and enlarge contemporary medical education.
- Western philosophical and medical perspectives on the "mind-body relationship."
- Philosophical bases, research literature, and clinical effectiveness of systems of healing from one's own and other cultures and with other parameters (e.g., Chinese, African, Indian, Native American, homeopathy, biofield therapeutics).
- Effects of social context—including family, socioeconomic status, culture, race, and gender—on health and illness. (Studies of this nature have been funded by NIH for many years; inclusion in a curriculum is needed now.)

Practical courses in an implementation plan could include the following:

- Experiential training in alternative medicine practices taught by skilled alternative medicine practitioners (e.g., biofeedback, meditation, guided imagery, manual therapies, hypnosis, yoga, tai chi, biofield therapeutics).
- Critical evaluation of the most current and significant data on alternative medical research.
- Use of case studies to illustrate the effects of clinical practices in alternative medicine.
- Examination of the ways alternative medical practices may be integrated into various training and teaching experiences and into comprehensive programs in different medical specialties.
- Implications of alternative medicine in our understanding of individual psychology and psychobiology, the physician's role and self-concept, and the doctor-patient (or patient-doctor) relationship; awareness of different cultural concepts concerning the relationship between mind and body; and interest in undertaking research studies of various alternative medical practices and the ways they might be fruitfully integrated with conventional practices.

Further steps can be taken in upgrading medical education:

- University-sponsored continuing medical education courses in alternative medicine can and should be made more broadly available to health care providers, including physicians, nurses, dentists, pharmacists, other allied health professionals, and medical school faculties. This education may take the form of consensus conferences, workshops and symposia, continuing medical education programs, tutorials, or lectures to be offered at annual meetings of selected medical societies and associations. For example, annual meetings of psychologists, neurologists, or endocrinologists could include guest lectures on the current state of science in the field of prayer healing or cognitive behavioral therapies. Conferences and symposia of this kind could facilitate communication and collaboration between the conventional medical community and practitioners of alternative medical therapies.

- The various centers proposed later in this chapter could also develop continuing medical education programs and assist OAM with the development of conferences and symposia to be held either at NIH or at individual research center sites.
- Implementation of this interdisciplinary training should be through research training fellowships.

Several funding options exist:

- Established faculty members at conventional medical institutions could spend several months or longer in settings where alternative medicine practices are taught and practiced. Doing so would familiarize the academic faculty members with the theory and practice of a given alternative medical technique and would enable them to participate in designing protocols with increased clinical insight.
- Individuals presently trained in alternative medical practice or conducting alternative medical research could receive grants to support several months or years of training in research methodology. These individuals could be supported to undertake master's, doctoral, or postdoctoral research fellowships and then participate in protocol development regarding alternative medical practices.
- OAM could identify existing fellowship training programs that may be receptive to pursuing research in alternative medicine. Fellows trained in this fashion would have the advantage of working in partnership with highly trained research scientists. For example, the Robert Wood Johnson Clinical Scholars Program or fellowship training programs administered by individual institutes within NIH may be willing to add fellowship slots earmarked for clinical or basic alternative medical science, relevant social sciences, or the biophysical sciences needed to pursue research in a field such as bioelectromagnetism. This approach would take advantage of expert faculty currently in existing training programs.

Funds could be made available to existing fellowship programs to ensure the additional positions in both intramural and extramural NIH research programs.

- OAM could support an annual or biennial competition for the best original research proposal by nonacademics on a presently unresearched idea.

References

Sherrill, K.A., and D.B. Larson. 1993. The anti-tenure factor in clinical research in clinical epidemiology and aging: diagnostic assessment and treatment recommendations. In J.S. Levin, ed. Religion in Aging and Health: Theoretical Formulations and Methodological Frontiers. Sage Publications, Thousand Oaks, Calif.

U.S. Department of Commerce. Bureau of the Census. 1989. Statistical Abstract of the United States 1989 (109th ed.). U.S. Department of Commerce, Washington, D.C.

Research Databases

PANEL MEMBERS AND CONTRIBUTING AUTHORS

Carola Burroughs—Chair
Jonathan Collin—Cochair

Gerald Bodeker, Ed.D.
Carlo Calabrese, N.D., M.P.H.
Aimee Carruth
Peter Chowka
Jonathan Collin, M.D.
Wayne B. Jonas, M.D.
David Larson, M.D., M.P.H.
Kevin McNamee, D.C., L.Ac.
Richard Pavek
Anne Phillips, J.D., M.S.L.
James P. Swyers, M.A.

Introduction

The first step in developing a research strategy is to study previously published research literature on the subject and related subjects. A centralized source of information on a medical system or particular therapy allows investigators to go directly to the most current and best research on a topic rather than wasting valuable time attempting to collect data from disparate sources. Thus, if investigators have access to a comprehensive research database, they can avoid repeating existing research and can obtain vital information for designing their own research.

Unfortunately, research into alternative medicine has been hampered because there is currently no easily accessible comprehensive database. Although a great deal of information can be found in the major medical databases on various aspects of alternative medicine, expert searching skills are needed to locate these materials. In addition, much of what has been collected on alternative medicine in the major medical databases has not been sufficiently indexed and cataloged. The problem is compounded if there are no journals available for a particular alternative discipline, if the relevant journals are not indexed and cataloged for inclusion in the databases, or if the data were not collected or reported properly. Further, other potentially valuable information is available only in foreign-language sources, such as the substantial bodies of literature on traditional Chinese and traditional Ayurvedic medicines. Consequently, a common complaint shared by the researchers of this report was the difficulty of tracking down material on alternative medicine that was known to exist but that nevertheless could not be located.

National Library of Medicine and MEDLINE

The premier source of medical science research information in the world is the U.S. National Library of Medicine (NLM). To make research information as accessible as possible, NLM has indexed much of its 16 million printed references into a computer-based bibliographic retrieval and publication system called MEDLARS (Medical Literature Analysis and Retrieval System). MEDLARS is accessible through more than 40 online electronic databases and databanks. The database of greatest interest to alternative medical researchers is MEDLINE (MEDLARS on Line). Most medical and health investigators in the United States turn first to MEDLINE for research materials.

MEDLINE contains more than 7.2 million records, with some 31,000 new citations added each month. Although the full text of each article is not in the database, approximately 60 percent of the citations contain author-generated abstracts or summaries of the articles. (Researchers may order copies of the full text of the articles that are indexed in MEDLINE from NLM.)

MEDLINE is readily accessible either through Grateful Med® search software (available from the National Technical Information Service) or by directly dialing NLM via standard online communications software, such as ProComm or Awremote. (For information on ordering Grateful Med and on using MEDLINE to conduct literature reviews, see "Information on the National Library of Medicine" in app. F.)

Current MEDLINE Indexing Terms for Alternative Medicine

MEDLINE uses a "controlled vocabulary," or "key words," indexing system called MeSH (Medical Subject Headings) to access information. There are now more than 18,000 MeSH headings and subheadings. MeSH also includes more than 20,000 chemical term records.

Inadequacies of MeSH Listings for Alternative Medicine

The 20 headings currently listed in MEDLINE that are relevant to alternative medicine are the following:

Acupuncture
Anthroposophy
Biofeedback
Chiropractic
Color therapy
Diet fads
Eclecticism
Electrical stimulation therapy
Homeopathy
Massage
Medicine—traditional
Mental healing
Moxibustion
Music therapy
Naturopathy
Radiesthesis
Reflexotherapy
Rejuvenation
Relaxation techniques
Tissue therapy

More specific titles and subjects are listed under those headings; for example, Ayurvedic and herbal medicines are both subheadings under traditional medicine. An April 1994 search of the available headings for alternative medicine brought up 29,080 citations (entries) dating back to 1966. Although NLM recently has made great strides in making more alternative medicine research literature more readily accessible, the MeSH headings used by NLM do not yet include many of the key words used in alternative medical therapies. For example, *craniotherapy* (a common term in chiropractic) and *therapeutic touch* (a practice in biofields therapeutics used by many nurses and others) are not indexed by NLM. A search for either of these terms will find nothing, even though there are articles on these subjects in NLM's database. Thus, although there are many articles relating to alternative medicine from conventionally focused peer-reviewed journals on MEDLINE, the researcher often has difficulty finding them. Such incompleteness in MeSH terms for alternative medicine is a major obstacle in implementing research on this subject.

NLM is aware of the increasing interest in alternative medicine and the need for adequate MeSH terms. NLM has contacted the Office of Alternative Medicine (OAM) and asked the office to review the current array of terms, make suggestions for new terms, and work with NLM to improve the indexing for alternative medicine.

Alternative Medical Journals Currently in MEDLINE

The list of alternative medical journals now being indexed by NLM is inadequate for current research needs. For example, MEDLINE at this time abstracts only 3 of the 16 journals available on chiropractic and carries no journals relating to homeopathy, naturopathy, or orthomolecular medicine.

The following are the journals relating to alternative medicine currently indexed in MEDLINE:

Acupuncture and Electro-Therapeutics Research
American Journal of Chinese Medicine
Biofeedback and Self Regulation
Chen Tzu Yen Chui (Acupuncture Research)
Chinese Medical Journal
Chung-Hua I Hsueh Tsa Chih (Chinese Medical Journal)
Chung-Kuo Chung Hsi I Chieh Ho Tsa Chih
Chung-Kuo Chung Yao Tsa Chih (China Journal of Chinese Materia Medica)
Journal of Manipulative and Physiological Therapeutics
Journal of Natural Products
Journal of Traditional Chinese Medicine
Planta Medica

In the NLM stacks are other related journals not indexed on MEDLINE (MEDLINE does not index all the journals related to any field).

The fact that MEDLINE does not include articles published before 1966 especially affects alternative medical research. Medical research literature before the 1960s contains a wealth of information on such practices as botanical medicine, homeopathy, hydrotherapy, nutrition, and manipulation. Research on these alternative processes slowed to a near standstill when medical focus shifted to manufactured drugs (before MEDLINE existed). Therefore, even though such information may still be available, possibly in the NLM stacks, it is largely out of print and unavailable to present-day researchers unless they know the information exists.

Other Alternative Medical Journals Proposed for Inclusion in MEDLINE

The following is a partial list of serials that alternative practitioners have proposed to OAM for inclusion in MEDLINE:

Acta Pharmacologica Sinica
Acta Pharmacutia Sinica
Advances, the Mind-Body Journal
Aktuelle Ernährungsmedizen
Alternatives
American Academy of Medical Acupuncture Review
American Chiropractor
Antha
Archives of Physical Medicine and Rehabilitation
Arzneimittel-Forschung
Australian Journal of Medical Herbalism
Biological Therapy
Birth Gazette
Brain/Mind and Common Sense
British Homeopathic Journal
British Journal of Clinical Pharmacology
British Journal of Midwifery
British Journal of Phytotherapy
Complementary Medicine Index
CP Currents & CP News
Current Medical Research Opinion
Economic Botany
Explore
Fitoterpia
Fortschritte der Medizin
Foster's Botanical and Herb Review
Frontier Perspectives
Gan To Kagaku Ryoho
Health Facts
Herbal Update and Natural Healthcare Quarterly
HerbalGram
Human Ecologist
Indian Journal of Homeopathic Medicine
Indian Journal of Medical Research
International Clinical Nutrition Review
International DAMS Newsletter
International Journal of Biosocial and Medical Research
IRCS Medical Science Library Compendium
Korean Biochemistry Journal
Journal of the Acupuncture Society of New York
Journal of Alternative and Complementary Medicine
Journal of the American Academy of Osteopathy
Journal of the American Institute of Homeopathy
Journal of Anthroposophic Medicine
Journal of Ethnopharmacology
Journal of Manual and Manipulative Therapy
Journal of Musculoskeletal Medicine
Journal of the National Academy of Acupuncture and Oriental Medicine
Journal of Naturopathic Medicine
Journal of Nurse Midwifery
Journal of Nutritional Medicine
Journal of Orthomolecular Medicine
Journal of Spinal Disorders
Journal of Traditional Acupuncture
Klinische Monatsblätter für Augenheilkunde
Massage Therapy Journal
Medical Anthropology
Medical Anthropology Quarterly
Medical Herbalism
Midwifery Today
New England Journal of Homeopathy
Onkologie
Orvosi Hetilap
Pharmacologic Biochemic Behavior
Phyto-Pharmica Review
Professional Journal of Botanical Medicine
Progressive Clinical Biological Research
Quintessence
Resonance
Simillimum
Social Science and Medicine
STEP Perspectives
Townsend Letter for Doctors
Veterinary and Human Toxicology
Vital Communications
Western Journal of Medicine
Zeitschrift für Phytotherapie

Other Indexes

Like MEDLINE, *Science Citation Index* (available at NLM but not available on line) and *Index Medicus* (a bound listing of references without abstracts) suffer from lack of early alternative medical articles and inadequate indexing.

If searches for alternative medical research focus on medical journals, some other reference sources that address relevant issues are likely to be overlooked. Among these are *Social Science Citation Index, Cumulative List of Nursing and Allied Health Literature, Agricola, National League of Nursing International Nursing Index,* and *Folklife Center Database.*

National Library of Medicine Selection of Journals

The NLM procedure for reviewing and accepting journals of current interest is appropriately rigorous; unfortunately, there are no alternative medicine investigators or practitioners on the Literature Selection Technical Review Committee at this time.

OAM should propose expert candidates for the NLM selection committee and submit their names to the Associate Director of Library Operations, NLM.

The NLM staff has expressed awareness of an increasing need for additional alternative medical journals and materials to be included in MEDLARS and MEDLINE and have indicated that when OAM submits materials, NLM will present them to its Literature Selection Technical Review Committee (Pavek, 1994).

Other Important Databases and Databanks

CATS, the British Library Medical Information Service's Current Awareness TopicS in allied and alternative medicine, is the next largest public database on alternative medicine after MEDLINE. (The British Library is the equivalent of the U.S. Library of Congress.) CATS currently lists more than 50,000 entries for such disciplines as Ayurvedic medicine, chiropractic, homeopathy, naturopathy, occupational therapy, oriental medicine, osteopathy, and physiotherapy. Arrangements are under way to make CATS commercially available on line through a U.S. company, probably in 1994.

It may be difficult, however, for clinical and basic sciences researchers to extract much useful material from CATS, because the database is a mixture of everything from peer-reviewed journal articles to newspaper clippings. Nevertheless, much material in CATS can benefit alternative medical researchers in this country when it becomes available.

NAPRALERT (Natural Products Alert), a database of the College of Pharmacy of the University of Illinois at Chicago, contains bibliographic and medicinal, pharmacologic, taxonomic, and chemical information on a great number of natural product extracts. This database contains more than 100,000 records, some dating as far back as 1650.

A growing number of alternative medical journals and publications carry research and clinical findings of varying levels of scientific rigor. The following databases are supported by or are specific to individual professions:

- CHIROLARS, a computer database (available on CD-ROM), contains 16,000 journal abstracts and conference proceedings in the field of chiropractic. Data are also available in book form in the *Index to Chiropractic Literature* and the *Chiropractic Research Abstracts Collection,* a compilation of more than 6,000 journals, journal articles, and books.
- A traditional Chinese medicine database at the American College of Traditional Chinese Medicine in San Francisco was begun with a small grant from the rock music group the Grateful Dead; lack of further funding has stalled the project.
- An electronic database of traditional Chinese medicine is available in Beijing.
- Ayurvedic databases are available in India.
- Alternative medical databases in various fields are available in Europe.

Research Database Enhancement

The role of OAM is pivotal in facilitating the needs of alternative medical researchers and meeting the information requirements of alternative medical health care practitioners. Enhancing the NLM national database, MEDLARS, should be one of the first steps.

Logic

Combining data from alternative medical journals and other research materials into the NLM's MEDLINE database and databanks—as opposed to developing a separate OAM-sponsored, comprehensive research database—is advisable for several reasons:

- A unified research database is consistent with the intent (as stated in the preface to this report) of incorporating the best of the alternative medical systems into the present U.S. medical health system rather than developing a separate medical health system.
- A separate database would continue the current subordination of alternative practices by making them appear unworthy of inclusion in MEDLINE.
- Having separate comprehensive databases would require that future researchers access at least two databases to complete their literature reviews.
- A separate research database would require considerable unnecessary duplication of effort, as well as additional OAM expense.
- Improving the NLM database is essential for communicating alternative medical treatment issues to conventional health care practitioners. These practitioners, who are responsible for the safety and efficacy of their health care practices, require guidance when a controversy exists about therapeutic or diagnostic options. Since they already use MEDLINE and other NLM resources, forcing practitioners to access a separate database would cause confusion and not serve alternative medicine's best interests.
- Often, materials on alternative medical systems from conventional medical journals that are referenced in MEDLINE are antagonistic to alternative medical research and practices. When offsetting information from alternative medical journals becomes available in MEDLINE, naive readers will not be left, as they are now, with the misleading impression that little research has been done and that the worth of the particular alternative medical practice is a negatively settled issue. When both sides of an issue are available, as is the case with most conventional issues, the responsible researcher is able to more fairly evaluate the situation.
- The insufficiency of alternative medical information on MEDLINE promotes the fiction that there is little research on alternative medicine; consequently, conventional researchers are unlikely to initiate investigatory efforts (Easterbrook et al., 1991; Kleijnen and Knipschild, 1992; Knipschild, 1993).

Though useful to researchers, MEDLINE is not suitable for use by the general public. A separate resource database is needed for consumer information (see the "Public Information Activities" chapter).

Directional Oversight

OAM should establish a standing research database committee to prepare materials for and to communicate with the NLM staff. This committee should be composed of knowledgeable alternative medical investigators and practitioners, historians, and other experts.

This undertaking will require scientific and technical competence so that information can be acquired, analyzed, and prepared in a timely, efficient, and cost-effective manner. The participation by experts in the various subjects will allow for thorough analysis of the range of alternative medical disciplines and literature. This will also help maintain the currency and vitality of the selected items and indexing terms.

Communications will be enhanced by having one member of the research database committee serve on the public information clearinghouse committee (this recommendation is proposed in "Public Information Activities").

Specific Objectives

The following specific objectives should be addressed:

- *Vocabulary.* The MeSH headings used by NLM in MEDLINE provide a meaningful hierarchy of indexing terms. An OAM research database committee should compile a list of additional alternative medical terms to enrich the MeSH headings now available. In doing so, the committee should follow accepted principles of NLM lexicography (in accordance with the MEDLARS *Indexing Manual,* parts I and II) and confer with the NLM staff.
- *Periodicals.* Many journals and other materials need critical and prompt evaluation to determine whether they should be recommended to NLM's selection committee for inclusion in MEDLARS and MEDLINE. Prescreening by an OAM research database committee using NLM's selection standards will speed up the process of inclusion.

- *Regular updating.* After the research database committee develops and initially applies a method of scanning literature for quality and inclusion, it should develop a process for regularly updating the list of included materials. Library professionals in health science from the academic and research communities should be invited to participate by submitting materials as they come to notice. The process should also include future listings that emerge from CATS and other major foreign electronic libraries.
- *Funding.* Funding possibilities for acquisition of presently uncataloged materials should be explored by the OAM research database committee in conjunction with NLM.

Data Collection and Dissemination

Data Collection

At this time, no centralized data collection process exists for gathering information on alternative medical practices, "anomalous healing events," and seemingly odd or extraneous sudden improvements in health and cure rates in individuals. To support both the research database and the consumer information clearinghouse detailed in this report, and to document evidence of improvements attributable to alternative medical practices, continual collection of a wide range of data will be needed.

Dissemination

Some research findings in alternative medicine will have immediate applicability to health care practices. OAM should implement a process to disseminate such research findings to the public and the biomedical community as they become available. The aim is to improve alternative medical health care treatment and prevention practices in a coordinated way as the knowledge base expands. This dissemination task falls under the aegis of the public information clearinghouse (see "Public Information Activities").

Specific Recommendations

The following can help significantly in building research databases:

- Enhancing databases should begin with a MEDLINE search for already indexed materials. Consideration should also be given to adding material currently carried in NLM stacks but not yet on-line.
- Methods should be selected or developed to scan the quality of information available to ensure the appropriateness of the material included. A mechanism to rate the quality of supporting scientific evidence could assist in identifying promising practices. Furthermore, such a search may well turn up areas of practice especially worthy of further investigation.
- Databases available from professional associations, schools, foundations, individuals, and corporations should be surveyed. The National Institutes of Health should solicit information on other information resources, which should include all alternative medical materials of note identified in publications in medical social science and medical humanities.
- Alternative medical literature currently available in foreign languages should be surveyed and then translated and included where appropriate. This is particularly important for those alternative medical therapies in use in the United States, such as the medicines of Asia, that have roots in other cultures. Early emphasis should be placed on Japanese, German, Chinese, and French literature.
- OAM should investigate the indexes of CATS for relevant materials.
- OAM should consult with State and national associations of various alternative health care professions and libraries for information and advice on key indexing words to be included from the various alternative disciplines. Continuing interaction with these groups will be necessary in order to ensure that the database is updated regularly.

References

Easterbrook, P.J., J.A. Berlin, R. Gopolan, and D.R. Matthews. 1991. Publication bias in clinical research. Lancet 337:867–872.

Kleijnen, J., and P. Knipschild. 1992. Review articles and publication bias. Arzneimittelforschung 42:587–591.

Knipschild, P. 1993. Searching for alternatives: loser pays. Lancet 341:1135–1136.

Pavek, R. 1994. Personal communication.

Research Methodologies

PANEL MEMBERS AND CONTRIBUTING AUTHORS

Barrie Cassileth, Ph.D.—Cochair
Wayne Jonas, M.D.—Cochair
Claire M. Cassidy, Ph.D.—Cochair

Robert Becker, M.D.
Berkley Beddell
Stephen Birch
Carlo Calabrese, N.D., M.P.H.
Harris L. Coulter, Ph.D.
Patricia Culliton, M.A., Dipl.Ac.
Etel E. DeLoach
Allen H. Frey, Ph.D.
James S. Gordon, M.D.
Elliott Greene, M.A.
Sandra Harner, Ph.D.
D. Warren Harrison, M.D.
George Kindness, Ph.D.
Kenneth A. Kivington, Ph.D.
Fredi Kronenberg, Ph.D.
Peter Lechner, M.D., F.A.C.A.
Kyriacos C. Markides, Ph.D.
Michael E. McGuinnis, Ph.D.
Patricia Muehsam, M.D.
Judith A. O'Connell, D.O.
Michael M. Patterson, Ph.D.
Richard Pavek
John C. Reed, M.D.
Kenneth M. Sancier, Ph.D.
Linda Silversmith, Ph.D.
Leanna Standish, N.D., Ph.D.
John Stegmaier
James P. Swyers, M.A.
Vernon M. Sylvest, M.D.
Jon D. Vredevoogd, Ph.D.
Jan Walleczek, M.D.
William S. Yamanashi, Ph.D.
Michael F. Ziff, D.D.S.

Introduction

In 1977 G. L. Engel, professor of psychiatry and medicine at the University of Rochester School of Medicine, wrote:

> The biomedical model assumes disease to be fully accounted for by deviations from the norm of measurable biological (somatic) variables. It leaves no room within its framework for the social, psychological, and behavioral dimensions of illness. . . . The biomedical model has thus become a cultural imperative, its limitations easily overlooked. In brief, it has now acquired the status of dogma. In science, a model is revised or abandoned when it fails to account adequately for all the data. A dogma, on the other hand, requires that discrepant data be forced to fit the model or be excluded.[1]

This chapter deals with methods of testing, strategies of validation, proofs of efficacy, and the application of these to alternative medical systems. The evaluation of alternative medical systems is no different from the study of conventional methods in that appropriate methods must be chosen to evaluate the system.[2] No medical system or method, alternative or otherwise, should be recommended for inclusion in the medical health system until it has been adequately tested. Data produced by incorrect or

---

[1]*From "The Need for a New Medical Model: A Challenge for Biomedicine,"* Science *(April 1977) 196:129.*

[2]*The following general points are relevant to alternative as well as conventional medical research for which funding is sought. A proposed basic research project should address a significant fundamental question; incorporate appropriate controls; employ appropriate tests of statistical significance and power; provide adequate characterization of the treatment used and the background context; present evidence to indicate how any results with nonhuman biological systems would apply to humans; and be based on testable hypotheses. Besides having similar characteristics, a proposed clinical study should address questions of effectiveness and/or safety; offer benefits commensurate with the risks involved for patients; allow questions of effectiveness to be decided within a predictable timeframe; and when appropriate, include comparisons to other medical approaches. Appendix F, "A Guide for the Alternative Researcher," provides additional material and references on how to plan and conduct research.*

inadequate research methods do not have validity and cannot contribute to knowledge.

Research Methodologies

The need to expand biomedical assumptions to include psychosocial and behavioral factors has become increasingly understood since Engel's 1977 comment. Indeed, the vast literature of studies that now includes psychosocial dimensions of disease outcomes, health, illness behavior, and correlates of well-being attests to wide acceptance of Engel's challenge. Many of these studies either encompass or cover aspects of some of the alternative therapies discussed in this report.

But other alternative systems and methods have not been adequately studied. One reason for this, according to various alternative medicine practitioners, is that conventional medicine researchers typically and inappropriately demand application of the "gold standard"—that is, prospective randomized clinical trials—when they are not appropriate. This demand occurs despite the availability of a range of suitable research methods from which to choose and the possibility that new methods will have to be identified to fit the situation. Sometimes the demand is for unusually large and complex designs intended to solicit multiple data rather than more appropriate, smaller designs that focus on first-step issues (Pavek, 1994).

Indeed, a review of published conventional research over the years indicates that prospective randomized clinical trials are not always possible or preferred. A 1990 report of the Institute of Medicine's Committee on Technological Innovation in Medicine supports this tacit reality and discusses methodological options:

> It has also become clear that randomized controlled clinical trials are not necessarily practical or feasible for answering all clinical questions. Therefore, a variety of other methods, such as nonrandomized trials or observational methods, have been adopted to provide complementary information. Traditionally these methods were regarded as weaker than randomized clinical controlled clinical trials for clinical evaluation. Recent methodological advances, such as the use of non-classical statistics and the ability to link large-scale automated databases for analysis . . . are strengthening these approaches.

Issues in Evaluating Alternative Medical Systems

Research design, even for conventional medicine, is a difficult and challenging process, even more so for alternative systems (Patel, 1987a). As should be abundantly clear from the introduction to the report, there is not one alternative medicine, but several. These consist of new approaches to patient care, new and unusual biomedical disease fighters, discrete methods of treatment, and systems of diagnostics and therapeutics that rely on and are governed by new paradigms.

Fortunately, helpful guidelines exist. The foremost guideline to keep in mind is that the basic goal of any investigation concerning a treatment for human beings is to determine whether the treatment makes a difference. Campbell and Stanley's classic monograph on experimental and quasi-experimental designs discusses lack of "internal validity"[3] as the most serious threat to answering that fundamental question, commenting that "internal validity is the basic minimum without which any experiment is uninterpretable: did in fact the experimental treatments make a difference?" (Campbell and Stanley, 1963). The monograph lists several types of threats to internal validity, including

- the possibility that events during the evaluation may unintentionally influence outcomes;
- the possibility that changes occurring naturally over time may be mistaken for treatment results; and
- the risk that subject self-selection, rather than the treatment under study, caused the result or lack of result.

Sophisticated experimental designs eliminate or control threats to internal validity. Many threats—though not all—are controlled when studies compare two or more treatments by randomly assigning subjects to each of those treatments. In designs lacking random assignment, additional efforts are needed to bolster as much as possible the validity of the evaluation.

The second major concern for designing evaluations is external validity—that is, the ability to generalize the results of the evaluation to other populations and settings.

---

[3] *Internal validity is the certainty that the treatment or regimen under study, rather than something else, produced the study results.*

Other methodological concerns that have been raised address certain problems that are typically advanced in discussions of alternative medical research. Indeed, research in alternative medicine often appears fraught with conditions that seem uncontrollable or impossible to study. In many instances, however, the technique or a comparable one has already been studied, and published results can provide both encouragement and specific guidance.

As examples, there are useful approaches for studying music therapy provided in papers on how to assess the effects of music therapy in Alzheimer's disease (Aldridge, 1993). Eisenberg and colleagues (1993) reviewed numerous controlled studies assessing the effectiveness of cognitive behavioral techniques in managing hypertension. Methods for controlling or dealing with unwanted influences of subject, practitioner, and environment in learning situations can be found in such general texts as *Complementary Methods for Research in Education* (Jaeger, 1988), *Research in Education* (Best and Kahn, 1986), and *Introduction to Educational Research* (Charles, 1988).

Additional examples of research concerns in alternative medicine, along with proposed solutions, are presented below.

Measuring the Perspectives of Patients

Systems of health, as well as individual health care practitioners, vary in their approaches to health care, patients' decisionmaking, and intended outcomes (end points). Some systems and practitioners focus on quality-of-life issues as being paramount to surgical operations and chemical treatments. This emphasis on quality of life—and on patients making their own decisions—often is considered typical of alternative medicine. There is also a large conventional medicine literature dealing with quality-of-life issues.

Sometimes, difficult decisions must be made that are influenced by the views of practitioner, patient, and health care system. The choice might involve enduring long-term minor discomfort by not electing surgery or choosing a surgical procedure that will eliminate the discomfort but that carries a 2-percent chance of death. Or the choice might concern electing to have or to forego artificial life-sustaining procedures and equipment, such as resuscitation and heart-lung machines in terminal stages of disease.

Breast cancer research is an example of research that led to choices for patients. Under many circumstances, women may elect treatment for their breast cancer: today's choices are lumpectomy plus radiation therapy versus mastectomy. Men diagnosed with advanced prostate cancer also have medically equivalent treatment choices—surgery (orchiectomy) versus subcutaneous injections—with both approaches achieving the same goal of halting the male hormone that promotes prostate tumor growth. In these two examples, patient choice became possible when careful clinical research produced treatment options and then documented that the old and new treatments were equivalent in their effects.

Patients have even more choice in the absence of major or potentially fatal disease. Faced with symptoms of an enlarged prostate, for example, many men elect to endure their symptoms rather than undergo surgery. Recent Agency for Health Care Policy and Research (AHCPR) guidelines made this choice explicit for patients with enlarged prostates and increased national awareness of the need for patient involvement and sensitivity to quality-of-life issues. The guidelines were developed by a panel that was required to include health care consumer representation. AHCPR advised doctors and men with enlarged prostates (not prostate cancer) to curtail the use of two widely used diagnostic tests that frequently led to surgery and to rely instead on a questionnaire that quantifies how severely the condition affects the patient's quality of life.

Because some patients are comfortable with symptoms that other patients consider unacceptable, and because an enlarged prostate is not life threatening, the recommended focus on the patient's view of symptoms—rather than clinical measurement of prostate enlargement—is expected to lead to more appropriate treatment and decreased costs for surgery. (In 1992, before the guidelines, some 220,000 medicare patients received corrective prostate surgery performed at a cost of more than $1 billion [see sidebar].) Alternative practitioners note that increased use of patient choice and quality-of-life decisionmaking—as exemplified by these guidelines—both encourage financial savings and address psychosocial concerns that should not be neglected.

US Issues Guidelines That May Lead to Less Surgery for Enlarged Prostate

By Ron Winslow

U.S. officials issued new guidelines for doctors and patients that could transform treatment for an enlarged prostate, a condition that afflicts about half of men over age 50.

If the guidelines are widely followed, they would likely lead to less surgery and fewer diagnostic tests than are now performed in managing the ailment. They call for patients to take a primary role in deciding whether surgery, medication, or just monitoring symptoms without treatment is the best course to follow.

Known as benign prostatic hyperplasia, or BPH, an enlarged prostate restricts or obstructs the flow of urine from the bladder through the penis, causing frequent and urgent urination and related symptoms. It isn't related to or a cause of prostate cancer. The most common treatment is surgery, which was performed on more than 220,000 Medicare patients in 1992 at a cost of more than $1 billion. Both the cost and the fact that doctors vary widely in prescribing treatments prompted U.S. health officials to consider BPH as a major candidate for an initiative to develop guidelines for a variety of common diseases. At the same time, new treatment alternatives, including drugs marketed by Merck & Co. and Abbott Laboratories have recently been approved by U.S. regulators, adding to options for both doctors and patients.

"There's been a tendency to intervene with surgery too quickly, rather than consider options," said Jarrett Clinton, administrator of the Agency for Health Care Policy and Research, a division of the Department of Health and Human Services, which announced the guidelines.

Surgery 'Most Effective'

"Our analysis clearly demonstrates that surgery is the most effective treatment for BPH," added Dr. John D. McConnell, chairman of urology at University of Texas Southwestern Medical Center, Dallas, and chairman of a 13-member expert panel that developed the guidelines. "But not all patients need or desire the most effective therapy."

The guidelines urge doctors to curtail use of two widely used diagnostic tests and rely instead on a new, seven-item questionnaire yielding a symptom score on a 35-point scale that indicates how severely BPH is affecting a patient's quality of life. Since some men live comfortably with symptoms that others consider severe, the guidelines say a focus on a patient's view of symptoms rather than clinical tests will lead to more appropriate treatment.

"The symptom score is a very pivotal part of the work-up and is one of the things that brings the patient into the process," said Dr. McConnell. "This is going to be a new concept for many physicians."

The new guidelines say patients with severe symptoms, including an inability to urinate, should be treated with surgery. But all others should fill out the questionnaire and use the results as a basis for discussing treatment strategies with their physicians.

"The best treatment is the one chosen by an informed patient," Dr. McConnell said. "A pill is less effective than surgery, but has less risk. We're trying to get doctors away from making that value judgment themselves. It's a patient's decision."

The guidelines also say that X-ray or ultrasound examination of the kidneys and cystoscopy, in which doctors look at the urinary tract through a scope, are of little use in deciding whether a patient needs treatment. A 1989 survey found that two-thirds of urologists routinely use those tests in examining a patient with BPH symptoms.

—*Wall Street Journal*, February 9, 1994, page B6

Disbelief

Disbelief is a factor not frequently addressed. Here, disbelief refers to the opinion of a physician, investigator, or research organization that a particular procedure or approach is ineffective. If this opinion is held by someone in a position to influence research funding or conduct, its impact can be widespread. In the view of alternative medicine researchers, the two typical ways in which they are affected include (1) outright, knee-jerk rejection of study proposals and (2) insistence on inappropriate and/or unnecessarily cumbersome study design.

A recent study provides corroboration concerning the alternative medicine researchers' perception of bias (Wilson et al., 1994). Wilson and his colleagues found that both medical and psychological researchers were more willing to overlook or disregard methodological flaws in studies that addressed "important" topics rather than "less serious" ones and to be more demanding in their standards for the latter.[4] In an analogous way, scientists with little knowledge of or interest in alternative medical subjects could be expected not to take them seriously or to demand additional proofs.

Indeed, a frequent complaint of alternative medicine practitioners is that they are often obliged to conduct later stage studies even before preliminary information is gathered (Pavek, 1994). They also report the strong tendency of research institutions and methodologists to insist that very stringent controls be included in beginning studies—controls that would never be considered for early investigation of more conventional subjects. In other words, alternative medicine researchers protest that the standards of proof are raised for research on alternative practices.

In *The Cancer Industry*, Ralph Moss provides another good example of such misdirection and misperception. Moss examined the American Cancer Society's (ACS's) list of unproven methods for the 1970s and 1980s, which mentioned 70 practitioners and 63 methods. Although ACS had described its "unproven" list as containing mostly unqualified practitioners and only a few researchers with appropriate degrees, Moss found that more than 70 percent held an M.D., Ph.D., or D.O. Further, more than 50 percent of the methods had never been investigated to prove whether or not they worked. Only 29 percent had received some investigation leading ACS to term them ineffective or "unproven" (Moss, 1989).

Perceiving these biases discourages alternative medicine researchers from attempting even preliminary studies. The discouraged investigator sees little point in proceeding if small, preliminary, information-gathering studies are so readily rejected. Likewise, large-scale, controlled trials demanded by those with such biases will likely not be funded.

Specific Testing Difficulties

The examples below serve to illustrate some of the controversy surrounding methodological decisionmaking for alternative medical systems.

Systematic therapeutic learning. Some alternative methods—such as biofeedback, meditation, imagery, and dance therapy—involve a learning process. With repetition, the person using them becomes more adept. Evaluating the benefit of such methods requires ensuring that a basic minimum of training is achieved by study subjects (i.e., the study must control for the amount of learning) and carefully selecting the appropriate research technique.

In studies of therapies involving learning, the research methodology usually includes appropriate control groups. Typically, the controls receive another intervention or none at all and would be students, patients, or clients of similar ages, talents, problems, interests, and whatever else is relevant to the process or technique under study. Many practitioners of alternative medicine consider the situation unethical if the control group receives no intervention. In addition, they note that subjects in the control group might be angry and frustrated (Goeble et al., 1993).

[4] *Wilson and his colleagues provided descriptions of six fictitious research studies to their research subjects. The studies were actually identical apart from the topic under investigation; noticeable methodological errors were included. One set of study subjects linked the effects of alcohol to heart disease (important) or heartburn (less serious), and another linked fast food to either cholesterol levels or acne. The persons reviewing "important" studies were considerably more likely to consider them publishable than those who reviewed "trivial" subjects.*

Furthermore, some alternative medicine practitioners are concerned about any research design involving a control group comparison, because they believe this test structure does not adequately evaluate certain alternative systems (Shellenberger and Green, 1986, 1987).

In contrast, methodologists are likely to insist that because research involving learning situations is influenced by the thoughts, feelings, intentions, and attitudes of both experimenter and subject, by practice effects, and often by the learning environment, this research requires control of these unwanted influences on results. For example, since the teacher cannot be blinded to the method or the results of the treatment in learning situations, methodologists propose as a solution that the contemplated research be conducted by someone other than the teacher or practitioner and that objective data (for example, physiological and laboratory measurements or subject self-report tests) be obtained.[5]

Before determining that new research methodologies might be needed, alternative medical investigators can look for guidance at the methods that have been used to research issues relevant to their own work and evaluate the resulting study. For example, those interested in biofeedback and similar self-training techniques can turn to studies published in periodicals such as the *Journal of Biofeedback and Self Regulation* and the *Journal of Behavior Therapy and Experimental Psychiatry* and can consult with members of the Association for Applied Psychophysiology and Biofeedback.

Similarly, problem-oriented journals provide illustrations for how to assess biofeedback and related techniques when applied to particular problems. Studies of the effectiveness of biofeedback, relaxation, or meditation in controlling epileptic seizures, for example, appear in journals such as *Neurological Clinics* and *Perceptual and Motor Skills*. Randomized clinical trials and other methods used to evaluate imagery training and migraine headaches are published in such journals as *Headache*.

Manual healing methods. Much like surgery on babies born with cleft palates, each manual healing procedure, no matter how well structured, is highly individualized. Even for one individual, the procedures in a treatment series may vary from session to session. Research methods must take this point into account. One possible approach is to conduct comparative studies of the effectiveness of one manual method versus another. Another approach is to compare outcomes with the results of standard medical therapy or no treatment.

Research and documentation are needed to objectively present the baseline status of the patients and measure actual changes in physiological function, work capacity, or functional activities induced by the manual healing method. Monitoring techniques like those developed for biofeedback studies (Goeble et al., 1993; Shellenberger and Green, 1986, 1987) and for orthopedic rehabilitation (gait analysis) (Harris and Wersch, 1994; Perry, 1992; Sutherland et al., 1988) may be adaptable to studies of manual healing methods.

An example of an approach applying monitoring methods and measuring an outcome is the following research strategy: Narula (1993) wanted to determine whether subjects with rheumatoid arthritis showed improvements after training in a manual healing method called the Feldenkrais method (see the "Manual Healing Methods" chapter). She applied video filming and "peak performance" software to examine whether subjects showed changes in their sit-to-stand movement pattern. Narula also measured grip strength with a dynamometer, walking speed by timing the number of seconds required to walk 50 feet, and pain and disease status with a quantifying questionnaire. (The treatment produced some improvements by all measures except grip strength.)

Another way that methodologists have proposed to deal with the problem of practitioner bias (and produce more accurate data on the merits of the procedure per se) would be to have subjects treated with their eyes closed or covered—in effect "blinded" to the individual therapist. Frequently, however, the subject is still able to recognize the therapist by other means. In addition, the subject's discomfort at being

[5] *The use of independent evaluators and objective data collection is relevant in all research studies of methods in which the teacher or practitioner plays a major role. Besides learning situations, these methods include, for example, biofeedback therapy and manual healing methods.*

"blindfolded" is likely to interfere with the treatment process.

Alternatively, and depending on the research question under study, a more useful approach would be to have more than one practitioner treat an individual, or the same practitioner could provide both the experimental and control treatments. However, when more than one practitioner provides treatment to the same subject, the subject is likely to have preferences and may therefore be uncomfortable with this process. In addition, difficulties may arise in transferring information from one practitioner to the next when much of that information involves physical sensing.

The use of independent observers who are not administering the therapy to gather and analyze results is another approach that can reduce practitioner bias. For example, in osteopathic research, this approach sometimes takes the form of having several practitioners independently assess the condition of patients before and after treatment, using a negotiated system of evaluation, then collating their results to determine whether significant changes have occurred (Beal et al., 1982). (This subject—inter-rater assessment—is discussed in another context in the osteopathic medicine section of the "Manual Healing Methods" chapter.)

Thus, although prospective, randomized, controlled clinical trials are not always feasible for studying manual healing methods, other methodologically sound studies can be constructed to evaluate these techniques.

New or unusual biochemical substances. Techniques for both laboratory and human testing of novel drugs or substances have been applied in conventional research for decades and also are applicable in alternative medical research. The research question dictates which methodology can and should be applied. For instance, to learn whether a new treatment increases length of remission (period without active disease) in lung cancer, patients receiving the new or alternative therapy and those on standard conventional treatment would be followed over time. The percentage of patients surviving after a given time, as well as the number of months to relapse or death, would then be compared for the two groups.

As another illustration, here are two possible ways to manage the apparent difficulty of studying iscador, a mistletoe extract used in alternative medicine as an anticancer treatment (see the "Pharmacological and Biological Treatments" chapter). Some alternative medicine practitioners have speculated that iscador cannot be studied with conventional methodologies. The reasoning is that since employing iscador produces a definite rash, blinding the investigator and the patient to the treatment used is impossible. One research approach avoiding this problem is to ask a question that does not require blinding: for example, "How much iscador is needed to produce a certain desired effect?" Another approach is to compare iscador treatment with a control procedure that has no effect against cancer but includes a (harmless) substance that also produces a rash. Patients would be randomly assigned to receive iscador or the control treatment.

Approaches that mix physics and biology. Standard methodological approaches can be used in researching interventions that invoke mechanisms that depend on physical properties. The essential step in such research—for example, in studying bioelectromagnetic applications—is to characterize the physical variable in greater detail than is common in clinical research. For example, artifacts caused by ambient electromagnetic fields in the laboratory environment (such as from power lines and laboratory equipment) must be avoided in bioelectromagnetics research. Furthermore, the bioelectromagnetic fields under study, which can involve very small quantities of energy, must be measured accurately in order to detect whether observed effects correlate with level of treatment. (A sample protocol for magnetic-field therapy is presented in the "Bioelectromagnetics Applications in Medicine" chapter.)

Systems with unconventional paradigms. Conventional research concepts and methods may not be capable of determining the mechanisms of action for systems that do not operate under conventional paradigms (Anthony, 1987; Bensoussan, 1991; Diamond and Denton, 1993; Patel, 1987b). Relevant examples include traditional Chinese medicine, with its concepts of an invisible *qi* moving through the body to organize it into balance and harmony; homeopathy, with extreme dilution rates that leave less than one molecule of a substance (too little for conventional science to study); and biofield therapeutics, which operate through application of an energy field that has not yet been fully characterized. Indeed, these situations are likely to lead to disbelief and claims of placebo effects.

For systems with unconventional paradigms, the question of clinical *effectiveness*—as opposed to *underlying paradigm, belief system,* or *mechanism of action*—can be readily studied. Indeed, many medical treatments have been implemented on the basis of evidence of safety and efficacy long before their mechanisms of action were detailed.

When unconventional paradigms are involved, it is particularly important that researchers trained in the biomedical model develop considerable knowledge of the alternative system under study and work jointly with an expert in that alternative field to design effective and valid research protocols.

Issues That Affect Both Conventional and Alternative Medical Systems

Effects on therapeutic outcome of patients' choices of treatment; participation by patients in their own care; and the relationship between the expectations of patients, cultural context, and lifestyle activities are examples of issues that are usually minor considerations in conventional medicine but are especially important in the alternative spectrum. Some alternative medical systems rely heavily on one or more of these issues.

Quality of Life

How one studies factors associated with quality of life depends on the research question being asked: this point makes generalization difficult.[6] The following are examples of research approaches when the attitudes of patients are under study:

- *Patients' expectations.* To answer the question of whether there is a correlation between patients' expectations for therapy, or hopelessness, and their clinical outcome, one research approach was to ask patients (who were part of a broader study) with newly diagnosed, prognostically poor cancers to complete a questionnaire concerning what they expected their treatment to accomplish. Patients checked one out of a choice of such response options as "Cure my disease"; "Hold my disease in check"; "Not much"; and "Don't know." Patients also completed a standardized "hopelessness" scale. (Patients were previously informed in detail through discussions with physicians, written consent forms, and other printed material about their diagnosis and prognosis.) The patients were followed over time. Data were analyzed to determine whether there was an association between length of survival and treatment expectations or hopelessness; none was found (Cassileth et al., 1985, 1988).
- *Patient choice.* Research on patient choice has ranged from questionnaire surveys of the preferences of patients for information about their illness and treatment and desire to participate in their own care (Cassileth et al., 1980) to intervention studies that address the later satisfaction of patients with the treatment option that they themselves had selected (Cassileth et al., 1989).

Additional suggested approaches can be gleaned from medical literature and other resources. Research on quality of life is common in conventional medicine; journals, annual meetings, international workshops, textbooks, and a project of the World Health Organization are devoted to quality-of-life research and measurement techniques.

Avoiding Patient Bias

The results of some studies may consist of patient or client reports of how they feel before versus after the treatment. Because people are likely to try to please or at least not insult their care givers, this is another situation in which to use independent observers (Kassirer, 1994). For example, the results could be collected by an investigator not involved in providing the therapy.

[6] *Potential alternative medical researchers can explore various approaches using the reference list provided in appendix F and using MEDLINE as a resource (see the "Research Databases" chapter as well as app. F section on the National Library of Medicine, which provides an introduction to MEDLINE). Relevant key terms can be selected for the MEDLINE search, such as* patient choice *and* patient participation.

General Procedural Issues

A sequence of steps defines the development and application of research, starting with the initial idea or hypothesis under consideration for testing (see app. F). Whether or not a research project should be carried out depends first on what is already known about the subject and then on the research questions posed and the proposed experimental design to answer those questions.

Before implementing new clinical investigations, the researcher conducts critical reviews of the literature. With assistance from certain methodology specialists, these reviews can include sophisticated systematic reviews and meta-analyses (see app. F) of existing studies of alternative medical practices. These reviews are useful to learn what others have done, obtain information about methods employed, and determine the shortcomings or missing information that the proposed study can redress. Such reviews are likely to

- summarize existing clinical information;
- identify methodologic inadequacies found in existing controlled experiments; and
- document evidence, or lack of evidence, of clinical effectiveness.

Whether researchers are using the newer analytical techniques or older ones, caution is always needed in determining whether the selected tools have been applied appropriately. When the tools are applied appropriately, the results can strengthen the believability of the alternative intervention under study.

After investigators review existing studies, they must establish appropriate methodologies for assessing their proposed research before the research commences. As indicated earlier in this chapter, there is a need to select appropriate methodologies for each alternative medical procedure or system being researched and to develop new ones if present methods are inadequate. Correspondingly, it is clear that alternative medical practitioners and researchers must interface directly with methodologists and experienced researchers to work out how to test the effectiveness of their systems.

Specific Recommendations

Implementation of the following recommendations would provide valuable methodological assistance for alternative medical research:

- OAM should sponsor, perhaps with the assistance of the National Institutes of Health Office of Medical Applications of Research, two or more methodology assessment conferences to begin the process of identifying or developing appropriate methodologies. These conferences should examine differing research assumptions and epistemological issues and should review available appropriate methodologies. Published proceedings from these conferences will be valuable to alternative and conventional investigators.
- Through the Field Investigations program, OAM should help practitioners to collect data in a scientifically valid manner, conduct retrospective reviews, assemble best case series, and conduct prospective pilot trials on existing therapies.
- OAM should implement systematic reviews, including meta-analyses, of the alternative medical therapies as necessary to assist in implementation of next-step clinical investigations in the various fields.
- OAM should develop and make available a list of research methodologists willing to collaborate or serve as resources for alternative medical investigators and for conventional investigators intending to study alternative practices.
- OAM should make resource materials to guide alternative researchers readily available, including guidelines on research methods and methodology bibliographies.

References

Aldridge, D. 1993. Music and Alzheimer's disease—assessment and therapy: a discussion paper. J. R. Soc. Med. 86(2):93–95.

Anthony, H.M. 1987. Some methodological problems in the assessment of complementary therapy. Stat. Med. 6:761–771.

Beal, M.C., J.P. Goodridge, W.L. Johnston, et al. 1982. Interexaminer agreement on long-term patient improvement: an exercise in research design. J. Am. Osteopath. Assoc. 81(5):322–328.

Bensoussan, A. 1991. Contemporary acupuncture research: the difficulties of research across scientific paradigms. Am. J. Acupunc. 19(4):357–365.

Best, J.W., and J.V. Kahn. 1986. Research in Education. Prentice Hall, New York.

Campbell, D.T., and J.C. Stanley. 1963. Experimental and Quasi-Experimental Designs for Research. Rand McNally, Chicago.

Cassileth, B.R., E.J. Lusk, D.S. Miller, et al. 1985. Psychosocial correlates of survival in malignant disease. N. Engl. J. Med. 312:1551–1555.

Cassileth, B.R., M.S. Soloway, N.J. Vogelzang, et al. 1989. Patients' choice of treatment in stage D prostate cancer. Urology 33 (Suppl.):57–62.

Cassileth, B.R., W.P. Walsh, and E.J. Lusk. 1988. Psychosocial correlates of cancer survival: a subsequent report 3–8 years after cancer diagnosis. J. Clin. Oncol. 6:1753–1759.

Cassileth, B.R., R.V. Zupkis, K. Sutton-Smith, et al. 1980. Information and participation preferences among cancer patients. Ann. Intern. Med. 92:832–836.

Charles, C.M. 1988. Introduction to Educational Research. Longman, Inc., White Plains, N.Y.

Diamond, G.A., and T.A. Denton. 1993. Alternative perspectives on the biased foundations of medical technology assessment. Ann. Intern. Med. 118:455–464.

Eisenberg, D.M., T.L. Delbanco, C.S. Berkley, et al. 1993. Cognitive behavioral techniques for hypertension: are they effective? Ann. Intern. Med. 118(12):944–972.

Goeble, M., G.W. Viol, and C. Orebaugh. 1993. An incremental model to isolate specific effects of behavioral treatments in essential hypertension. Biofeedback Self Regul. 18(4).

Harris, G.F., and J.J. Wersch. 1994. Procedures for gait analysis. Arch. Phys. Med. Rehabil. 75:216–225.

Jaeger, R., ed. 1988. Complementary Methods for Research in Education. American Educational Research Association, Washington, D.C.

Kassirer, J.P. 1994. Incorporating patient's preferences into medical decisions [editorial]. N. Engl. J. Med. 330(26):1895–1896.

Moss, R. 1989. The Cancer Industry. Paragon House, New York.

Narula, M. 1993. Effect of the six week Awareness through Movement Lessons—the Feldenkrais method on selected functional movement parameters in individuals with rheumatoid arthritis (M.S. thesis, Oakland University, Rochester, Mich.) (abstract).

Patel, M.S. 1987a. Evaluation of holistic medicine. Soc. Sci. Med. 24(2):169–175.

Patel, M.S. 1987b. Problems in the evaluation of alternative medicine. Soc. Sci. Med. 25(6):669–678.

Pavek, R. 1994. Personal communication.

Perry, J. 1992. Gait Analysis: Normal and Pathological Function. SLACK Inc., Thorofare, N.J.

Shellenberger, R., and J.A. Green. 1986. From the Ghost in the Box to Successful Biofeedback Training. Health Psychology Publications, Greeley, Colo.

Shellenberger, R., and J.A. Green. 1987. Specific effects and biofeedback vs. biofeedback-assisted self-regulation training. Biofeedback Self Regul. 12(3):185–209.

Sutherland, D.H., R.A. Olshen, E.W. Biden, et al. 1988. The Development of Mature Walking. Mackeith Press, London.

Wilson, T., et al. Psychological Science 4:322–325, cited in April 1994 in "Study of 'studies' reveals surprising science bias" in Brain-Mind, A Bulletin of Breakthroughs, Interface Press, Los Angeles, Calif., April 1994, 19(7).

Peer Review

PANEL MEMBERS AND CONTRIBUTING AUTHORS

Carlton F. Hazlewood, Ph.D.—Cochair
Edward H. Chapman, M.D.—Cochair

R. James Barnard, Ph.D.
Myrin Borysenko, Ph.D.
Rosalin L. Bruyere, D.D.
James A. Caplan
Effie Poy Yew Chow, Ph.D., C.A.
Winston Franklin
Carol Hegedus, M.S., M.A.
Darrcy A. Loveland, J.D.
Gladys T. McGarey, M.D.
Richard Pavek
William H. Philpott, M.D.
David M. Sale, J.D., LL.M.
Savely L. Savva
Marilyn Schlitz, Ph.D.
Gertrude Schmeidler, Ph.D
Jeremy Waletzky, M.D.

Introduction

Peer review is the process of allowing the researcher's peers to evaluate the research credibility and potential value of researchers' work. Peers are chosen to participate in the evaluation process on the basis of their knowledge of or expertise in the area of scientific investigation being considered. The peer review process is widely used in such areas as education, publication, state licensing, and review of clinical outcomes on a case-by-case basis by physician review organizations mandated by Federal law. Though these areas all have tremendous relevance to alternative medicine, this report will chiefly focus on the National Institutes of Health (NIH) evaluation process for applications for research grants and research contracts.

Structure of the Peer Review System

Intake of Applications

At NIH, the peer review process is administered by the Division of Research Grants (DRG), to which the grant application is submitted.[1] An initial administrative review by the division leads to the assignment of the application to one of the various institutes within NIH—such as the National Cancer Institute or the National Heart, Lung, and Blood Institute—and also to 1 of some 100 standing initial review groups (IRGs), or study sections, within DRG. Each study section has a scientific review administrator plus 20 or so scientists, each of whom is a specialist in a given area.

If the application does not fit the scope of any of the established study sections, the scientific review administrator in the DRG, in consultation with the science administrator in the institute to which the application has been assigned, may convene a "special" (one-time) study section or an "ad hoc" (temporary) study section to undertake the review.

Review of Applications

In the review process, each grant is reviewed in detail by a primary and a secondary reviewer within the study section, who then present their findings to the entire study section. (The findings of these two reviewers are likely to shape the study section's decision.) After their review, study section members vote whether or not to recommend for further consideration and assign to the application a funding "priority score" ranging from 100 to 500. A "perfect " score is 100. The applicant receives a written response called a summary statement ("pink sheet") that briefly

[1] *Some institutions have their own panels for grants review. These standing study sections are usually concerned with evaluating training grants, center grants, and requests for applications that bear directly on specific missions of the institute.*

discusses the decision of the study section and the numerical score assigned to the application.

The actual funding of grants is made after a secondary review of the application by an advisory council or board of those NIH centers and institutes that have funding authority. With current levels of funding, it is likely that only grants with scores lower than 150 will receive funding.

Appeals

An applicant may investigate an unfavorable recommendation by contacting the science administrator within the institute to which the application was assigned and the scientific review administrator of the regular study section. The applicant may request additional information and even appeal. If sufficient reasons are identified by the applicant, he or she may request that the appropriate branch chief within the institute review the decision. The appeal may then be carried up the chain of command to the director of the institute.

This appeals process is, however, not frequently employed. A major concern for applicants who choose to appeal is the potentially negative effect that requesting an appeal may have on their professional reputations. Furthermore, as it currently stands, the appeal process is perceived by a number of scientists that have actively used it to be an exercise in futility (Hazelwood, 1992, 1993; Ling, 1992).

Potential Concerns

The NIH peer review process in alternative medicine is not expected to raise methodological issues substantially different from those encountered with other emerging fields of scientific endeavor with which this division may have been initially unfamiliar. Rather, the major challenges are intellectual ones for the reviewers involved in the peer review process.

Alternative medicine challenges established scientists and institutions by proposing models and patterns that differ from what is medically familiar. Peer review in alternative medicine will require reviewers to confront issues of potential bias stemming from differences in basic assumptions about health and disease that may reflect the limitations of current scientific knowledge (Ling, 1992).

Historically, new ideas in science have rarely been readily accepted by proponents' peers. In fact, established scientists are major contributors to the resistance to new ideas. The peer review system, which matured during the latter half of this century, may be contributing to the resistance to acceptance of legitimate scientific discoveries that are out of the mainstream (Horrobin, 1990). This is particularly so in the case of alternative medical practices.

In general, there are two approaches to research: innovations, which directly challenge existing models and patterns; and improvements, which refine and advance the results stemming from innovative research. For example, Thomas Edison's research in the 19th century led to an innovation, the light bulb, while later research resulted in various improvements of the light bulb, such as the "Miser." Alternative medicine usually involves innovative research, particularly because research developments in this field are so new. Some peer review bodies may inadvertently fail to recognize innovative research in study proposals they review (Horrobin, 1990).

Inherent resistance to innovative research must be recognized and acknowledged before much can be done to install a peer review system that supports innovation and shortens the time between scientific discovery, creation of new effective treatments, and availability to the general public (Ling, 1992).

Because many alternative medical applications do not fit within the scope of existing study sections, the ad hoc review mechanism must be used until enough experience has been obtained with these applications to allow the formation of new standing review groups. Moreover, since standing study sections primarily serve NIH institutes and centers, the status of OAM as an office, rather than a center or institute, complicates the review process.

The following points summarize specific concerns that are likely to arise in an examination of the peer review process:

- Grant proposals are usually evaluated in terms of established priorities. Peers are chosen to review established categories of specialization, and proposals must generally fit into one of those categories. This process tends to promote research in long-established directions and discourages efforts toward new synthesis and new concepts.

- Peer reviewers are not neutral parties; rather, they are specialists in specified areas, and they also may have vested interests. Reviewers may make their living teaching or practicing the very ideas that are called into question by the new research thinking or the new practices being proposed.
- It appears that NIH does not consider it a conflict of interest for a scientist to serve on an appeal board when he or she holds a perspective that conflicts with the premises of an appellant. Proponents of alternative medicine are concerned that this practice presents the greatest difficulty of the NIH review process. The issue is especially important for approaches such as homeopathy and biofield therapeutics, whose basic assumptions challenge conventional scientific assumptions.
- Shortages of research funds intensify the problem of bias against innovative research and alternative medical approaches.
- The appeals system as it now functions is not viewed as effective. There is a belief that too few win appeals without repercussions on their careers; this, in turn, discourages others from participating.

1993 Grant Review Process

Grant applicants have made various complaints about the grant review process resulting from OAM's first RFA (see sidebar). Some complaints concerned misassignments, category and procedural errors, and possible violations by the peer review groups of the rules of the RFA process.

Recommendations

The optimal peer review process for proposed alternative medical research projects would rely on one or more standing study sections that meet regularly and are made up of experts from a

The 1993 Research Grants Application and Review Experience*

The purposes of the request for applications (RFA) sponsored by the Office of Alternative Medicine (OAM) and released in spring 1993 were to foster alternative medicine-researcher collaborations and provide opportunities to obtain preliminary or pilot data that might justify additional support for research. NIH received some 800 letters expressing interest in the RFA and 463 applications for the 30 grants for which there was funding. Only 10 or fewer applications did not meet the RFA's requirements. DRG deemed the response overwhelming.

Several senior staff members of DRG who participated in the application review process attended an orientation seminar presented by OAM. Eight review panels were set up for the six categories of subjects to which applications were assigned: Diet/Nutrition/Lifestyles; Mind/Body Control; Traditional and Ethnomedicine; Structural and Energetic Therapies; Bioelectromagnetic Applications; and Pharmacological and Biological Therapies. The division worked with OAM to identify alternative medical practitioners to serve, along with more conventional scientists, on the panels. The division also kept statistics on the nature of the applicants, noting, for example, that nearly two-thirds held a Ph.D. or an M.D. and that very few applicants were members of underrepresented minority groups, even though some members of these groups do use alternative medical practices.

The eight panels conducted the initial review of the grant applications. OAM originally intended that the applications then be reviewed by members of the Ad Hoc Advisory Panel on Alternative Medicine; however, this step turned out to be disallowed by Government regulations. Instead, the second review was carried out by OAM staff members. OAM then submitted a list of recommended grantees to the National Advisory Research Resources Council; this is the advisory council of NIH's National Center for Research Resources, which has grantmaking authority and which is accustomed to dealing with a broad range of subjects. The advisory council accepted OAM's recommendations, and the 30 grant awards were announced in fall 1993.

**Based on presentations by D. Eskinazi (OAM) and F. Calhoun (DRG) to the July 14–15, 1993, meeting of the Ad Hoc Advisory Panel to the Office of Alternative Medicine, and on followup interviews.*

broad spectrum of alternative medicine practices, and basic and clinical scientists who have balanced perspectives and can offer an objective opinion on methodological issues related to applications from practitioners of alternative medicine. Consequently, DRG should be asked to set up a model for the peer review process that allows a balanced evaluation of science that is outside of traditional or mainstream thinking.

Specific steps to improve the review process include the following:

- OAM should recruit experts within the alternative medical community who are willing to review and give advice on applications prior to their being formally submitted.
- Ad hoc study section members should be selected by the criteria already established by NIH for regular review groups, with these additional provisions:
  - For alternative medicine practitioners the "equivalent" to a doctoral degree can include board certification in their field.
  - Where there is no board, special approval on the basis of expertise and experience may be needed.
  - The presence of healthy skeptics is essential to adequate review, but it is necessary to screen out obviously antagonistic reviewers.
- During the initial phases of OAM's operation, its staff should participate in decisions concerning the referral process. To achieve this, OAM and DRG staffs will need to cooperate in deciding either to send each proposal to the OAM initial peer review panel or, if feasible, to route it through the regular NIH grant process. When a program analyst sends the alternative medical grant proposal to DRG, the analyst could assist the process within the division—for instance, by making recommendations for appropriate reviewers to participate in the ad hoc study section.
- For the first few years, an initial OAM review panel (i.e., a special or ad hoc study section) should function to review grant applications that do not fit the criteria for existing DRG study sections.
- On the basis of the experience of the initial review section, NIH should then establish an official ad hoc panel within either DRG or OAM. It is anticipated that the ad hoc panel would function for up to 5 years.
- Ultimately, an initial review group (or study section) should be established for OAM within DRG. If the OAM evolved to center status, initial review groups could be established within the Center for Alternative Medicine to review training grants, center grants, RFAs, and so on.
  - The reviewers of any application should include at least one expert in the discipline specified in the application.
  - The entire review section should be at least 50 percent composed of clinicians or researchers from the various types of alternative medical practice groups, such as bioelectromagnetics, acupuncture, homeopathy, and lifestyle interventions.
- Because it is possible that some errors did occur in the 1993 RFA review process, it is recommended that an ad hoc review committee be drawn from members of OAM's new mandated advisory council and from methodologists knowledgeable in alternative practices to review a randomized sample of the studies that were proposed. If this effort reveals that errors did occur, the committee should then develop guidelines to help future peer review committees dealing with alternative medical subjects.
- Since the problem of appropriate peer selection is ongoing, a select committee should be established to continually review the makeup of the peer review panels. (This committee is a logical outgrowth of the ad hoc review committee proposed in the preceding paragraph.)
- OAM should encourage DRG to develop a *workable* and effective NIH appeals process—one that allows due process.

References

Hazelwood, C.F. 1992. Personal communication.

Hazelwood, C.F. 1993. Personal communication.

Horrobin, D.F. 1990. The philosophical basis of peer review and the suppression of innovation. JAMA 263(10):1438-1441.

Ling, G.N. 1992. A Revolution in the Physiology of the Living Cell. Krieger Publishing Co., Melbourne, Fla.

Public Information Activities

by Richard Pavek

According to Section 404E (d) (1) of the June 1993 amendments to the Public Health Service Act, the Office of Alternative Medicine (OAM) is to "establish an information clearinghouse to exchange information with the public about alternative medicine." This chapter of the report deals with implementation of that directive and other public information activities.[1]

As vital as research databases are to the researcher, information libraries are of equal importance to the clinician, physician, and patient; without information there is no way a physician or patient can make truly informed choices. (Obviously, databases for consumers and practitioners differ from research databases in scope, language, complexity, and intent even though they may share many of the same materials.) An accessible database of alternative medicine information is a vital need for the American public. Except for current efforts at OAM, the National Institutes of Health (NIH) does not currently maintain a special information service for consumers wanting information on alternative medicine.[2]

Nevertheless, several institutes at NIH, as well as some other Federal agencies, include alternative medical practices in some of their information. The National Institute of Neurological Disorders and Stroke includes acupuncture and psychological techniques; the National AIDS Information Clearinghouse, information on nutrition strategies; the National Institute of Mental Health, information on biofeedback; and the National Cancer Institute, information on chaparral tea and other medicinal herbs. Outside NIH auspices, the Science and Technology Division, Reference Section, of the Library of Congress has reference guides to acupuncture and medicinal plants, among others.

A national clearinghouse would provide a clear, concise message for the broader health care community, as well as interested members of the lay public, about the benefits of alternative medicine based on a body of scientific information that is current, accurate, and complete. Thus, a National Library of Medicine (NLM) alternative medicine clearinghouse would provide a gateway for knowledge transfer to several audiences: health care practitioners, policymakers, educators, and the public at large.

Current Information Sources on Alternative Medicine

Doctor's Office

Unfortunately, most health information currently available to consumers comes from the conventional medical practitioner's office in the form of leaflets provided as a "public service" by the American Medical Association or by drug companies. The rare citation of any alternative medical practices usually mentions biofeedback or massage. A few medical practitioners with alternative interests do provide a range of relevant material.

Health Newsletters

Some major medical schools publish "health newsletters," which are sold by subscription to the public. Although these newsletters often carry prestigious faculty names under the masthead, the newsletter is usually edited and published by independent publishing houses. If alternative medical practices are mentioned, it is usually in the context of urging caution in using them because they are unresearched. Some newsletters are stridently against alternative medicine.

---

[1]*This report recognizes that researchers in alternative medicine have different information needs from the general public. Recommendations to address these needs are discussed in the "Research Databases" chapter.*

[2]*OAM has begun to conduct an informal clearinghouse, responding to the hundreds of phone call inquiries it receives each week requesting information about alternative therapies and research.*

Directories and Guides

A number of books available on the retail market index and describe alternative medical practices. These books vary in comprehensiveness and usability.[3]

Magazines and Newspapers

Consumer Reports recently published a three-part 1994 series, "Alternative Medicine: The Facts" (volume 59, January, March, and June). Other magazines of general interest frequently publish similar articles, and certain specialty magazines are even more likely to do so, including, for example, *New Age Journal, East West Journal,* and *Yoga Journal.* The *New York Times* and other newspapers sometimes publish articles on alternative medicine, especially on diet, supplements, and mind-body approaches.

Private Sector Databases

Several private sector databases in use in the United States cover alternative medical practices. The databases are organized in different formats. Some of the best known are listed here:

- Wellnet is an electronic allied health professional database.
- IBIS is a hypertext database that includes information on conditions and treatment approaches used by alternative practitioners in such fields as homeopathy, naturopathy, nutrition, oriental botanicals, osteopathy, physical medicine, psychosocial therapies, Western botanicals, and biofield therapies.
- Herbalgram is a consumer- and physician-oriented reference library on herbal botanicals.
- The *Brain-Mind Bulletin* maintains a reference library that includes listings on a wide range of subjects, most of which are alternative medicine issues.
- *Alternative Medical Connection* is a new journal of alternative medicine with an online database available to consumers and clinicians.

Inappropriate Regulations

Regulations sometimes keep important information about the potential benefits of alternative agents from consumers. For example, the present policy of the Food and Drug Administration (FDA) is to allow the sale of herbal medicines provided that no information is included on the conditions for which they are to be used. Although this policy addresses the technicality of current laws, it leaves the consumer vulnerable to misapplication of herbal medications.

Development of an Information Clearinghouse

OAM will have to collaborate with appropriate NIH agencies as well as others, such as the Agency for Health Care Policy and Research and the National Center for Health Statistics, to collect information on the extent and pattern of utilization and on cost-effectiveness of alternative medical practices. This cooperation may be implemented by adding alternative medical questions to existing statistical instruments, or it may involve a separate effort.

Information will have to be gathered from a wide range of sources. To assess the extent of consumer use of, and satisfaction with, over-the-counter interventions, practitioner-independent approaches may be helpful. For example, patients fill out questionnaires to assess treatments offered through "buyers clubs," such as those operated for persons with HIV and AIDS and chronic fatigue syndrome (also known as chronic fatigue immune dysfunction syndrome). Practitioner-independent approaches may be in widespread use in the community but have never received investigation in controlled clinical trials.

---

[3]*Examples of recent books: (1) British Holistic Medical Association. 1986–1990.* Holistic Medicine, *5 vols. Wiley, Sussex, England. (2) Burroughs, K., and M. Kastner. 1993.* Alternative Healing: The Complete A–Z Guide to Over 160 Different Alternative Therapies. *Halcyon, La Mesa, Calif. 356 pp. (3) Drury, N. 1981.* The Healing Power: A Handbook of Alternative Medicine and Natural Health. *Frederick Muller, London. 231 pp. (4) Hafen, B.Q., and K.J. Frandsen. 1983.* From Acupuncture to Yoga: Alternative Methods of Healing. *Prentice-Hall, Englewood Cliffs, N.J. 135 pp. (5) Linde, S., and D.J. Carrow, eds. 1985.* Directory of Holistic Medicine and Alternate Health Care Services in the U.S. *Health Plus, Phoenix, Ariz. 262 pp. (6) Lyng, S. 1990.* Holistic Health and Biomedical Medicine: A Countersystem Analysis. *State University of New York Press, Albany, N.Y. 268 pp. (7) Olsen, K. 1991.* The Encyclopedia of Alternative Health Care. *Platkus, London. 330 pp. (8) Weil, A. 1983.* Health and Healing: Understanding Conventional and Alternative Medicine. *Houghton Mifflin, Boston. 296 pp.*

Accessing Information

Information will have to be made available to consumers through various means. Electronic access through America OnLine, CompuServe, Genie, and Prodigy will likely be very useful.

However, since not all consumers have access to home computers, other means will be required to provide information to the general public—for example, through print information, CD-ROM disks at public libraries, and other community outlets.

Media Activities

A noteworthy shift in media attitudes toward alternative medicine since the early 1990s is attributable to the establishment of OAM. NIH should be supported in its endeavors in this area, and OAM should be encouraged to continue its efforts to increase awareness of alternative medicine among the scientific and lay media.

Among other duties, the OAM public information officer should

- initiate and maintain regular mailings of worth to selected medical journals of note;
- notify interested associations and groups of impending OAM activities;
- promptly circulate minutes of the meetings of the OAM Advisory Council to interested associations and individuals; and
- function as a speakers bureau by maintaining and coordinating a list of available speakers, including members of the OAM staff, members of the OAM Advisory Council, and other known alternative medicine spokespersons.

Recommendations

OAM should convene a committee of advisory panel members; OAM staff members; experts on database development; technical, organizational, and legal experts; and others to develop a workable plan to implement the public information clearinghouse mandated by Congress. To coordinate efforts and avoid expensive redundancy, the committee should include a member of the parallel committee that will plan the research database associated with NLM.

Since many institutes at NIH have clearinghouses, it is advisable to survey several of them to discover the methods they have found appropriate. Representatives from appropriate ones should be invited to meet with the committee.

The committee should address issues such as the following:

- Scope of available resources.
- Inclusion of future data.
- Search and indexing mechanisms suitable for the general consumer (for electronic databases).
- Intellectual property and copyright issues.
- Fees for inclusion of material.
- User fees.
- Hard-copy retrieval methods.
- Electronic access routes.
- Comparative costs of possible approaches.
- Ethical issues.
- Qualitative review for inclusion.
- Costs of qualitative reviews.

Specifically, OAM should do the following:

- Develop a consumer-oriented computerized inquiry system devoted to alternative medicine. This system would be similar to health consumer subsections of America OnLine and CompuServe, such as the Cancer Forum. Initially it might be based on an existing public information database, such as that operated by *Brain-Mind Bulletin*.
- Develop hard-copy (i.e., printed) materials for distribution to the public.
- Maintain a source within OAM to disseminate alternative medical materials and to field questions from the media and others.
- Supply treatment information for herbal medicinals, which (in accordance with current FDA policy) are currently packaged without use instructions. (Including use information on the package is a violation of current FDA rules.) Such a reference document, which is legal, would be of considerable benefit to the public.

Part III
Conclusion, Appendixes, Glossary, and Index

Conclusion

This report has covered a broad spectrum of alternative medical therapies and systems of medicine. Some of these medical systems, such as Ayurvedic medicine and traditional oriental medicine, are centuries old and are still in extensive use in other nations and cultures of the world. Others, such as osteopathy and naturopathy, evolved in the United States in the not-too-distant past but were relegated to the fringes of medicine because they differed from conventional biomedicine in the concepts of health and illness they embraced. Still others, such as some of the mind-body and bioelectromagnetic approaches, are on the frontier of scientific knowledge and understanding.

Many alternative practitioners face numerous economic, political, and scientific barriers that block their acceptance by mainstream biomedicine. On the other hand, some alternative medical practitioners do not expect to be brought into the fold. Rather, they just want the opportunity to coexist peacefully with mainstream medical practitioners and to be allowed to offer consumers alternative health care options. Consumers, however, are not waiting for mainstream science to give them a "green light" on many alternative treatments before using them. The fact is that today alternative medicine constitutes a significant and growing portion of the Nation's health care expenditures.

Recent surveys have demonstrated that most people who opt to use alternative treatments or systems of medicine believe that conventional medicine has not adequately addressed their needs, or they want to supplement and thus improve on their conventional treatment. This is especially true of people with chronic, debilitating illnesses such as arthritis, pain, cancer, and AIDS. People often are attracted to alternative medicine practitioners who emphasize the patient's role in the healing process as well as the importance of the patient-practitioner interaction.

Studies also show that individuals who seek out and use alternative medical treatments tend to be the better educated and the more affluent. Thus the stereotype of the alternative medicine consumer as an uneducated, poor person succumbing to the sideshow lures of quacks and charlatans appears to be greatly overblown. The reality is that because patients, in general, are demanding more health care options at a lower cost, a growing number of conventionally trained American physicians have already begun incorporating alternative medical modalities into their everyday medical practices.

The dominant biomedical U.S. health care system has made countless technological discoveries and innovations in the past half century, revolutionizing the way the body, the mind, and the environment are viewed. By all measures, however, it is an extremely expensive system offering limited accessibility. In other words, the patients who have the most money and live nearest the best health care facilities often receive the best care. Increasingly, this situation will dictate that the elderly, the disadvantaged, people with chronic illnesses, and the very young go without adequate health care—the populations that need health care most.

One of the simplest and most effective ways to significantly lower health care costs and thus increase access is through a major focus on preventive medicine. In this clinical arena, many of the alternative health care systems may have much to offer. Homeopathic and naturopathic physicians, for example, strongly advise their patients about diet and other health-promoting lifestyle choices as a matter of routine care. In contrast, many conventional physicians do not routinely give such advice until a patient has already become chronically ill, by which time the patient may need expensive high-tech surgery and face a lifetime of expensive drug therapy.

Another major factor contributing to the skyrocketing health care costs in this country is the amount of time involved in officially certifying a drug or medical intervention as clinically effective and safe. Millions of dollars may be spent, and years may pass, before a potentially lifesaving drug, instrument, or intervention winds its way through the complex Federal approval process. That same process too often ignores or discounts related, potentially valuable Canadian,

European, and Asian data that could significantly shorten the assessment process.

In addition, standards of testing drugs and therapies in the United States are inconsistent with standards in many other technologically developed countries. For example, U.S. regulations on testing herbal medicines require a much more circuitous testing process than is required overseas. There, evidence of prior use without adverse side effects may be accepted by medical authorities without data from extensive clinical trials; preliminary clinical trials can therefore focus immediately on the *effectiveness* of the herbal remedy. In the United States, however, Phase I trials focus solely on safety issues, and effectiveness is not dealt with until much later.

Furthermore, in many European and Asian countries it is completely acceptable to test an herbal extract as a single drug rather than require every potentially active ingredient in the plant to be tested, as is the rule in the United States. Thus in other developed countries significantly less time and cost often are involved in bringing a potentially beneficial herbal or naturally occurring remedy to market.

As U.S. consumers continue to use alternative medicine, the challenge for health care policymakers and Federal regulators is not only to protect the public from unscrupulous medical practitioners but also to ensure the public's access to the most effective treatments available. Certainly, patients should have recourse if it can be shown that their practitioners or the treatments they offer have no clinical or psychological benefit. By the same token, patients with debilitating severe or chronic illnesses should have the right to have access to—as well as insurance to cover—an alternative therapy they believe offers them relief.

Many of the alternative therapies described and discussed in this report—hypnosis, art therapy, music therapy, chiropractic, massage therapy, acupuncture, and many herbal and nutritional supplementations, to name a few—have already received extensive and positive clinical evaluations. However, no critical mass of researchers, clinicians, and policymakers has formed to give them more exposure and recognition. Therefore, many of these therapies should be included in any serious discussions about developing a truly comprehensive health care system. Others, as the report has indicated, need to be quickly and thoroughly evaluated before any judgment can be passed. However, they still may represent a great and largely untapped resource for improving the Nation's health.

Appendix A
Participants at the Unconventional Medical Practices Workshop

Westfields International Conference Center
Chantilly, VA

September 14–16, 1992

Jeanne Achterberg, Ph.D.
Professor of Psychology
Saybrook Institute
San Francisco, CA

Irene Ansher, M.A.
Executive Director
Employee Assistance Coordination Organization
Potomac, MD

L. Eugene Arnold, M.D.
Special Expert
National Institute of Mental Health
Los Angeles, CA

Raymond Bahor, Ph.D.
Associate Chief
Division of Research Grants, NIH
Bethesda, MD

Becky Barbatsis, M.P.H.
Bethesda, MD

Ellen Barlow
Movement Therapist
Association for Body-Mind Centering
New York, NY

R. James Barnard, Ph.D.
Professor and Vice Chair
Department of Physiological Science
University of California, Los Angeles

Feneydoon Batmanghewidj, M.D.
Global Health Solutions

Robert Becker, M.D.
Lowville, NY

Berkley Bedell
Former Congressman
Spirit Lake, IA

Barbara Bemie, L.Ac.
President
American Foundation of Traditional Chinese Medicine
San Francisco, CA

Katy Benjamin, S.M., M.S.W.
Social Science Analyst
Agency for Health Care Policy and Research
Rockville, MD

Brian M. Berman, M.D.
Director
University of Maryland Pain Center
University of Maryland School of Medicine
Baltimore, MD

Robert Beutlich
President
U.S. Psychotronics Association
Chicago, IL

Stephen Birch
Research Director
New England School of Acupuncture
Watertown, MA

Richard A. Bloch
R.A. Bloch Cancer Foundation
Kansas City, MO

Gerard Bodeker, Ed.D.
Director of Research
Lancaster Foundation
Fairfield, IA

Dean Bonlie, D.D.S.
President
Magnetico, Inc.
Calgary, Alberta
Canada

Jay P. Borneman, M.S., M.B.A.
American Association of Homeopathic Pharmacists
Bryn Mawr, PA

Myrin Borysenko, Ph.D.
Executive Director
Mind Body Health Sciences
Scituate, MA

Jane B. Brady, M.S.
Well Mind Association
Silver Spring, MD

Carol Brenholtz, M.S.S.W.
Center for Mind-Body Studies
Washington, DC

Barbara A. Brennan, M.S.
Founder
Barbara Brennan School of Healing
East Hampton, NY

Seymour Brenner, M.D.
Radiation Oncologist
Director
Radiation Therapy
Peninsula Hospital
Brooklyn, NY

Robert Brink, Ph.D.
Psychologist
Sykesville, MD

Dannion H. Brinkley
Director
Theater of the Mind
Anniston, AL

Beverly Britton-Elkashef
Biofeedback Therapist
Behavioral Science Association
Association for Applied Psychophysiology and Biofeedback
Baltimore, MD

Rosalyn L. Bruyere, D.D.
Director
Healing Light Center Church
Sierra Madre, CA

Carola Burroughs
Health Educator
Brooklyn AIDS Task Force
Brooklyn, NY

Stanislaw Rajmund Burzynski, M.D., Ph.D.
President
Burzynski Research Institute, Inc.
Houston, TX

Dwight Byers
President
International Institute of Reflexology
Saint Petersburg, FL

Al Bymanis
Director of Public Relations
National Association for Music Therapy
Silver Spring, MD

Carlo Calabrese, N.D., M.P.H.
Chair
Research Department
Bastyr College
Seattle, WA

Faye J. Calhoun
Deputy Chief for Review
Division of Research Grants, NIH
Bethesda, MD

James A. Caplan
President
CAPMED/USA
Bryn Mawr, PA

Aimee L. Carruth
Partner-Cofounder
Wellness Design
Evergreen, CO

Claire Cassidy, Ph.D.
Director
Social Research
Traditional Acupuncture Institute
Bethesda, MD

Barrie R. Cassileth, Ph.D.
Consulting Professor
Community and Family Medicine
Duke University Medical Center
Chapel Hill, NC

Edward H. Chapman, M.D.
President
American Institute of Homeopathy
Newton, MA

Deepak Chopra, M.D.
Author
South Lancaster, MA

Effie Poy Yew Chow, Ph.D., C.A.
President
East West Academy of Healing Arts
San Francisco, CA

Peter Chowka
San Diego, CA

George V. Coecho, Ph.D.
Chief
International Activities
Alcohol, Drug Abuse, and Mental Health Administration
Rockville, MD

Roger B. Cohen, M.D.
Staff Fellow
Division of Cytokine Biology
Center for Biologics Evaluation and Research
Food and Drug Administration
Bethesda, MD

Mary Colligan-Stiff, B.A.
Legislative Analyst
Food and Drug Administration
Rockville, MD

Jonathan Collin, M.D.
Editor
Townsend Letter for Doctors
Physician, Private Practice
Port Townsend, WA

Serafina Corsello, M.D.
Executive Medical Director
Corsello Centers for Nutritional-Complementary Medicine
Huntington, NY

Jerry Cott, Ph.D.
Chief, Psychotherapeutic Drug Discovery and Development Program
National Institute of Mental Health
Rockville, MD

Martha Clayton Cottrall, M.D.
Kushi Institute
Becket, MA

Harris L. Coulter, Ph.D.
President
Center for Empirical Medicine
Washington, DC

Jim Cox, D.Th.
Bethesda, MD

Michael L. Culbert, D.Sc.
Vice President/Information
American Biologics-Mexico SA
Chula Vista, CA

E. Morgan Culliton
Alexandria, VA

Patricia D. Culliton, M.A., Dipl.Ac.
Acupuncture Researcher
Hennepin County Medical Center
Minneapolis, MN

Jonathan Davidson, M.D.
Director
Anxiety and Traumatic Stress Program
Duke University Medical Center
Durham, NC

Etel E. DeLoach
President
Aesculapian Institute for Healing Arts, Inc.
Lilburn, GA

Alan Demmerle, M.S.E.E.
Director
Rolf Institute
Chevy Chase, MD

Patrick M. Donovan, N.D.
Academic Faculty
John Bastyr College
Seattle, WA

Larry Dossey, M.D.
Dallas Diagnostic Association
Santa Fe, NM

Robert Duggan
President
Traditional Acupuncture Institute, Inc.
Columbia, MD

Sherry Dupere, Ph.D.
Health Scientist Administrator
Fogarty International Center, NIH
Bethesda, MD

Michael Eck, M.S.
Consumer Safety Officer
Food and Drug Administration
Rockville, MD

David Eisenberg, M.D.
Instructor in Medicine
Department of Medicine
Harvard Medical School
Beth Israel Hospital
Boston, MA

Jacquelyn Eisenberg, M.D.
President
Mind-Body Medicine Engineering Research Institute
Madison, VA

John M. Ellis, M.D.
Medical Director of Clinical Research
Titus County Hospital
Mt. Pleasant, TX

Judy Epstein
Nurse Massage Therapist
National Association of Nurse Massage Therapists (NANMT)
Tucson, AZ

Mary Lee Esty, M.S.W.
Center for Mind-Body Studies
Chevy Chase, MD

Helga Fallis
Publisher/Producer
"Health Links"
Arlington, VA

Mary A. Foulkes, Ph.D.
Mathematical Statistician
National Institute of Allergy and Infectious Diseases, NIH
Bethesda, MD

Winston Franklin
Executive Vice President
Institute of Noetic Sciences
Sausalito, CA

Allan H. Frey, Ph.D.
Chairman of the Board
Randomline, Inc.
Potomac, MD

Viola M. Frymann, D.O.
Director
Osteopathic Center for Children
La Jolla, CA

Adriane Fugh-Berman, M.D.
Taoist Health Institute
Washington, DC

Alan Gaby, M.D.
Board of Trustees
American Holistic Medical Association
Pikesville, MD

Marie Galbraith, B.A.
Gerson Clinic
People Against Cancer
New York, NY

Nath Gary
Attorney
Mueller Medical International
Toronto, Canada

Satip Ghosh, B.S.
Center for Mind-Body Studies
Bethesda, MD

Natalie Golos
Associate Fellow
American Academy of Environmental Medicine
Derwood, MD

James S. Gordon, M.D.
Clinical Professor
Department of Psychiatry and Community and Family Medicine
Georgetown University School of Medicine
Director, Center for Mind-Body Studies
Washington, DC

Richard J. Grable, E.E., M.B.A.
Vice President
Research and Development
Lintronics Technologies, Inc.
Tampa, FL

Elliott Greene, M.A.
President
American Massage Therapy Association
Silver Spring, MD

Howard C. Greenspan
Annandale, NJ

Mary Gregg, M.S., M.B.A.
Cancer Program Specialist
National Cancer Institute, NIH
Bethesda, MD

M. Linden Griffith
Director
Washington Seniors Wellness Center
Washington, DC

Stephen Groft, Pharm.D.
Acting Director
Office of Alternative Medicine, NIH
Bethesda, MD

Debra Grossman, M.A.
Project Officer
National Institute on Drug Abuse, NIH
Silver Spring, MD

Barry L. Gruber, Ph.D.
Psychologist
Medical Illness Counseling CT
Annapolis, MD

John Hammel
Member
Health Resources Council
Morristown, NJ

Pat Hancock
Tai Chi Teacher
Body Balance
Clarksburg, MD

Sandra Harner, Ph.D.
Director of Health Research
Foundation for Shamanic Studies
Westport, CT

Thomas E. Harries, Ph.D.
National Manager, TQI R&D
National VA Chaplain Center
Department of Veterans Affairs
Veterans Affairs Medical Center
Hampton, VA

D. Warren Harrison, M.D.
Director
African Basic Food (Uganda) Limited
National Nutrition Program
AIDS Research
Hedgesville, WV

Carlton Hazlewood, Ph.D.
Professor
Molecular Physiology and Biophysics
Baylor College of Medicine
Houston, TX

Carol Hegedus, M.S., M.A.
Director of Institutional Relations
Fetzer Institute
Kalamazoo, MI

Max Heirich, Ph.D.
Associate Professor and Associate Research Scientist
University of Michigan
Ann Arbor, MI

Mimi Herrmann
President
Quanta Dynamics
Research Investigator
University of Louisville Medical School
Louisville, KY

Mary Hessler, Ph.D.
President
Lintronics Technologies, Inc.
Tampa, FL

Yong Hi, M.D., M.P.H.
President
International Chinese Traditional Medicine Exchange Association
Baltimore, MD

Richard Z. Hicole
Rockville, MD

Gar Hildenbrand
Executive Director
Gerson Research Organization
San Diego, CA

Peter Hinderberger, M.D.
President
Physicians' Association for Anthroposophical Medicine
Baltimore, MD

Sandy Hoar
Physician Assistant
George Washington University
Mind Body Center
Hyattsville, MD

Judith Ann Horman
National Foundation for Cancer Research
Bethesda, MD

David B. Howe
Executive Vice President
Lintronics Technologies, Inc.
Tampa, FL

Paul Hower, M.S.
President
ESS, Inc.
Atlanta, GA

Tori Hudson, N.D.
Associate Academic Dean
National College of Naturopathic Medicine
Portland, OR

Morgan Jackson, M.D.
Medical Officer
Agency for Health Care Policy and Research
Rockville, MD

Jennifer Jacobs, M.D.
Department of Epidemiology
University of Washington School of Public Health
Edmonds, WA

Joseph J. Jacobs, M.D.
Director–designate
Office of Alternative Medicine, NIH
Bethesda, MD

Norma Jennings
Light and Living Series
Silver Spring, MD

Gary Johnson
Spring Valley, NY

Wayne B. Jonas, M.D.
Training Director
Medical Research Fellowship
Walter Reed Army Institute of Research
Walter Reed Army Medical Center
Washington, DC

C.B. Scott Jones, Ph.D.
President
Human Potential Foundation
Vienna, VA

George W. Jones, M.D.
Professor
Urology
American University
American Cancer Society—Unproven Methods Committee
Washington, DC

Judi Jones
University of Michigan Medical School
Ann Arbor, MI

William Kammerer, M.D.
Anesthesia Section
Clinical Center, NIH
Bethesda, MD

Paul Kanofsky, Ph.D.
Systems Analyst
University of Medicine and Dentistry of New Jersey
Newark, NJ

Ted Kaptchuk
Research Associate
Beth Israel Hospital
Cambridge, MA

Patrice Keane
Executive Director
American Society for Psychical Research
New York, NY

George Kindness, Ph.D.
Laboratory Director/Immunologist
Great Lakes Association of Clinical Medicine
Bluffton, OH

M. Lucille Kinlein
Founder
Profession of Esca
Hyattsville, MD

Dorothy A. Kinzey, Ph.D.
Psychologist
Self-employed
Arlington, VA

Kenneth A. Klivington, Ph.D.
Assistant to the President
Salk Institute for Biological Research
La Jolla, CA

Fredi Kronenberg, Ph.D.
Assistant Professor
College of Physicians and Surgeons
Columbia University
New York, NY

Midge Krowiz
President
Taylor Associates
Fielding Institute
Vienna, VA

James R. Kuperberg, Ph.D.
Principal
Kuperberg Consulting Group
Reston, VA

Jody F. Kusek
Food and Drug Administration
Rockville, MD

Joseph S. Latino, Ph.D.
Director
Special Hematology/Oncology Laboratories
Brooklyn Hospital Center
Brooklyn, NY

Floyd E. Leaders, Jr., Ph.D.
President
The Leaders Group
Gaithersburg, MD

Peter Lechner, M.D., F.A.C.A.
Second Department of General Surgery
Public Hospital of Graz
Austria

David Yue-Wei Lee, Ph.D.
Senior Scientist
Research Triangle Institute
Research Triangle Park, NC

Rachel Levinson
Office of Science Policy and Legislation, OD, NIH
Bethesda, MD

Spafford Lewis, B.A., M.S.
Healer
Center at Center Valley
Center Valley, PA

Abraham R. Liboff, Ph.D.
Professor of Physics
Director of Medical Physics
Oakland University
Rochester, MI

Christeene Lindsay-Hildenbrand
Research Associate
Gerson Research Organization
San Diego, CA

Wayne A. Little, B.S.
Writer
National Institute of Dental Research, NIH
Bethesda, MD

Nancy Lonsdorf, M.D.
Medical Director
Maharishi Ayur-Veda Medical Center
Washington, DC

Darrcy A. Loveland, J.D.
Legislative Counsel
American Art Therapy Association
American Dance Therapy Association
Laguna Beach, CA

Carl D. Lytle, Ph.D.
Research Biophysicist
Food and Drug Administration
Rockville, MD

Kyriacos C. Markides, Ph.D.
Professor
Department of Sociology
University of Maine
Orono, ME

Linda Markush, M.P.H.
Silver Spring, MD

Reverend Phyllis B. Martin
Maryland State Representative and Tri Area Coordinator
National Federation of Spiritual Healers of America
Clinton, MD

Robert S. McCaleb
President
Herb Research Foundation
Boulder, CO

Gladys Taylor McGarey, M.D.
President
Beth Taylor Foundation
Scottsdale Holistic Medical Group
Scottsdale, AZ

Michael E. McGinnis, Ph.D.
Assistant Professor
Department of Biology
Spelman College
Atlanta, GA

Kevin McNamee, D.C., L.Ac.
Director
Center for Oriental Medical Research and Education
San Diego, CA

Ted D. Miller, D.O.
Osteopathic Physician
Private Practice
Silver Spring, MD

Kaiya Montaocean
Co-Director
Center for Natural and Traditional Medicine
Washington, DC

Jay Moskowitz, Ph.D.
Associate Director for Science Policy and Legislation
Office of the Director, NIH
Bethesda, MD

Ralph W. Moss, Ph.D.
Editor
The Cancer Chronicles
New York, NY

Patricia Muehsam, M.D.
Bioelectrochemistry Laboratory
Department of Orthopaedics
Mt. Sinai School of Medicine
New York, NY

Laura Nader, Ph.D.
Professor of Anthropology
Department of Anthropology
University of California, Berkeley
Berkeley, CA

Avery Nelson, Ph.D.
Bethesda, MD

Eta R. Nelson, B.S.
Researcher
Taste and Smell Clinic
Falls Church, VA

Roger Nelson, Ph.D.
Research Staff
Princeton Engineering Anomalies Research
Princeton University School of Engineering
Princeton, NJ

Sandra Occhipinti, B.S.
Technical Information Specialist
National Institute of Child Health and Human Development, NIH
Bethesda, MD

Judith A. O'Connell, D.O.
President
American Academy of Osteopathy
Dayton, OH

Bonnie B. O'Connor, Ph.D.
Assistant Professor
Community and Preventive Medicine
Medical College of Pennsylvania
Philadelphia, PA

Kathern H. Oddenino
President and Director
LIFEFORCE Corporation
A Holistic Health Retreat Center
Annapolis, MD

Anthony Paul Ortega
PHA-Traditional Medicine Specialist
Indian Health Services
Public Health Service
Rockville, MD

A. Michael Parfitt, M.D.
Bone and Mineral Research Laboratory
Henry Ford Hospital
Detroit, MI

Michael M. Patterson, Ph.D.
Professor of Osteopathic Medicine
College of Osteopathic Medicine
Ohio University
Athens, OH

Sally J. Phillips, Ph.D.
Professor
Department of Kinesiology
University of Maryland at College Park
College Park, MD

William H. Philpott, M.D.
Chairman
Institutional Review Board
Bio Electro Magnetic Institute
Reno, NV

Kenneth Pittaway, N.D., Ph.D.
President
National Institute of Natural Health Sciences
De Pere, WI

Curt Pospisk
Program Analyst
National Institute of Neurological Disorders
and Stroke, NIH
Bethesda, MD

Vera Pratt
Co-Director
Center for Natural and Traditional Medicines
Washington, DC

Peter Preuss
President
Preuss Foundation for Brain Tumor Research
Solana Beach, CA

R.E. Prumphrey, M.D.
Clinical Professor
George Washington University
Washington, DC

John C. Reed, M.D.
American Academy of Medical Acupuncture
Phoenix, AZ

Mary Faith Rhoads, B.A.
The Center at Center Valley
Center Valley, PA

Teresa Simons Robinson
Writer
Arlington, VA

Anthony L. Rosner, Ph.D.
Director of Research
Foundation for Chiropractic Education and Research
Arlington, VA

Beverly Rubik, Ph.D.
Director
Center for Frontier Sciences
Temple University
Philadelphia, PA

John B.K. Rutayuga, Ph.D.
Co-Director
Center for Natural and Traditional Medicines
Washington, DC

Helen M. Ryan
Representative
American Indian Health Clinic
La Jolla, CA

David M. Sale, J.D., LL.M
Reiki Foundation
Arnold, MD

Nelda Samarel, R.N., Ed.D.
Associate Professor
William Paterson College of New Jersey
Wayne, NJ

Kenneth M. Sancier, Ph.D.
Vice President
Qigong Institute of
East West Academy Healing Arts
Menlo Park, CA

Savely L. Sawa
Executive Director
Monterey Institute for the Study of Alternative
Healing Arts
Monterey, CA

Sharon Scandrett-Hibdon, Ph.D.
President-Elect
American Holistic Nurses' Association
Associate Professor
University of Tennessee, Memphis
Collierville, TN

Paul Scharff, M.D.
Medical Director
Rudolf Steiner Fellowship Foundation
American College of Anthroposophically
Extended Medicine
Spring Valley, NY

Marilyn Schlitz, Ph.D.
Department of Anthropology
University of Texas, Austin
Mico, TX

Gertrude Schmeidler, Ph.D.
Professor Emeritus, City College
City University of New York
Hastings-on-Hudson, NY

Dorothy R. Schultz
President
Hypoglycemia Association, Inc.
Ashton, MD

Mangala Searles
Director
Natural Therapeutics
Austin, TX

Pam Selle, Ph.D.
Planning Office
Office of the Director, NIH
Bethesda, MD

Grace Shen, Ph.D.
Program Director
National Cancer Institute, NIH
Bethesda, MD

Oscar Carl Simonton, M.D.
Medical Director
Simonton Cancer Center
Pacific Palisades, CA

Janet I. Smith
President
National Wellness Coalition
Washington, DC

Sheleyh Smith, M.P.H.
Public Health Educator
National Institute of Mental Health, NIH
Rockville, MD

Sharon Snider
Public Affairs Specialist
Press Office
Food and Drug Administration
Rockville, MD

Edward Sopcak
Howell, MI

Robert F. Spiegel
Director
Psycho-Medical Chirologists
Silver Spring, MD

Leanna Standish, N.D., Ph.D.
Director of Research
Bastyr College of Natural Health Sciences
Seattle, WA

Daphne Stegmaier, B.A.
New Hope
Wheaton, MD

John Stegmaier
New Hope
Wheaton, MD

Vernon M. Sylvest, M.D.
Director
Institute of Higher Healing
Richmond, VA

James Tanner, P.D.
Chief
Nutrient Surveillance Branch
Food and Drug Administration
Washington, DC

Liz Tarr, B.A.
Baltimore, MD

Jack O. Taylor, D.C.
Dr. Taylor's Wellness Center
Arlington Heights, IL

Jack Thomas, S.T.M.
Editor
Maryland Bodywork Reporter
Thurmont, MD

Virginia Thompson, D.C.
Chiropractor
Countryside, VA

James C. Torgersen, M.D., D.Sc.
Dean, Wellness College
Director, Wellness Center
Hawthorne Foundation
Hawthorne University
Salt Lake City, UT

Wayne Trainer, B.A.
Health-Fitness Pioneer
Healthy Frameworkes
Garner, NC

Eleanor M. Vogt, Ph.D.
Vice President
National Pharmaceutical Council
Reston, VA

Jon D. Vredevoogd
Associate Professor
Michigan State University/ Upledger Institute
East Lansing, MI

Jeremy Waletzky, M.D.
Associate Clinical Professor
George Washington University
Washington, DC

Morton Walker, D.P.M.
Medical Journalist
Freelance Communications
Stanford, CT

Jan Walleczek, Ph.D
Staff Scientist
Research Service-151
Veterans Administration Medical Center
Loma Linda, CA

Jennifer Warburg, M.S.W.

George Washnis
President
PDC
Wheaton, MD

David Weiss, B.S.
Co-Founder
Wellness Design
Brookline, MA

Judith M. Whalen, M.P.A.
Chief
Office of Science Policy
National Institute of Child Health and Human Development, NIH
Bethesda, MD

Gale White, M.S.
Senior Public Health Advisor
Food and Drug Administration
Rockville, MD

Virginia Wiese
Lanham, MD

Frank Wiewel
Founder and President
People Against Cancer
Otho, IA

Angela Wozencroft
Osteo-Myofascial Therapist
Rockville, MD

William S. Yamanashi, Ph.D.
Adjunct Professor and Assistant Director of Research
Research Section
Department of Surgery
University of Oklahoma College of Medicine, Tulsa
Tulsa, OK

Cynthia Yockey
President
Ayurveda Health Education Services, Inc.
Silver Spring, MD

Michael F. Ziff, D.D.S.
Executive Director
International Academy of Oral Medicine and Toxicology
Orlando, FL

Marvin C. Ziskin, M.D.
Professor of Radiology and Medical Physics
Department of Diagnostic Imaging
Temple University Medical School
Philadelphia, PA

Appendix B
Comments of the Panel on Mind-Body Interventions on the National Research Council's Reports on Alternative Medicine

In 1991 the National Research Council (NRC) issued an evaluation of some of the therapies examined herein (Druckman and Bjork, 1991). The NRC in 1988 also reviewed certain human-performance technologies designed to enhance human abilities beyond normal levels, which are also the concern of the Panel on Mind-Body Interventions (Druckman and Swets, 1988). Because the conclusions of the NRC reports differ from our own, and because these reports have been influential in shaping public opinion about the effectiveness and benefits of certain mind-body interventions, we believe it is important to comment on these discrepancies.

We shall focus on the NRC's treatment of meditation, one of the approaches we have closely examined, and parapsychology, an indirectly related area, to illustrate these differences of opinion and describe how they have taken shape.

Meditation

The 1991 NRC report stated, "Overall, our assessment of the scientific research on meditation (primarily, transcendental meditation [TM]) leads to the conclusion that it seems to be no more effective in lowering metabolism than are established relaxation techniques; it is unwarranted to attribute any special effects to meditation alone" (Druckman and Bjork, 1991). The NRC report reached this conclusion by drawing primarily on two previous narrative reviews. One of these, by Holmes, covered less than half the relevant studies on TM available at the time it was prepared (Holmes, 1984). The other, by Brener and Connally (1986), also appears to have ignored much of the available and relevant research.

A meta-analysis by TM researchers Dillbeck and Orme-Johnson on the effects of meditation, published in *American Psychologist*, came to a different conclusion but was ignored in the NRC report. Their quantitative approach showed that the effect size for TM was more than twice that of resting quietly on basal skin resistance, respiration rate, and plasma lactate (Dillbeck and Orme-Johnson, 1987).

Furthermore, Eppley, Abrams, and Shear, addressing psychological and physiological measures of anxiety, showed that TM typically produces two to three times the reductions in effects of chronic stress compared with other meditation and relaxation techniques (Eppley et al., 1989). Yet the NRC report said "no evidence supports the notion that . . . meditation permits a person to better cope with a stressor."

Meta-analysis allows quantitative analysis of various aspects of the literature. For instance, it allows one to compare the results of studies done by experimenters who are cordial, neutral, and negative toward TM. The Eppley meta-analysis demonstrated that the distribution of effects was normal, indicating that the positive conclusions reached in studies of TM are not the result of selective reporting, and that the NRC's characterization of researchers who are practitioners of meditation as subjectively biased "devotees" is without merit. The Eppley meta-analysis also contradicted the Brener and Connally claim that meditation research suffered from "weak design" by providing quantitative demonstration that the results cannot be accounted for by subject selection, experimenter bias, expectancies, or atmospheric effects.

The NRC report embodies some faulty assumptions about meditation. It expresses the expectation that meditation should "[lower] reactivity to challenge"—that is, to make one less responsive to stressors, perhaps through "distracting a person" or providing a "quiet place." But this is neither the traditional nor the express purpose of TM, which is to achieve "restful alertness, a state of unifying capacity." These misunderstandings may be due to the fact, acknowledged by the NRC, that no one on their committee was personally familiar with the *experience* of any of the meditation practices they reviewed. The difficulties this created were also acknowledged by the committee: "It seems appropriate to be mindful of the constraints that science, as well as culture, background, and personal life experience, place on how the committee views the field of meditation."[1]

The most glaring omission in the NRC report is a large database (more than 40 published reports) of societal impact studies on what the TM researchers call the consciousness field. The theory underlying this research is that the field, when supported by a sufficient number of meditators, produces the effects and benefits of meditation in the larger population. This is a nonlocal effect, a type of action-at-a-distance, and the TM researchers describe a correspondence to aspects of quantum nonlocality in their efforts to explain the results of these studies.

On the positive side, the NRC report makes a number of very sensible recommendations for research. In a general observation, they state that "learning to relax and enjoy good feelings may prompt a person to make positive changes in his or her work and personal situation. . . . [I]t may be that meditation and relaxation . . . effect cognitive change."[2] Their overall conclusion restates a question about relative efficacy and constitutes an implicit recommendation for more incisive research, but they do not dispute the potential therapeutic effects of meditation broadly defined.

Parapsychology

In its 1988 report the NRC is strongly critical of parapsychology, a field that studies, from an independent perspective, the nonlocal events exemplified in prayer and mental-spiritual healing that we have reviewed earlier. The NRC emphasized their belief that more than 130 years of research have failed to find any evidence of parapsychological phenomena. Because of the relevance of this research to issues addressed by the Panel on Mind-Body Interventions, the literature was examined, revealing impressive evidence in clear disagreement with the NRC's conclusion.

In the December 1989 issue of *Foundations of Physics*, Radin and Nelson reported the largest meta-analysis of parapsychological findings ever done—a total of 832 studies from 68 investigators, involving the influence of human consciousness on microelectronic systems (Radin and Nelson, 1989). The results: "Radin and Nelson's meta-analysis demonstrates that the . . . results are *robust* and *repeatable*. Unless critics want to allege wholesale collusion among more than 60 experimenters or suggest a methodological artifact common to . . . hundred[s of] experiments conducted over nearly three decades, there is no escaping the conclusion that [these] effects are indeed possible" (Broughton, 1991; Jahn and Dunne, 1987).

Meta-analysis has also been applied to research studies in precognition, which typically involve card-guessing by a subject *before* the targets are even prepared. Honorton and Ferrari found 309 studies in English-language publications by 62 investigators, involving more than 50,000 subjects who participated in nearly 2 million trials. Their findings were as follows:

- Thirty percent of the studies produced statistically significant results (where 5 percent was expected by chance). The odds of this result happening by chance are approximately 1 in 1,024.
- The results could not be explained by the failure of researchers to report negative studies (the "file drawer" effect).
- Studies with the most rigorous methodology tended to produce *better* results (exactly the opposite of critics' claims).
- The effect size remained constant over the more than 50 years under consideration (Honorton and Ferrari, 1989).

---

[1]*The data show that the TM-trained body operates at a lower baseline level of activity and has more adaptive reserves; hence, the meditator may respond more powerfully and recover more rapidly when challenged by stressors.*

[2]*The above observations on the NRC report on meditation are based on Orme-Johnson and Alexander's "Critique of the National Research Council's Report on Meditation" (1992).*

An excellent summary of the techniques of meta-analysis applied to several parapsychological databases was published in 1991 by Jessica Utts in *Statistical Science* (Utts, 1991).

A charge frequently made about parapsychology and the nonlocal therapies we have examined is that the quality of research in these areas is low or substandard. In its 1988 report, the NRC commissioned psychologist Robert Rosenthal of Harvard University to prepare an evaluation of all the controversial areas of interest to the NRC committee. Parapsychology researcher Richard S. Broughton describes this undertaking:

> Rosenthal is widely regarded as one of the world's experts in evaluating controversial research claims in the social sciences and has spent much of his career developing techniques to provide objective assessments of conflicting data. Neither Rosenthal nor his coauthor, Monica Harris, had taken any public position on parapsychology. . . . The report by Harris and Rosenthal determined that the "research quality" of the parapsychology research was the best of all the areas under scrutiny. . . . Incredibly . . . [the] committee chairman . . . asked Rosenthal to withdraw the parapsychology section of his report. Rosenthal refused. In the final document, the Harris and Rosenthal report is cited only in the several sections dealing with nonparapsychological topics; there is no mention of it in the parapsychology section (Broughton, 1991).

The Panel on Mind-Body Interventions believes it is necessary to acknowledge and document our differences of opinion with the NRC reports. At the same time, we do not wish to overemphasize or dwell on these conflicting points of view.

If the field of alternative medicine is to progress, it is vital that any evaluation of mind-body practices be comprehensive, rigorous, and unbiased.

References

Brener, J., and S.R. Connally. 1986. Meditation: Rationales, Experimental Effects, and Methodological Issues. Paper prepared for the U. S. Army Research Institute for the Behavioral and Social Sciences, European Division, Department of Psychology, University of Hull, London.

Broughton, R.S. 1991. Parapsychology: The Controversial Science. Ballantine Books, New York, p. 291.

Dillbeck, M.C., and D.W. Orme-Johnson 1987. Physiological differences between transcendental meditation and rest. American Psychologist 42:879–881.

Druckman, D., and R.A. Bjork, eds. 1991. In the Mind's Eye: Enhancing Human Performance. National Academy Press, Washington, D.C.

Druckman, D., and J.A. Swets, eds. 1988. Enhancing Human Performance: Issues, Theories, and Techniques. National Academy Press, Washington, D.C.

Eppley, K.R., A.I. Abrams, and J. Shear. 1989. Differential effects of relaxation technique on trait anxiety: a meta-analysis. J. Clin. Psychol. 45:957–974.

Holmes, D.S. 1984. Mediation and somatic arousal reduction: A review of the experimental evidence. American Psychologist 39:1–10.

Honorton, C., and D.C. Ferrari. 1989. Future telling: a meta-analysis of forced-choice precognition experiments, 1935–1987. J. Parapsychol. 53:281–308.

Jahn, R.G., and B.J. Dunne. 1987. Precognitive Remote Perception. In Margins of Reality: The Role of Consciousness in the Physical World. Harcourt Brace Jovanovich, pp. 149–191.

Orme-Johnson, D.W., and C.N. Alexander. 1992. Critique of the National Research Council's report on meditation. Manuscript available from the first author. Maharishi International University, Fairfield, Iowa.

Radin, D.L., and R.D. Nelson. 1989. Consciousness-related effects in random physical systems. Foundations of Physics 19:1499–1514.

Utts, J. 1991. Replication and meta-analysis in parapsychology. Statistical Science 4:363–403.

Appendix C
WHO Guidelines for the Assessment of Herbal Medicines

Introduction

For the purpose of these guidelines "HERBAL MEDICINES" should be regarded as:

Finished, labelled medicinal products that contain as active ingredients aerial or underground parts of plants, or other plant material, or combinations thereof, whether in the crude state or as plant preparations. Plant material includes juices, gums, fatty oils, essential oils, and any other substances of this nature. Herbal medicines may contain excipients in addition to the active ingredients. Medicines containing plant material combined with chemically defined active substances, including chemically defined, isolated constituents of plants, are not considered to be herbal medicines.

Exceptionally, in some countries herbal medicines may also contain, by tradition, natural organic or inorganic active ingredients which are not of plant origin.

The past decade has seen a significant increase in the use of herbal medicines. As a result of WHO's promotion of traditional medicine, countries have been seeking the assistance of WHO in identifying safe and effective herbal medicines for use in national health care systems. In 1989, one of the many resolutions adopted by the World Health Assembly in support of national traditional medicine programmes drew attention to herbal medicines as being of great importance to the health of individuals and communities (WHA 42.43).

There was also an earlier resolution (WHA 22.54) on pharmaceutical production in developing countries; this called on the Director-General to provide assistance to the health authorities of Member States to ensure that the drugs used are those most appropriate to local circumstances, that they are rationally used, and that the requirements for their use are assessed as accurately as possible. Moreover, the Declaration of Alma-Ata in 1978 provided for inter alia, the accommodation of proven traditional remedies in national drug policies and regulatory measures. In developed countries, the resurgence of interest in herbal medicines has been due to the preference of many consumers for products of natural origin. In addition, manufactured herbal medicines from their countries of origin often follow in the wake of migrants from countries where traditional medicines play an important role.

In both developed and developing countries, consumers and health care providers need to be supplied with up-to-date and authoritative information on the beneficial properties, and possible harmful effects, of all herbal medicines.

The Fourth International Conference of Drug Regulatory Authorities, held in Tokyo in 1986, organized a workshop on the regulation of herbal medicines moving in international commerce. Another workshop on the same subject was held as part of the Fifth International Conference of Drug Regulatory Authorities, held in Paris in 1989. Both workshops confined their considerations to the commercial exploitation of traditional medicines through over-the-counter labelled products. The Paris meeting concluded that the World Health Organization should consider preparing model guidelines containing basic elements of legislation designed to assist those countries who might wish to develop appropriate legislation and registration.

The objective of these guidelines, therefore, is to define basic criteria for the evaluation of quality, safety, and efficacy of herbal medicines and thereby to assist national regulatory authorities, scientific organizations, and manufacturers to undertake an assessment of the documentation/submission/dossiers in respect of such products. As a general rule in this assessment, traditional experience means that long-term use as well as the medical, historical and ethnological background of those products shall be taken into account. Depending on the history of the country, the definition of long-term use may vary, but would be at least several decades. Therefore, the assessment shall take into account a description in the medical/pharmaceutical literature or similar sources, or a documentation of knowledge on the application of a herbal

GUIDELINES FOR THE ASSESSMENT OF HERBAL MEDICINES

Programme on Traditional Medicines

World Health Organization

Geneva, 1991

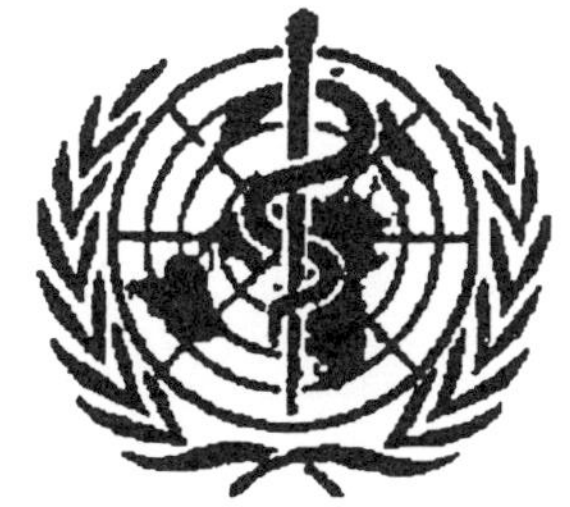

In both developed and developing countries, consumers and health care providers need to be supplied with up-to-date and authoritative information on the beneficial properties, and possible harmful effects, of all herbal medicines.

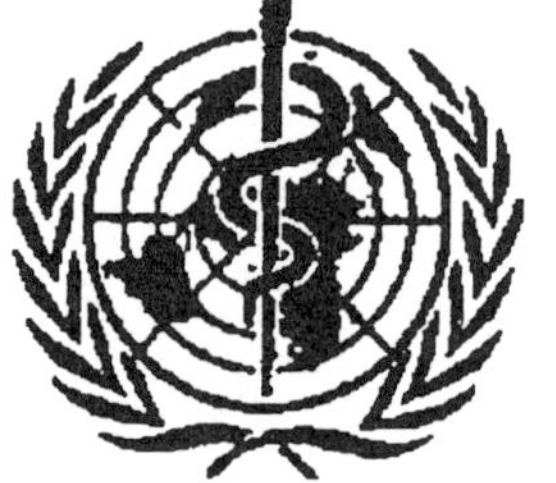

medicine without a clearly defined time limitation. Marketing authorizations for similar products should be taken into account.

The foregoing guidelines for the Assessment of Herbal Medicines were finalized at a WHO Consultation in Munich, Germany, from 19-21 June 1991. The request for WHO to prepare these guidelines came from the Fifth International Conference of Drug Regulatory Authorities (ICDRA) held in Paris in 1990. The finalized guidelines were presented to the Sixth ICDRA in Ottawa in 1991. These efforts concentrate on herbal medicines, but might at a later stage be the basis for the assessment of other traditional medicines not covered by these guidelines. In the meantime, it is up to the national authorities to adapt the guidelines for assessment of traditional medicines and other herbal drugs.

Prolonged and apparently uneventful use of a substance usually offers testimony of its safety. In a few instances investigations of the potential toxicity of naturally occurring substances widely used as ingredients in these preparations have revealed previously unsuspected potential for systematic toxicity, carcinogenicity and teratogenicity. Regulatory authorities need to be quickly and reliably informed of these findings. They should also have the authority to respond promptly to such alerts, either by withdrawing or varying the licences of registered products containing the suspect substance, or by rescheduling the substance in order to limit its use to medical prescription.

Assessment of quality, safety, and efficacy and intended use

Pharmaceutical assessment

This part should cover all important aspects of the quality assessment of herbal medicines. However, if a pharmacopoeia monograph exists it should be sufficient to make reference to this monograph. If no such monograph is available, a monograph must be supplied and should be set out in the same way as in an official pharmacopoeia.

All procedures should be in accordance with Good Manufacturing Practices (GMP).

Crude plant material

The botanical definition, including genus, species, and authority should be given to ensure correct identification of a plant. A definition and description of the part of the plant from which the medicine is made (e.g., leaf, flower, root) has to be provided as well as an indication as to whether fresh, dried, or traditionally processed material is used. The active and characteristic constituents should be specified and, if possible, content limits defined. Foreign matter, impurities and microbial content should be defined or limited. Voucher specimens, representing each lot of plant material processed, should be authenticated by a qualified botanist and should be stored for at least a ten -year period. A lot number should be assigned and this should appear on the product label.

Plant preparations

Plant preparations include comminuted or powdered plant materials, extracts, tinctures, fatty or essential oils, expressed juices and preparations whose production involves a fractionation, purification, or concentration process. The manufacturing procedure should be described in detail. If any other substance is added during the manufacture to adjust the plant preparation to a certain level of active or characteristic constituents or for any other purpose, the added substances should be mentioned in the procedure description. A method for identification and, where possible, assay of the plant preparation should be added. If the identification of an active principle is not possible, it should be sufficient to identify a characteristic substance or mixture of substances (e.g., "chromatographic fingerprint") to ensure consistent quality of the preparation.

Finished product

The manufacturing procedure and formula including the amount of excipients should be described in detail. A finished product specification should be defined. A method of identification and, where possible, quantification, of the plant material in the finished product should be defined. If the identification of an active principle is not possible, it should be sufficient to identify a characteristic substance or mixture of substances (e.g., "chromatographic finger-print") to ensure consistent quality of the product. The finished product should comply with general requirements for particular dosage forms.

For imported finished products, confirmation of the regulatory status in the country of origin should be required; the WHO Certification Scheme on the Quality of Pharmaceutical Products Moving in International Commerce should be applied.

Stability

The physical and chemical stability of the product in the final marketing container should be tested under defined storage conditions and the shelf-life should be established.

Safety assessment

This part should cover all relevant aspects of the safety assessment of a medicinal product. A guiding principle should be that if the product has been traditionally used without demonstrated harm no specific restrictive regulatory action should be undertaken unless new evidence demands a revised risk-benefit assessment.

A review of the relevant literature should be provided with original articles or references to the original articles. If official monograph/review results exist, reference can be made to them. However, although experience on long-term use without any evidence of risks may indicate harmlessness of a medicine, it is not certain in some cases to what extent reliance can be placed solely upon long-term usage to provide assurance of innocuousness in the light of concern generated in recent years over long-term hazards of some herbal medicines.

Reported side effects should be documented according to normal pharmaco-vigilance principles.

Toxicological studies

If any toxicological studies are available, they should be part of the assessment. Literature should be indicated as above.

Documentation of safety based on experience

As a basic rule, documentation of a long period of use should be taken into consideration when safety is being assessed. This means that, when there are no detailed toxicological studies, documented experience on long-term use without evidence of safety problems should form the basis of the risk assessment. However, even in cases of long-used drugs, chronic toxicological risks may have occurred, but may not have been recognized. If available, the period of use, the health disorders treated, the number of users, and the countries with experience should be specified. If a toxicological risk is known, toxicity data have to be submitted. Risk assessment, whether it is independent of dose (e.g., special danger or allergies), or whether it is a function of dose, should be documented. In the second instance the dosage specification must be an important part of the risk assessment. An explanation of the risks should be given, if possible. The potential for misuse, abuse, or dependence has to be documented. If long-term traditional use cannot be documented, or doubts on safety exist, toxicity data should be submitted.

Assessment of efficacy and intended use

This part should cover all important aspects of the efficacy assessment. A review of the relevant literature should be carried out and copies provided of the original articles or proper references to them. Research studies, if they exist, should be taken into account.

Activity

The pharmacological and clinical effects of the active ingredients and, if known, their constituents with therapeutic activity should be specified or described.

Evidence required to support indications

The indication(s) for the use of the medicine should be specified. In the case of traditional medicines, the requirements for proof of efficacy shall depend on the kind of indication. For treatment of minor disorders and for nonspecific indications, some relaxation is justified in the requirements for proof of efficacy, taking into account the extent of traditional use; the same considerations may apply to prophylactic use. Experience with individual cases recorded in

In 1989, one of the many resolutions adopted by the World Health Assembly in support of national traditional medicine programmes drew attention to herbal medicines as being of great importance to the health of individuals and communities.

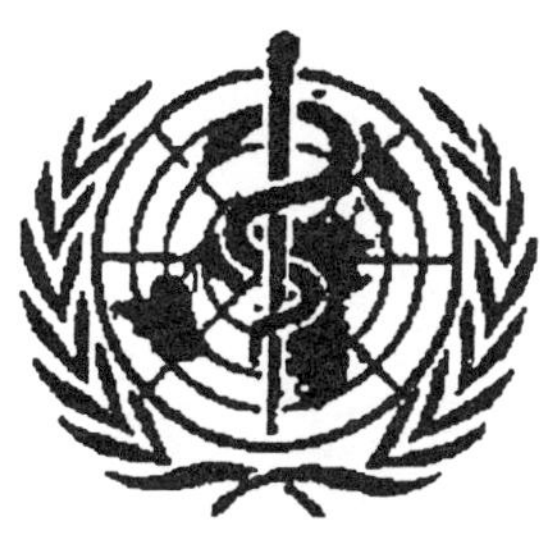

WHO guidelines for the assessment of herbal medicines are intended to facilitate the work to be carried out by regulatory authorities, scientific bodies, and industry in the development, assessment, and registration of such products.

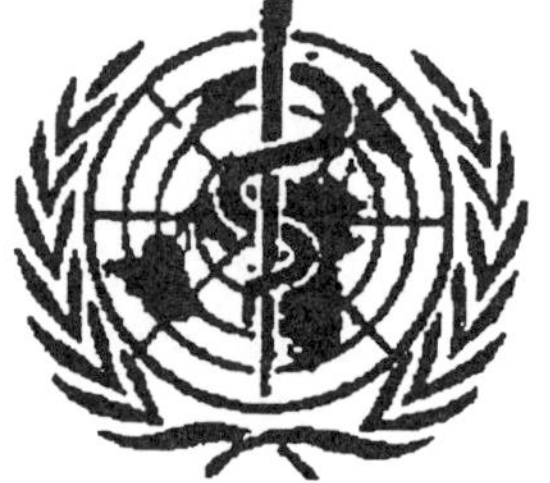

reports from physicians, traditional health practitioners, or treated patients should be taken into account.

Where traditional use has not been established, appropriate clinical evidence should be required.

Combination products

Because many herbal remedies consist of a combination of several active ingredients, and experience on the use of traditional remedies is often based on combination products, the assessment should differentiate between old and new combination products. Identical requirements for the assessment of old and new combinations would result in an inappropriate assessment of certain traditional medicines.

In the case of traditionally used combination products, the documentation of traditional use (classical texts such as Ayurveda, Traditional Chinese Medicine, Unani, Sida) and experience may serve for documentation of efficacy.

An explanation of a new combination of well-known substances including effective dose ranges and compatibility should be required in addition to the documentation of traditional knowledge of each single ingredient. Each active ingredient must contribute to the efficacy of the medicine.

In order to justify the efficacy of a new ingredient and its positive effect on the total combination, clinical studies may be required.

Product information for the consumer

The labelling of the products and the package insert should be understandable to the consumer/patient. The package information should cover all necessary information on the proper use of the product.

The following elements of information usually suffice:

- name of the product
- quantitative list of active ingredient(s)
- dosage form
- indications
- dosage (if appropriate, specified for children and the elderly)
- mode of administration
- duration of use
- major adverse effects, if any
- overdosage information
- contraindications, warnings, precautions and major drug interactions
- use during pregnancy and lactation
- expiration date
- lot number
- holder of the marketing authorization

Identification of the active ingredient(s) by the Latin botanical name, in addition to the common name in the language of preference of the national regulatory authority, is recommended.

Not all information that is ideally required may be available. Therefore, drug regulatory authorities should determine their minimum requirements.

Promotion

Advertisements and other promotional activities to health personnel and the lay public should be fully consistent with the approved package information.

Utilization of guidelines

WHO guidelines for the assessment of herbal medicines are intended to facilitate the work to be carried out by regulatory authorities, scientific bodies and industry in the development, assessment and registration of such products. The assessment should reflect the scientific results gathered in past years in that field that could be the basis for the future classification of herbal medicines in different parts of the world. Other types of traditional medicines in addition to herbal products may be assessed in a similar way.

The effective regulation and control of herbal medicines moving in international commerce also require close liaison with appropriate national institutions that are able to keep under regular review all aspects of their production and use, as well as to conduct or sponsor evaluative studies of their efficacy, toxicity, safety, acceptability, cost, and relative value compared with other drugs used in modern medicine.✤

Appendix D
Plant Sources of Modern Drugs

Species	Family	Type of Drug/Product
Acacia senegal (L.) Willd.	Leguminosae	Gum acacia
Agathosma betulina (Berg.) Pillans (Syn.: *Barosma betulina* (Berg.) Bartl. et Wendl. f.)	Rutaceae	Buchu leaf
Ammi majus L.	Umbelliferae	*Xanthotoxin*
Ananas comosus (L.) Merr.	Bromeliaceae	Bromelain
Aralia racemosa L.	Araliaceae	Aralia extracts
Arctostaphylos uva-ursi (L.) Spreng.	Ericaceae	Uva ursi
Atropa belladonna L.	Solanaceae	Belladonna extract
Avena sativa L.	Gramineae	Oatmeal Concentrate
Berberis vulgaris L.	Berberidaceae	Berberine
Calendula officinalis L.	Compositae	Calendula oil
Camellia sinensis L. (Syn.: *Theasinensis* L.)	Theaceae	Caffeine
Capsicum annuum L.	Solanaceae	Capsicum oleoresin
C. baccatum L. var *pendulum* (Willd.) Eshbaugh	Capsicum oleoresin	
C. chinense Jacquin	Capsicum oleoresin	
C. frutescens L.	Capsicum oleoresin	
Capsicum pubescens R. et P.	Solanaceae	Capsicum extract
Carica papaya L.	Caricaceae	Papain
Cassia senna L. (Syn.: *C. acutifolia* Delile, senna leaf, *C. angustifolia* Vahl)	Leguminosae	Sennosides A + B, senna pods
Catharanthus roseus (L.) G. Don	Apocynaceae	*Leurocristine* (vincristine) and *incaleukoblastine* (vinblastine)
Cephaelis ipecacuanha (Brot.) A. Richard	Rubiaceae	Ipecac fluid extract, ipecac syrup
Chrysanthemum cinerariaefolium (Trev.) Vis.	Compositae	Pyrethrins
Cinchona calisaya Wedd.	Rubiaceae	*Quinine, quinidine*
C. ledgeriana Moens		*Quinine, quinidine*
C. pubescens Vahl		*Quinine, quinidine*
Cinnamomum camphora (L.) J. S. Presl	Lauraceae	Camphor

Species	Family	Type of Drug/Product
Citrus limon (L.) Burm. f.	Rutaceae	Pectin
Citrus sinensis (L.) Osbeck	Rutaceae	Citrus bioflavonoids
Colchicum autumnale L.	Liliacae	*Colchicine*
Commiphora abyssinica Engl.	Burseraceae	Myrrh gum
C. molmol Engl. ex Tschirch	Myrrh gum	
Digitalis lanata Ehrh.	Scrophulariaceae	*Digoxin, lanatoside C,* and *acetylgitoxin*
D. purpurea L.		*Digitoxin*, and *digitalis* whole leaf
Dioscorea composita Hemsl.	Dioscoreaceae	*Diosgenin*
D. floribunda Mar. et. Gal.		*Diosgenin*
D. deltoidea Wallich		*Diosgenin*
Duboisia myoporoides R. Br.	Solanaceae	*Atropine, hyoscyamine, scopolamine*
Eucalyptus globulus Labill.	Myrtaceae	Eucalyptol (cineole), eucalyptus oil
Fagopyrum esculentum Moench	Polygonaceae	Rutin
Frangula alnus P. Miller (Syn.: *Rhamnus frangula* L.)	Rhamnaceae	Frangula bark
Gaultheria procumbens L.	Ericaceae	Wintergreen oil
Gelsemium sempervirens (L.) St. Hil.	Loganiaceae	Gelsemium extract
Glycine max (L.) Merr.	Leguminosae	Sitosterols
Glycyrrhiza glabra L.	Leguminosae	Licorice extract
Gossypium hirsutum L.	Malvaceae	Cottonseed oil
Guarea rusbyi (Britton) Rusby	Meliaceae	Cocillana extract
Hamamelis virginiana L.	Hamamelidaceae	Witch hazel extract
Lavandula officinalis P. Miller (Syn.: *L. officinalis* Chaix)	Labiateae	Lavender oil
Linum usitatissimum L.	Linaceae	Linseed oil
Malus sylvestris P. Miller	Rosaceae	Pectin
Melaleuca leucadendron L.	Myrtaceae	Cajeput oil
Mentha arvensis L.	Labiatae	Menthol
M. piperita L.	Peppermint oil	
M. spicata L.	Spearmint oil	
Myristica fragrans Houtt.	Myristicaceae	Nutmeg oil
Myroxylon balsamum (L.) Harms	Leguminosae	Tolu balsam

Species	Family	Type of Drug/Product
M. balsamum var. *pareirae* (Royle) Harms (Syn.: *M. pareirae* (Royle) Klotzsch)	Peru balsam	
Olea europaea L.	Oleaceae	Olive oil
Papaver somniferum L. (Paregoric)	Papaveraceae	Opium extract *codeine, morphine, noscapine,* and *papaverine (33)*
Pausinystalia yohimba Pierre ex Beille	Rubiaceae	Yohimbine
Physostigma venenosum Balf.	Leguminosae	*Physostigmine* (eserine)
Pilocarpus jaborandi Holmes	Rutaceae	*Pilocarpine*
Pimpinella anisum L.	Umbelliferae	Anise oil
Piper cubeba L. f.	Piperaceae	Cubeb oil
Plantago indica L.	Plantaginaceae	Psyllium husks
P. ovata Forsk.	Psyllium husks	
P. psyllium L.	Psyllium husks	
Podophyllum peltatum L.	Berberidaceae	Podophyllin
Polygala senega L.	Polygalaceae	Senega fluid extract
Populus balsamifera L. (Syn.: *P. candicans* Ait., *P. tacamahacca* P. Miller)	Salicaceae	Poplar bud
Prunus domestica L.	Rosaceae	Prune concentrate
P. virginiana L.	Wild cherry bark	
Quercus infectoria Olivier	Fagaceae	Tannic acid
Rauvolfia serpentina (L.) Benth. ex Kurz	Apocynaceae	*Reserpine* alseroxylon fraction, powdered whole root
Rauvolfia R. vomitoria Afzel.		*Deserpidine, reserpine, rescinnamine*
Rhamnus purshiana DC.	Rhamnaceae	Cascara bark, casanthranol, danthron*(33)*
Rheum emodi Wallich	Polygonaceae	Rhubarb root
R. officinale Baill.		Rhubarb root
R. palmatum L.		Rhubarb root
R. rhaponticum L.		Rhubarb root
Ricinus communis L.		Castor oil, *ricinoleic acid*
Rosa gallica L.	Rosaceae	Rose petal infusion
Salix alba L.	Salicaceae	Saligenin
Sanguinaria canadensis L.	Papaveraceae	Sanguinaria root
Santalum album L.	Santalaceae	Sandalwood

Species	Family	Type of Drug/Product
Sassafras albidum (Nutt.) Nees	Lauraceae	Sassafras extract
Serenoa repens (Bartr.) Small	Palmae	Saw palmetto berries
Sesamum indicum L.	Pedaliaceae	Sesame oil
Sterculia urens Roxb.	Sterculiaceae	Sterculia gum (karaya gum)
Strychnos nux-vomica L.	Loganiaceae	Strychnine
Styrax benzoin Dryand.	Styracaceae	Benzoin gum
S. paralleloneurus Perkins		Benzoin gum
Symphytum officinale L.	Boraginaceae	Allantoin
Syzygium aromaticum (L.) Merr.	Myrtaceae	Clove oil et Perry
Theobroma cacao L.	Sterculiaceae	Theobromine
Thymus vulgaris L.	Labiatae	Thymol
Urginea maritima (L.) Baker	Liliaceae	Squill extract
Veratrum viride Ait.	Liliaceae	*Veratrum viride* extract, cryptennamine
Zea mays L.	Graminae	Cornsilk

Appendix E
The 20 Most Popular Asian Patent Medicines That Contain Toxic Ingredients

1. Product Name: Ansenpunaw Tablets
   Manufacturer: Chung Lien Drug Works, Hankow, China
   Toxic Ingredients: cinnabar (mercury chloride)

2. Product Name: Bezoar Sedative Pills
   Manufacturer: Lanzhou Fo Ci Pharmaceutical Factory, Lanzhou, China
   Toxic Ingredients: cinnabar 2% or 10%

3. Product Name: Compound Kangweiling
   Manufacturer: Wo Zhou Pharmaceutical Factory, Zhe Jiang, China
   Toxic Ingredients: centipede (scolopendra) 10%

4. Product Name: Dahuo Luodan
   Manufacturer: Beijing Tung Jen Tang, Beijing, China
   Toxic Ingredients: centipede (scolopendra)

5. Product Name: Danshen Tabletco
   Manufacturer: Shanghai Chinese Medicine Works, Shanghai, China
   Toxic Ingredients: borneol

6. Product Name: Fructus Persica Compound Pills
   Manufacturer: Lanzhou Fo Ci Pharmaceutical Factory, Lanzhou, China
   Toxic Ingredients: cannabis indica seed (℞)

7. Product Name: Fuchingsung-N Cream
   Manufacturer: Tianjin Pharmaceuticals Corp., Tianjin, China
   Toxic Ingredients: fluocinolone acetanide (℞)

8. Product Name: Kwei Ling Chi
   Manufacturer: Changchun Chinese Medicines & Drugs Manufactory, Chang Chun, China
   Toxic Ingredients: cinnabar

9. Product Name: Kyushin Heart Tonic
   Manufacturer: Kyushin Seiyaku Co., Ltd., Tokyo, Japan
   Toxic Ingredients: toad venom, borneol

10. Product Name: Laryngitis Pills
    Manufacturer: China Dzechuan Provincial Pharmaceutical Factory, Chengtu Branch
    Toxic Ingredients: borax 30%, toad-cake 10%

11. Product Name: Leung Pui Kee Cough Pills
    Manufacturer: Leung Pui Kee Medical Factory, Hong Kong
    Toxic Ingredients: dover's powder (opium powder) (℞)

12. Product Name: Lu-Shen-Wan
    Manufacturer: Shanghai Chinese Medicine Works, Shanghai, China
    Toxic Ingredients: toad secretion

13. Product Name: Nasalin
    Manufacturer: Kwangchow Pharmaceutical Industry Co., Kwangchow, China
    Toxic Ingredients: centipede 5%

14. Product Name: Nui Huang Chieh Tu Pien
    Manufacturer: Tung Jen Tang, Beijing, China
    Toxic Ingredients: borneo camphor

15. Product Name: Niu Huang Xiao Yan Wan
    Bezoar Antiphlogistic Pills
    Manufacturer: Soochow Chinese Medicine Works, Kiangsu, China
    Toxic Ingredients: realgar 19.23%

16. Product Name: Pak Yuen Tong Hou Tsao Powder
    Manufacturer: Kwan Tung Pak Yuen Tong Main Factory, Hong Kong
    Toxic Ingredients: scorpion 10%

17. Product Name: Po Ying Tan Baby Protector
    Manufacturer: Po Che Tong Poon Mo Um, Hong Kong
    Toxic Ingredients: camphor 20%

18. Product Name: Superior Tabellae Berberini HCl
    Manufacturer: Min-Kang Drug Manufactory, I-Chang, China
    Toxic Ingredients: berberini HCl (℞)

19. Product Name: Watson's Flower Pagoda Cakes
    Manufacturer: A.S. Watson & Co., Ltd., Hong Kong
    Toxic Ingredients: piperazine phosphate (℞)

20. Product Name: Xiao Huo Luo Dan
    Manufacturer: Lanzhou Fo Ci Pharmaceutical Factory, Lanzhou, China
    Toxic Ingredients: aconite 42%

Source: Oriental Herb Association, State of California Department of Health Services. January 28, 1992.

℞: requires doctor's prescription.

Appendix F
A Guide for the Alternative Researcher

by Claire Cassidy, Ph.D., Barrie Cassileth, Ph.D., Wayne B. Jonas, M.D., Richard Pavek, and Linda Silversmith, Ph.D.

The guidelines in this appendix are provided to assist the alternative researcher. The topics presented were selected from a broader array of methodologies and approaches. There is no intention to be all-inclusive. Topics that were omitted may nevertheless be appropriate tools for conducting alternative research.

General Methodological Guidelines

Research studies on alternative medical therapies should be held to the same rigorous scientific and ethical standards that are applied to research on conventional therapies. The guidelines in this appendix represent a summary of major principles for new investigators as they begin to develop research protocols or grant applications. It is recommended that at least one investigator in each study of alternative medicine be experienced in the therapy or research area to be investigated.

It takes as many years to learn how to conduct good research as to become an accomplished practitioner of alternative medicine. Alternative practitioners who wish to do research need to increase their understanding of good research design, but they should also seek out experienced researchers to guide them as collaborators or resources.

Approaches for conducting research must follow a logical sequence for gathering useful data. Typically, research on a given topic is first *exploratory*, then *descriptive* and *qualitative*, then *correlative* and *comparative*, and finally *experimental* and *quantitative*. Interviews and surveys are examples of descriptive research or possibly correlative/comparative research; best case series fit the correlative/comparative category; and clinical trials are experimental.[1]

Once a decision has been made that a topic is worthy of investigation and not duplicative of previous work, preliminary or pilot studies (exploratory-descriptive) generally are carried out to determine whether there are any promising effects worthy of further investigation and to detect any negative side effects or practical difficulties. These studies may consist of anecdotal case reports, systematic case studies, or uncontrolled single-group studies. Questions are then formulated for use in controlled comparisons (correlative-comparative) using controls such as the best available "other techniques" or a placebo. A large enough group of patients and sufficient time are necessary to provide enough data to suggest whether the treatment is really working and what conditions seem most practical. If effectiveness is reported, then large studies (experimental-quantitative), such as clinical trials, should be organized to find out whether the earlier observations hold true with a more detailed examination using a greater number of participants.

Whatever the research approach, the following procedure generally applies:

1. Identify the paradigm, model, or pattern and explanatory strategies that underlie the intervention under consideration for testing and evaluation.

2. Carefully develop one or two precise research questions to form the basis of the study. The research questions are crucial

[1]*The subsequent sections of this appendix present several types of research in the same sequence in which they are usually applied, providing guidelines to literature reviews, descriptive and cross-cultural studies, "best case" screening, clinical trials, and outcomes research. These are followed first by introductions to two sophisticated approaches to analyzing research—meta-analysis and systematic reviews—and then by a selected bibliography, information on the National Library of Medicine, and useful contact information.*

because they lead directly to the study's objectives, methods, implications, and so on.

3. Ensure that all components of the research plan relate logically to one another. Research questions, goals, subject groups, therapies (regimens, products, etc.) to be studied, and methodologies must be mutually consistent and appropriate. When conceptualizing study objectives, make them consistent with research questions and assumptions of the intervention; in turn, make the study design (the strategy for conducting the study) consistent with research objectives. For all procedures that are operator dependent, identify the skills training and experience of the operator (e.g., teacher or deliverer of treatment). Clarify the nature of the population to be studied; in particular, identify whether the entry criteria lead the study population to be different from the spectrum of people being treated by practicing clinicians.

4. Conduct a library search and gather a comprehensive collection of previous research in the specific area to be studied. Because of incomplete archiving and indexing, computer database searches are currently inadequate to capture the information needed. It may be necessary to read published articles in their entirety and to speak with representatives of alternative medical organizations to locate some references and information. Literature reviews should be comprehensive and systematic (see the "Guidelines for Conducting Literature Reviews" section below).

5. Explain explicitly the methods used to obtain the literature. Simple citation of publications is not adequate. Literature obtained through library search serves as the basis for the "Background" section of grant applications or manuscripts. Background sections should incorporate accurate, high-quality summary evaluations of existing literature. If a systematic review (see the "Introduction to Systematic Reviews" section) or meta-analysis (see the "Introduction to Systematic Reviews" section) has been conducted to quantitatively evaluate the literature, this point should be noted.

6. Clearly define (not just label) the intervention to be tested or evaluated.

7. Include in the study any special diagnostic or outcome aspects of the alternative medicine practice that can be reliably measured.

8. Thoroughly and objectively document all procedures and events that occur during the research study, from subject accrual through data collection, data analysis, and reporting of results.

9. In clinical research (studies involving humans), include adequate control groups and provide followup of subjects over time, with appropriate monitoring of both the intervention group and the control group.

10. In clinical research, consider and minimize any potential risks to subjects. Along with other required information, these risks must be explained to potential subjects in an informed consent document, provided by the sponsoring institution's human subjects committee or institutional review board.

11. Before research begins, decide and indicate in the research proposal what will be considered sufficient evidence to recommend inclusion of the intervention in clinical practice (if relevant).

12. Where appropriate, use standard comparative outcome measures that will allow the new data to be compared with previous and future information on the same topic.

13. Obtain expert guidance on computerizing and analyzing research data. Biostatistics and computer programming assistance will ensure proper management and analysis of data.

Guidelines for Conducting Literature Reviews

Summary information about previous work in a given field is necessary for grant applications and publications. In addition, literature reviews in and of themselves often are useful additions to the literature.

Overview of Goals of the Review

The literature review must address a clearly focused question. It should specify the particular population, intervention or treatment, subject or diagnostic group, or the like, on which the review will focus. A summary table of all studies in-

Some Helpful References for New Investigators*

Altman, D.G. 1991. *Practical Statistics for Medical Research.* Chapman & Hall, London.

Bernard, H.R. 1993. Research Methods in Cultural Anthropology (2nd ed.). Sage Publications, Newbury Park, Calif.

Brink, P., and M. Wood. 1988. *Basic Steps in Planning Nursing Research* (3rd ed.). Jones and Bartlett, Boston.

Briscoe, M.E. 1990. *A Researcher's Guide to Scientific and Medical Illustrations.* Springer-Verlag, New York.

Educational Testing Service. Undated. Test Collection Catalog No. 3 (a source for standard test and evaluation forms; available from ETS, PO Box 7234, San Diego, CA 91207).

Gehlbach, S.H. 1993. *Interpreting the Medical Literature.* McGraw-Hill, New York.

Haley, R.W. 1994. "Designing clinical research". In Y.C. Pak and P.M. Adams, eds. *Techniques of Patient Oriented Research.* Raven Press, New York.

Hulley, S.B., and S.R. Cummings, eds. 1988. *Designing Clinical Research—An Epidemiological Approach.* Williams & Wilkins, Baltimore.

Leede, P.D. 1992. *Practical Research: Planning and Design* (5th ed.). McMillan, New York.

Lewitt, G.T., and D. Aldrich. 1993. Clinical Research Methodology for Complementary Therapies. Hodder & Stoughton, London.

Lincoln, Y., and E. Guba. 1985. Naturalistic Inquiry. Sage Publications, Beverly Hills, Calif.

Marshall, C., and G. Rossman. 1989. Designing Qualitative Research. Sage Publications, Newbury Park, Calif.

McCracken, G. 1988. *The Long Interview.* Sage Publications, Newbury Park, Calif.

Pocock, S.J. 1983. *Clinical Trials: A Practical Approach.* Wiley, Chichester, England.

Schwartz, S.M., and M.E. Friedman. 1992. *A Guide to NIH Grant Programs,* Oxford University Press, New York.

Yin, R.K. 1994. *Case Study Research, Design, and Methods* (2nd ed.). Sage Publications, Thousand Oaks, Calif.

Zeiger, M. 1991. *Essentials of Writing Biomedical Research Papers.* McGraw-Hill, New York.

**These references were selected as basic guides. An extensive methodological bibliography is provided at the end of this appendix.*

cluded in the review, along with their data, may be appropriate. The review should address a specific and pragmatic issue.

Literature Search

The process of collecting relevant articles must be comprehensive and thorough. The search should use bibliographic databases such as MEDLINE, *Science Citation Index, Social Science Citation Index,* references from relevant articles, personal communications with authors, and manual searches of databases such as *Index Medicus.* Note that currently this approach may locate only 25 to 50 percent of articles on alternative medicine because most such articles do not appear in standard medical journals (see the "Research Databases" chapter).

Search methods must be systematic and clearly described. Possible selection bias must be addressed when articles are obtained through personal contact. Negative studies should be described along with others; their exclusion suggests possible bias.

Selection of Articles for the Study

The chosen method for selecting articles must be clear, systematic, and appropriate. Inclusion and exclusion criteria should be preestablished in the form of a protocol to be followed when reviewing articles for inclusion; the selection process should then be followed systematically.

The selection protocol should address major criteria that are relevant to the therapy or system under review, including whether the population is adequately defined, whether the exposure or intervention is clearly described, and whether outcomes are detailed and comparable.

Articles should be reviewed in random order and selected as they meet the preestablished criteria. The reliability of the selection process can be measured by comparing articles collected by at least two independent selectors (expert and nonexpert). The extent of selection disagreement can then be evaluated, and a method can be developed to deal with discordant selections.

Research Quality

The quality of the methodology of each study under review is evaluated according to a single set of standards applied to all studies, whether or not the studies have been published. Literature evaluation must be reproducible. It should be conducted by evaluators who are blind with respect to authors, institutions, and study results. These methods of assessment should be described in the introduction to the literature review.

Combining of Results

Results across studies may be combined only when the studies are adequately similar. Study designs, populations, exposures, outcomes, and direction of effect should be similar enough to warrant combining. If studies are methodologically similar, it is less likely that chance influences their results. Analysis of numerous subgroups matched between studies should be avoided, as spurious statistical significance is likely to result. Comparisons are more likely to be valid if variation in the primary studies is considered when results are combined. Differences in study design and components (e.g., population, exposure or intervention, outcomes) should be addressed. Any nonstatistical criteria used for comparison should be explained.

Meta-Analysis and Systematic Reviews

A statistical review method that combines data from several studies is termed meta-analysis (or statistical meta-analysis). These quantitative analyses, which require similar study samples, interventions, and outcomes, can evaluate the magnitude of treatment effect (percentage risk reduction) and the possibility that the differences were due to chance. Meta-analyses can be used to determine the frequency (i.e., quantity) and the quality of the research method employed in studying a specific factor or issue within a single research field or across several fields of study.

Systematic reviews are another orderly approach to reviewing research literature. Like meta-analysis and other quantitative review methods, systematic reviews use clearly specified methods to avoid the introduction of bias in the selection and interpretation of the research literature being reviewed. Clearly defined criteria for including or excluding specific journals and articles are applied; additional criteria are used to evaluate the quality of the measures applied in the reported research to assess the topic of interest. Systematic reviews differ from meta-analyses in that the studies selected for review need not use strictly similar study samples, interventions, or outcome measures.

For additional information, see the "Introduction to Meta-Analysis" and "Introduction to Systematic Reviews" sections.

Significance of Results

The importance of the results can be determined by calculating an *odds ratio* (the odds of the effect occurring in the exposure group divided by the odds of the effect occurring in the control or comparison group). The resultant number should be large to have any significance. The results should be reported in a clinically meaningful manner such as the absolute difference or the number needed to treat. The results also should be reproducible and generalizable, with similar effects on different types of subject groups. (The level of significance of results could become a criterion for including studies in an alternative medicine research database; such a database is proposed in the "Research Databases" chapter.)

All clinically important consequences should be considered, including other outcomes from the intervention or treatment; these results should be discussed in the context of those analyzed in the review.

Guidelines for Descriptive and Cross-Cultural Studies Using Qualitative Research Methods[2]

Overview

Many alternative medical systems and practices derive from other cultures or reflect models of health and dysfunction that differ substantively from those current in conventional medicine. As a result, research on alternative medical systems often is in effect, if not explicitly, cross-cultural. The fundamental issue of cross-cultural research is that people who have different views of what constitutes reality also experience reality differently. This means that questions, concepts, dis-

[2]*Descriptive research is sometimes called "qualitative research," but descriptive research actually uses a mixture of qualitative and quantitative techniques.*

eases, treatments, and research protocols that "make sense" in one setting may not make sense in another.

Before conventional quantitative techniques can be validly applied to the scientific analysis of alternative medical systems, enough must be known of these systems to understand how their beliefs (conscious and unconscious) and behaviors differ from those of conventional systems. These differences can then be taken into account in research design. Failure to know about and account for differences leads to uninterpretable or inaccurate research, raises the potential for misapplying findings to the care of patients, and violates the criterion of model fit.[3]

Methods for cross-cultural research—adjusting for the existence of different models of reality—are most highly developed in the social sciences, especially anthropology and communications, and have been incorporated into medical outcome studies. These methods are mostly categorized as qualitative, but quantitative versions of some techniques are available. In practice, most cross-cultural descriptive research demands the use of qualitative methodologies or a mixture of qualitative and quantitative techniques.

The focus of qualitative research is the individual practitioner or patient, and the community. This form of research is respondent centered, and researchers must take care not to impose their own assumptions or biases on data collection. Qualitative research requires the use of open-ended research techniques or instruments. The research team should include investigators who have had prior experience with qualitative methods and have produced publications that provide evidence of relevant expertise.

Methodological issues of clarity, validity, and the testing of hypotheses are similar in qualitative and quantitative research (see the "Guidelines for Clinical Trials" section for a summary). Correspondingly, in qualitative research as in quantitative research, concepts are detailed, theory is constructed by the testing of hypotheses, data are collected systematically, and criteria of soundness are applied to design, data collection, and interpretation.

Uses of Qualitative Research

Qualitative research is a body of techniques and assumptions concerning how to gather and analyze complex real-world data so that they can be applied to real-world problems (Bernard, 1993; Denzin and Lincoln, 1994; Marshall and Rossman, 1989). All qualitative research shares a set of assumptions or concepts about the research field (Marshall and Rossman, 1989):

- To find out about people's behavior, it is best to immerse oneself in the actual setting chosen for study.
- The participants in the study have values that researchers must honor.
- The researcher's task is to discover these values and perspectives and how they affect the participants' behavior and experience.
- Research is an interactive process.
- Research relies on people's words, stories, and actions as the primary data.

Accordingly, in qualitative or field research, the investigator has direct contact with research subjects and is directly and personally involved in data collection and analysis, with the aim of generating realistic descriptions and explanations. The choice of data collection methods, sampling procedures, and analytic approaches during the research process evolves into a question-specific research design (Crabtree and Miller, 1992). As data are collected and analyzed, this iterative process affects future decisions for additional sampling, collection, and analysis.

Data collection in field research is accomplished primarily through the use of observation, interviewing, and recordings. The researcher may be required to make relatively "unstructured" observations or "structured" observations that depend on a particular knowledge base. Observation is formalized in many ways, including studying proxemics (how people use space) and kinesics (how people move to communicate), participant observation, and various unobtrusive observational measures in which participants are unaware that they are being observed.

[3]*The design and methods chosen for conducting research must be consistent with the assumptions of the model used in generating the hypothesis under study. Model fit is explained more fully in the "Guidelines for Clinical Trials" section.*

The basic approach for data collection usually consists of interviews with individuals or groups. Focus-group interviews are appropriate in some settings and for some purposes but should not replace individual indepth interviews (McCracken, 1988). Sometimes questionnaires can be administered as interviews. Interviews may be conducted at several levels—unstructured (guided everyday conversation), semistructured (more focused but still open-ended), or structured (like spoken questionnaires). Conversations and events may be recorded with audio or video equipment.

Surveys can be constructed on the basis of interview data and, though not administered in a face-to-face setting, can be personalized by offering respondents opportunities to expand on their answers or to contact the researcher for an interview if they want to say more than the survey form permits.

Qualitative researchers have also developed various projective instruments that elicit respondents' unconscious knowledge and beliefs. For example, anthropologists use card-sort and triad-sort techniques, geographers use "mental map" techniques, and psychologists use various picture-response instruments. Preexisting instruments are rarely appropriate for studies across cultures or medical systems.

Much qualitative research also uses secondary sources, such as films, videotapes, texts, and photos. Historical, proxemic, and content analyses of these materials can reveal the unstated values and assumptions of the producers and participants.

To analyze the data collected, the researcher must develop an organizing system, segment the data accordingly, and then determine connections. If the data do not sort well into the categories first selected, the organizing system must be revised. Connections among the sorted data may be made either statistically or interpretively.

Analytical goals

The goal of any analysis is to bring order to what are often extremely complex data. Qualitative researchers try to discover classes of behavior or responses, themes that guide interpretation of events, and differing patterns of response. The first step is descriptive—simply to disentangle the data. Researchers then try to generalize, that is, to find and name the rules under which a particular result may be expected and to explain why this should be so. Much qualitative research eventually is applied in efforts to improve the quality of life, for example, by delivering health care in ways that make sense to the target population.

To be considered useful, qualitative research must fulfill certain criteria of soundness. It must be clear under which circumstances a particular finding applies and whether a finding works consistently. Another demand is that this research be objective. Traditional criteria, such as reliability and validity (see the "Guidelines for Clinical Trials" section), are applied (Kirk and Miller, 1986). However, some authors have defined different criteria of soundness for qualitative research (Lincoln and Guba, 1985; Marshall and Rossman, 1989):

- *Credibility.* The conduct of inquiry must enable the subjects of the research to say, "Yes, that question (or that interpretation) sounds right to me." This demand can be met because qualitative research deals directly with research subjects.

- *Transferability.* A researcher samples a population and makes generalizations about the whole population. If another researcher thinks this generalization applies to a different population, tests it, and finds it to be true, then the criterion of transferability has been met. Note that the underlying concepts are transferred, not the specific data.

- *Dependability.* Rather than assume that observed events can be replicated (the reliability assumption in quantitative research), qualitative researchers want to be able to account for events as they arise and change. When they do so successfully, the criterion of dependability has been met.

- *Confirmability.* This criterion is met when the findings of one researcher can be confirmed by another. Qualitative researchers can easily bias their data collection by becoming subjectively involved with the research field; this criterion helps to ensure that excessive subjectivity is not biasing the data, that is, that the data are objective.

Although analytical procedures in qualitative research are not necessarily statistical (as they are in quantitative research), some distinct statistical methods can be applied to qualitative research

(Bernard, 1993; Miles and Huberman, 1994); software programs such as Anthropac, Ethnograph, and NUDIST, are available to apply these analyses.

Qualitative Versus Quantitative Methods

Research design often requires a combination of qualitative and quantitative approaches. Qualitative and quantitative research differ in the underlying assumptions that researchers make (Cassidy, 1994). In quantitative research, scientists are likely to detail (and often count) particularities and therefore focus on strategies that limit the view, even if they must do so artificially. The randomly assigned, blinded, controlled clinical trial is an important example of this approach; it is not like the real world, because patients normally do not choose practitioners or treatments randomly, and both practitioner and patient usually know what is going on.

Quantitative methods are useful for answering the following types of questions: How many? How much? How often? What size? What are the measurable associations? What will happen if . . .? Does one variable cause the other? Is A more effective than B? The quantitative approach serves to isolate variables so that their influence on outcome can be separated from other factors that might otherwise cloud the interpretation.

In contrast, qualitative researchers are interested in complexity and pattern—the interactions among variables—and purposely avoid approaches (such as the use of controls) that simplify and focus. Qualitative methods are useful for answering the following types of questions: What is going on? What is the nature of the phenomenon? What variations occur? How does it work? How did something happen? What patterns can be identified? Is the original theory or hypothesis correct? Does the original theory fit other circumstances? What difference does this program or intervention make? Why does this intervention work or not work?

In a real-world medical setting, these questions might address the following issues:

- Differences in therapeutic effectiveness when patients are assigned or freely choose their health care.
- How patient and practitioner interact, and how this interaction affects the medical outcome.
- How the design of the health care delivery setting affects patient or practitioner satisfaction.
- How patients compare care in two different medical systems.
- How patients become acclimated in a new (e.g., alternative) system of medical care.

There is another important difference between qualitative and quantitative approaches. Quantitative research depends on an assumption that a certain commonality or unchangingness underlies how materials interact. This assumption translates to a demand that a hypothesis be tested the "same way" and "as planned" in different research settings. Once the research has begun, the protocol cannot be changed, for doing so introduces new variables that would invalidate the work.

Qualitative research depends on the opposite assumption, namely that the real world always involves flux and change. Qualitative research protocols outline the goal and approaches, but they are based on the assumption—indeed, the expectation—that unpredictable events will occur and that the research protocol can be changed as one means of dealing with these events (Marshall and Rossman, 1989). Such changes do not invalidate the qualitative research so long as researchers recognize that change is necessary, document the reasons, and create a logical means to deal with the novel event.

Qualitative methods can explain the real world of alternative health care delivery. The qualitative approach is an ideal way to elucidate outcomes issues (as in cost and clinical effectiveness studies) and can be used in settings where little is known about a practice and its theory, techniques, practitioners, or users. When qualitative and quantitative methods are linked, researchers are able to gather fruitful data suitable for use in improving the delivery of health care.

Guidelines for Screening Best Cases

Introduction

Many practitioners of unconventional therapies for cancer and other illnesses have not documented the effects of their treatments, yet they claim positive results. A process is needed to screen such claims to determine whether each patient, or case, provides enough information to qualify as part of a *best case series* and then to determine whether there are enough cases to meet criteria for a best case series.

The guidelines summarized below were adapted from a National Cancer Institute publication (NCI, 1991) produced to assist the development and reporting of best case series for unconventional cancer treatments. These guidelines retain references to cancer therapies, but a similar approach could also be applied to some other unconventional treatments. Applying this simple and reliable best case evaluation system should enable many unconventional therapies to be screened for adequate information. If available information were not found to be adequate, further attempts to evaluate the therapy would be postponed until better information could be obtained.[4]

With sufficient information to create a best case series, cases that meet NCI's criteria (or other designated criteria for other health problems) can be determined. Necessary information includes documentation—using standard measures—of the patient's diagnosis, staging (severity of illness), treatment, outcome, and so on. The procedure for determining adequate best case information includes six steps.

Conclusion

NCI's best case criteria represent a specific and reliable means of uncovering therapies worthy of study. This approach uses a single standard to detail the amount of information available and the response achieved.

This method is used to screen charts for adequate information, estimate clinical response, and evaluate practitioner judgment about clinical response. It provides a systematic method for determining which one or ones of the numerous unconventional approaches to cancer warrant further evaluation through clinical trials. The method is applicable to therapies for other problems besides cancer when appropriate evaluators are available.

Guidelines for Clinical Trials

The following guidelines address major methodological issues relevant to designing and conducting clinical trials. The final guideline addresses how interactions between the subject and the health care practitioner may affect study results.

Model Fit

The basic assumptions about health and disease intrinsic to the system under study should be noted, as should the model for classifying and treating patients by that system. For example, if clinical acupuncture care is under investigation, a description of qi and meridians (see the glossary) and the criteria for patient classification and outcome changes must be presented.

The study population should be selected and classified in a way that reflects the assumptions of the model under consideration. For example, if the study addresses disease outcomes, proper diagnostic categories must be used. If the study involves assumed changes in energy patterns, pulses, or symptoms, patients must be classified according to these criteria from the outset. Outcome measures used must be consistent with these assumptions.

The design and methods to explore the intervention must be selected in a way that is consistent with the model's assumptions and with the objectives of the study. Methodologic goals include efforts to (1) demonstrate any effect, (2) assess relative effects between therapies or therapeutic systems, (3) test the utility of an intervention in actual practice, (4) evaluate a possible mechanism of action, (5) examine an assumption that underlies a practice, (6) examine patient reports of satisfaction and relevant explanatory models, (7) examine practitioner explanations of what happened and why, and (8) examine the character of the practitioner-patient relationship and how it affects the delivery and receipt of care.

The goals of the investigation in relation to the system under study must be clearly delineated in the protocol. The study's title and conclusions

---

[4]*Since preparing the best case screening guidelines in response to a request from Congress, NCI has reviewed three series of best cases—for nutritional therapy (Nicholas Gonzales), antineoplastons (Stanislaw Burzynski), and insulin potentiation therapy (Steven Ayre). As a result of these reviews, NCI determined that antineoplaston therapy is a suitable candidate for clinical trials (see also the "Pharmacological and Biological Treatments" chapter); clinical trials began in winter 1993–94.*

NCIs Suggested Steps for Screening Best Cases

1. Chart Selection

The practitioner or another individual in the alternative medicine setting reviews clinic charts and selects those that are believed to represent the best examples of successful treatment. These charts are copied and brought or sent to NCI, where an independent evaluator reviews them. Alternatively, the evaluator may visit the clinic and review the best case charts on site.

2. Chart Review

The evaluator judges the charts acceptable if the needed information is present and rejects them if it is lacking. The reason for either decision is documented. The evaluator's specific criteria for adequacy of information also can guide the practitioner to select best cases.

When a specified proportion of submitted charts contains adequate information, outcome evaluation can be considered. Charts that provide adequate evidence of response or lack of response are then evaluated according to outcome criteria.

3. Inclusion Criteria

Evidence for the diagnosis of cancer (or another illness under treatment) and details of the treatment regimen are documented. Clinical information that demonstrates the status and course of the illness, such as the malignancy and the sites of metastatic disease, must be detailed. Minimum evidence includes the following:

a. The diagnosis of cancer must be documented by one of the following:*

- A pathology report.
- Radiological, surgical, or blood evaluation, and a specialist's written report diagnosing cancer or indicating that it has recurred.
- A specialist's written report that standard treatment is unlikely to be helpful or has failed, or that the disease severity prior to alternative medicine treatment indicated extremely poor prognosis.

b. The patient must have received the unconventional treatment according to the alternative medicine practitioner's regimen. Information about the treatment must include the following:

- Detailed description of treatment source, doses, method, and delivery frequency.
- Chart documentation of patient compliance, such as pill counts and completion of at least 70 percent of followup visits.
- Complete documentation of any other previous or ongoing therapies, medications, and so on.

4. Exclusion Criteria

The following problems invalidate a chart for inclusion in a best case analysis. If any of these are present, the chart information is inadequate:

- No evidence of the disease under study when the patient began alternative medical treatment.
- No pathology diagnosis or objective evidence of disease recurrence as defined above when alternative medical treatment began.
- Inadequate delivery (insufficient dosage or treatment time) of the therapy under study, or current or recent delivery of another therapy that could affect the disease.

The diagnosis of any other illness must be similarly documented with measures appropriate to that illness.

- Followup less than 6 months from the start of therapy, or less than 2 standard deviations beyond the patient's expected survival, as determined by current estimates of life expectancy for the same diagnosis and stage of the disease when treatment was started.

5. Outcome Criteria

If criteria for adequate information as described above are met, cases can be reviewed according to outcome (clinical response) criteria. If outcome criteria also are met, it can be concluded that the therapy is producing positive results and that further study may be warranted. Outcome criteria consist of complete or partial clinical response as determined by the following standard oncology definitions:

- *Complete tumor remission.* Complete disappearance of all evidence of tumor (all sites of measurable disease) for a minimum number of weeks.
- *Partial tumor response.* Fifty percent decrease in the size of the tumor. This is calculated as the sum of the perpendicular diameters of all measured lesions, with no progression of disease at any site and no appearance of new lesions for a specific number of weeks.
- *Prolonged quality-of-life expectancy.* Evidence that the patient has experienced good quality of life (increased energy, improved appetite, greater mobility, and reduced pain) since the start of treatment for longer than expected by at least 2 standard deviations.
- *Complete or partial tumor response.* Determined either by a pathology report of a biopsy showing no evidence of disease, or by radiological, surgical, or blood evaluation and a specialist's written opinion that evaluation indicates disease reduction or elimination.

6. Tabulation

Using forms available from NCI, a specific procedure is followed to record all patient data:

a. Information is carefully tabulated on a standard Best Case Series Form.

b. Each chart selected is evaluated and results are recorded on a Score Sheet.

c. All reasons for inclusion or exclusion are noted on the Score Sheet and recorded on a Spread Sheet.

d. If a chart displays adequate information, outcome criteria also are recorded on the Score Sheet and Spread Sheet.

e. The proportion of cases submitted to cases included in the best case series is calculated by dividing the accepted cases by the total number of cases submitted. This calculation provides a "discrepancy index," which is an estimate of the accuracy of practitioners' judgments about the success of their treatment. The amount of discrepancy due to inadequate information or faulty outcome estimation can be determined.

should reflect the assumptions of the relevant model and the study goals that were actually investigated.

Hypothesis

Clearly established hypotheses should be contained in the research description or grant application. These should identify or predict the main results so that analyses can test the hypotheses.

Patient Selection Bias

The means by which people are identified and accrued to the study, as well as the numbers of potential subjects who decline participation, must be carefully recorded. For example, did subjects come to the study through advertisements? Were they recruited from clinical practices? By random dialing?

Eligibility and selection (inclusion/exclusion) criteria should be clearly stated. Criteria used to diagnose or classify subjects must be valid and reliable. A reference should be given to document the established reliability of the classification system used. In cancer studies, for example, detailed and specific classifications are established (see the "Guidelines for Screening Best Cases" section).

If no generally accepted classification system exists, the system used in the study must itself be detailed and defended in the methods of the current trial.

Randomization or Matching

Comparison groups are developed through a specific process such as randomization, matching, or stratification. Randomization (or a related procedure) applied to a large enough group should distribute differences in the control and treatment groups in a random fashion. In this way the two groups are "equalized" and made as similar as possible except for the intervention to be studied. The method used to create the comparison group should be clearly described. The method should be balanced at least by age, gender, specific diagnosis and stage of disease, important prognostic factors, and other factors relevant to the particular study.

Control Subjects

To obtain comparative data that will shed light on results found in the treatment (or experimental) group of subjects under study, an appropriate control group is needed. Data from control and treatment group subjects are gathered simultaneously by the researchers. Ideally, the groups are identical except for the treatment or intervention to be studied. However, because no two people are identical in every way that may relate to the illness or therapy to be studied, subjects are randomized or matched.

Blinding

Evaluators of the condition of subjects should be blind with respect to (1) whether subjects receive the intervention or a placebo treatment, (2) how the outcome will be measured, and (3) how results will be analyzed.

Crossover Bias

There should be no dilution or co-intervention, that is, the treatment group should not receive any other therapy or intervention in addition to that evaluated in the study. There should be no contamination, that is, control subjects must not receive the same treatment or one that is similar to the treatment received by the experimental subjects.

Confounding Factors

Possible confounding variables (factors that may influence the study's results) must be addressed adequately. The study groups should be comparable on important prognostic factors. All funding sources should be disclosed, and reports should indicate whether these sources were independent of potential profit from the type of treatment under study.

Sample Size

Estimates of the required number of subjects must be made before the study begins and must be discussed in the research proposal. The statistical basis for selecting the number should be given, and the calculations that led to that number should be described. The research proposal also should provide information about how the researchers plan to attain the desired sample size.

Outcomes and Measurement Errors

Outcome and measurement criteria must be clearly defined and explicit. The validity of the outcome measurements used should be established by references and by verification within the study (against a "gold standard" or parallel outcome measures). The measurement methods used must be sensitive enough to detect the outcome or change to be investigated. All important outcomes must be reported.

The duration of effects must be considered in evaluating outcomes. For example, if subjects of a treatment are crossed over to a control group, consideration must be given to whether they were still experiencing effects from their treatment after the crossover. Statistical mechanisms for handling this type of problem exist.

Loss to Followup

At least 80 percent of subjects brought into the study should be shown to remain with the study long enough for necessary followup to occur. Subjects who withdraw from the study must be fully described. For the study results to be acceptable, subject characteristics (including age, gender, diagnosis, stage of disease, and other important factors) must be similar for those who withdrew and those who remain in the study.

Statistical Methods

Descriptive statistics (data) are presented on all prognostic and outcome factors. Inferential and hypothesis-testing statistics (p-values) are calculated and reported for all major treatment-outcome links. Confidence intervals or probability distributions also are reported for primary treatment-outcome links.

Multiple Measures

When more than one measure, variable, or comparison group is assessed, appropriate analyses are applied. Examples of such analyses include analysis of variance with multiple comparison groups, post hoc analyses, subgroup analyses, multiple hypothesis testing with serial *t*- or *z*-tests, and serial dependent measures.

Clinical Significance

Clinical (versus statistical) significance indicates whether research effects are important or meaningful. Patient or physician satisfaction with treatment is an example. Results that achieve statistical significance are not meaningful unless they are also clinically important or meaningful in clinical practice. For example, a very small difference in the effectiveness of two treatments would not be likely to change clinical practice or to influence physicians or patients to adopt the new treatment.

The new treatment should have a low risk of causing direct harm in comparison to the risks of not treating the disease. If risks associated with the treatment are low, the treatment is more likely to be used.

Generalizability

Results cannot be generalized beyond the type of illness or patient studied. Any other studies that addressed the same research questions should be discussed in the protocol. If intervention X is shown to work for patients with diabetes, for example, it cannot also be said to work for people with other illnesses. If intervention Y produces good results in breast cancer, it cannot be claimed to work in lung cancer. Broader generalizability is possible only with very large research projects that include adequate numbers of men and women of different age groups, disease severity categories, and stages of the illness.

As a general guideline, there should be at least 40 people in each group for each treatment-outcome link examined.

Disclosure Issues

The sources of funding for the research should be disclosed, as should any additional sources of funding for the participating investigators when these sources have the potential to influence their work. Reports on the research should indicate whether any of these sources might potentially profit from the type of treatment under study or might profit from an alternative treatment if the treatment under study were discredited.

Patient and Practitioner Beliefs and Interactions

Often in clinical trials, the beliefs of and interactions between investigators and subjects are assumed not to be important, but in alternative medicine these are valid concerns. This guideline addresses such personal considerations.

One consideration is bias, which is not usually intentional in research. The differences that could introduce interference or bias in the conduct of the research should be identified and evaluated. Among these are (1) whether the treatment is delivered in the usual method and style used in health care practice, (2) whether the health care practitioner and patient have expectations about the treatment results, (3) whether the patient has complied with the treatment regimen, and (4) whether interference with normal spontaneity and flexibility in patient-therapist interactions has been avoided or noted.

Utility of the treatment involves the question of whether the treatment, as reported, could be applied by practitioners other than those who participated. The investigators' belief in the efficacy of the treatment should also be assessed, and any idiosyncratic responses or beliefs should be described.

Study subjects must be adequately prepared for their participation. The view of each subject on the need for treatment should be evaluated. For example, does the subject regard the problem as a major or minor condition?

The possibility of transpersonal phenomena should also be considered. Such phenomena might include cultural or spiritual perceptions of the study's importance; cultural disparities in treatment delivery; events that might affect outcome, such as direct observer and evaluation effects[5]; and possible field—that is, nonlocal—effects.

Introduction to Outcomes Research

Outcomes research evaluates the ultimate effects of treatment systems on patients. This evaluation usually involves a retrospective examination of records or databases accumulated by health care practitioners, hospitals, insurers, and government health programs in order to identify which medical interventions produced the best outcomes (Wennberg, 1990). It is also possible to conduct prospective research by tracking clinical practices concurrently into the future. Outcomes research has been described as the use of natural experiments to find what works in medicine.

The databases under examination in outcomes research may be developed by using various kinds of research methods—descriptive (qualitative), best case (mixed qualitative and quantitative), or quantitative. Clinical case records and insurance claims data are often perused.

Advocates of outcomes research claim that it is potentially cheaper and faster than clinical trials and can provide data on treatments that would not otherwise be evaluated. In fact, retrospective database analysis may be the only way to obtain data on treatments with rare complications. Outcomes research is also useful when dealing with "soft" results such as effects on the quality of life. Consequently, some advocates of alternative medical practices consider outcomes research ideal for examining aspects of alternative medicine.

Outcomes research has other inherent advantages. It does not interfere with the doctor-patient relationship, does not require informed consent or permission from an institutional review board (as do clinical trials), and includes groups (such as the elderly, children, the poor, and minorities) that might not be widely represented in clinical trials.

Critics point out that any research based on retrospective analysis of clinical records is flawed by hidden biases in the data. They claim that researchers cannot correct for the subtle reasons why doctors choose one treatment over another for a given patient (or why patients choose their doctors). Furthermore, the records under examination were made for a different purpose and are likely to be incomplete in describing all relevant conditions that may affect the patients whose records are being analyzed.

Proponents and opponents of outcomes research agree that some aspects of the research are useful—that it is important to learn what doctors are actually doing in clinical practice and that this knowledge can provide a basis for further studies, including clinical trials.

One government agency, the Agency for Health Care Policy and Research (AHCPR), was created in 1989 largely to conduct outcomes research. However, in a recent article in *Science*, Anderson (1994) reported that "after spending nearly $200 million on outcomes research (about one-third of the agency's budget . . .), AHCPR cannot point to a single case in which its database studies have changed general clinical practice." Anderson further noted that even the agency's most definitive result—a guideline to physicians that "watchful waiting" is more appropriate for some patients than surgery for benign prostate disease (see the "Research Methodologies" chapter)—was accompanied by a recommendation for a clinical trial to confirm these findings.

Increasingly, it appears that AHCPR will use its database analyses of outcomes to supplement and complement other tools, including case control studies, meta-analyses of previous studies, and clinical trials. Two new references are expected to help researchers rank the value of outcomes research: (1) the proceedings of a March 1993 conference sponsored by the New York Academy of Sciences that analyzed the relative merits of outcomes research and clinical trials (Warren and Mosteller, 1994); and (2) the results of an 18-month study by the Office of Technology Assessment (OTA) analyzing AHCPR's outcomes research (publication due September 1994).[6]

---

[5]*An example is the Hawthorne effect, the observation that experimental subjects who are aware that they are part of an experiment often perform better than totally naive subjects.*

[6]*The working title of the OTA report is* Searching for Evidence: The Effort to Identify Health Care Technologies That Work.

Introduction to Meta-Analysis

The term *meta-analysis* was first coined by G.V. Glass, in a 1976 study of the efficacy of psychotherapy, as "the statistical analysis of a large collection of results from individual literature, for the purpose of integrating the findings." Although meta-analytic procedures have been widely employed in the social sciences since the early 1970s, many did not consider it a valid tool for the natural sciences until numerous retrospective studies accumulated that used meta-analysis to analyze data that had previously been studied with other statistical tools. As these studies illustrated both the statistical power and the increased information provided by meta-analysis, interest in its medical applications began to increase significantly. Since then, meta-analysis has been applied to questions of efficacy (e.g., chemotherapy in breast cancer, patient education interventions in clinical medicine, spinal manipulation); questions of cause and effect (e.g., effect of exercise on serum lipid level); and, increasingly, public health problems. Today meta-analysis is being used in a variety of settings to draw conclusions from results collected from literature or narrative reviews and from data pooled from independent studies (often clinical trials).

In general, meta-analysis is a systematic method that uses statistical analysis for extracting, comparing, and combining results from independent studies to obtain quantifiable outcomes. Meta-analysis also can help detect gaps in knowledge in the published literature and thus can help provide guidance for future research. Although there have been several approaches to meta-analysis, each follows the same basic procedure:

1. Define the problem and criteria for admission of studies.
2. Locate research studies.
3. Classify and code study characteristics.
4. Measure study characteristics quantitatively on a common scale.
5. Aggregate findings to study characteristics (analysis and interpretation).
6. Report the results.

Problem formulation includes explicit definition of outcomes and potentially confounding variables. Carefully done, this step enables the investigator to focus on the relevant measures in the studies under consideration and to specify the relevant methods for classifying and coding study characteristics. The literature search uses a systematic approach to locating studies. First, information is obtained from colleagues in a particular discipline. Second, the various indexes, abstracting services, and electronic databases are searched. Third, references from the primary articles are used to find secondary sources of information. Finally, information is gathered from academic, private, and government sources, including unreferenced reports and unpublished data.

In order to measure results across disparate studies, several methods are used. The most common method is to measure the effect size (i.e., an index of both the direction and the magnitude of the effect of a procedure under study). One estimate of the effect size for quantitative data is the difference between the two group means, divided by the control group standard deviation, $(X_t - X_c)/S_c$, where X_c is the mean of the control group and S_c is the standard deviation of the control group. Effect size expresses differences in standard deviation units so that, for example, if a study has an effect of 0.2 standard deviation units, the overall effect size is only half that of another study that has an effect size of 0.4 standard deviation units. The appropriate measure of effect across the research literature varies according to both the nature of the problem being assessed and the availability of published data. Pooling of data from controlled clinical trials, for example, has been more widely used in the medical literature than for other subjects.

Effect size for proportions has been calculated in cohort literature as either a difference, $P_t - P_c$, or as a ratio, P_t/P_c. The latter has the advantage of considerable change relative to the control percentage; in epidemiological studies, it is equivalent to the concept of risk ratio.

Whatever combination statistic is used, a systematic quantitative procedure to accumulate results across studies should include the following:

1. Summary descriptive statistics across studies, and the averages of those statistics.
2. Calculation of variance of a statistic across studies.
3. Correction of the variance by subtracting sampling error.

4. Correction in the mean and variance for study artifacts other than sampling, such as measurement error.

5. Comparison of the corrected standard deviation to the mean to assess the size of the potential variation across studies.

The value of meta-analysis is that as evidence begins to accumulate, meta-analysis forces systematic thought about methods, outcomes, categorizations, populations, and interventions. In addition, it offers a mechanism for estimating the magnitude of the effect in terms of a statistically significant effect size or pooled odds ratio. Furthermore, the combination of data from several studies increases generalizability and potentially increases statistical power, thus enabling more complete assessment of the impact of a procedure or variable. Quantitative measures across studies also can give insight into the nature of the relationships among variables and can provide a mechanism for detecting and exploring apparent contradictions in research results. Further, because meta-analysis is less subjective than other analytical methods, it has the potential to decrease investigator bias.

However, like the value of all review methods, the value of meta-analysis can be limited by a number of factors. For example, the current use of parametric statistical methods for meta-analysis is the subject of intense theoretical study. Other methodological issues of concern include bias, variability between studies, and the development of models to measure variability across studies. One major concern about qualitative reviews of the literature is that although meta-analysis is more explicit, it may be no more objective than a narrative review. Both critics and advocates of meta-analysis are concerned that an unwarranted sense of scientific validity, rather than true scientific understanding, may result from quantification. More simply stated, use of sophisticated statistics will not improve poor data but could lead analysts to an unwarranted level of comfort with their conclusions.

Introduction to Systematic Reviews

The systematic review is an orderly approach to reviewing research literature that minimizes the problems that can arise with less scientifically rigorous review methods (Larson et al., 1992). To avoid introducing bias in the selection and interpretation of the literature under study, systematic reviews spell out in advance the approach to be taken. Systematic review entails defining criteria for (1) the selection of journals and articles to include and exclude, (2) the quality of the measures used in the selected literature to assess the factor being reviewed, and, (3) the quality of each study's research methodology. The technique also looks at the frequency of assessment of a particular research question, variable, or measure.

Advantages

Systematic reviews, like meta-analyses and unlike standard literature reviews, are replicable from one reviewer to the next. This point is particularly important when a potentially controversial research topic is being evaluated.

Systematic reviews differ from meta-analytical reviews in two major ways. First, the systematic review costs much less—only 10 to 20 percent of the expense of a similarly sized meta-analysis. Second, systematic reviews can consider single factors of interest within an inadequately developed research field. In contrast, meta-analyses require a well-developed research field with a large amount of experimental or quasi-experimental research; they also require that an adequate number of studies address essentially the same research question using comparable study samples.

While systematic reviews can examine the key or central findings in studies, they also permit analysis of noncentral or peripheral factors. Thus systematic reviews are particularly useful in examining an underdeveloped or infrequently studied research issue.

Method

There are five key steps in conducting a systematic review: (1) selecting the factor or factors to be studied; (2) deciding whether to use an exhaustive review or field review approach; (3) assessing the frequency and quality of measurement of the factor of interest; (4) evaluating the studies that contain the factor of interest; and (5) determining and maintaining reviewer reliability.

Selecting the factor or factors to be studied. This first step involves formulating research questions based on the topic the reviewer wishes to study. Each systematic review should address clear research questions. For example, several systematic reviews have focused on whether the quantity or quality of research containing religious variables was substandard in certain clinical scientific literatures (Larson et al., 1986). Another review concerning the effects of pornography asked whether existing research demonstrated harm—or lack of harm—in assessing the associations in each literature report between exposure to pornographic materials and changes in attitudes concerning rape or aggression toward women.

Deciding whether to use an exhaustive review or field review approach. Both types of systematic reviews use research reports that have undergone a peer review process of critique and revision prior to being published. However, criteria for what to include and exclude are defined differently for the two types of reviews.

The *exhaustive review* method involves identifying every possible peer-reviewed study from every relevant field of study that includes information about the factor of interest. This review is carried out in three steps. (1) First, an initial list of articles is prepared, based on a multiple, overlapping, computerized literature search that uses multiple key-word terms and indexes. (2) Next, other potentially relevant articles are identified in the reference sections of the articles obtained in the initial search, and these new articles are also searched for relevant references. This repeated reference review continues until no new articles can be identified for addition to the master list. (3) The final step is the circulation of the list of articles to identified experts, such as the three to five researchers with the most publications on the research study list; these researchers are asked to identify additional relevant articles.

In contrast, *field reviews* involve selecting only one field of study, the leading peer-reviewed journals in that field, and the period to be reviewed (usually 5 to 10 years). The leading journals are identified as the ones most frequently cited in a particular research field, by using the *Science Citation Index* or the *Social Science Citation Index* as a citation source. (These indexes provide ratings of journals in various research fields based on the frequency with which their articles are cited). If the goal is to define the most accurate and up-to-date research in a specific field, then the field review is the more appropriate type of systematic review to use.

The field reviewer obtains a proper sample by manually searching through every journal issue and every article in the journal to identify studies that include the review factor of interest. Some topics of previous systematic reviews include mental health factors in nursing home studies, AIDS research in general medical journals, and religious factors in psychiatry, family medicine, and pastoral care journals. The total numbers of articles scanned and articles selected should be tracked. Editorial articles, commentaries, and other nonquantifiable opinion articles should be excluded.

Assessing the frequency and quality of measurement of the factor of interest. In this step the factor of interest is examined across the reviewed articles to determine whether it is of major or minor importance—that is, whether it is frequently or infrequently assessed. Additional information is tabulated concerning whether the factor is being assessed through use of one or several questions and—if through several questions—whether reliability was reported or demonstrated.

Evaluating the studies that contain the factor of interest. Next the research quality of the studies that include the factors of interest is assessed. If a study is poorly designed, its findings may be questionable.

Assessing the quality of the methods used requires clearly defining each study factor, including such variables as the response rate, size of the study population, use of a control or comparison population, type of sampling method used, and whether study measures demonstrated reliability. For example, defining the response rate might entail grouping rates in categories: low, less than 50 percent; medium, 50 to 69 percent; and high, 70 percent and more. Similarly, other factors require some definition and grouping.

Determining and maintaining reviewer reliability. Reproducibility of systematic reviews depends on training multiple reviewers to appropriately assess the factors of interest. The goal here is statistical reliability, so that reviewers reviewing the same articles achieve the same assessments. Training reviewers has been found to produce replicable results with reliabilities above 0.90 (Larson et al., 1992).

High reliability can be maintained through periodic checks—especially if a large number of studies and a large number of reviewers are involved—and, if necessary, retraining of reviewers.

Usefulness

The kinds of information that systematic reviews can provide about a specific research field or topic include the following:

- Number of studies assessing the factor of interest.
- Statistical reliability of measures assessing the factor of interest.
- Approach most often used for assessing the factor of interest.
- Frequency of assessing the factor as a variable of major versus minor study relevance.
- Quality of the research studies that include the factor of interest.

Selected Bibliography for Researchers

Abramson, J.H. 1988. Making Sense of Data. A Self-Instruction Manual on the Interpretation of Epidemiologic Data. Oxford University Press, Oxford.

Aldridge, D. 1987. Clinical assessment of acupuncture in asthma therapy: discussion paper. J. Royal Soc. Med. 80:222–224.

Aldridge, D. 1989. A guide to preparing a research application. Comp. Med. Res. 3(3):31–37.

Altman, D.G. 1991. Practical Statistics for Medical Research. Chapman & Hall, London.

Anderson, C. 1994. Measuring what works in health care. Science 263:1080–1082.

Anthony, H.M. 1987. Some methodological problems in the assessment of complementary therapy. Stats. Med. 6:761–771.

Anthony, H.M. 1989. Clinical research: questions to ask and the benefits of asking them. Comp. Med. Res. 3(3):3–6.

Bailar, J.C., and K. Patterson. 1986. Journal peer review: the need for a research agenda. In J.C. Bailar III, and F. Mosteller, eds. Medical Uses of Statistics. NEJM Books, Waltham, Mass.

Battista, R.M., and S.W. Fletcher. 1988. Making recommendations on preventive practices: methodological issues. Am. J. Prev. Med. 4 (suppl):53–67.

Bauer, H.H. 1992. Scientific Literacy and the Myth of the Scientific Method. University of Illinois Press, Urbana, Ill.

Baum, M. 1989. Rationalism versus irrationalism in the care of the sick: science versus the absurd. Med. J. Aust. 151:607–608.

Baum, M. 1991. Rationalism versus irrationalism in the treatment of cancer—quack cures or scientific remedies? Surgery 1:2223a–2223c.

Bensoussan, A. 1991. Contemporary acupuncture research: the difficulties of research across scientific paradigms. Am. J. Acupunc. 19(4):357–365.

Bernard H.R. 1993. Research Methods in Cultural Anthropology (2nd ed.). Sage Publication, Newbury Park, Calif.

Bracken, M.B. 1987. Clinical trials and the acceptance of uncertainty. BMJ 294:1111–1112.

Brink, P., and M. Wood. 1988. Basic Steps in Planning Nursing Research (3rd ed.). Jones & Bartlett, Boston.

Briscoe, M.E. 1990. A Researcher's Guide to Scientific and Medical Illustrations. Springer-Verlag, New York.

Canter, D. 1987. A research agenda for holistic therapy. Comp. Med. Res. 2:104–121.

Cassidy, C. 1994. Unraveling the ball of string: reality, paradigms, and the study of alternative medicine. Advances, the Journal of Mind-Body Health 10:5–31.

Cassileth, B.R. 1984. Contemporary unorthodox treatments in cancer medicine. Ann. Intern. Med. 101:105–112.

Cassileth, B.R., E.J. Lusk, D. Guerry, et al. 1991. Survival and quality of life among patients on unproven versus conventional cancer therapy. N. Engl. J. Med. 324:1180–1185.

Chalmers, T.C., P. Celano, H.S. Sachs, et al. 1981. Bias in treatment assignment in controlled clinical trials. N. Engl. J. Med. 309:1358–1361.

Chalmers, T.C., H.J. Smith, B. Blackburn, et al. 1981. A method for assessing the quality of a randomized control trial. Controlled Clin. Trials 2:31–49.

Colditz, G.A., J.N. Miller, and F. Mosteller. 1989. How study design affects outcomes in comparisons of therapy. I: Medical. Stat. Med. 8:441–454.

Coulter, H.L. 1991. The Controlled Clinical Trial: An Analysis. Center for Empirical Medicine, Washington, D.C.

Crabtree, B.F., and W.L. Miller, eds. 1992. Doing Qualitative Research. Sage Publications, Newbury Park, Calif.

Crichton, N.J. 1990. The importance of statistics in research design. Comp. Med. Res. 4(2):41–49.

Denzin, N., and Y. Lincoln, eds. 1994. Handbook of Qualitative Research. Sage Publications, Thousand Oaks, Calif.

DerSimonian, R., L.J. Charette, B. McPeek, et al. 1982. Reporting on methods in clinical trials. N. Engl. J. Med. 306:1332–1337.

Detsky, A.S., C.D. Naylor, K. O'Rourke, et al. 1992. Incorporating variations in the quality of individual randomized trials into meta-analysis. J. Clin. Epidemiol. 45(3):255–265.

Diamond, G.A., and T.A. Denton. 1993. Alternative perspectives on the biased foundations of medical technology assessment. Ann. Intern. Med. 118:455–464.

Dickerson, K. 1990. The existence of publication bias and risk factors for its occurrence. JAMA 263:1385–1389.

Druckman, D., and R.A. Bjork, eds. 1991. In the Mind's Eye: Enhancing Human Performance. National Academy Press, Washington, D.C.

Easterbrook, P.J., J.A. Berlin, R. Gopalan, et al. 1991. Publication bias in clinical research. Lancet 337:867–872.

Eddy, D.M. 1990. Should we change the rules for evaluating medical technologies? In A.C. Gelijns, ed. Modern Methods of Clinical Investigation? National Academy Press, Washington, D.C.

Eddy, D.M. 1992. Assessing Health Practices & Designing Practice Policies: The Explicit Approach. American College of Physicians, Philadelphia.

Eddy, D.M., V. Hasselblad, and R. Shachter. 1992. Meta-Analysis by the Confidence Profile Method. Academic Press, Boston.

Eisenberg, D.M., R.C. Kessler, C. Foster, et al. 1993. Unconventional medicine in the United States—prevalence, costs, and patterns of use. N. Engl. J. Med. 328:246–252.

Emerson, J.D., E. Burdick, D.C. Hoaglin, et al. 1990. An empirical study of the possible relation of treatment differences to quality scores in controlled randomized clinical trials. Controlled Clin. Trials 11:339–352.

Ernst, E., T. Saradeth, and K.L. Resch. 1993. Drawbacks of peer review. Nature 363:296.

Feinstein, A.R. 1983. An additional basic science for clinical medicine: II. The limitations of randomized trials. Ann. Int. Med. 99:544–550.

Feinstein, A.R. 1985. Clinical Epidemiology: The Architecture of Clinical Research. W.B. Saunders, Philadelphia.

Fisher, P. 1990. Research into homeopathic treatment of rheumatological disease: why and how? Comp. Med. Res. 4(3):34–40.

Flay, B.R. 1986. Efficacy and effectiveness trials (and other phases of research) in the development of health promotion programs. Prev. Med. 15:451–474.

Fricke, R., and G. Treinis. 1985. Einführung in die Metaanalyse. Verlag Hans Huber, Berlin.

Fuchs, V.R., and A.M. Garber. 1990. The new technology assessment. N. Engl. J. Med. 323(10):673–677.

Ganiats, T.G. 1993. Are all outcomes created equal? Fam. Pract. Res. J. 13(1):1–5.

Gehan, E.A. 1982. Progress of therapy in acute leukemia:1948–1981. Controlled Clin. Trials 3:199–207.

Gelband, H., et al. 1990. Unconventional Cancer Treatments. U.S. Government Printing Office, Washington, D.C.

Gelijns, A.C., and S.O. Thier. 1990. Medical technology development: an introduction to the innovation-evaluation nexus. In A.C. Gelijns, ed. Modern Methods of Clinical Investigation. National Academy Press, Washington, D.C.

Gerbarg, Z.B., and R.I. Horwitz. 1988. Resolving conflicting clinical trials. J. Clin. Epidemiol. 41(5):503–509.

Gevitz, N., ed. 1988. Other Healers: Unorthodox Medicine in America. Johns Hopkins University Press, Baltimore.

Glass, E.V. 1976. Primary, secondary, and meta-analysis of research. Educational Researcher. 5:3-8.

Greenberg, R.P., R.F. Bornstein, M.D. Greenberg, et al. 1992. A meta-analysis of antidepressant outcome under "blinder" conditions. J. Consult. Clin. Psychol. 60(5):664–669.

Guyatt, G.H., J.L. Keller, R. Jaeschke, et al. 1990. The n–of–1 randomized control trial: clinical usefulness—our three-year experience. Ann. Intern. Med. 112: 293–299.

Haley, R.W. 1994. Designing clinical research. In Y.C. Pak and P.M. Adams, eds. Techniques of Patient Oriented Research. Raven Press, New York.

Hauser, S.P. 1991. Unproven methods in oncology. Eur. J. Cancer 27(12):1549–1551.

Haynes, R.B. 1991. ACP Journal Club's Modus Operandi [Editorial]. Ann. Intern. Med. 115, suppl 3:A14.

Heron, J. 1986. Critique of conventional research methodology. Comp. Med. Res. 1(1):10–22.

Hill, C., and F. Doyon. 1990. Review of randomized trials of homeopathy. Rev. Epidemiol. 38:139–142.

Hinkle, L.E., and H.G. Wolff. 1958. Ecological investigations of the relationship between illness, life experiences and the social environment. Ann. Intern. Med. 49:1373–1388.

Hornung, J., and K. Linde. 1991. Guidelines for the exact description of the preparation and mode of application of serial dilutions and potencies on ultra low dose effects and homeopathic research—a proposal. Berlin Journal of Research in Homeopathy 1(2):121–123.

Hufford, D.J. 1988. Contemporary folk medicine. In N. Gevitz, ed. Other Healers: Unorthodox Medicine in America. Johns Hopkins University Press, Baltimore.

Hulley, S.B., and S.R. Cummings, eds. 1988. Designing Clinical Research. Williams & Wilkins, Baltimore.

James, I. 1989. Tactics and practicalities. Comp. Med. Res. 3(3):7–10.

Jenicek, M. 1989. Meta-analyses in medicine—where we are and where we want to go. J. Clin. Epidemiol. 42(1):35–44.

Jingfeng, C. 1987. Toward a comprehensive evaluation of alternative medicine. Soc. Sci. Med. 25(6):659–667.

Jonas, W.B. 1992. Evaluation of studies involving non-mainstream medicine. Presented at the 7th Annual Primary Care Research and Statistics Conference, University of Texas Health Science Center, San Antonio.

Kiene, H. 1993. Kritik der klinischen Doppelblindstudie. MMV Medizin Verlag, München.

Kirk, J., and M. Miller. 1986. Reliability and Validity in Qualitative Research. Sage Publications, Newbury Park, Calif.

Kleijnen, J. 1991. Food supplements and their efficacy. CIP-Gegevien Koninklijke Bibliotheek, Den Haag, Netherlands.

Kleijnen, J., and P. Knipschild. 1992. Review articles and publication bias. Arzneimittelforschung 42:587–591.

Kleijnen, J., P. Knipschild, et al. 1991. Clinical trials of homeopathy. BMJ. 302:316–323.

Kleijnen, J., G. ter Riet, and P. Knipschild. 1991. Acupuncture and asthma—a review of controlled trials. Thorax 46(11):799–802.

Kleinman, A., L. Eisenberg, and B. Good. 1978. Culture, illness, and care. Ann. Intern. Med. 88:251–258.

Knipschild, P., J. Kleijnen, et al. 1990. Zur Glaubwirdigkeit alternativer Medizin. Skeptiker 3(3):4–8.

L'Abbé, K.A., A.S. Detsky, and K. O'Rourke. 1988. Meta-analysis in clinical research. Ann. Intern. Med. 107:224–233.

Larson, D.B., L.E. Pastro, J.S. Lyons, et al. 1992. The systematic review: an innovative approach to reviewing research. Paper prepared for the Department of Health and Human Services, Assistant Secretary for Planning and Evaluation, by the Family and Community Policy Division.

Larson, D.B., E.M. Pattison, D.G. Blazer, et al. 1986. Systematic analysis of research on religious variables in four major psychiatric journals, 1978–1982. Am. J. Psychiatry 143:329–334.

Leede, P.D. 1992. Practical Research: Planning and Design (5th ed.). McMillan, New York.

Leibrich, J. 1990. Measurement of efficacy: a case for holistic research. Comp. Med. Res. 4(1):21–25.

Lewitt, G.T., and D. Aldrich. 1993. Clinical Research Methodology for Complementary Therapies. Holder & Stoughton, London.

Lincoln, Y., and E. Guba. 1985. Naturalistic Inquiry. Sage Publications, Beverly Hills, Calif.

Little, J.M. 1993. Eupompus gave splendour to art by numbers. Lancet 341:878–880.

Lyne, N. 1989. Theoretical and empirical problems in the assessment of alternative medical technologies. Scand. J. Soc. Med. 37:257–263.

Marshall, C., and G. Rossman. 1989 Designing Qualitative Research. Sage Publications, Newbury Park, Calif.

McCracken, G. 1988. The Long Interview. Sage Publications, Newbury Park, Calif.

Miles, M., and H. Huberman. 1994. Qualitative Data Analysis (2nd ed.). Sage Publications, Thousand Oaks, Calif.

Moher, D., et al. 1993. Proceedings of Assessing the Quality of Randomized Controlled Trials (RCTs): The Development of a Consensus. Ottawa, Ontario, Canada, October 7–8, 1993.

Mulow, C.D. 1987. The medical review article: state of the science. Ann. Int. Med. 106:485–488.

Murray, R.H., and A.J. Rubel. 1992. Physicians and healers: unwitting partners in health care. N. Engl. J. Med. 326:61–64.

National Cancer Institute. 1991. Preparation of Best Case Series and the Conduct of Pilot Clinical Trials Using Unconventional Cancer Treatments. (Informal publication, available from NCI's Clinical Trials Evaluation Program).

Naylor, C.D. 1988. Two cheers for meta-analysis: problems and opportunities in aggregating results of clinical trials. CMAJ 138:891–895.

Nishiwaki, R., A. Morton, et al. 1990. Perceived health quackery use among patients. West. J. Med. 152:87–89.

Orme-Johnson, D.W., and C.N. Alexander. 1992. Critique of the National Research Council's Report on Mediation. Maharishi International University, Fairfield, Iowa.

Ottenbacher, K.J. 1986. Evaluating Clinical Change. Williams & Wilkins, Baltimore.

Oxman, A.D., and G.H. Guyatt. 1988. Guidelines for reading literature reviews. CMAJ 138:697–703.

Patel, M.S. 1987a. Evaluation of holistic medicine. Soc. Sci. Med. 24(2):169–175.

Patel, M.S. 1987b. Problems in the evaluation of alternative medicine. Soc. Sci. Med. 25(6):669–678.

Patton, M. 1986. Qualitative Evaluation Methods. Sage Publications, Beverly Hills, Calif.

Pocock, S.J. 1977. Randomized clinical trials. BMJ 1(6077):1661.

Pocock, S.J. 1983. Clinical Trials: A Practical Approach. Wiley, Chichester, England.

Ravnskov, U. 1992. Cholesterol lowering trials in coronary heart disease: frequency of citation and outcome. BMJ 305:15–19.

Reilly, D.T. 1987. Strategy for research in homeopathy. Br. Hom. J. 77:52–54.

Reilly, D.T., and M.A. Taylor. 1988. The difficulty with homeopathy: a brief review of principles, methods and research. Compl. Med. Res. 3:70–78.

Reilly, D.T., M.A. Taylor, C. McSharry, et al. 1986. Is homeopathy a placebo response? Controlled trial of homeopathic potency, with pollen in hayfever as model. Lancet 2(8512):881–886.

Riegelman, R.K., and R.P. Hirsch. 1989. Studying a Study and Testing a Test: How to Read the Medical Literature. Little, Brown & Co., Boston.

Rietter, G., J. Kleijnen, et al. 1989. Nawoord en aanbevelingen de effectiviteit van acupunctuur. Huisarts en Wetenschap 32:308–312.

Rubik, B. 1992. The Interrelationship Between Mind and Matter. Center for Frontier Sciences, Temple University, Philadelphia.

Sackett, D.L., R.B. Haynes, and P. Tugwell. 1991. Clinical Epidemiology: A Basic Science for Clinical Medicine. Little, Brown & Co., Boston.

Sacks, H.S., J. Berrier, D. Reitman, et al. 1987. Meta-analyses of randomized controlled trials. N. Engl. J. Med. 316:450–455.

Sacks, H.S., T.C. Chalmers, et al. 1983. Randomized versus historical assignment in controlled clinical trials. N. Engl. J. Med. 309:1353–1361.

Sacks, H.S., T.C. Chalmers, and H. Smith, Jr. 1983. Sensitivity and specificity of clinical trials: randomized versus historical controls. Arch. Intern. Med. 143:753–755.

Saks, M., ed. 1992. Alternative Medicine in Britain. Clarendon, Oxford.

Schwartz, D., and J. Lellouch. 1967. Explanatory and pragmatic attitudes in therapeutical trials. J. Chronic Dis. 20:637–648.

Schwartz, S.M., and M.E. Friedman. 1992. A Guide to NIH Grant Programs. Oxford University Press, New York.

Sermeus, G. 1987. Alternative medicine in Europe: a quantitative comparison of alternative medicine and patient profiles in nine European countries. Belgian Consumers' Association, Brussels.

Shapiro, D.A., and D.S. Shapiro. 1982. Meta-analysis of comparative therapy outcome studies: a replication and refinement. Psychol. Bull. 92:581–604.

Singleton, R., D. Straits, M. Straits, et al. 1988. Approaches to Social Research. Oxford University Press, New York.

Spiegelhalter, D.J., and S.L. Lauritzen. 1990. Techniques for Bayesian analysis in expert systems. Annals of Mathematics and Artificial Intelligence 2:353–359.

Strauss, A., and J. Corbin. 1990. Basics of Qualitative Research, Grounded Theory Procedures and Techniques. Sage Publications, Newbury Park, Calif.

Thacker, S.B. 1988. Meta-analysis: a quantitative approach to research integration. JAMA 259:1685–1689.

Vaskilampi, T., P. Merilaimen, et al. 1992. The use of alternative treatments in the Finnish adult population. Compl. Med. Res. 6(1):9–20.

Visser, J. 1990. Alternative medicine in the Netherlands. Compl. Med. Res. 4:28–31.

Warren, K.S., and F. Mosteller, eds. 1994. Doing More Harm than Good: The Evaluation of Health Care Interventions. Academy of Sciences, New York.

Wennberg, J.E. 1990. What is outcomes research? In A.C. Gelijns, ed. Modern Methods of Clinical Investigation. National Academy Press, Washington, D.C.

Wiegant, F.A.C., C.W. Kramers, et al. 1991. Clinical research in complementary medicine: the importance of patient-selection. Comp. Med. Res. 5(2):110–115.

Wilkin, D., L. Hallam, and M-A Doggett. 1992. Measures of Need and Outcome for Primary Health Care. Oxford University Press, Oxford.

Williamson, J.W., P.G. Goldschmidt, et al. 1992. The quality of medical literature: an analysis of validation assessments. In J.C. Bailar III and F. Mosteller, eds. Medical Uses of Statistics. NEJM Books, Boston, Mass.

Woolf, S.H. 1991. Manual for Clinical Practice Guideline Development. AHCPR Pub. No. 91-0007. U.S. Department of Health and Human Services, Washington, D.C.

World Health Organization. 1990. Report of the WHO Consultation on AIDS and Traditional Medicine: Clinical Evaluation of Traditional Medicines. Geneva.

World Health Organization. 1991. Report from the Program on Traditional Medicines. Guidelines for the Assessment of Herbal Medicines. Geneva.

Zeiger, M. 1991. Essentials of Writing Biomedical Research Papers. McGraw-Hill, New York.

Information on the National Library of Medicine

The following Fact Sheets on the library and its services are available from the Public Information Office, National Library of Medicine, 8600 Rockville Pike, Bethesda, MD 20894; telephone 301-496-6308; E-mail publicinfo@occshost.NLM.NIH.gov.

- Assistance for Research Investigators
- DIRLINE (Directory of Information Resources)
- DOCLINE
- Grateful Med®
- HISTLINE (History of Medicine Online)
- History of Medicine Division
- LOANSOME DOC™
- Medical Subject Headings (MeSH)
- The National Library of Medicine
- National Network of Libraries of Medicine
- NLM Online Databases and Databanks
- Online Indexing System
- Public Services Division

Grateful Med® may be ordered from the National Technical Information Service, 5285 Port Royal Road, Springfield, VA 22161; 703-321-8547.

Order number PB92-105444/GBB (for IBM PC, includes tutorial) $29.95 plus shipping.

Order number PB93-502433/GBB (for Macintosh, includes tutorial) $29.95 plus shipping.

A list of other NLM Searching Tools (books and software), item number MMS 3/94, is available from NTIS at 703-321-8547, or fax your request to 703-321-8547/9038.

Contact References

Office of Alternative Medicine

Executive Plaza South
6120 Executive Boulevard
Suite 450
Rockville, MD 20892-9904

Phone 301-402-2466
Fax 301-402-4741

NIH Guide for Grants and Contracts *(a weekly publication)*

Contact person:

Myra Brockett (as of 5/94)
Institutional Affairs Office

Phone order: 301-496-5366

Written order:

Building 1, Room 328
National Institutes of Health
9000 Rockville Pike
Bethesda, MD 20892

E-mail address: q2c@cu.nih.gov

This publication is available electronically to institutions via Bitnet or Internet and is also on the NIH Gopher. Alternative access is through the NIH grant line using a personal computer (data line 301-402-2221). Contact (as of 5/94) Dr. John James at 301-594-7270 for details.

Grants Information Office, Division of Research Grants

National Institutes of Health
Westwood Building, Room 449
Bethesda, MD 20892

Phone: 301-594-7248

Request: *Preparing a Research Grant Application to the National Institutes of Health: Selected Articles,* revised October 1993.

Abbreviations and Glossary

Abbreviations

AA — Alcoholics Anonymous

AC — alternating current

ACS — American Cancer Society

AHCPR — Agency for Health Care Policy and Research

AIDS — acquired immunodeficiency syndrome

AMA — American Medical Association

AMTA — American Massage Therapy Association

BEM — bioelectromagnetics

BRM — biological response modifier

CCE — Council of Chiropractic Education

CHD — coronary heart disease

CoQ_{10} — coenzyme Q_{10}

DC — direct current

DMT — dance/movement therapy

D.O. — doctor of osteopathy

DRG — Division of Research Grants

ECT — electroconvulsive therapy

EDTA — ethylene diamine tetraacetic acid

EEG — electroencephalogram

ELF — extremely low frequency

EM — electromagnetic

EMG — electromyographic

EMS — eosinophilia myalgia syndrome

FDA — Food and Drug Administration

FDCA — Food, Drug, and Cosmetic Act

FTC — Federal Trade Commission

G — gauss

GSR — galvanic skin response

HDL — high-density lipoprotein

HIV — human immunodeficiency virus

HPA — hypothalamic-pituitary-adrenocortical

Hz — Hertz, (see hertz)

IgA — immunoglobulin A

IgE — immunoglobulin E

IND — investigational new drug

INF–A — interferon alpha

INF–G — interferon gamma

IU — international units

LDL — low-density lipoprotein

MEDLARS — Medical Literature Analysis and Retrieval System

MEDLINE — MEDLARS on Line

MHz — megahertz

MRI — magnetic resonance imaging

NAMT — National Association for Music Therapy

NCI — National Cancer Institute

NCNM — National College of Naturopathic Medicine

NCSA — Network Chiropractic Spinal Analysis

NHLBI — National Heart, Lung, and Blood Institute

NIOSH — National Institute for Occupational Safety and Health

NLM — National Library of Medicine

NRC — National Research Council

NSAID — nonsteroidal anti-inflammatory drugs

NSF — National Science Foundation

OAM — Office of Alternative Medicine

OTA — Office of Technology Assessment

PEMF — pulsed electromagnetic field

PET — positron emission tomography

PRC — People's Republic of China

RF — radio frequency

RFA — request for applications

SD — standard deviation

SHBG — sex hormone binding globulin

TCES — transcranial electrostimulation

TENS — transcutaneous electrical nerve stimulation

TIMPs — (proteins that are) tissue inhibitors of metalloproteinases

TM — transcendental meditation

TNF — tumor necrosis factor

USAID — United States Agency for International Development

WHO — World Health Organization

Glossary

adiposity: the state of being fat.

adjustment: the chiropractic adjustment is a specific form of direct manipulation of joint (articular) areas, using either long or short leverage techniques with specific contacts. It is characterized by a dynamic thrust of controlled velocity, amplitude, and direction (see **thrust**). Colloquially referred to as "bone cracking."

adrenergic: activated by, characteristic of, or secreting adrenaline (scientific name, epinephrine) or similar substances that constrict blood vessels and raise blood pressure, preparing the body for "fight or flight."

adrenochrome: a red oxidation product of epinephrine that slows the blood flow because of its effect on capillary permeability. It is currently being tested as a psychomimetic drug (a drug that imitates natural substances that can affect a person psychologically).

allergic rhinitis: hay fever; significant nasal drainage and inflammation of the eyes in susceptible subjects, caused by inhaling allergens (usually pollens).

allopathy: substitutive therapy; a therapeutic system in which a disease is treated by producing a second condition that is incompatible with or antagonistic to the first. May be used to describe Western medicine as currently practiced.

amide: an organic compound in which the hydroxyl (-OH) of a carboxyl group (-COOH) of an acid has been replaced by the nitrogen-containing group $-NH_2$. For example, $O{=}C{-}NH_2$.

amine: an organic compound containing nitrogen, equivalent to replacing one or more atoms of hydrogen in ammonia by an organic hydrocarbon. For example, $-NH_2$.

amyotrophic lateral sclerosis: a disease marked by progressive degeneration of the nerve cells that conduct electrical impulses, leading to degeneration of the motor cells of the brain stem and spinal cord and resulting in a deficit of motor skills among other symptoms; it usually ends fatally within 2 to 3 years. Also called Lou Gehrig's disease.

anabolism: constructive metabolic processes in which new substances are built.

anaphylaxis: a major type of allergic reaction to a substance, resulting in difficulty breathing and followed usually by shock and collapse of the blood system.

angina pectoris: a spasm with sudden chest pain, accompanied by a feeling of suffocation and impending death, most often due to lack of oxygen to part of the heart wall, and caused by excitement or activity.

angiography: the study of the cardiovascular system (heart and blood) by radioscopy after the introduction of a contrasting material, such as radioactive iodine, into the body.

anthropology: the study of human beings and their origin in relation to social, cultural, historical, environmental, and developmental aspects.

antipsychotic drug: a substance effective in the treatment of psychosis, a severe type of mental disorder involving total disorganization of the personality.

apoenzyme: the protein portion of an enzyme that can be separated from any cofactor but needs the cofactor present to function properly as an enzyme.

arrhythmia: any variation from the normal rhythm of the heartbeat.

ascorbyl palmitate: a derivative of vitamin C that is being tested as a preventive agent.

autism: a condition characterized by preoccupation with inner thoughts, daydreams, fantasies, delusions, and hallucinations; egocentric, subjective thinking lacking objectivity and connection with reality; a disorder of currently unknown origin characterized by such activities.

benzopyrene: a highly carcinogenic organic chemical that is produced when carbon compounds are incompletely burned.

bind: an increasing resistance to motion in the problem area (in manual therapy the practitioner uses feedback obtained by touching the problem area to guide the medical procedure). See also **ease**.

bioelectromagnetics: the scientific study of interactions between living organisms and electromagnetic fields, forces, energies, currents, and charges. The range of interactions studied includes atomic, molecular, intracellular up to the entire organism.

biofeedback: the process of furnishing an individual with information, usually in an auditory or visual mode, on the state of one or more physiological variables such as heart rate, blood pressure, or skin temperature; it often enables the individual to gain some voluntary control over the physiological variable being sampled.

biofield: a massless field (not necessarily electromagnetic) that surrounds and permeates living bodies and affects the body. Possibly related to qi. See **qi**.

bioflavonoid: a generic term for a group of anti-oxidant compounds that are widely distributed in plants and involved in animals in maintaining the walls of small blood vessels in a normal state. See **flavenoids**.

biogenesis: Thomas Huxley's theory that living matter always arises by the agency of preexisting living matter. The opposing theory is spontaneous generation.

biomechanics: the study of structural, functional, and mechanical aspects of human motion.

biophoton: a small amount of electromagnetic energy emitted by molecules in living organisms. Biophoton emission is associated with processes, such as mitosis (cell division), and possibly with the vibrations of certain large molecules; It may also be used to communicate information over relatively large distances, as the firefly does.

biorhythm: the cyclic occurrence of body processes, such as in daily, or circadian, rhythm. Other rhythms may be monthly or yearly.

biostatistics: the science of applying statistics in biology, medicine, and agriculture.

botanical medicine: another term for herbal medicine.

cardiac catheterization: the passage of a small fluid-gathering tube through a vein in the body into the heart to gather blood samples, to measure internal blood pressure, or to obtain other intracardiac information.

catabolism: destructive metabolic processes in which substances are broken down.

catecholamine: chemical messengers, such as dopamine and norepinephrine, that stimulate various receptors in the sympathetic and central nervous systems in the body.

catechu: an extract from the heartwood of the *Acia catechu* tree that contains catechin, a crystalline, contraction-causing chemical. Formerly used as an antidiarrheal agent.

cell proliferation: growth by the reproduction of similar cells.

cellular metabolism: the sum of the chemical processes of a cell, including the transformation of sugars into energy and related processes.

cervical dysplasia: deviations in the cells that cover the uterine cervix, which may begin as unusual increased cell growth and progress to the loss of the unique characteristics of a cell; tends to lead to a tumor.

chakra: one of the areas of rotation in the biofield, first elaborated in ancient Indian metaphysics.

chelation: formation of a complex molecule involving a metal ion and two or more polar groupings of a single molecule. Chelation can be used to remove an ion from participation in biological reactions, causing a change in the reaction.

chemopreventive: the attempt to prevent disease through the use of chemicals, drugs, or food factors, such as vitamins.

chemotherapy: treatment of disease by chemical compounds selectively directed against invading organisms or abnormal cells.

chiropractic practice: a discipline of the scientific healing arts concerned with the development, diagnosis, treatment, and preventive care of functional disturbances, disease states, pain syndromes, and neurophysiological effects related to the status and dynamics of the locomotor system, especially of the spine and pelvis.

chiropractic science: the investigation of the relationship between structure (primarily of the spine) and function (primarily of the nervous system) in the human body.

cholecystectomy: surgical removal of the gall bladder.

chronic fatigue syndrome: an illness characterized by long periods of fatigue, often accompanied by headaches, muscle pain and weakness, and elevated antibody titers to some herpesviruses. The cause or causes are unknown.

chronic hepatitis: a persistent inflammation of the liver.

circadian: a phenemenon being, having, characterized by, or occurring in approximately 24-hour periods or cycles (as of biological activity or function).

clairsentience: the ability to use touch to sense subtle variations in the biofield.

clairvoyance: the ability to perceive things that are out of the range of normal human senses.

closed system: a field or system that does not react with other fields or anything outside that system.

cochlear reflex: a contraction of the cochlea—a spirally wound tube that forms part of the inner ear—when a sharp, sudden noise is made near the ear.

cofactor: a non-protein chemical that is not an enzyme in its own right but must be present for an apoenzyme (i.e., the protein component of the enzyme) to function.

collagen: an insoluble, fibrous protein that occurs in bones as the major portion of the connective tissue fibers. Yields gelatin and glue on prolonged heating with water.

complementary medicine: another term for *alternative medicine*; frequently used in Europe.

congenital: something that exists at, and usually before, birth.

corpus callosum: the mass of white matter in the brain that connects the two hemispheres, linking the "creative" (or left-brained) side with the "raw intelligence" (or right-brained) side.

coumarin: an odorous material found in tonquin beans, sweet clover, and woodruff; used for scenting tobacco and as an anticoagulant to prevent excessive blood clotting.

cryosurgery: the application of extreme cold to destroy tissue.

cyclotron resonance: the resonant coupling of electromagnetic power into a system of charged particles undergoing orbital movement in a uniform magnetic field.

cytokine: a generic term for various small proteins that are released by cells and that act as intercellular communicators to elicit an immune response. Examples include the interferons and the interleukins.

cytokinesis: the contraction of a belt of cytoplasm, bringing about the separation of two daughter cells during cell division in animal tissues.

cytotoxicity: the degree to which a chemical is toxic, or lethal, to a cell, such as how toxic a chemotherapy agent may be to cancer cells.

Delphi method: a consensus procedure in which participating experts are polled individually and anonymously, usually with self-administered questionnaires. The survey is conducted over a series of "rounds." After each round, the results are elicited, tabulated, and reported to the group. The Delphi process is considered complete when there is convergence of opinion or when a point of diminishing return is reached.

diabetes mellitus: a disorder of metabolism in which the lack of available insulin causes an excess of sugar in the blood and urine, as well as excessive thirst and loss of weight. Various long-term problems can result.

diagnosis: the art of distinguishing one disease from another; the use of scientific and skillful methods to establish the cause and nature of a person's illness.

dietetics: the study and regulation of the diet.

direct technique: any manual medical method or maneuver that engages and passes through and beyond an area of increasing tissue or joint motion resistance, commonly called a "direct barrier." (Physical penetration of the body surface is not involved.)

dosimetry: the process of measuring doses of radiation (e.g., x rays).

double-blind: a term pertaining to a clinical trial or other experiment in which neither the subject nor the person administering treatment knows which subjects are receiving actual treatment and which are receiving a placebo.

dysfunction: a term used in medicine to describe abnormal, impaired, or incomplete functioning of an organ or part.

dysmenorrhea: a condition characterized by difficult and painful menstruation.

ease: a region of decreasing resistance to movement. In manual therapy the practitioner uses feedback obtained by touching the problem region to guide the medical procedure. See **bind**.

echocardiography: a method of graphically recording the position and motion of the heart walls or the internal structures of the heart and neighboring tissue by the echo obtained from beams of ultrasonic waves directed through the chest wall.

eczema: an inflammatory skin condition characterized by itching and the secretion of liquids from subdermal pockets of pus and water.

electroencephalogram (EEG): a recording of the electrical potentials on the skull generated by currents emanating spontaneously from nerve cells in the brain.

electromagnetic field: the force or energy associated with electromagnetic interactions, charges, and currents. EM fields include electrostatic, magnetostatic, radiation, induction, vector-potential, and scalar-potential fields, and Hertz and Fitzgerald potentials. The EM field is usually said to comprise two components: an "electric field" and a "magnetic field." However, according to apparently well-established theorems (e.g., Maxwell's equations), these two components are closely coupled and not truly independent of each other.

electromagnetic radiation: one type of EM field, namely, an oscillating EM field that has free motion in space at a distance from its source.

electromagnetism: the magnetism produced by an electric current.

electrophysiology: the study of the mechanisms and consequences of the production of electrical phenomena in the living organism.

electropollution: EM fields produced by sources that may have harmful effects on humans, such as electric power transmission and radio transmission.

electrosurgical excision: surgical removal of an organ or tissue by electrical methods.

embolism: the blocking of a blood vessel, usually by a blood clot or thrombus originating from a remote part of the circulatory system.

emission tomography: a computer-constructed image of the body, created by measuring radioactive presences in the body.

end play: discrete, short-range movements of a joint, independent of the action of voluntary muscles, determined by springing each vertebra or extremity joint at the limit of its passive range of motion; also called "joint play."

endocrine: a material that is secreted internally in the body, most commonly through the bloodstream rather than through the various ducts; of or pertaining to such a secretion.

endorphin: any of three compounds found naturally in the brain that may have adrenaline-like effects, such as a burst of energy or an analgesic effect.

endoscopy: visual inspection of any cavity of the body by means of an endoscope (an instrument to examine the interior of a hollow cavity inside the body, such as the bladder).

enzymes: proteins that catalyze many biochemical reactions, necessary in all life forms.

epidemiology: the medical study of the incidence, distribution, and control of disease in a population; the conditions controlling the presence or absence of a disease or pathogen.

esophageal motility: the muscular movements of the esophagus, the tube that carries food from the mouth to the stomach. Orderly and rhythmic esophageal motility is necessary for swallowing; any disorder in this process may result in pain and dysfunction.

ethnobotany: the science of plants in relation to ethnic groups of humans.

etiology: the medical study of causes of disease.

faith healing: healing that occurs because of the patient's belief in a supernatural being or the healer.

fascia: a sheet of fibrous tissue that envelops the body beneath the skin; it also encloses muscles and groups of muscles, and separates their several layers or groups.

fibromyalgia: a poorly understood illness characterized by fibrous muscular pain.

fibrositis: an inflammation of fibrous tissue.

flavonoids: a large group of metabolic byproducts of mosses and other plants, based on 2-phenylbenzopyran (a particular type of organic compound with a ring structure); for example, the chemicals that give yellow, red, and blue colors to plants.

forensic: evidence or material gathered for or used in legal proceedings or in public debate.

free radical: a molecule or atom in which the outermost ring of electrons is not complete, making it extremely chemically reactive.

galvanic skin response: a change in the electrical resistance of the skin, recorded by a polygraph; widely used as an index of autonomic (involuntary) nervous system reactions.

gastroenteritis: an inflammation of the mucous membrane of the stomach and the intestines.

gauss: a unit of magnetic flux density. In colloquial terms, the strength of a magnetic field is specified in terms of gauss; for instance, the strength of a typical household magnet that holds papers on a refrigerator is about 200 G.

glycyrrhetinic acid: a derivative of vitamin A that is being tested for its disease preventive activity.

Hawthorne effect: the observation that experimental subjects who are aware that they are part of an experiment often perform better than totally naive subjects.

heavy metal: a metal of high atomic number; may be used to measure electron density in electron microscopy; high concentrations of heavy metals can harm plant and animal growth.

hematology: the medical specialty that pertains to the anatomy, physiology, pathology, symptomatology, and therapeutics of blood and blood-forming tissues.

Hertz (Hz): the unit of measure used to specify the frequency of complete waves of electromagnetic radiation, such as light, radio waves, and x rays; expressed as cycles per second. These waves take on the property of a sinusoid (see **sinusoidal**). Table 1 in the "Bioelectromagnetics Applications in Medicine" chapter shows the electromagnetic spectrum ranging from 0 Hz to over 10^{20} Hz.

heuristic: anything that encourages or promotes investigation; that which is conducive to discovery.

high sense perception: a system of diagnosis based on **clairsentience** and **clairvoyance**.

hippocampus: a particular part of the gray matter of the brain; in humans, it extends from the olfactory lobe to the posterior end of the cerebrum.

homeopathy: an alternative medical system that treats the symptoms of a disease with minute doses of a chemical. In larger doses, the compound would produce the same symptoms as the disease or disorder that is being treated.

homeostasis: the maintenance of a static, constant, or balanced condition in the body's internal environment; the level of physiological well-being of an individual.

humoralism, humorism: an ancient theory that health and illness are related to a balance or imbalance of body fluids or "humors."

hydrocortisone: a complex chemical secreted by the human adrenal cortex which has life-maintaining properties and is important to sustaining blood pressure and the balance of fluids and electrolytes in the body.

hydrotherapy: treating a disease with water, externally or internally.

hypercholesterolemia: an excess of cholesterol in the blood.

hyperlipidemia: an excess of lipids (fatty components, such as cholesterol or triglycerides) in the blood.

hypertension: a persistent state of high arterial high blood pressure.

hypothalamic-pituitary-adrenocortical axis: the interaction involving chemical and neuronal signals between the hippocampus, pituitary gland, and the cortex (outer layer) of the adrenal glands, with significant impacts on the body's state of health.

iatrogenic: an illness, injury, disease, or disorder induced inadvertently by physicians or their treatments.

ichthyosis: a group of skin disorders characterized by increased or aberrant development of keratin, resulting in noninflammatory scaling of the skin.

immunocompromising: anything that interferes with the healthy function of the immune system.

impedance: the state of resistance in electrical circuits.

incontinence: the inability to control one or both excretory functions (i.e., defecation and urination).

indirect technique: any manual medical method or maneuver that engages and passes through and beyond an area of decreasing resistance, commonly called an "indirect barrier." (Physical penetration of the body surface is not involved.)

indole: a type of nitrogen-containing organic compound with a double ring structure; a breakdown product of the amino acid tryptophan and related biologically active compounds.

infrasonic energy: energy waves transmitted at a frequency lower than the frequency at which humans are normally aware of sound.

innate: something that inborn or hereditary.

innate intelligence: the intrinsic biological ability of a healthy organism to react physiologically to the changing conditions of the external and internal environment.

interferon: one of a group of small immune system stimulating proteins produced by viral-infected cells or by noninfected white blood cells; it is used as an anticancer agent in some clinical trials because of its ability to inhibit further viral replication.

interleukin: one of a group of small proteins that are involved in communication among white blood cells and that activate and enhance the immune system's disease-fighting abilities.

internal validity: the certainty that the treatment or regimen under study, rather than something else, is responsible for producing study results.

irritable bowel (spastic colon) syndrome: a condition characterized by sudden, involuntary contractions of the colon.

ki: the Japanese term for *qi*.

kinesthetic senses: the senses by which movement, weight, and position are perceived; commonly used to refer specifically to the perception of changes in the angles of joints.

L-dopa: the naturally occurring form of the amino acid dopa, which is a precursor of epinephrine and other biologically active compounds. It is used in the treatment of Parkinson's disease.

leukocytes: a group of blood cells that have a nucleus but lack hemoglobin and that are involved in fighting disease; also known as "white blood cells."

limbus: a general term for describing border structures, such as the limbic region of the brain.

lipids: a generic term for organic compounds based on fatty acids, such as fats, waxes, fat- soluble vitamins, and steroids.

local healing: biofield healing that uses the practitioner's hands on the subject's body.

lymph: a clear, transparent, or yellowish-opaque liquid found in the vessels of the lymphatic system; this liquid returns proteins and other substances from tissues to the blood.

lymphatic system: the system of the lymph, including the lymph nodes, and the vascular channels that transport lymph.

lymphocyte: a white blood cell formed in lymphatic tissue; in normal adults, lymphocytes comprise approximately one-quarter of the white blood cells.

macrophage: a class of white blood cells, found in tissues, that are scavengers. Macrophage can wander the system or migrate to points of infection in the body.

magnetic resonance imaging: the use of nuclear magnetic resonance of protons to produce proton density maps or images of tissues or organs in the human body.

magnetite: a spinel (metal oxide) of iron (Fe_3O_4); a naturally occurring magnet.

manipulation: a term used in connection with the therapeutic application of manual force. Spinal manipulation, broadly defined, includes all procedures in which the hands are used to mobilize, adjust, manipulate, apply traction, massage, stimulate, or otherwise influence the spine and nearby (paraspinal) tissues with the goal of positively influencing the patient's health.

materia medica: a collection of descriptions of products that are usable medically as drugs. In homeopathy, substances are included that may not be in the official pharmacopoeia (drug registry), as are descriptions of how to physically prepare the substances as drugs.

mental healing: a process whereby one individual endeavors to bring about the healing of another by using conscious intent, without the intervention of any known physical means. The term is often used synonymously with *spiritual healing*.

meridian: In Asian traditional medicine, the body has a channel with 12 portions, or meridians, which loop through the body in an endless circuit, connecting the principal organs and other body parts. The meridians are said to carry *ching qi*, which regulates the relationship between, and the functioning of, the various body structures.

meta-analysis: a method for combining the results of several or many studies to see if the combined results provide significant information that was not obtainable by examining individual studies.

metabolism: the sum total of the chemical and physical changes constantly occurring in a living body.

metaphysics: the branch of philosophy that systematically investigates first causes and the ultimate nature of the universe. Such investigations are generally of insubstantial elements and are outside physics, thus difficult to measure.

metastasis: the movement of cancerous cells in the body from a primary site to a distant site, usually through the blood or lymph system, with the subsequent development of secondary cancers.

mobilization: the process of making a fixed part movable; a form of manipulation characterized by nonthrust, passive joint manipulation.

modulation: the change of amplitude or frequency of a carrier signal of given frequency.

molecular biology: the study of the structure and function of macromolecule in living cells.

morbidity: the state or condition of being diseased, for an individual or community.

mortality: the death rate within a given population.

motion palpation: a term used in connection with using touch to diagnose passive and active segmental joint ranges of motion.

motor hand: the hand the practitioner uses to induce passive movement in the subject. See **bind**.

mucosal: a term for cells of or pertaining to the mucous membrane, a tissue layer that lines various tubular cavities of the body, such as the viscera, uterus, trachea, and nose.

multivariate analysis or **multivariate statistical treatment:** a method of statistical analysis that employs several measurements of various characteristics on each unit of observation.

musculoskeletal manipulation: a hands-on procedure to physically correct or reset abnormalities of joint muscle and connective tissue function.

mutagenic: an agent that causes change or induces genetic mutation in the DNA of cells.

myocardial infarction: a sudden shortage of arterial or venous blood supply to the heart due to blockage or pressure; it may produce a sizable area of dead cells in the heart.

myofascial: of or relating to the sheets of fibrous tissue (that is, fasciae) that surround and separate muscle tissue.

necrosis: death of cells or groups of cells in a living body.

neurodegenerative disease: a disease that involves deterioration in the function and form of nerves and related structures. Alzheimer's disease and multiple sclerosis are examples.

neuropeptide: a small chain of linked amino acids with neurological activity.

neurotransmitter: a chemical messenger used by nerves.

neutrophil: a granular white blood cell having a nucleus with three to five lobes connected by slender threads of chromatin and cytoplasm containing fine, inconspicuous granules.

nocebo effects: a toxic or negative placebo event.

noetic: a thought process based on pure intellect or reasoning ability, (e.g., a noetic doctrine).

noninvasive: not involving physical penetration of the skin (e.g., a noninvasive diagnostic or therapeutic technique).

nonlocal: something that occurs at a distance; in physics a nonlocal effect is a form of influence that is unmediated, unmitigated, and immediate. Nonlocal healing is healing that occurs at a distance.

oncology: the study of all aspects of cancer.

open system: a system that interacts with other fields or systems, giving off or receiving energy or materials. The opposite is a closed system.

orthomolecular medicine: a system of medicine aimed at restoring the optimal concentrations and functions at the molecular level of certain substances normally present in the body, such as vitamins.

osteopathic: a system of therapy that emphasizes normal body mechanics and manipulation to correct faulty body structures.

otitis media: inflammation of the middle ear.

oxidation: the addition of oxygen to a compound or the removal of electrons from a compound.

***p*-value:** the probability that the observed outcome of a particular experiment is due to random chance. Also known as uncertainty level.

Paleolithic: of or belonging to the period of human culture beginning with the earliest chipped stone tools, about 750,000 years ago, until the beginning of the Mesolithic period, about 15,000 years ago.

palpation: the physical examination of the body using touch.

paradigm: an explanatory model, especially one of outstanding clarity; a typical example or archetype. See Introduction of this report.

parapsychology: the field of study concerned with the investigation of evidence for paranormal psychological phenomena, such as telepathy, clairvoyance, and psychokinesis.

pathogen: any disease-producing microorganism or substance.

pathogenesis: the cellular events and reactions and other pathologic mechanisms occurring in the development of disease.

pathology: the medical study of the causes and nature of disease and the body changes wrought by disease.

pellagra: a clinical syndrome due to deficiency of niacin, characterized by inflammation of the skin and mucous membrane, diarrhea, and psychic disturbances.

peptide: any of various amides that are derived from two or more amino acids when the amino group of one acid is combined with the carboxyl group of another; peptides are usually obtained by partial breakdown of proteins.

peroxidation: the process by which enzymes activate hydrogen peroxide and induce reactions that hydrogen peroxide alone would not effect.

person-years: a unit of time used in various statistical measurements of the aggregate effects of agents or events on people, as in epidemiology.

phagocyte: a cell (e.g., a white blood cell) that characteristically engulfs foreign material and consumes debris and foreign bodies.

pharmacology: the science that deals with the origin, nature, chemistry, effects, and uses of drugs.

pharmacopeia: a book describing drugs, chemicals, and medical preparations, especially one issued by an officially recognized authority and serving as a standard for the preparation and form of drugs; a collection or stock of drugs.

phenomenology: the study of phenomena; in psychiatry, it is the theory that behavior is determined by the way the person perceives reality rather than by external reality.

physics, classical: the branch of physics that studies mechanics and electromagnetism. It includes kinetics, optics, hydraulics, aerodynamics, and astrophysics.

physics, quantum: the branch of physics that deals with atomic and subatomic particles.

placebo: an inert substance that is given to the control group of patients in a blinded trial. A placebo is used to distinguish between the actual benefits of the medication and the benefits the patients think they are receiving.

platelet: a disk-shaped structure found in the blood of all mammals, chiefly known for its role in blood coagulation.

plethysmography: the recording of the changes in size when an organ or other structure is modified by the circulation of blood through it.

polarity: the differences between portions of a biofield, similar to the polarity or directionality of magnet fields; a form of manual healing that incorporates this feature.

positron emission tomography: a form of diagnostic imaging that makes use of the electromagnetic energy transitions of "excited" molecules to indicate changes in the function of tissues under investigation.

postoperative: something that occurs after a surgical operation.

potentized: in homeopathic pharmacy, a substance that is prepared by dilution while the diluting fluid is being agitated in a standard fashion; widely believed by practitioners to impart additional medical value to higher dilutions.

propranolol: a chemical that decreases heart rate and output, reduces blood pressure, and is effective in the preventive treatment of migraine.

proprioceptive: stimuli produced by movement in body tissues. Proprioceptive nerves are the sensory nerves in muscles and tendons that detect such movements.

prospective study: a scientific study that is planned in advance, as opposed to looking back at previous situations to collect data for analysis.

psoriasis: a chronic disease of the skin in which red scaly papules and patches appear, especially on the outer aspects of the limbs.

psychic healing: a term for biofield and mental healing, used especially in England.

psychogenic: anything that is produced or caused by psychic or mental factors rather than by organic factors.

psychoneuroimmunology: the study of the roles that the mind and nervous system play in various phenomena of immunity, induced sensitivity, and allergy.

psychopathology: the medical study of the causes and nature of mental disease.

psychosomatic medicine: the branch of medicine that stresses the relationship of bodily and mental happenings, and combines physical and psychological techniques of investigation.

pulmonary: anything pertaining to the lungs.

qi (chi, ki): in Eastern philosophies, the energy that connects and animates everything in the universe; includes both individual qi (personal life force) and universal qi, which are coextensive through the practice of mind-body disciplines, such as traditional meditation, aikido, and tai chi.

qigong (qi gong): the art and science of using breath, movement, and meditation to cleanse, strengthen, and circulate the blood and vital life energy.

quantum domain: the atomic and subatomic dimension dealt with in the science of quantum physics.

Raynaud's disease/phenomenon: a disorder characterized by intermittent, bilateral attacks in which a restriction of blood flow occurs in the fingers or toes and sometimes the ears or nose. Severe paleness, a burning sensation, and pain may be brought on by cold or emotional stimulation; these symptoms sometimes are relieved by heat. The condition is due to an underlying disease or anatomical abnormality.

reduction: any chemical process in which an electron is added to an atom or an ion, or an oxygen is removed. The opposite process is oxidation.

retrospective study: a scientific study that collects data for analysis after events, rather than during events.

rheumatoid arthritis: a chronic inflammation of the joints, which may be accompanied by systemic disturbances such as fever, anemia, and enlargement of lymph nodes.

sacrum: the part of the vertebral column (backbones) that is directly connected with or forms a part of the pelvis; in humans it consists of five united vertebrae.

secretory immunoglobulin A (IgA): the predominant immune system protein in body secretions such as oral, nasal, bronchial, urogenital, and intestinal mucous secretions as well as in tears, saliva, and breast milk.

sensing hand: the hand used by the practitioner in manual therapy to detect changes (see **bind**); the sensing hand is used to assess the subject's increasing and decreasing resistance to the passive motion demands of the practitioner's motor or operating hand.

serial *t*- or *z*- tests: various types of statistical measurements that are used to determine whether data have significance.

serotonin: a naturally occurring body chemical that can cause blood vessels to contract; it is found in various animals, bacteria, and many plants. Serotonin acts as a central neurotransmitter and is thought to be involved in mood and behavior.

short leg: an anatomical, pathological, or functional leg deficiency leading to dysfunction.

sinusitis: the inflammation of any of the air-containing cavities of the skull, which communicate with the nose.

sinusoidal: of, relating to, shaped like, or varying according to a sine curve or sine wave, which is a waveform of single frequency and infinite repetition in relation to time.

sleep latency: the interval before sleep.

sociogenic: anything arising from or imposed by society.

somatic: pertaining to or characteristic of the body; distinct from the mind.

somatic dysfunction: impaired or altered function of related components of the somatic system (the skeleton, joints, and muscles; the structures surrounding them; and the related circulatory and nerve elements).

spiritual energy: energy that comes from a supernatural being or the cosmos.

structural diagnosis (osteopathic): an osteopathic physician's use of hands and eyes to evaluate the somatic system, relating the diagnosis of somatic dysfunction to the state of a patient's total well-being, according to osteopathic philosophy and principles.

subatomic: something pertaining to the constituent parts of an atom.

subluxation: a situation in which two adjacent structures involved in joints have an aberrant relationship, such as a partial dislocation, that can cause problems either in these and related joints or in other body systems that are directly or indirectly affected by them.

symptomatology: the study of symptoms.

syndrome: the signs and symptoms associated with a particular disease or disorder.

synergistic: entities working together or cooperating to produce a positive effect greater than the sum of the contributing individual entities.

systemic review: a method of analyzing a group of scientific studies that may individually be weak, producing results with more significance than the individual studies may have.

theosophy: a doctrine concerning a deity, the cosmos, and the self that relies on mystical insights by unusually perceptive individuals; it teaches that its practitioners can master nature and guide their own destinies.

thromboembolism: an obstruction of a blood vessel with clotting material carried by the bloodstream from the site of origin to plug another vessel.

thrombus: an aggregation of blood factors that creates an obstruction; more severe than a clot.

thrust: the sudden manual application of a controlled directional force on a suitable part of the patient's body, the delivery of which effects an adjustment (see **adjustment**).

transcranial electrostimulation: a method of clinical treatment involving electrical stimulation of the brain through the skull.

transcutaneous electrical nerve stimulation: a clinical treatment modality involving electrical stimulation of nerves through the skin.

trigger points: specific points in the muscular and fascial tissues that produce a sharp pain when pressed; may also correspond to certain types of traditional acupuncture points.

triplet states: a state in which there are two unpaired electrons.

turnover: the movement of a substance into, through, and out of a place; the rate at which a material is depleted and replaced.

vascular system: the system formed by the blood vessels.

visceral: pertaining to the soft interior organs in the cavities of the body.

Index

U.S. GOVERNMENT PRINTING OFFICE : 1996 O - 169-663 : QL 3

To order additional copies of this book use the convenient order form below.

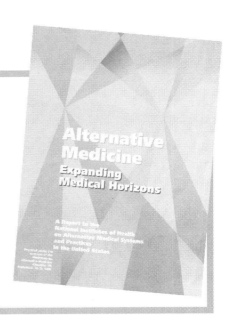

RUSH DELIVERY: Delivery within 48 hours via Fed Ex is available for credit card telephone orders by calling (202) 512–1800. For a flat rate of $8.50 per order you can get delivery within 48 hours on an order of up to 10 titles or 100 copies if the order is placed before 12:00 noon eastern time.

Superintendent of Documents Order Form

Order Processing Code:

* 7578

Charge your order. It's easy! VISA MasterCard

To fax your orders (202) 512–2250

To phone your orders (202) 512–1800

❑ **YES,** send me ____ copies of **Alternative Medicine: Expanding Medical Horizons**, 017–040–00537–7 for $25 each ($31.25 foreign).

The total cost of my order is $_______. Price includes regular shipping and handling and is subject to change.

Company or personal name (Please type or print)

Additional address/attention line

Street address

City, State, Zip code

Daytime phone including area code

Purchase order number (optional)

Check method of payment:

❑ Check payable to Superintendent of Documents

❑ GPO Deposit Account

❑ VISA ❑ MasterCard

(expiration date)

Authorizing signature 1/95

Mail to: Superintendent of Documents
P.O. Box 371954, Pittsburgh, PA 15250–7954

Thank you for your order!